# *Chemical and Biological Properties of Food Allergens*

# Chemical and Functional Properties of Food Components Series

SERIES EDITOR

## Zdzisław E. Sikorski

**Chemical and Biological Properties of Food Allergens**
Edited by Lucjan Jędrychowski and Harry J. Wichers

**Food Colorants: Chemical and Functional Properties**
Edited by Carmen Socaciu

**Mineral Components in Foods**
Edited by Piotr Szefer and Jerome O. Nriagu

**Chemical and Functional Properties of Food Components, Third Edition**
Edited by Zdzisław E. Sikorski

**Carcinogenic and Anticarcinogenic Food Components**
Edited by Wanda Baer-Dubowska, Agnieszka Bartoszek and Danuta Malejka-Giganti

**Methods of Analysis of Food Components and Additives**
Edited by Semih Ötleş

**Toxins in Food**
Edited by Waldemar M. Dąbrowski and Zdzisław E. Sikorski

**Chemical and Functional Properties of Food Saccharides**
Edited by Piotr Tomasik

**Chemical and Functional Properties of Food Lipids**
Edited by Zdzisław E. Sikorski and Anna Kolakowska

**Chemical and Functional Properties of Food Proteins**
Edited by Zdzisław E. Sikorski

# Chemical and Biological Properties of Food Allergens

EDITED BY

## Lucjan Jędrychowski
Institute of Animal Reproduction & Food Research
Olsztyn, Poland

## Harry J. Wichers
Wageningen University and Research Centre
Netherlands

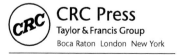

CRC Press
Taylor & Francis Group
Boca Raton London New York

CRC Press is an imprint of the
Taylor & Francis Group, an **informa** business

CRC Press
Taylor & Francis Group
6000 Broken Sound Parkway NW, Suite 300
Boca Raton, FL 33487-2742

First issued in paperback 2019

© 2010 by Taylor & Francis Group, LLC
CRC Press is an imprint of Taylor & Francis Group, an Informa business

No claim to original U.S. Government works

ISBN-13: 978-1-4200-5855-0 (hbk)
ISBN-13: 978-0-367-38513-2 (pbk)

---

**Library of Congress Cataloging-in-Publication Data**

---

Chemical and biological properties of food allergens / editors, Lucjan Jedrychowski,
　　Harry J. Wichers.
　　　　p. ; cm. -- (Chemical and functional properties of food components series)
　　Includes bibliographical references and index.
　　ISBN 978-1-4200-5855-0 (hardcover : alk. paper)
　　1. Food allergy. 2. Allergens. I. Jedrychowski, Lucjan. II. Wichers, Harry. III. Title. IV.
Series: Chemical and functional properties of food components series.
　　[DNLM: 1. Allergens--chemistry. 2. Food Hypersensitivity--immunology. WD 310
C517 2010]

QR188.C47 2010
616.97'5--dc22　　　　　　　　　　　　　　　　　　　　　　　　　　2009028070

---

**Visit the Taylor & Francis Web site at**
**http://www.taylorandfrancis.com**

**and the CRC Press Web site at**
**http://www.crcpress.com**

# Contents

# Preface

Hypersensitivity, including a hypersensitive response to foodstuffs, is one of the major health problems nowadays. Symptoms of food hypersensitivity cause acute discomfort for patients and are becoming an increasing social and economic problem, although much progress has been made in recent years in many areas related to food allergies. Many food allergens have been characterized at a molecular level, their spatial structure has been determined, and allergen fragments (epitopes) responsible for reactions with IgE antibodies have also been characterized. A deeper understanding of the mechanism of the immunopathogenesis of food allergies has been reached, and this may soon lead to novel diagnostic and therapeutic approaches. Many informative books have been published on this subject. However, we need to constantly update ourselves to keep abreast of the latest developments in the many sciences related to food hypersensitivity. On the other hand, the advances in research on food hypersensitivity open a wide range of potential new solutions and possibilities. International teams of scientists committed to research in fields such as medicine, molecular biology, food biotechnology, and foodstuff assays have achieved remarkable results.

This book should help in understanding the problems related to the occurrence of allergies, particularly food allergies. It contains up-to-date information on the mechanisms involved in hypersensitive responses and threats caused by ingesting foodstuffs and their components that are often associated with modern food-processing technologies. It provides in-depth knowledge on allergens and related disciplines. It also responds to the need for popular social education, which aims to instruct potential patients on methods of avoiding harmful allergens. This objective is aided by the presentation of the problems, which consists of a detailed characterization of the major groups of allergens, a description of their behavior during various technological and biotechnological processes, as well as an indication of potential reactions with other allergens. Due to its educational value, this book may also be of interest to general consumers, allergic consumers, representatives of the agro-food industry (including primary producers, manufacturers, and retailers), and health professionals and regulators. It should also be a dependable reference for researchers (clinicians, food scientists, dieticians, and nutritionists) and students of molecular biology (particularly the up-to-date characterizations of mechanisms causing allergies and genetic modifications aimed at decreasing allergenic activity of food products), food technology (mainly health risks related to particular food components and the effect of technological processes on allergenic activity of food products as well as foodstuff assays), biotechnology (primarily allergenic threats caused by microorganisms and microbial metabolites), and food safety, as well as medical studies connected with diagnostic methods (elimination diets and food challenges) and allergy therapies.

This book draws its material from existing databases on allergens and from Web pages devoted to this issue. Hence, it encourages the readers to expand their knowledge on their own—it can be especially beneficial for college students. It should be present on the shelves of libraries at all universities, especially universities and scientific institutes that specialize in biological research.

**Lucjan Jędrychowski**

# Acknowledgments

I would like to thank my wife and children for being so understanding and patient while I was absent from home writing this book. I am also grateful to all the co-authors and my co-workers for their assistance and kindness.

**Lucjan Jędrychowski**

# Editors

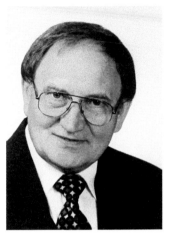

**Lucjan Jędrychowski** is a researcher in biotechnology, food sciences, and food allergies, and is the head of the Department of Food Enzymes and Allergens at The Polish Academy of Sciences' Institute of Animal Reproduction and Food Research in Olsztyn. His research interests include the investigation and determination of radionuclide contamination of food, exploring possibilities for the decontamination and application of radionuclides S-35 and P-32 by incorporation into chlorella for inducing mutations, the evaluation of properties of enzymes and applications of enzyme preparation in the food industry and in food analysis, food allergens, the application of immunological methods (ELISA, ELISPOT) for investigating biologically active compounds in food (mainly allergens), and the investigation of biologically active compounds in food for both their positive and negative effects in an organism. He is a coauthor of 365 publications, 5 books, and 2 patents.

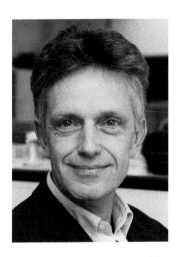

**Harry J. Wichers** is a biochemist by training. He received his PhD on the topic "Biotechnological production of pharmaceuticals with plant cell cultures" from the University of Groningen.

After working for five years at the TNO-Zeist, Department of Biotechnology, he joined the Wageningen University and Research Centre in the early 1990s, where he worked on the biochemical characterization of food quality parameters.

Wichers has been program leader of research on the relationship between food and health. In this research, data on the physiological effects of food constituents are integrated with data of their characteristics in the raw materials and their behavior during processing in order to develop foods that are attractive to the senses and have a positive impact on human health.

Wichers is one of the founders of the Allergy Consortium Wageningen; in this expertise center, research teams from each science group of Wageningen-UR cooperate to develop strategies for allergy management.

He has held a chair entitled "immune modulation by food" since April 2005. Through this chair, the interactions between food (constituents) and the (human or animal) immune system are studied in order to contribute to the development of foods, feed, or ingredients that can aid in balancing, fortifying, or sustaining an appropriate immune response. In this research, structure–activity relationships of immune-modulating natural compounds are studied. The immunological readout systems include receptor-binding studies, and gene expression through expression array–based analyses.

# Contributors

**Sabine Baumgartner**
Department for Agrobiotechnology,
    IFA-Tulln
University of Natural Resources and
    Applied Life Sciences
Vienna, Austria

**Joanna Bober**
Department of Medical Chemistry
Pomeranian Medical University
    of Szczecin
Szczecin, Poland

**Merima Bublin**
Department of Pathophysiology
Medical University of Vienna
Vienna, Austria

**Beata Cudowska**
IIIrd Department of Pediatrics
Medical University of Bialystok
Bialystok, Poland

**Matthias Egger**
Department of Molecular Biology
Christian Doppler Laboratory for
    Allergy Diagnosis and Therapy
University of Salzburg
Salzburg, Austria

**Anja Maria Erler**
Department of Molecular Biology
Christian Doppler Laboratory for
    Allergy Diagnosis and Therapy
University of Salzburg
Salzburg, Austria

**Michael Faltlhansl**
Department of Molecular Biology
Christian Doppler Laboratory for
    Allergy Diagnosis and Therapy
University of Salzburg
Salzburg, Austria

**Fátima Ferreira**
Department of Molecular Biology
Christian Doppler Laboratory for
    Allergy Diagnosis and Therapy
University of Salzburg
Salzburg, Austria

**Gabriele Gadermaier**
Department of Molecular Biology
Christian Doppler Laboratory for
    Allergy Diagnosis and Therapy
University of Salzburg
Salzburg, Austria

**Anna Halász**
Department of Biology
Central Food Research Institute
Budapest, Hungary

**Andrea Harrer**
Department of Molecular Biology
Christian Doppler Laboratory for
    Allergy Diagnosis and Therapy
University of Salzburg
Salzburg, Austria

**Michael Hauser**
Department of Molecular Biology
Christian Doppler Laboratory for
    Allergy Diagnosis and Therapy
University of Salzburg
Salzburg, Austria

**Martin Himly**
Department of Molecular Biology
Christian Doppler Laboratory for
    Allergy Diagnosis and Therapy
University of Salzburg
Salzburg, Austria

**Karin Hoffmann-Sommergruber**
Department of Pathophysiology
Medical University of Vienna
Vienna, Austria

**Geert Houben**
Department of Food and Chemical
    Risk Analysis
TNO Quality of Life
Utrecht, Netherlands

**Lucjan Jędrychowski**
Department of Food Enzymes
    and Allergens
Institute of Animal Reproduction
    and Food Research
Polish Academy of Sciences
Olsztyn, Poland

**Maciej Kaczmarski**
IIIrd Department of Pediatrics
Medical University of Bialystok
Bialystok, Poland

**Elżbieta Korotkiewicz-Kaczmarska**
University Children's Hospital
Bialystok, Poland

**Elżbieta Kucharska**
Department of Human Nutrition
Faculty of Food Sciences
    and Fisheries
West Pomeranian University of
    Technology
Szczecin, Poland

**Samuel Lehrer**
Section of Allergy, Rheumatology, &
    Clinical Immunology
Health Science Center
Department of Medicine
Tulane University Medical School
New Orleans, Louisiana

**Joanna Leszczynska**
Faculty of Biotechnology and Food
    Sciences
Technical University of Lodz
Lodz, Poland

**Andreas Lopata**
College of Science, Engineering and
    Health
School of Applied Sciences
Royal Melbourne Institute of
    Technology
Melbourne, Victoria, Australia

**Niels Lucas Luijckx**
Department of Food and Chemical
    Risk Analysis
TNO Quality of Life
Utrecht, Netherlands

**András Nagy**
Department of Biology
Central Food Research Institute
Budapest, Hungary

**Edina Németh**
Faculty of Veterinary Science
Department of Pharmacology and
    Toxicology
Szent Istvána University
Budapest, Hungary

**Christina Oberhuber**
Biomay AG
Vienna, Austria

**Tadeusz Ogoński**
Faculty of Biotechnology and Animal
  Breeding
Department of Physiological Chemistry
West Pomeranian University of
  Technology
Szczecin, Poland

**Angelika Paschke**
Department of Chemistry, Food
  Chemistry
University of Hamburg
Hamburg, Germany

**André H. Penninks**
Department of Toxicology and Applied
  Pharmacology
Experimental Immunology
TNO Quality of Life
Zeist, the Netherlands

**Georg Schmidt**
Department of Molecular Biology
Christian Doppler Laboratory for
  Allergy Diagnosis and Therapy
University of Salzburg
Salzburg, Austria

**Patricia Schubert-Ullrich**
Department for Agrobiotechnology,
  IFA-Tulln
University of Natural Resources and
  Applied Life Sciences
Vienna, Austria

**Marielle Spanjersberg**
Department of Food and Chemical
  Risk Analysis
TNO Quality of Life
Utrecht, Netherlands

**Agata Szymkiewicz**
Department of Food Enzymes
  and Allergens
Institute of Animal Reproduction
  and Food Research
Polish Academy of Sciences
Olsztyn, Poland

**Michael Wallner**
Department of Molecular Biology
Christian Doppler Laboratory for
  Allergy Diagnosis and Therapy
University of Salzburg
Salzburg, Austria

**Patrick Weber**
Department of Food Chemistry
Institute of Biochemistry and
  Food Chemistry
University of Hamburg
Hamburg, Germany

**Nicole Wopfner**
Department of Molecular Biology
Christian Doppler Laboratory for
  Allergy Diagnosis and Therapy
University of Salzburg
Salzburg, Austria

**Barbara Wróblewska**
Department of Food Enzymes
  and Allergens
Institute of Animal Reproduction
  and Food Research
Polish Academy of Sciences
Olsztyn, Poland

# Abbreviations

**ADCC**—antibody-dependent cytotoxicity
**AEDS**—atopic eczema/dermatitis syndrome
**AFM**—atomic force microscopy
**AOAC INTERNATIONAL**—Association of Analytical Communities
**AP 1**—activating protein 1
**APC**—antigen-presenting cells
**ATP**—atopy patch test
**ATR**—attenuated total reflection
**AUC**—analytical ultracentrifugation
**B10A**—strain of the mouse
**Balb/c**—albino strain of laboratory mouse
**BALT**—bronchus-associated lymphoid tissue
**BHA**—butylated hydroxyanisole (antioxidant)
**BHR**—bronchial hyperreactivity
**BHT**—butylated hydroxytoluene (antioxidant)
**BN rats**—Brown Norway (BN) rats
**BRs**—brassinosteroids
**BSA**—bovine serum albumin
**C3H/hej**—strain of the mouse
**CCD**—cross-reactive carbohydrate determinants
**CCDs**—cross-reactive carbohydrates
**CD**—circular dichroism
**CD**—cluster of differentiation
**Cd**—parameter introduced by authors expressing the product of temperature and time
**CLA**—cutaneous lymphocyte antigen
**CM**—cow's milk
**CMA**—cow's milk allergy
**CmM**—camel milk
**CMPA**—cow milk protein allergy
**CMPI**—cow milk protein intolerance
**cns**—central nervous system
**CRIE**—crossed radioimmunoelectrophoresis
**CTACK**—cutaneous T-cell-attracting chemokine
**CTLA4**—cytotoxic T lymphocyte associated antigen 4
**DAG**—diacylglycerol
**DAO**—diaminooxidase
**DBA/2**—strain of the mouse
**DBPCFC**—double-blind placebo-controlled food challenge method—the golden standard in food allergy determination
**DC**—dendritic cell

**DDBJ**—*see* EMBL

**DLS**—dynamic light scattering

**DM**—donkey's milk

**DNA**—deoxyribonucleic acid

**DNCB**—2,4-dinitrochlorobenzene

**DSC**—differential scanning calorimetry

**DTH**—delayed cellular hypersensitivity

**DXMS**—deuterium exchange mass spectrometry

**EAACI**—European Academy of Allergology and Clinical Immunology

**EAR**—early anaphylactic phase

**ECFA**—eosinophil chemotactic factors of anaphylaxis

**ECP**—eosinophil cationic protein

**EDN**—eosinophil-derived neurotoxin

**eHF**—extensively hydrolyzed formula

**ELISA**—enzyme-linked immunosorbent assay

**EMBL**—European Molecular Biology Laboratory (Heidelberg) Nucleotide Sequence Database (also known as EMBL-Bank). The database is produced in an international collaboration with GenBank (USA) and the DNA Database of Japan (DDBJ). The EMBL nucleotide sequence database is part of the Protein and Nucleotide Database Group (PANDA)

**EPO**—eosinophil peroxidase

**ESI**—electrospray ionization

**EU**—European Union

**FA**—food allergy

**FACS**—Facial Action Coding System

**FAO**—Food and Agriculture Organization

**FEV1**—forced expiratory volume in 1 s

**FLAG–tag**—polypeptide protein tag that is added to a recombinant expressed protein

**FTIR spectroscopy**—Fourier transform infrared spectroscopy

**GALT**—gut-associated lymphoid tissue

**GI**—gastrointestinal

**GITR**—glucocorticoid-induced tumor necrosis factor receptor

**GITR**—glucocorticoid-induced tumor necrosis factor receptor of TNF

**GITR-L**—glucocorticoid-induced tumor necrosis factor receptor ligand

**GM**—goat's milk

**GMCSF**—granulocyte-macrophage colony stimulating factor

**GMP**—Good Manufacturing Practice

**GRAS**—generally regarded as safe

**HLA**—human leukocyte antigen

**HP**—hypersensitivity pneumonitis

**HPLC**—high-performance liquid chromatography

**Hsp70**—the 70 kDa heat-shock proteins

**HT-29**—designations of the cell line—synonym ATCC® Number HTB-38™

**i.p.**—intraperitoneal

**ICAM-1**—intracellular adhesion molecules-1

**IDO**—indoleamine 2,3-dioxygenase

**IFNγ**—interferon-gamma

**IgA**—immunoglobulin A

**IgE**—immunoglobulin E

**IgG**—immunoglobulin G

**IL**—interleukin

**IP3**—inositol 1,4,5-triphosphate

**ISP**—ice structuring protein

**IT**—informatic technology

**ITAM**—immunoreceptor tyrosine-based activation motif

**IUIS**—International Union of Immunological Societies

**JAK**—Janus kinases

**JNK**—Jun N-terminal kinases

**kDa**—kiloDalton

**LAB**—lactic acid bacteria

**LAR**—late anaphylactic phase

**LIC technology**—The strategy for ligation independent cloning (LIC) is a special technique used to amplify the gene of interest employing gene-specific primers that include complementary linearized vectors. This method can also be easily adapted for high-throughput cloning. The main advantage of the LIC protocol is that it completely avoids restriction digestion and ligation of the inserted DNA that is particularly significant for large genes.

**LOAEL**—lowest observed adverse effect level

**LOD**—limit of detection—defined as the analyte concentration interpolated from a standard curve at a response level equivalent to zero concentration plus three standard deviations

**LOQ**—limit of quantitation—the lowest and highest standard used in the analysis

**LPS**—lipopolysaccharide

**LTB$_4$**—leukotriene B (4)

**LTP**—lipid-transfer protein

**MALDI**—matrix-assisted laser desorption ionization

**MALT**—mucosa-associated lymphoid tissue

**MAO**—monoaminooxidase

**MAPK**—mitogen-activated protein kinases

**MBP**—major basic protein

**MC**—mucosal cell

**MCP 1**—monocyte chemoattractant protein 1

**MDC**—macrophage-derived chemokine

**MED**—minimal eliciting dose

**MHC**—major histocompatibility complex

**MIF**—macrophage inhibitory factor

**MIP 1**—macrophage inflammatory protein 1

**MIP 2**—macrophage inflammatory protein 2

**MM**—mare's milk

**MMC**—mucosal mast cells

**MoM**—mother's milk

**MS**—mass spectrometry

**MW**—molecular weight synonym of the molecular mass (abbreviated M)—is the mass of one molecule

**NALT**—nose-associated lymphoid tissue

**nanoLC-MSMS**—nanoliquid chromatography–tandem MS

**NCF**—neutrophil chemotactic factors

**NFA**—nuclear factor of activated T-lymphocytes

**NF-kappaB**—nuclear factor kappa B

**NK**—cells natural killer cells

**NMR**—nuclear magnetic resonance

**NOAEL**—the highest tested dose without adverse effects (no-observed-adverse-effect level)

**NOE**—nuclear Overhauser enhancement

**nsLTPs**—nonspecific lipid-transfer protein

**OAS**—oral allergy syndrome

**OFC**—oral food challenge

**OVA**—ovalbumin

**PAF**—platelet activating factor

**PAMP**—pathogen-associated molecular patterns

**PANDA**—*see* EMBL

**PBMCs**—primary blood mononuclear cells

**PCR**—polymerase chain reaction

**PDB codes**—Protein Data Bank codes (*see also* wwPDB)

**PDDF**—pair distance distribution function

**PFS**—pollen-food syndrome

**pHF**—partially/moderately hydrolyzed formulae

**PKC**—protein kinase C

**PPV**—positive predictive value

**PR**—pathogenesis-related proteins

**PST**—prick skin tests

**RANTES**—factor regulated on activation normal T cells expressed and secreted

**RAST**—radioallergosorbent test

**RBL**—functional rat-basophil assay

**RIVM**—public health and environment

**s.c.**—subcutaneous

**SALT**—skin-associated lymphoid tissue

**SAXS**—small-angle x-ray scattering

**SCF**—stem cell factor

**SCS**—spent culture supernatant

**SDS-PAGE**—sodium dodecyl sulfate polyacrylamide gel electrophoresis

**SEC**—size exclusion chromatography

**SF**—soy formulae

**SIT**—specific immunotherapy

**SLIT**—sublingual immunotherapy

**SM**—sheep's milk

**SNP**—single nucleotide polymorphism

**SPT**—skin prick test

**STAT**—signal transducer and activator transcription

**STI**—soybean trypsin inhibitor

**TARC**—thymus activation-regulated chemokine

**TCC**—T-cell clones

**TCL**—T-cell line

**TCR**—T-cell antigen receptor

**TGF-β**—transforming growth factor-β

**TLPs**—thaumatin-like proteins

**TLR**—toll-like receptors

**TMV**—tobacco mosaic virus

**TNF**—tumor necrosis factor

**TNF-α**—tumor necrosis factor-α

**TNO**—Netherlands Organisation for Applied Scientific Research

**TROSY**—transverse relaxation-optimized spectroscopy

**UHT**—ultrahigh temperature—food prepared during partial sterilization by heating it for a short time, around 1–2 s, at a temperature exceeding 135°C

**VC**—Netherlands Nutrition Centre

**VCAM-1**—vascular cell adhesion molecule-1

**VEGF**—vascular endothelial growth factor

**VIP**—vasoactive intestinal peptide

**VPAC$_1$ and VPAC$_2$**—vasoactive intestinal peptide (VIP) receptors

**WDEIA**—wheat-dependent exercise-induced anaphylaxis

**WHO**—World Health Organization

**wwPDB**—Worldwide Protein Data Bank (group which joined the wwPDB in 2006) consists of organizations that act as deposition, data processing, and distribution centers for PDB data. The founding members are RCSB PDB (USA), PDBe (Europe) PDBj (Japan), and BMRB (USA). The mission of the wwPDB is to maintain a single protein data bank archive of macromolecular structural data that is freely and publicly available to the global community

**α-la**—α-lactalbumin (alfa-lactalbumin)

**β-lg**—β-lactoglobulin (beta-lactoglobulin)

# 1 Molecular, Cellular, and Physiological Mechanisms of Immunological Hyporesponsiveness/ Sensitization to Food

*Elżbieta Kucharska, Joanna Bober, and Tadeusz Ogoński*

## CONTENTS

## 1.1 PUTATIVE MECHANISM SUGGESTED FOR INTESTINAL INDUCTION OF ORAL TOLERANCE ACCORDING TO LUMINAL ANTIGEN DOSE

It is a fascinating quality of the gastrointestinal tract to generate an immunological response to bacteria and food components taken in. In a healthy state, the immune response is adequate to the degree of hazard. Inflammatory reaction is not triggered by the case of food components and microorganisms which are constantly present in the gastrointestinal tract flora. They are treated as self. This is possible due to the anatomy and histology of their structure and to the functional diversification of the gastrointestinal tract cells. It also results from the capacity to develop a food tolerance phenomenon. This phenomenon is necessary in protecting a macroorganism against overstimulation of the immune system.

The estimated area of the gastrointestinal tract is approximately $300\,m^2$ and the estimated amount of food taken in is many tons. Reduced food tolerance could result in developing chronic and then autoimmunological inflammations.

The balance between induction and inhibition processes is maintained, thanks to specific and nonspecific immunity. One of the basic factors is the normal structure of the gastrointestinal tract.

From the intestinal lumen, the esophagus, stomach, and intestines are covered with two layers of mucus—mobile and static. Mucus creates gel containing mucopolysaccharides and glycoproteins which isolate a cylindrical-epithelium-covered surfaces. The nondissolving mucus layer is covered by the mobile dissolving layer. They don't demonstrate any chemical difference from each other (Mowat, 2003).

Humans are protected against physiological and pathogenic flora invasion by means of nonspecific humoral response factors. These include low pH of gastric juice, proteolytic enzymes, lactoferrin, lysozyme, and defensins. Another crucial element is physiological bacterial flora, whose content changes throughout the human life cycle, and that hinders the development of pathogenic flora; moreover, it also has immunoregulative functions.

Specific humoral response depends mainly on secretory IgA that are found in mucus on the surface of intestinal epithelium. They are responsible for blocking adhesive receptors against pathogenic bacterial flora and hindering protein molecule absorption (Macpherson et al., 2000). Low concentration of secretory IgA in the mucus membranes of gastrointestinal tract, upper airways, or urinogenital system leads to recurring inflammations or developing allergies in humans and animals (Hidvegi et al., 2002; Frossard et al., 2004).

The surface of the small intestine is covered with cylindrical epithelium consisting mainly of enterocytes, among which there are goblet cells and intraepithelial lymphocytes that are especially numerous above lymphatic papules. Desmosomes are responsible for attachment and adhesion of the cells constituting epithelium. Moreover, in the peak parts epithelial cells are additionally linked creating zonulae occludentes formation. They attach chemidesmosomes to the stroma thus connecting the cells with basilar membrane. During the first months of human life, intestinal epithelium does not render a hermetic barrier against micromolecules. Excessive penetration of the mucous membrane by protein compounds is now considered responsible for the development of food allergy in infants.

An important role in the nonspecific cellular response is played by Paneth cells which line the bottom of the intestinal glands. Their granules contain compounds that can damage bacteria. These include a lysozyme which damages peptidoglycan, the basic structure of Gram positive bacterial cellular membrane; secreted phospholipase A2 involved in lipopolysaccharide metabolism; and α-defensins, cryptydins, which decompose bacterial proteins.

Under the epithelial stratum, the lamina propria of mucous membrane is located and it contains elements directly involved in immunological response, i.e., phagocytes—granulocytes, macrophages, T and B lymphocytes, plasmatic cells, and mucosal mast cells (MMCs). The main part is constituted by T lymphocytes 40%–60%, then B lymphocytes and plasmatic cells 20%–40%, macrophages 10%, eosinophils 5%, and mast cells 1%–3%. MMCs contain vasoactive compounds, so they indirectly influence cellular content by means of decreasing their inflow. Moreover, they regulate cytokine release in the normal and inflammatory environment. Within mucosal lamella serous IgA can be found that form complexes with antigens in intercellular spaces. The complexes are phagocytosed or moved reversely into the intestinal lumen (Van Egmond et al., 2001).

The gastrointestinal tract is considered the largest systemic lymphatic organ. It contains numerous lymphocytic groups which create appendix, sometimes referred to as "abdominal tonsil," lymphatic nodes of gastrointestinal tract, solitary lymphatic follicles, and Peyer's patches at the base of intestinal villi.

Peyer's patches are the tiniest of the above structures, but due to their vast numbers they account for a significant group of lymphocytes in gastrointestinal system. They develop in the prenatal stage and their number gradually decreases as the aging process progresses. Peyer's patches have a characteristic structure. They are mainly formed by groups of B lymphocytes surrounded by T lymphocytes. Peyer's patches form domes. From the side of the intestine, the dome is covered in cylindrical epithelium containing numerous enterocytes transformed into microfold cells.

Contrary to prior concepts, the intestinal epithelium is not a hermetic barrier for most micro-particles. The food reaching the ileum is, to a large extent, metabolized by digestive enzymes. A part of antigens, however, remains unchanged. Selecting antigens from the environment is facilitated by glycocalyx which covers the epithelium.

It forms lectin bindings with antigen proteins or antigen–antibody complexes, in most cases and IgA is the antibody.

In a healthy state, antigens enter through M cell pathways. M cells are crescent-shaped, arching toward the intestinal lumen. In the concave part, there is a niche filled with B and T lymphocytes and macrophages as well as dendritic cells. M cells owe their name to the numerous folds on the surface, through which antigens reach the inside. M cells are responsible for delivering antigens to macrophages for "preliminary treatment" or to dendritic cells or B lymphocytes so that they can generate and present immunological responses to other elements. Dendritic cells may also be attached to antigens without the use of M cells, via long projections with which they reach the intestinal lumen (Brandtzaeg, 2001).

Stimulated lymphocytes are transported via lymphatic cells to the nearest mesenteric lymph nodes, and next to systemic immunological organs, and via the blood stream to other tissues. Stimulation or expiration of immunological responses occurs. Some lymphocytes return to the intestines, thanks to integrin $\alpha4\beta7$ and CCR9 chemokine receptors.

### 1.1.1 MOLECULAR AND CELLULAR MECHANISMS OF FOOD ALLERGY

#### 1.1.1.1 Allergens

According to Johansson, allergens are antigens that trigger allergy. Most of them have a protein, they are usually glycoproteins (Johansson et al., 2001) dissolved in water and resistant to digestion. The immune system recognizes them, and as a result specific IgE are produced, type I allergy develops, or specific T-cell antigen receptor (TCR) are produced and type IV allergy develops according to Gell Coombs. Symptoms of type II and type III food allergies occur much more rarely.

A common feature of allergens is that they comprise a fairly broad range of particle of sizes ranging from 3 to 160 kDa, usually 20–40 kDa. Some of them show enzymatic activity which enables passage through the mucous membrane barrier (Rolland and O'Hehir, 2001). Similar immunological phenomena are triggered by haptens.

Until recently it was believed that haptens, since their particles are tiny, must be combined with peptides to gain antigenic properties. It is now believed that there is a group of simple compounds, including mannitol, which directly induces IgE-dependent reactions, thanks to the similarity of alcohol particles to sugar bound with protein (Venkatesh and Venkatesh, 2003). Haptens enter the body via mucous or serous membranes, or the skin; they are sometimes introduced to tissues during surgical procedures and induce inflammatory-allergic reactions. Examples of haptens include metal ions or simple chemical compounds found in drugs, cosmetics, preservatives, pigments, and food formulations. Some haptens may be released in the body during the process of complex compound (e.g., medicines) metabolism in the gastrointestinal system.

#### 1.1.1.2 Anaphylaxis

The term "anaphylaxis" was introduced by Paul Portier and Charles Richet in 1902 (in Greek *ana-* reverse, *phyl-* protection).

It is a potentially lethal immediate hypersensitivity reaction, in whose pathomechanism the main role is played by IgE antibodies. Mediators released in the process are responsible for tissue reactions, which may involve the respiratory system, gastrointestinal system, and the skin or cardiovascular system.

The probability of occurrence of sudden death due to the food anaphylaxis has been calculated over 10 years' retrospective research at 0.06 deaths in 1,000,000; in children aged 0–15 per year based on results of 10 years' retrospective studies. The most frequent allergen was cow's milk accounting for approximately 50% of deaths. Also, severe anaphylactic reactions were observed following the consumption of nuts. That estimated probability of death occurrence is 1 in 800,000 children per year, assuming that 5% of the population exhibits symptoms of food allergy (Macdougall et al., 2002).

According to Pirquet, an allergy is the changed reactivity of the system to a reintroduced antigen. This scenario also includes anaphylactic reactions, which result from multiple contact of the system with allergen or hapten, especially if they are introduced parenterally. Chronic immunization leads to the production of IgE antibodies, which show cytophylaxis. They bind their Fc fragment with the surface of mast cells and basophils. An excessive amount of antibodies appearing in blood serum indicates an increase in IgE ratio.

The number of IgE receptors on the surface of mast cells and basophils is different and varies from one organism to another. MacGlashan thought that the number of IgE particles bound with the surface determines the level of cell sensitivity (MacGlashan and Lichtenstein, 1981). Releasability, i.e., a spontaneous non-IgE-dependent capacity to degranulate, is a factor affecting the level of anaphylactic reaction involvement, and it also varies in particular organisms (MacGlashan, 1993). IgE binds with the surface of mast cells by means of receptors. Cells are equipped with the following:

- FcεRI is a high-affinity receptor. Apart from mast cells and basophils, it may be found on Langerhans cells, eosinophils, and monocytes.
- FcεRII (CD23) receptor plays an important role in regulation of IgE synthesis. In comparison to FcεRI, it shows low affinity to IgE. It is found on dendritic cells, macrophages, monocytes, platelets, T and B lymphocytes, and eosinophils. In its soluble form, it sometimes activates B lymphocytes to produce IgE.

Mac-2 receptor is found on mast cells, macrophages, and neutrophils. It is a lectin, so when it is bound with a cell or when it is released to the environment, it binds with carbohydrates. Thus an intolerance reaction may occur—without IgE participation. It may also trigger lectinophagocytosis through phagocytes (Valenta, 1994). IgE may also bind with FcγII i FcγIII—receptors of low IgE affinity. What is more, FcγIIIR receptors in the form of FcγIIIRB have an oligosaccharide structure, so they bind bacterial lectins, and are present on neutrophils (Sokal, 1995).

In the submucosal layer of the gastrointestinal tract, there are numerous $MC_T$ mucosal cells. They are equipped with granules and contain biogenic amines, chemotactic factors, and as far as proteases are concerned, tryptase.

$MC_T$ cells are sensitive to cromoglycates. The cytokines, they secrete include, mainly IL 5 and IL 6 in considerable concentrations, when stroma contains IL 4 as well as IL 1, 3, 8, 10, 13, 16, MIP-1$\alpha$, MIP-2$\alpha$, and TGF$\beta$.

In the anaphylactic processes, bridging of allergen-specific IgEs (bound with the surface of a mast cell by the allergen) induces cell degranulation. This is a process which cells undergo not only due to allergen effect, but also when toll-like receptors (TLR) bind with bacteria, thermal shock proteins, or viruses (Patella et al., 2000; Malaviya and Abraham, 2001). First the compounds in preformed granules are released and later derivatives of arachidonic acid, i.e., generated compounds and cytokines are released.

Histamine is a biogenic amine in human $MC_T$s. In the inactive form, it produces complexes with proteoglycans in mast cells. When it is secreted by preformed granules, it exhibits pathogenetic and proinflammatory effect. It is in the system within 15–30 min. Its role in the patomechanism is then overtaken by hydrolases and leukotriens generated from arachidonic acid, acting with histamine, but 1000 times stronger and lasting 6–10 h longer. Release of histamine by stimulating the receptors in various cells results in the following:

- Dilating vessels, manifested with local reddening; generally, an increase in the volume of vascular placenta, and consequently, decrease of blood pressure and arrhythmia
- Increased permeation to intracellular spaces leading to blistering or oral mucosal urticaria, swelling of the lips, tongue, throat—oral allergy syndrome (OAS); or generally urticaria occurrence, swelling of the larynx, and pulmonary edema
- Contraction of smooth muscles and increased mucus secretion in bronchi—leading to worsening expiratory dyspnea
- Accelerated gastrointestinal peristalsis and increased amount of mucus resulting in nausea, vomiting, paroxysmal abdominal pain, and diarrhea

In the most severe cases, a shock develops at various severity levels, including an irreversible shock. Anaphylactic shock is usually developed within a few to 30 min after contact with food allergen.

With less severe symptoms in the early anaphylactic phase (EAR), after 6–10 h, the late anaphylactic phase (LAR) occurs, which is triggered by mast cells releasing chemokines, cytokines, and leukotriens—massive chemoattractants for neutrophils and eosinophils.

Leukotriens are mainly produced in mast cells, basophils, eosinophils, pulmonary macrophages, and neutrophils as a result of lipooxigenation of arachidonic acid. These compounds show a strong immunomodulating effect. $LTB_4$ is the strongest chemoattractant in the system. It is released by macrophages and neutrophils, thus increasing the flow of cells to the site of inflammation. Leukotriens cause a chronic bronchial contraction, increased intestinal peristalsis, and mucus secretion.

Neutral and acidic serine proteases released from mast cells-tryptase $MC_T$ may damage type IV collagen and the intercellular matrix. Eosinophil chemotactic factors of anaphylaxis (ECFA) and neutrophil chemotactic factors (NCFs) are directly responsible for late cell phase development.

Eosinophils and neutrophils are highly enzymatically equipped (Rothenberg et al., 2001). Eosinophils are widely presented as main anaphylactic cells due to the fact that they contain compounds which exacerbate and extend an allergic reaction process. Such compounds include major basic protein (MBP), eosinophil cationic protein (ECP), eosinophil peroxidase (EPO), and eosinophil-derived neurotoxin (EDN). The effects of these compounds lead to lymphocyte (especially Th2) chemotaxis, which (by means of IL 3, IL 5, and granulocyte-macrophage colony stimulating factor [GMCSF]) increases eosinophilopoesis, and next—due to increased chemokine concentration—the flow of cells to tissues contributing to eosinophilic oesophagitis, gastroenteritis, vasculitis, and carditis.

- Stimulated expression of adhesion molecules: VCAM-1 and ICAM-1; increased release of cytokines and mediators (GMCSF, TNFα, PAF, $PGE_2$, $PGF_{2\alpha}$), and consequently damaging the cells of intestinal epithelium.
- Facilitated permeation through the walls of granulocyte vessels, thanks to increased expression of integrins and selectins.
- Release of TGFα from eosinophils, which triggers the proliferation of fiberblasts, while ECP stimulates collagen synthesis, which contributes to the development of fibrosis.

Neutrophil granulocytes contain approximately 100 enzymes in their lysosomal granules. The digestion process leads to releasing

- Free radicals, which damage tissues and disturb the balance between proteolytic enzymes and their inhibitors
- Elastase degrading elastin and other proteins
- G cathepsin which degrades proteoglycans and depolymerize collagen fibers

It is known that the progress of allergic inflammation is significantly severe if accompanied by a bacterial infection. Apart from the lectin mechanism, the stimulation of TLR receptors increases the flow of cells and the released cytokines mix. It has been recently proved that eosinophils are also equipped with this type of receptors. Potential participation of eosinophils in the exacerbation of allergic diseases observed while developing a concomitant microorganic infection has thus been proved (Cheung et al., 2008).

After first 24 h and during following days, LAR may transfer into a late-type allergy. It is an infiltration of (mainly) T lymphocytes CD4 and CD8, and macrophages from Peyer's patches and it shows the properties of a contact allergy, in comparison to lymphocytes from blood (Nagata et al., 2000). Gell–Coombs type IV hypersensitivity may develop as the continuation of type I allergy. The sites in which the infiltration forms may include bronchi, skin, and various parts of the gastrointestinal tract.

### 1.1.1.3  Type II Allergy

Type II allergy develops as a result of haptens on the surface of cells (usually blood cells) binding with IgM or IgG antibodies directed to act against haptens. These may include medicines, bacterial elements, viruses, chemicals, and food components—the latter rather rarely, in comparison with type I and IV allergies. Classical complementary activation leads to damaged blood cells and to the occurrence of hemolytic anemia, leukopenia, or thrombocytopenia symptoms. According to Barr, apart from hypochromic anemia—the iron deficiency—anemia caused by red and white cells damaged by the complement may develop. It is a system of enzymatically active proteins which bind with antibodies acting against allergens connected to the surface of the cells (Barr et al., 1958). Cytotoxicity may occur in the systems which can be complement and noncomplement dependent. The flow of phagocytes and increased phagocytosis of the damaged erythrocytes may efficiently eliminate cells from the blood stream. Antibody-dependent cytotoxicity (ADCC) is another possible mechanism. The cells covered in haptens and antibodies which hardly bind the complement or do not bind it at all, are destroyed by other cells equipped with Fc fragment antibody, by means of exocytosis.

In a number of cases the reason for blood cell deficiency is unknown. It is then referred to as "spontaneous, idiopathic." Perhaps more detailed diagnostic methods will solve the problem.

The reason for hyperactivity or hypoactivity of a hormonally active organ is also very often unknown. The immunology-related background is screened in tests. Finding the antibodies against tissue-specific antigens or nonspecific ribonucleic acids, microsomes, endoplasmatic net enables recognition of autoimmunization mechanisms. This, however, is the result not the cause. It seems that food haptens may also participate in this allergy type.

### 1.1.1.4  Type III Allergy

Allergic, leukoclastic vasculitis is etiologically related to allergen and hapten hypersensitivity. These may include microorganisms, medicines, various chemical substances, and food compounds. When antigens appear in intercellular spaces and blood stream they induce first IgM and next IgG antibodies production. Excessive antigen or excessive antibodies appear in blood system complexes, which set *in situ*, or in small skin vessels, kidneys, and joints. Classic complement activation leads to increased granulocyte flow and fagocytosis results in releasing numerous proteases, hydrolases, and lipases, which damage vessel walls leading to leukoclastic inflammation (Roszkiewicz et al., 2007). It is a nonhomogenous group of systemic vasculitides caused by exogenic factors such as medicines, microorganisms, and food; there are also endogenic factors, e.g., DNA in collagenoses. As the vessels are damaged due to complexes setting as deposits, vessels become less hermetic and so morphotic elements penetrate tissues. Hemorrhagic eruptions appear on the skin. Granulocytic infiltration may lead to further damage to tissues, due to the release of elastase, collagenase, and other enzymes. In the late phase of inflammation, lymphocytes and macrophages also take part in forming infiltrations and, as a result of vascular damage, symptoms of thrombosis and reduced blood flow occur. So type III allergy is transformed into Gell–Coombs type IV hypersensitivity.

## 1.1.2 MECHANISMS OF CELL-MEDIATED DELAYED HYPERSENSITIVITY REACTIONS (TH1)

Delayed cellular hypersensitivity (DTH) occurs fairly often, involving approximately 18% of patients with food allergy. An effect of triggering the specific cellular response is the development of enteropathy, enterocolitis, and proctitis, usually as a result of allergy to cow milk proteins. Another allergen which may cause a DTH response is gluten, which is connected to coeliac disease. Considering various diseases or syndromes, it is fairly difficult to determine one Gell–Coombs allergy type. Most often overlapping syndromes occur, which are initially manifested by IgE-dependent allergy symptoms occurring within 30 min of contact with an allergen; next they are dominated by cellular infiltrations occurring after 6–8 h with predominant presence of eosinophils and granulocytes; then after 24–48–72 h they transform into symptoms dependent on predominantly T lymphocyte infiltrations. Therefore, in the analysis of temporal changes at the site of contact with an allergen, early IgE-dependent anaphylactic phase and late IgE-independent T-lymphocyte-dependent phase have been determined. Thus, two questions can be asked:

1. Which factors are critical in selecting and developing a T-lymphocyte-dependent response?
2. Why does a Th2-dependent response switch into a Th1-dependent response, instead of regression or consolidation of symptoms?

T lymphocytes are called "the conductors of the immunological orchestra." Twenty years ago Th and Ts lymphocytes were described, and then based on the released cytokines within the Th type, Th1 was determined, which releases IFNγ and α lymphotoxin, and Th2, which releases IL 4, IL 5, IL 10, and IL 13. Soon it became evident that there was a third subpopulation of lymphocytes—Th17—involved in infectious immunity and autoimmunological processes. T lymphocytes need to be presented with an antigen in order to activate their functions. Therefore, it seems that the character and volume of stimulation are determined by the type and dose of an antigen, the mode of presentation in terms of costimulatory molecules, and finally the concentration and content of cytokines contained in stroma, as well as the stage in mechanism processes.

The antigens that stimulate DTH-type response are usually the conservative pathogen associated molecular patterns (PAMPs) or nonmethylated CpG of bacterial origin which react with appropriate toll-like receptors (TLRs) on antigen presenting cells (APCs) (Ulevitch, 1999). They may also include proteins, glycoproteins from virus surfaces or allergens contained in food, e.g., β-lactoglobulin and cow milk caseins, gluten, and gliadin (Bjorksten et al., 2001).

Dendritic cells (DCs) are responsible for the recognition and presentation of antigens; it was believed that there were two types of these cells, which underwent differentiation in the development from CD34 cells in bone marrow. They included dendritic lymphoidal and dendritic cells stemming from monocytes. The former ones were supposed to be responsible for activating Th2 lymphocytes and the latter ones, for stimulating Th1. This categorization was widely discussed. It was proved that, depending on cytokine concentration in stroma, immature DCs developed in the direction determined by the type of antigen, thus becoming functionally diversified. Apart from the level of cell maturity, antigen concentration is of vital importance. It has been shown that large doses of antigen induce clonal deletion and anergy, while small, often repeated doses induce active suppression through Treg lymphocytes.

DC differentiation is stimulated by the presence of IL 4, granulocyte-macrophage colony stimulating factor (GMCSF), transforming growth factor (TGFβ), tumor necrosis factor (TNF), and stem cell factor (SCF) in the stroma. The inhibiting factors include IL 10 and vascular endothelial growth factor (VEGF). After an antigen is detected and caught in the intestinal lumen either directly or indirectly through M cells, DCs are transported to the nearest lymph nodes and then—in the blood—to other organs (Bjorksten et al., 2001).

The next stage is the mode of presentation of the antigen to Th0 cells and biochemical and functional changes lead to the switch from Th0 to Th1. One possibility is a formation of an immunological synapse between APCs and Th lymphocytes. The presentation and recognition process is a dynamic reaction leading to changes in tubuline fibers, and next to the transposition of molecules in a cell, which results in varying expression of surface elements.

The process begins with the recognition of peptides in the context of class II major histocompatibility complex (MHC) on the DC surface, then intracellular signals, i.e., protein kinase C (PKC), calcium ions, and the nuclear factor, κB. At the early stage of transmitting the signal from the TCR receptor, it is also important that there is phosphorylation of both tyrosines in CD3 cell parts in the cytoplasm, i.e., immunoreceptor tyrosine-based activation motif (ITAM). This process progresses with the participation of activated Fyn kinase. Moreover, an activating Lck kinase noncovalently connected to CD4 or CD8 is necessary. The dominant role of Lck kinase is emphasized in transmitting the signal in peripheral lymphocytes. Phosphorylated ITAMs are the loci for attaching ZAP-70 kinase previously phosphorylated by SRC-like kinases. Then, active ZAP-70 kinase undergoes autophosphorylation. This is proceeded by attaching phosphorylated tyrosines, adaptor proteins, responsible for signal transduction to the cell (Zhang et al., 1998). Adaptor proteins mediate in activating the cascade of serine and threonine kinases known as mitogen-activated protein kinases (MAPKs), which contribute to activating protein 1 (AP 1) engaged in cell proliferation (Fraser et al., 1999). Second messengers are compounds produced as a result of cellular membrane phospholipid catabolism induced by activated phophorylated phospholipase C. They include inositol 1,4,5-triphosphate (IP3) and diacylglycerol (DAG). IP3 is transported in the cytoplasm and combines with the receptor on the endoplasmic reticulum thus inducing the release of calcium. As a result of the influence of this element, a transcription factor, which is a nuclear factor of activated T lymphocytes (NFAT), is transported into the nucleus, which then leads to the expression of a number of cytokine genes (Myung et al., 2000).

DAG directly activates serine-threonine kinases, whose role is to activate transcription factors—NF-AT, NF-κB, and AP-1.

In order to stimulate the transformation of lymphocytes, another signal is needed, which will be delivered from the interaction between costimulatory molecules; on the surface of DCs and CD40, which is a ligand. Examples for costimulatory molecules include ICAM 1 or ICAM 2; B7.1 or B7.2., CD40, CD70, and ICOS–L; on the surface of lymphocytes, e.g., LFA-1, CD28, and CD154. Particular proteins should appear in a fixed order so that the stimulation signal can be transmitted and so TCR and CD80/86 activation induces a sudden CD40L expression and cytokine, especially IL 12 release, as shown by Cella and Koch (Cella et al., 1996; Koch et al., 1996). Moreover IL 1, IL 18, and TNF are also released. Cytokines are factors of immunological response affecting the functions of a number of cells, not only in the system of two indirectly bound cells. The condition for interaction is the cell must be equipped with a cytokine-specific receptor.

Incorporation of cytokine in a naïve Th lymphocyte receptor activates the route of Janus kinases (JAK1, JAK2, JAK3), transmission proteins for intracellular signals, and activating transcriptions—Signal Transducer and Activator Transcription (STAT)—consequently phosphorylation of receptor tyrosine results.

As a result of binding phosphorylated STAT with phosphorylated receptor tyrosine, cytokines move into the nucleus becoming DNA transcription factors. It has been observed that, e.g., cytokine IFNγ, IL 12, IL 4, IL 10 bind with various receptors and activate various JAK proteins leading to the activation of various STAT, which accounts for the interchange ability of T-lymphocytes depending on the cytokine saturation of stroma. Bird et al. have shown that by modifying the content of cytokines pharmacologically, mice may exhibit nonnuclear changes in most lymphocytes, and development of cells in Th2 direction (Bird et al., 1998). The phenotype that is generated is hereditary because chromatin rearrangement is irreversible. Noble showed that triggering calcium release in lymphocytes in mice or inhibiting PKC causes cell polarization in Th1 direction, otherwise Th2 are formed (Noble et al., 2000).

Th1 lymphocytes condition specific immunity against intracellular microorganisms. In this type of infection, APC cells are usually stimulated by TLR receptors, and as a result, IL 12 is released. Moreover, IFN.γ. concentration in stroma increases because dendritic cells activate NK cells. Then, triggered by the cytokine caused by the activation of JAK1 and JAK-2 following the STAT1 and T-bet expression, a ligand appears for IL 12, and STAT 3, STAT 4, and nuclear factor kB are activated. Consequently, Th1 characteristic cytokines are released, and due to IFNγ effect, transformation is induced in the surrounding Th0 lymphocytes in Th1 direction. Also, receptor expression increases for IL 18, which is released by DCs, and acts synergetically with IL 12, as Stoll observed (Stoll et al., 1998). Yoshimoto showed that IL 12 increases IL 18 receptor concentration in Th1 and B lymphocytes (Yoshimoto et al., 1998).

Induced chemokines play an important role in inflammatory and allergic processes, in contrast to constructive chemokines, whose tissue concentration is constant. Chemokines are responsible for managing the flow of various populations of lymphocytes, macrophages, as well as the migration of dendritic cells from tissues to lymph nodes and organs. The participation of cytokines in Th1 lymphocytes activation and differentiation in the process of development was researched and proved by Karpus when he incubated naïve T lymphocytes with macrophage inflammatory protein 1 α (MIP 1 α) and as a result obtained an increase in IFNγ production, while incubation with monocyte chemoattractant protein 1 (MCP 1) lead to an increase in IL 4 release, and, consequently, Th2 stimulation (Karpus et al., 1997).

The central DTH cell is Th1 lymphocyte. In the course of Gell Coombs type IV allergy the following have been observed:

1. Release of larger amounts of macrophage inhibitory factor (MIF) by homogeneous suspensions of DCs isolated from patients with colitis ulcerosa, due to the effect of Th1 lymphocyte cytokines, in comparison with healthy human DC. It was observed that in an *in vitro* test MIF blocks the flow of mononuclear cells and granulocytes, while in *in vivo* it is released not only by lymphocytes but also by dendritic cells and leads to cell accumulation—occurrence of inflammatory infiltration. Disease development is also the result of the effect of TNFα, IL 1, IL 6, IL 8, and other cytokines released by macrophages and lymphocytes (Murakami et al., 2002). Thus, it has been proved that DCs can release MIF.

2. Extended life expectancy of activated Th1 lymphocytes and increased release of Th1 phenotype cytokines is due to inhibited apoptosis of these cells (Romagnani, 2000), as a result of stimulating macrophages and TCRγδ lymphocytes to develop an inflammatory condition due to the accumulation of macrophages within 24–48 h of contact with an allergen. In the stimulated macrophages, the number of oxygen and nitrogen compounds increases, and surface expression of MHC class II antigens as well as monokine IL 1 and TNFα release occurs. Activation of fibroblasts with cytokines, particularly with TNFα, leads to the release of metalloproteases by cells, causing collagen, proteoglycan, and glycoprotein degradation, thus damaging intercellular matrix (Romagnani, 2000).

### 1.1.2.1   Gluten-Sensitive Enteropathy (Celiac Disease)

Celiac disease is the result of the development of inflammatory-allergic condition due to gluten intolerance. The disease occurs both in adults and in children in a number of countries all over the world. Its occurrence is fairly frequent, it is estimated that approximately 1% of the population suffers from it. Patients manifest not only gastrointestinal symptoms, but also symptoms which are the consequence of malabsorption syndrome, such as osteoporosis, hypochromic anemia, hypoproteinaemia, hypocalcemia, short stature in children, vitamin deficiency, secondary polysensibilization, and emotional disturbances. Moreover, it has been observed that the occurrence of autoimmunological diseases and neoplasms in patients who are not treated with gluten-free diet doubles (Swinson et al., 1983; Ventura et al., 1999).

Gluten-sensitive enteropathy is a congenital disease, linked with the occurrence of MHC II DQ-2 and DQ-8 locus in immunocompetent cells. At an early stage of the disease, specific IgE are observed after intake of grain containing gluten with gliadin, in the form of hordein (barley), secalin (rye), or avenin (oats) (Bischoff and Crowe, 2005).

These proteins contain considerable amounts of glutamine—an amino acid which is a transglutaminase 2 substrate. In the process of celiac disease development, glutamine undergoes deamination, and next the product is bound with HLA DQ8 or HLA DQ2, due to affinity 25 times higher than in the form containing glutamine

(Kim et al., 2004). The complex formed in this way strongly activates T CD4+ lymphocytes (Arentz-Hansen et al., 2000). Transglutaminase 2 triggers an increase in the activity of phospholipase A2, indirectly by means of glutamic acid derived from glutamine. Active phospholipase A2 catalyzes the release of arachidonic acid from phosphatidylcholine. It is also a substrate in cyclo- and lipoxygenation synthesis of leukotrienes and prostaglandins, as well as other eicosanoids responsible for the development of an extended inflammatory-allergic process at the site of product accumulation (Schuppan, 2000). Cellular infiltration of nonproliferating CD4 TCRαβ lymphocytes and the proliferating CD8 TCRαβ and TCRγδ, as well as macrophages is the exponent. Their cumulative effect is the release of numerous cytokines, including IFNγ and TNFα.

It has been proven that it is mainly TNFα that stimulates fibroblasts to release metalloproteases—compounds leading to the degradation of proteoglycans, collagen, and glycoproteins, and consequently damage the substance of basic connective tissue. As a result, the mucous barrier becomes less hermetic and a subsequent atrophy of intestinal villi and reduction of absorption surfaces occurs (Schuppan, 2000).

B lymphocytes also take part in the inflammatory processes, as they are stimulated to transform into plasmatic cells by gliadin and glutein native peptides, then by transglutaminase and transglutaminase-gliadin complexes (Ventura et al., 1999). In this way, specific IgA are produced, which are directed against the above antigens. Anti-transglutaminase antibodies are widely considered as the most specific disease marker (Hill and Mc Millan, 2006). As the disease progresses, antibodies characteristic of autoaggression develop that is a result of the fact that larger amounts of damaged cell fragments reach the blood stream. These include anti-ssDNA, anti-dsDNA, and anti-cardiolipin antibodies; however, frequent concomitant occurrence of celiac disease and autoimmunological diseases, such as collagenoses, type I diabetes, autoimmunological thyroiditis, or cholangitis have been reported (Szaflarska-Szczepanik, 1997).

Another crucial factor in the course of gluten-sensitive enteropathy is the process of quick enterocyte recovery observed as early as 24h (the normal rate is approximately 6 days), as well as increased cell apoptosis, which is dependent on both INFγ and TNFα. Both apoptosis and the recovery of intestinal epithelial cells are balanced after introducing a gluten-free diet, according to Moss et al. (1996). Also the occurrence of mastocyte inflow has been observed in the course of the development of an inflammatory-allergic condition. It is known that, apart from considerable granule content, they also release proinflammatory cytokines. As the inflammatory condition subsides, a decrease in mastocyte numbers has been observed both in villi and at their base. Thus, mastocytes have become one of the most significant recovery markers in treatment with a gluten-free diet (Elson et al., 1986).

### 1.1.2.2 Enteropathy Induced by Cow Milk Proteins and Other Allergens

Allergy to cow milk protein is frequent in infants aged 3 and below and it occurs in approximately 3% of them. The reason for the occurrence of symptoms is sometimes the lack of possibility to breastfeed an infant in the first 4 months of its life, and if an infant is breastfed, human milk may also cause allergy. As the mother applies an elimination diet or provides the child with highly hydrolyzed diary products, with time, most children cope with the allergy well. The estimated number of children developing tolerance is approximately 70%–90%. Prognosis is worse if a child manifests symptoms of allergy to other allergens. In most cases, allergy to milk develops in children with atopy, especially if labor was concluded with a cesarean section (Eggesbø et al., 2003; Salam et al., 2006). A different content of bacterial flora and a different length period in which Gram negative rods settled in the child's gastrointestinal tract are given as the explanation for the fact (Renz-Polster et al., 2004). Additionally, the bacteria strains are "incidental," they do not come from the mother but usually from the hospital environment (Magalhaes et al., 2007). A child develops nettle rash, symptoms of gastrointestinal disturbances, spastic bronchitis or asthma, thus Gell–Coombs type I allergy develops. Second, there is a possibility that the development of type IV allergy will lead to enteropathy development. Occasionally, there are conditions which progress according to Gell–Coombs type II and III mechanisms.

In the case of enteropathy induced by cow milk, allergens—usually β-lactoglobulin, which is not found in human milk, or α-lactoalbumine—are not hydrolyzed in an infant's gastrointestinal tract. In newborns, acidity in the stomach is lower than in adults. For most of the day, pH is approximately 4, while in adults the figure is 1 (Knapczyk and Lauterbach, 2001). Moreover, enzymes in the gastrointestinal tract are not as active as in adults; they are secreted in smaller amounts as an infant's gastrointestinal tract is still under development after labor. Both small and large peptides may penetrate intestinal walls. Physiologically, whole IgG molecules from the mother pass through. That is why milk proteins may easily penetrate the mucous membrane without any obstacles (Warner and Warner, 2000). Following the absorption of allergens, most dendritic cells are APC cells. They are responsible for stimulating Th1 lymphocytes or developing food tolerance (Bohle, 2004). The effect of the panel of released cytokines (described above) is maturation and differentiation of Th1 lymphocytes toward milk-specific allergens CD4 and CD8, and the increased homing receptor expression, including integrin $\alpha4\beta7$, accounts for the inflow of lymphocytes to the intestinal walls (Kohno et al., 2001). The increase in Th1-specific cytokines results in the inflow and stimulation of macrophages. The released lysosomal enzymes damage intestinal walls. Cow milk protein allergy (CMPA) develops, which may be accompanied by cow milk protein intolerance (CMPI) with exacerbated symptoms of chronic inflammation and severity of disease progress.

Food enteropathy may also be accompanied by atopic dermatitis (AD). AD patients do not always manifest increased blood serum IgE (Lugović et al., 2005). It is believed that the location of atopy in skin results from increased number of cutaneous lymphocyte antigen (CLA+) for T lymphocytes, found in atopic patients who have had contact, e.g., with casein. TCD4 lymphocytes travel to skin locations because there is an increased production of chemokines by stromal cells and lymphocytes themselves. Increased cutaneous T cell-attracting chemokine (CTACK/CCL27)—a T lymphocyte chemoattractant—concentration triggers the release of TNFα by macrophages, and then by keratinocytes. Thymus activation-regulated chemokine (TARC/CCL17) and macrophage-derived chemokine (MDC/CCL22) release more monocytes and DCs. CCL27 concentration increases, particularly at the sites where skin is damaged, which corresponds to the severity of AD progress (Nakazato et al., 2008). Initially, an increase in the number of Th2 lymphocytes is observed with chemokine CCR3 + and CCR4 + receptor expression. Gradually stromal IL 4 and IL 13 concentration is reduced, but there is a significant increase in INFγ, IL 5, and IL 12 (Schröder and Mochizuki, 1999), as well as GMCSF, TNFα and chemokine CCL5 (RANTES) (Giustizieri et al., 2001). Apart from IFNγ, the remaining cytokines are released by the eosinophils and macrophages in the cellular infiltration, as well as skin keratinocytes. The inflow of both types of cells is driven by an increase in the concentration of MDC/CCL22 (Vulcano et al., 2001) and eotaxines (Leung and Soter, 2001). Rearrangement in the panel of cytokines and cellular stroma is a result of the fact that they are joined by Th1 lymphocytes and cytotoxic TCD8 (Brand et al., 1999). The exacerbation of the inflammatory process increases as contaminations occur, which happens easily as a result of keratinocyte apoptosis Fas-LFas (ligand Fas) (Trautmann et al., 2000), skin is thinner and more permeable. A symptom characteristic of AD is itch, then excoriation, thus vulnerability increases to *Staphylococcus*, *Streptococcus*, fungal and viral infections, as well as further immunity superantigens.

A similar pathomechanism of infection may be induced by other allergens or allergen groups contained in food, e.g., profilins, cross-compatible allergens, etc.

### 1.1.3 ROLE OF THE DELETION, ENERGY SUPPRESSION, "IGNORANCE," AND APOPTOSIS MECHANISMS IN FOOD ANTIGEN TOLERANCE

Food tolerance is a notion within a broader issue of immunological tolerance, the core of the lack of inflammatory response from the immune system to one's own systemic antigens. Selection of cellular clones in prenatal period and developing suppression mechanisms lead to maintaining a good health state. Despite nearly 100 years of research, the phenomena have still not been fully explained. In-depth understanding would perhaps enable solving the problem of allergy related to allergens penetrating mucous membranes or skin, and preventing demyelinization conditions, type I diabetes, collagen arthritis, and other autoaggressive diseases. This would be especially valuable since treatment methods so far, involving cytostatic treatment, radiotherapy, and immunosuppresive medicines, destroy immunity to a number of antigens and, often, create a temporary malfunction of other immunity mechanisms.

Food tolerance is a state of no immunological response to antigens constantly penetrating the system through the gastrointestinal pathway, or those which a system permanently encounters, with maintained response to other antigens. The status depends on a number of variables: antigen dose, its type, frequency of intake, and maturity of the cells involved in immunological expression of surface molecules—MHC antigens, costimulatory molecules CD, cytokine concentration in stroma, or on the cell surface. Tolerance develops as a result of clonal deletion, anergy, or suppressive (regulative) cell activation in the system. It has been noticed that the type of activated immunity response depends on the dosage of the oral antigen intake. Positive clinical effects achieved, thanks to specific immunotherapy (SIT), is justified by triggering the mechanisms participating in the process (Fontenot and Rudensky, 2004).

Dendritic cells are the main APCs of the gastrointestinal system and they release a number of cytokines which have an immunomodulating effect on other cells. DC maturity is the critical factor in T lymphocyte stimulation or anergy. The correct expression of MHC antigens and differentiation molecules induces immunity and leads to an increase in stromal inflammatory cytokine, including IL 2, concentration. Low expression of antigens for class II MHC or costimulatory molecules CD80 and CD86 is the reason for T lymphocytes failing to detect the presented antigens. This may be caused by high stromal IL 10 concentration.

It is interesting that dendritic cells from Peyer's patches may produce IL 10, which can increase the percentage of Th2 lymphocytes releasing IL 4 and IL 10.

Also epithelial cells—enterocytes may be APC cells; in humans—present antigens to T CD8 lymphocytes, which produce antigen nonspecific TCR (Mayer and Shlien, 1987). In rats, on the other hand, selective immunosuppression has been observed which was dependent on antigen-specific T lymphocytes (Bland and Warren, 1986) releasing TGFβ, present in Peyer's patches as soon as within 24–48 h of the intake of small antigen doses (Lider et al., 1989). Occurrence of food tolerance may be due to some haptens, e.g., DNCB (2,4-dinitrochlorobenzene) administered to mice orally, according to Galliaerde et al. (1995).

Presentation of antigens to T lymphocytes by APC cells necessitates the participation of costimulatory molecules, including, above all, CD40 on DCs binding with ligand CD154 on T lymphocytes and CD80/86 (B7-1/B7-2) with CD28 on T lymphocytes, which are necessary in order to trigger further stages of immunological response. Lack of binding of CD40 with ligand inhibits the interaction of CD80/86 with CD28, which prevents T lymphocyte activation, but stimulates Treg lymphocytes to release IL 1. In IgE-dependent allergies, however, it is emphasized that stimulation is necessary, especially by B7.2 to release IL 4.

CTLA4 present on T lymphocytes, which also binds with CD80/86, is considered most important in activating suppression. It has been observed that activating this transmitting path for Treg lymphocytes involves increased release of INFγ by DCs, which induces the production of indoleamine 2,3-dioxygenase (IDO) and degradation of tryptophan in T lymphocytes. As a result, proliferation of these cells is blocked.

The process of differentiation from Th0 to Th1 lymphocytes depends on IL 12 concentration value, and further stages on the availability of an antigen and release of IFNγ (Yamamoto et al., 2007). The process of differentiation from Th0 to Th2 determines lymphocytes. The differentiation from Th0 to Th2 is determined by the presence of monokine 12, and next IL 4 in tissues. Also the type of stimulated TLR is important. In the situation of allergic disease and Th2-sensitive response, TLR 2 and 4 are stimulated, and on DCs Delta and Jagged ligands appear due to the effect of prostaglandins, Jagged 1 binds with Notch 1 on Th2 lymphocyte surface. This triggers the production of IL 4 production and potentiation of Th2-sensitive response. An increase in IL 4 concentration leads to the suppression of Th1-sensitive specific cellular response, and it is widely known that the two populations remain in balanced proportions in good health status.

Tolerance following the intake of a large dose of antigen develops through clonal deletion of specific Th1 lymphocytes or increase in the number of antigen nonspecific

Ts CD4. According to the findings of Watanabe, characteristic Ts CD4 lymphocyte features include high Fas molecule ligand expression, and the release of interleukins with a suppressor effect: IL 10, IL 4, and TGFβ. Thus, increasing Fas molecule expression leads to apoptosis of the cells which have FasL on the surface (Watanabe et al., 2002).

Administering large doses of antigen leads to a decrease of specific TCR and consequently, reduced release of cytokines characteristic of Th1 and Th2 lymphocytes, i.e., IL 2, IFNγ, IL 5, and IL 4, as a result of clonal deletion. Among other persisting T CD4 lymphocytes, reduced IL 2 receptor expression and failure to release some cytokines (IL 2, 4, 10, and/or TGFβ) is observed. As a result their response to the antigen is weaker (Cohn, 2001).

In the process of food tolerance development, the presence of other cell populations have been observed, namely Treg lymphocytes (CD4+ CD25+), Ts CD8, Th3 CD4 CD25, and atypical cells of hepatic origin which may participate in immunoregulation processes—the so-called double-marked lymphocytes, scarce in the system in order to avoid negative selection in the thymus.

CD4 Tαβ lymphocytes are a diverse population of cells releasing a variety of cytokines. In mice two types of CD4 lymphocytes have been determined: Th3 (CD4+ CD25−) and regulatory lymphocytes—Tr 1 (CD4+ CD25+).

Th3 lymphocytes are mainly found in mucous membranes, they release TGFβ and cytokines: IL 4 and IL 10. They are sometimes referred to as CD4+ CD25− since they do not demonstrate CD25 expression. They can be obtained after oral administration of myelin to mice. Their presence has been observed in mesenterial lymph nodes. Th3 lymphocytes may inhibit the development of allergic encephalitis in mice, if they are administered peritoneally. Administering anti-TGFβ monoclonal antibodies to mice reversed the immunosuppression effect (Chen et al., 1994).

CD4+ CD25+ lymphocytes referred to as natural regulatory cells (Trn), or Tr 1 lymphocytes account for not more than 2% in human peripheral blood. They acquire suppressor properties when activated by an antigen, and then show antigen non-specific effects (Thorton and Mshevach, 2000). They manifest a high expression of adhesive molecule ICAM 1 and CD25, i.e., subunit α of L-selectin and IL 2 receptor, in contrast to activated CD4 and CD8 manifesting transient and low CD25 expression and low L-selectin expression. Moreover, in humans these cells present a phenotype of memory cells CD45RB + CD45RO + (Taams et al., 2001). Initially, it was believed that the thymus is the only locus for production of CD4 + CD25 + lymphocytes, but after recording their presence in the system of thymectomized mice, it became apparent that they can mature in the liver following contact with immature DCs presenting CD8α + (Thomson et al., 1999).

Tr 1(CD4+ CD25+) lymphocytes have been obtained in *in vitro* conditions in the breeds of naïve T lymphocytes in the presence of IL 2. It has been recorded that, in contrast to Th3, Tr 1 lymphocytes do not release considerable amounts of IL 4, TGFβ, and IL 2, but mainly IL 10. Tr 1 cells show poor proliferation and it is believed that their *in vivo* life expectancy is short; Tr1 cells however, exhibited an effect by inhibiting the proliferation of incidental cells. When implanted in mice, they inhibited enteritis progression (Groux et al., 1997). Moreover, Zhang has observed that while breeding with CD4+ CD25− cells, the proliferation of the latter reduced (Zhang et al., 1998). Additionally, it has been noted that on CD4+ CD25+ cells, a reduced expression of a surface element cytotoxic T-lymphocyte associated antigen 4 (CTLA4) occurs. This is produced, as Samoilova has shown, as a result of stimulation with a large antigen dose (Samoilova et al., 1998). Research of primitive CD4+ CD25− cells following contact with CD4+ CD25+ lymphocytes produced an interesting explanation of the participation of cytokines IL 10 and TGFβ in suppression modification. The term "contagious" tolerance was created to refer to a phenomenon manifesting itself with generating subsequent populations of CD4+ CD25+ lymphocytes by CD4+ CD25− cells with both cytokines acting as agents (Zheng et al., 2004).

The assumption made about the nature of cytokine was controversial. Thorstenson et al. obtained CD4+ CD25+ lymphocytes from mice which had been parenterally immunized with ovoalbumin and received the same allergen orally in order to induce tolerance. It has been observed that adding anti-TGFβ antibodies to the breed does not inhibit suppression. More to that, thanks to the development of lymphocyte CD4+ CD25+ sensitive food tolerance *in vivo* inhibition of delayed-type hypersensitivity has been achieved.

A probable tolerance mechanism behind this would be transporting TGFβ by means of either *in vitro* or *in vivo* indirect contact of suppressive cell and regulatory cell. The reason for that is assumed to be a new CD4 lymphocyte clone which does not produce IL 2 (Thorstenson and Khoruts, 2001). The observed effect is suppression of Th1 lymphocytes which release mainly INFγ and lymphotoxin. Thus it has been concluded that TGFβ is the most involved cytokine in the food tolerance process, which is confirmed by Nakamura (Nakamura et al., 2001).

CD4 lymphocyte population is under the supervision of hepatic cells. Blood is transported to the liver from the abdominal organs, except for the urinogenital system. The liver is involved in food tolerance development due to the constant presentation of antigens from Browicz–Kupfer cells which form the sinus walls. Liver Browicz–Kupfer cells are sedentary macrophages whose role is analogical to that played by stromal cells in the thymus with regard to T lymphocytes. Apart from conventional CD4 and CD8 lymphocytes, NKT cells, Tγδ lymphocytes, T lymphocytes with β chain expression for IL 2(CD122), there are the following atypical cells in the liver: CD3+ CD56+ (31.5%), NKT (approximately 30%), CD8αα (15.4%), CD3+ CD4-CD8-(14.5%), CD3+ CD4+ CD8+ (5.5%), and TCRγδ(2.7%). Their participation in contributing to the tolerance phenomenon consists of stimulating naïve CD4 lymphocytes to transform into suppressor lymphocytes and release a range of cytokines, mainly IL 4, IL 10, and TGFβ (Akdis et al., 2005).

Treg lymphocytes may have an effect on the number of other cell populations, inhibiting activation, proliferation, and—finally—effector functions. The reasons behind this wide range of capacity were assumed to be related to Tregs being equipped with A and B granzymes, perforins, and Fas. Ramsdel has proved that Tregs are capable of killing CD4 and CD8 lymphocytes, immature and mature marrow dendritic cells and macrophages by means of perforins and granzymes (Ramsdell, 2003). A problem that remains is an answer to the question about the way in which target cells are recognized. Like other researchers, the author believes that it is very likely that lymphocytes are detected by TCR in the context of class II MHC antigens, macrophages—by CD14—and dendritic cells—by CD80/86 (Levings et al., 2002; Misra et al., 2004). Tregs also control the number of B lymphocytes by triggering an apoptosis process through the Fas pathway.

There have been attempts to link the properties of particular subpopulations with the expression of surface molecules. It has been noted that transcriptive factor Foxp3, which is an activator for the production of scurfin, a protein found both on CD25+ and CD25− lymphocytes, may deprive cells of suppressive properties, as they may lead to reduced cytokine release and T-lymphocyte proliferation (Schubert et al., 2001; Ramsdell, 2003). Consequently, food allergy or autoimmunological conditions may develop.

The next surface molecule is CTLA-4, whose expression increases following Trn activation. The molecule can be blocked with monoclonal antibodies, which also significantly reduce Trn suppressor effect. A probable way of reducing CTLA-4 immunological response is binding DCs with CD80–86 presented above and blocking the transmittal of the signal which disables Trn lymphocyte suppressive properties. What is also worth noting is an increase in TGFβ release (Levings et al., 2001).

GITR molecule, which is a TNF receptor induced by glucocorticosteroids, is worth mentioning as transmitting a signal with it as an agent reduces Trn suppressor properties. In genetic tests a lack of messenger RNA for IL 2 has been found, yet its presence for IL 4, IL 10, and TGFβ, while cytokines are not secreted outside cells *in vitro* tests. Potential release capacity *in vivo* is suggested especially for IL 10 (Hara et al., 2001).

Treg cells are equipped with TLR 4, TLR 5, TLR 7, and TLR 8 receptors. Bacterial LPS (lipopolysaccharide) may act on TLR 4, either directly or not, through APC cells. Indirect stimulation with the use of *Bordetella pertussis* leads to the release of IL 10 (Higgins et al., 2003), while the use of *Candida albicans* additionally extends life expectancy of CD4+ CD25+ lymphocytes (Netea et al., 2004)

The phenomenon of tolerance can be reversed by stimulating TLRs with PAMP molecules, which are structures of grouped microorganisms usually immune to mutations. Therefore, it is a mechanism which changes the anergy of T lymphocytes and tolerance to its own tissues and antigens, e.g., saprophytic bacteria into stimulation of the immune system.

In order to explain self-tolerance to one's own gastrointestinal flora, mononuclear colon cells with LPS isolated from *Bacteroides vulgatus, Bacteroides fragilis,* and *Salmonella minesota* were bred *in vitro*. The findings included: increase in gene expression of Fox p3 marker on lymphocytes, increase in CD25 expression, and an increase in IL 10 synthesis. At the same time, reduced synthesis was observed in macrophages MD-2 surface molecule and no increase in inflammatory cytokine concentration was observed (Shirai et al., 2004). The phenomenon of suppression may be overcome by means of activating dendritic cells to release IL 6, or by *in vitro* stimulation of TLR 4 and TLR 9 receptors on CD4+ CD25+ cells, as discussed by Passare (Pasare and Medzhitov, 2003, 2004). Also, viral PAMPs may be used to block CD4+ CD25+ lymphocyte activity. Overcoming suppression is referred to as contrasuppression. It is known that certain viral diseases (*Myxovirus* infections) increase the likelihood of respiratory airway allergy in infants.

The presence of regulatory cells is necessary to maintain systemic homeostasis. It has been observed that their contact with commensal flora of mucous membranes in the first days of life is the condition for their development. In germfree animals it is impossible to induce food tolerance mediated by Th2 lymphocytes. Perhaps this is the answer to the question "Why is the number of allergic diseases on the increase, although the exposure to allergens is decreasing?"

### 1.1.4 Mechanism and Symptoms of Individualistic Adverse Reactions to Foods

Nonallergic hyperreactivity corresponds to the traditional notion of food intolerance. It is a syndrome in which dysfunctions are similar to those observed in the course of allergic diseases, induced by various mechanisms, excluding immunology-related factors. Nonallergic hyperreactivity occurs more frequently than allergy. Morbidity rate in children is approximately 20%–50%, while in adults it is estimated to be approximately 20%. Attention is drawn to the fact that the enzymatic system in children is less mature, so the capacity to bind chemical compounds by plasma proteins is poorer, and so is the blood–brain barrier permeability by low molecular weight compounds.

Biogenic amines are often mentioned but they are not the only mechanism. The indirect systemic effect of vasoactive amines not degraded in the gastrointestinal tract occurs if the release of enzymes by enterocytes—mono and diaminooxidase (MAO and DAO, respectively)—is lacking or if it is blocked by medicines or alcohol (Tuormaa, 1994).

Vasoactive amines include

- Tyramine contained in Cheddar, Emmental, and Roquefort cheese; marinated and canned fish; and walnuts.
- Histamine found in foods which undergo a fermentation process, e.g., blue cheese, beer, sourkraut, and pickles. What is more, tomatoes and strawberries also contain a large amount of this biogenic amine. Both types can induce nettle rash in small children and elderly people.

Symptoms of histamine poisoning can also occur as a result of consuming mackerel-type fish. The condition is referred to as "scombrotoxic fish poisoning" and results from the fact that bacterial flora develops on the surface of a product—the flora most often includes *Enterobacteriaceae*, which generate large amounts of histidine transformed into histamine. Poisoning symptoms, depending on the degree to which the gastrointestinal tract is filled, occur within 2 min to 2 h of consumption. They include reddening of the skin, headache, vomiting, diarrhea, a burning sensation in the mouth and throat, and increased heart rate (Jansen et al., 2003).

Histamine may also be released from mastocytes in the gastrointestinal tract induced by aspartame, sodium benzoate, sodium glutamate—which causes "Chinese Restaurant Syndrome"—and sulfites, which mainly occur in dried fruit and vegetables, marinated vegetables, fruit juices, and low-quality wines (Landete et al., 2005).

The amines which are also worth noting include

• Phenylethylamine, which is found in chocolate and is also the reason for migraine (Millichap and Yee, 2003)
• Serotonine in bananas, whose amount accumulates as the fruit ripens, especially when it is overripe—octopamine in lemons

In children who drink juices containing aspartame, hypersensitivity has been observed and an increased tendency toward aggressive behavior has been observed. It has been found that aspartame intake leads to doubling phenylalanine concentration in the central nervous system. Also an increase in tyrosine has been observed, followed by a decrease of tryptophan—a serotonine precursor. Low CNS serotonine in children has been found to be responsible for neurosis symptoms.

Tartazine (yellow pigment), on the other hand, may cause typical histamine poisoning symptoms, such as: reduced blood pressure, increased heart rate, skin hyperemia, itching, nettle rash, and runny nasal discharge. The symptoms occur due to degranulation of a large number of mastocytes as a result of ion imbalance, such as tartazine chelates zinc ions.

The reason for gastrointestinal tract symptoms, such as fermentative diarrhea or acidic stools may be in the deficiency or lack of enzymes which break down disaccharides, with the most frequent occurrence of lactase deficiency. The deficiency may be congenital, or acquired as a result of rotavirus infection, antibiotic-induced diarrhea, coeliac disease, enteropatic diabetes, and reduced lactase release, developing as the aging process progresses. In the case of a genetic lack of lactase, symptoms are sustained throughout the lifetime. Acquired deficiency is temporary, often dependent on the amount of milk consumed. The reason for the symptoms may be the process of anaerobic fermentation of lactose by bacterial flora. Organic acids are produced, especially lactic acid—as a result intestinal mucous membrane is irritated, peristalsis accelerates, and carbon dioxide content leads to gushing stool (Tuormaa, 1994; Jansen et al., 2003).

Symptoms of nonallergic hyperreactivity may also be of Pavlov's conditional reflex character—in that intolerance is coded in CNS, e.g., children vomiting at the sight of food which once caused poisoning.

## 1.2 INFLUENCE OF SEVERAL FACTORS: GENETIC BACKGROUND; AGE DEPENDENCE IN FOOD ALLERGY, FIRST EXPOSURE; FOOD ALLERGY IN CHILDREN AND ALLERGY MARCH; NATURE, DOSE, AND BALANCE BETWEEN TOLERANCE (SUPPRESSION) AND SENSITIZATION (PRIMING)

### 1.2.1 GENETIC BACKGROUND

Allergic diseases are often related to patients' genotypes. It is known that the likelihood of their occurrence is as much as 70% when both parents are affected with the disease, or 40% if one parent, usually the mother, is affected (Ruiz et al., 1992; Oddy et al., 2002). These conditions manifest themselves in consecutive generations. Boys are affected with such conditions 1.5 times more often than girls (Mandhane et al., 2007).

Allergy is a multigenetic condition, therefore with the current status of research development, vaccines which might prevent the occurrence of these syndromes are not known. Moffatt proved that asthma is often related to the occurrence of histo-compatibility antigens HLA DRB1, which corresponds with the increased number of total IgE, however, it is particular genes that are responsible for increased specific IgE concentration (Moffatt et al., 2001).

Recently research has progressed, which has made it possible to link allergies to certain antigens with mutations in antigen-specific genes, or with a more fre-quent occurrence of genes which code class II HLA antigens. Senechal observed an increase in the occurrence of allergy to birch and apple pollen in people who have DR 4 or DR 7 in their genotype (Senechal et al., 1999).

Allergy to nuts has been found to co-occur with DRB1*08/12, or DQB1 *0301 and DPB1 according to Howell (Howell et al., 1998). Moreover, the risk of nut allergy is increased by polymorphism within chromosome 1, which codes for the production of STAT6 protein (Amoli et al., 2002).

Camponeschi has linked allergy to cow milk with HLADQ7 (Camponeschi et al., 1997). Mutation has been observed within IgE receptor gene in the course of inhala-tion and food allergy to profilins, which are found in tree pollen and fruit, as well as allergy to domestic dust. It is a gene for the receptor subunit of high FcεR1-β affinity on 11q13 chromosome (Hage-Hamsten et al., 2002).

In screening tests a positive correlation was observed between cord blood Ig E concentration in an infant at birth, and atopic symptoms in the mother (Jonhsson et al., 1996).

Chromosome 5 contains some genes responsible for immunological response. It has been observed on the grounds of population tests conducted in families with atopy that an increased IgE concentration in subjects is of hereditary character, although it is not certain if the only responsible genes are the ones located in chro-mosome 5—q31 and q32. It has been reported that gene polymorphism within chro-mosome 5 is not always an allergy exponent as it may co-occur with an increased Ig E concentration in atopy-free individuals (van Herverden et al., 1995). Moreover, chromosome 5 contains genes for IL 13 and IL 4. The presence of genes correlates, to a various extent, with bronchial hyperreactivity (BHR) genes, high IgE serum concentration, and IL4Aα receptor, which is common for both cytokines. Howard tested the interactions between these genes and he compared them with CTLA4 gene located in chromosome 2, in order to determine which parts of the genome are most responsible for potential asthma or BHR occurrence (Howard et al., 2003). Research into polymorphism of IL 4 genes, receptors for IL 4 and IgE, was yet another stage of research development (Takabayashi et al., 2000). It was observed that severe AD is frequently related to mutations within SPINK5, a gene coding serine protease inhibitor responsible for skin biochemical transformations (Kusunoki et al., 2005).

Finally, genes responsible for high IgE concentration, atopy, and asthma were localized in chromosome 13q14 as single nucleotide polymorphism (SNP) at the site of IL 21 receptor (Hecker et al., 2003). Moreover, a link was observed between TcR complex of Tγ/δ lymphocytes and chromosome 14, and the synthesis of IgE-specific antibodies (Moffatt et al., 1994). Shin observed that 6p21 mutations lead to increased production of proinflammatory TNF and TNFα, and increased IgE concentration (Shin et al., 2004).

Eotaxins are compounds with chemotactic effect on eosinophils, basophils, and mastocytes. Mutations were observed in the loci of eotaxin 2 genes in patients with asthma and high IgE (Shin et al., 2003).

Potential reasons for allergy development are being researched with regard to reduced production of cytokines of suppressive effect. Mutations have been observed within chromosome 19q13 coding TGFβ1 and chromosome 1 containing the gene for IL 10 (Hobbs et al., 1998).

### 1.2.2 AGE DEPENDENCE IN FOOD ALLERGY, FIRST EXPOSURE

The co-occurrence of genetic and environmental factors has been proved by a number of researchers. The relation between a history of atopy in the family, prenatal exposure to tobacco smoke (passive smoking), and the effects of an elimination diet applied by pregnant women was analyzed. Prophylactic diets during pregnancy apparently do not contribute to prevention of allergy development, but eliminate allergens from the diet in the period of breastfeeding. This has been proven to be effective (Kramer and Kakuma, 2006).

Exposure of children to tobacco smoke has been found to increase IgE concentration and the tendency to develop eosinophilia, it also increased the percentage of children allergic to indoor allergens (Kabesch and Mutius, 2000).

For years the method based on elimination of allergens from the surroundings of the potential patients was not undermined. It was believed that one of the reasons for developing an allergy might be early contact of mucous membranes with allergic substances. It was pointed out that bacteria and viruses contributed to the exacerbation of the existing atopic diseases and the general guideline was to bring up children in an environment with a limited number of microorganisms.

A few years ago the first findings appeared which undermined this concept. It was noticed that the children who did not develop diseases in childhood, develop allergies more often. Moreover it was reported that children who stayed in rural areas, where exposure to allergens and bacterial endotoxins was greater than in urban areas, less frequently developed diseases (Braun-Fahrlander, 2000; Von Mutius et al., 2000; Remes et al., 2003; Gehring et al., 2004).

A few authors even expressed the belief that rural conditions offer protection from atopy (Von Mutius et al., 2000; Upham and Holt, 2005), although there were also papers which showed no difference (Schulze et al., 2007). Additionally, an assumption was made that staying in a rural area over a number of years reduced the risk of allergy, also in adults (Chen et al., 2007). In research published in 2007 a relation was shown between allergen type and class of antibodies generated in children who drink milk and stayed in a rural area. Exposure to endotoxins in a rural environment sometimes provided protection regarding allergy to grass or feline allergens, but was of no influence regarding hyperreactivity to saprophytes (Stern et al., 2007).

Th1 cells are considered to be responsible for reducing the number of allergy occurrences. In order to confirm the thesis, the frequency of atopic conditions in children with positive and negative tuberculin reactions was compared. In the group vaccinated against tuberculosis, morbidity was lower (Matricardi et al., 2000). Recent study results are not unambiguous. A problematic influence of BCG vaccinations in allergy development prevention (Nuhoglu et al., 2003; Townley et al., 2004); however, the capacity is indicated to inhibit rhinitis, asthma, and AD development, with lack of influence in the case of rhinoconjunctivitis (Miyake et al., 2008).

Infections, e.g., *infectious liver inflammation type A*, *Toxoplasma gondii*, *Helicobacter pylori*, or an orofecal infection in childhood, have been reported to reduce the percentage of disease occurrences in children with an allergy of upper airways and increased IgE (Matricardi et al., 2000). In a recent study, lack of this relation has been found for *Helicobacter* (Kolho et al., 2005). Gereda emphasized the value of stimulating Th1 lymphocytes with endotoxins (Gereda et al., 2000). It has been reported that stimulating TLR receptors prevents allergic disease development in childhood. Romagnani believes that both mechanisms—Th1 and Toll receptor stimulation—are triggered by bacteria which are found in rural environment (Romagnani, 2004a,b). The upshot is an increase in IL 12 and IFNγ release induced by contact with bacteria (Mowat, 2003).

TLRs are found everywhere in the human body—in the epithelium, APC cells, eosinophils, mastocytes, neutrophils, B lymphocytes, vascular endothelial cells, keratinocytes, adipocytes, cardiomyocytes, and fibroblasts. Most of them are present on the cell surface, some are present in the cytoplasm, as they bind with antigens of endocellular microorganisms, which have undergone degradation in proteasome and lysosomes.

In humans, 10 TLRs have been determined that detect—either individually or in groups—PAMP sequences which are stable structures of microorganisms. It has been reported that LPS (lipopolysaccharide) is detected by TLR2, from *Porphyromonas gingivalis*; and TLR4, from *E. coli*. DNA fragments from lactic acid rods are detected by TLR 9. It is a receptor on the surface of cytoplasmatic vesicles which connect with phagolysosomes in the phagocytosis process. TLR9 has been observed to be induced by bacterial nonmethylated oligonucleotides DNA-CpG sequences, which leads to the development of Th1 and Treg CD25 lymphocyte, and genes for IL 10 and TGFβ-sensitive response (Hemmi et al., 2000). It is interesting that TLR9 activation also leads to a decrease of expression of FcεRI receptors on dendritic cells. Cross-binding of these receptors consequently results in decreasing the amount of TLR9 (Schroeder et al., 2005).

Also, the role of dendritic cells activated by LPS, CpG sequences, or peptidoglycan is emphasized in releasing IL 12 and stimulating the response of Th1 lymphocytes in the desensitization process. Moreover, stimulating TLR4 and TLR2 by LPS may increase the production of cytokines dependent on Th2 lymphocytes and thus intensify allergic reactions. It has also been reported that the effect of LPS on immature dendritic cells accelerates their maturation as the kinase pathway is stimulated (c-Jun N-terminal kinases (JNK)) (Nakahara et al., 2004). Cells have more potential to present an antigen. On their surface costimulatory molecules appear, and the concentration of the released proinflammatory cytokines TNFα, IL 6, 12, and 18 in stroma increases. Since TLR receptors are also found on mastocytes and basophils, their activation leads to increased release of compounds from preformed and generated granlues, i.e., to the development of an inflammatory-allergic response. Apart from TLRs, which constitute an integral element of a cell, serum and other systemic fluids contain soluble forms of TLRs, which are also involved in immunological processes. Numerous studies have shown that suppression is induced by LPS stimulating Treg CD4+ 25+ with the use of TLR4 and also by means of increased IL 10 production. Toll receptors are also responsible for contributing to recovery processes in damaged intestinal epithelium.

Modifying primary and secondary immunological response by *Bifidobacterium* and *Lactobacillus* probiotics is linked with their structures being recognized by TLR 9 present on monocytes and lymphocytes, as well as with TLR expression on dendritic cells. As a result, release of IL 12 and IFNγ is increased. Also preferential recruitment of Th1 lymphocytes has been observed. Saito made a hypothesis that individually selected TLR ligand doses might be administered as a medicine to infants at risk of allergy (Saito et al., 2003).

TLR2 and 4 receptors participate in preapoptic transmission. It has been reported that thermal shock proteins stimulate TLR 4 and TLR2 on their own, or after they are linked with an allergen. Immunomodulative effect is manifested by *Mycobacterium vaccae*, which stimulates TLR 2 through lipoarabinomannan, an integral component of vaccines that contain allergen proteins (Tighe et al., 1998). It also seems justified to include lipoproteins and lipopolysaccharides in vaccines as they stimulate TLR2 and TLR4 (Tlaskalova-Hogenova et al., 2002), like *L. plantarum* (Karlsson et al., 2002).

In order to reduce the risk of allergy, use of medicines has been tested. It seems an interesting idea to use tetracyclines deprived of antibiotic properties (mino and doxycyklines), administered orally to mice to reduce Ig E concentration. An inversely proportional relationship to the dose has been reported (Durkin et al., 2007).

On the other hand, it is known that

1. *Helicobacter pylori* infections lead to chronic inflammatory condition of mucous membrane in the stomach and duodenum, thus they may contribute to allergization (Matysiak-Budnik et al., 2003).
2. Infections with *Clostridium* anaerobes also lead to damage to mucous membranes due to toxins released (e.g., *C. difficile*).
3. Treatment of gastrointestinal system inflammations may lead to damage to delicate structures within the system by antibiotics and to physiological bacterial flora selection.
4. Most medicines are haptens, so an antibiotic therapy may have an allergizing effect.
5. Frequent and early use of antibiotics in the course of infection may extend the period in which an appropriate pool of memory cells is generated and thus an appropriate level of immunity may not be ensured.

Having stated the above, what becomes particularly significant is physiological intestinal flora in infants when the system is learning to detect antigens and determine self and nonself. Bacteria, usually from the mother, or from the child's immediate environment, settle in the child's gastrointestinal tract in the first days of birth. It is important that they mainly include nonpathogenic colibacilli and lactic acid rods. During pregnancy Th2 sensitive immunity predominates. Stimulation with nonmethylated CpG sequences from physiological flora results in an increase in Th1, thus leading to increased release of cytokines by Th1 and macrophages.

A double role is played by lipopolysaccharides of Gram negative rods. The polysaccharide part stimulates B lymphocytes and humoral response, while lipid A stimulates Th1 lymphocytes (Weiner et al., 1997). Apart from Gram negative bacteria, immunity is also modified by Gram positive rods and cocci. Gram negative rods cause a less significant increase in IL 12 and TNFα concentration than Gram positive cocci, which, however, are relatively less numerous in the gastrointestinal tract of young children.

The immunomodulative effect of lactic acid rods is invaluable. It has been observed that administering Lactobacillus GG to women during pregnancy and after labor increased milk IL 10 and TGFβ concentration and in breastfed children decreased the occurrence of atopic eczema (Isolauri et al., 2000).

Also increased release of IL 12 by macrophages has been observed with a parallel decrease of release of allergen-specific IgE as a result of *L. casei* effect (Shida et al., 1998).

It has been known for a long time that apart from their immunomodulative effect, lactic acid rods have a beneficial effect on the content of bacterial flora in the gastrointestinal tract, thus reducing the percentage of anaerobes. More lactic acid rods were bred in the cultures from the gastrointestinal tract of 1 year old infants from Estonia. Atopic conditions were less frequent in those children than in children from Sweden, who often presented *Clostridium* rods in the gastrointestinal tract (Sepp et al., 1997).

An interesting issue which has recently become apparent is the influence of physical exercise on allergic reaction processes. It has been observed that allergy to food allergens combined with significant exertion is linked with rhinorrhoea, spastic symptoms in upper airways, nettle rash with considerable eruptions, angioedema, syncope often referred to as short-term loss of consciousness, vomiting, diarrhea, and headache lasting up to 3 days. The reason is yet unknown. Patients manifested high allergen specific IgE concentration. Physical activity probably increases a mastocyte cellular membrane fluidity, intensives degranulation. As a consequence one can observe high levels of histamine (Johansson et al., 2001).

### 1.2.3 ALLERGY MARCH

Research conducted by Moneret-Vautrin has shown that allergy in children aged from 6 months to 14 years initiates with allergy to milk, then eggs, fish, and hazelnuts. They account for 74.2% of symptoms. In 63% of adults, apples, hazelnuts, vegetables (carrots, celeriac), seafood, eggs, fish, and milk are allergens (Moneret-Vautrin et al., 1998).

Allergy affects only 2% of subjects in the adult age and 6%–10% of children. The figures indicate that most children "outgrow" allergy (Brandzeg, 2002). The remaining ones, unfortunately, may experience exacerbation of symptoms, which may cause allergy march. The condition often initiates on contact with cow milk, due to the presence of allergens in breast milk or as a result of contact with peptides—hydrolysis remnants in infant formulas. Symptoms of enteritis appear, then they are accompanied by atopic dermatitis and—at the same time, or soon after that—wheezing, next—sometimes at the age of seven, sometimes earlier—asthma (Illi et al., 2004).

These symptoms may subside spontaneously at the age of 3 or 4, or at puberty. Expression may be intensified, or the affected site may change. The exacerbation of disease can be caused by accompanying viral or bacterial infections and expansion of the panel of allergens leading to polysensibilization (Böhme et al., 2002).

## 1.2.4 BALANCE BETWEEN TOLERANCE (SUPPRESSION) AND SENSITIZATION (PRIMING)

One method of regaining the balance between induction and inhibition processes is the application of sublingual immunotherapy (SLIT). The oral cavity is a particularly predisposed gastrointestinal site as mucous membranes contain relatively few cells presenting antigens. They are usually dendritic cells resembling Langerhans cells and macrophages which transport antigens to the nearest lymph nodes to introduce them to Th0 lymphocytes (Noirey et al., 2000). As a result, the T-lymphocyte pool is stimulated. It is an effect of exposure to inhaled or food allergens, everyday, even for several years, under the tongue.

The mode of administration is safe. Complications were very rare and included asthma, nettle rash, angioedema, local changes sometimes. If a reaction occurred in the form of itch and oral cavity oedema, the dose was reduced. Passalacque has found that symptoms of intolerance occurred at the rate of 1 in 1000 doses, both in children (even under 5), and in adults (Passalacqua et al., 2006). Positive and long-term effects of desensitization have been recorded in the case of conjunctivitis, rhinitis, and asthma (Andre et al., 2000). A research paper which is a meta-analysis of all double-blind studies so far, presents the view that SLIT is moderately effective in the treatment of asthma, but can counteract allergy to an extending panel of allergens. The background of such an opinion is unambiguous test results in particular analyzed programs (van Wijk, 2008).

In general, SLIT is said to be a safe and cheap method in extended treatment, and it is not always necessary to select allergens individually.

The immunological mechanism of tolerance formation has not been not fully explored. It has been noted that during SLIT period the following may occur: reducing the severity of symptoms relating to upper airway allergy (Ciprandi et al., 2006); increase in IL 10, but reducing T-lymphocyte proliferation in adults (Fanta et al., 1999), lack of T-lymphocyte number in children, and lack of change in the concentrations of the following cytokines IL 2, 4, 10, TgFβ, INFγ (Dehlink et al., 2006), decrease of allergen-specific IgE concentration, reducing degranulation, and decreasing eosinophil life expectancy as well as increase in IgA concentration (Bahceciler et al., 2005). In order to fully discover SLIT mechanisms, more tests are necessary.

It is an attractive treatment model which has a potential of extending adjuvants and the allergen panel, and, involving other areas of mucous membranes and immunization through the skin.

## 1.3  APPLICATION OF FUNCTIONAL GENOMICS AND PROTEOMICS IN ALLERGY AND CLINICAL IMMUNOLOGY

### 1.3.1  FUNCTIONAL PROTEOMICS AND GENOMICS

The development of new technologies within functional (and structural) genomics is considered to be an indispensable factor in the development of personalized medicine, which is based on individual approach to a patient. It is assumed that determining an individual genetic profile of a patient will enable safe and efficacious treatment.

Functional genomics consists of research into functions of particular genome elements and transcription process regulation. Recognizing the functions of each genome is determined at several levels, which include: the analysis of gene expression on mRNA level (transcriptomics), the analysis of proteome (proteomics), analysis of metabolome (metabolomics), and the analysis of mutant phenotypes (phenomics). DNA microarray method is among those used more and more frequently; it enables global assessment of gene expression in normal and pathological conditions, which makes it possible to determine the profile of gene expression in a given clinical situation.

Progress in sequencing human genes has contributed to proteomics development. There is functional, structural, and expressional proteomics. Functional genomics is a study of mutual interactions between proteins, it describes the types of these interactions and helps determine the functions of those proteins, as well as showing the manner in which they form complexes, thus providing the basis for direct understanding of health and disease processes which may consequently support the efforts to develop targeted therapies, new diagnostic methods, and new medications.

Successful progress in functional genomics has contributed to the development of its more detailed subdiscipline, namely functional immunomics, which consists in researching mechanisms of action for (chemical and biological) factors connected to immunological processes via various specific cellular and humoral responses induced by antigens presented to the cells of immunological system. It has contributed notably to the understanding of the very immunological system, diagnosing and prognosing diseases, generating vaccines, and fighting other conditions occurring in humans, from infections to allergies and neoplasms (Braga-Neto and Marques, 2006).

Progress in functional genomics is related to combining its methods with applications for automatic analysis of protein enzymatic activity and occurrence, accompanied by detection of protein products by means of 2D electrophoresis and mass spectrometry. This will enable detection of mRNA and protein as gene expression product, as well as comprehensive research of the relationship between genetic polymorphism, and individual and environmental factors (such as allergen or treatment exposure).

Comprehensive genomic research therefore necessitates a combination of several advanced techniques (technologies) which would form more complex technological lines. An example of such solutions may be found in recent scientific papers (Pawliczak and Shelhamer, 2003; Braga-Neto and Marques, 2006):

1. Cell line studies
   - Material collection → 2D electrophoresis → Mass spectrometry
   - Material collection → 2D electrophoresis → Protein sequencing → Data mining tools ↔ Drug Discovery
   - Material collection → mRNA microarray (GeneChip or CDNA) → Data mining tools ↔ Drug Discovery
2. Clinical studies
   - Clinical evaluation and material collection → SNP detection (DNA)
   - Clinical evaluation and material collection → ELISA microarray → Data mining tools ↔ Drug Discovery
   - Clinical evaluation and material collection → ELISA microarray → Protein sequencing → Data mining tools ↔ Drug Discovery
   - Clinical evaluation and material collection → mRNA microarray (GeneChip or CDNA) → Data mining tools ↔ Drug Discovery
   - Clinical evaluation and material collection → Protein sequencing → Data mining tools ↔ Drug Discovery

### 1.3.2  FUNCTIONAL GENOMICS IN CLINICAL IMMUNOLOGY AND ALLERGOLOGY

It is assumed that soon complete information on human genome will open the door to recognizing and classifying individual differences in genomic DNA and searching for the links between polymorphism, in particular, single nucleotide polymorphism (SNP), and disease pathogenesis as well as response to medications and xenobiotics. Detailed information on genome will also be the starting point for recognizing transcriptomes (sets of metabolically active mRNA copies), and further in the future, proteomes (sets of proteins undergoing a given metabolic pathway), as well as searching for pathology background on molecular level. Once this is possible, treatment side effects can be eliminated or reduced to a minimum, and diseases of allergic origin can be classified on the grounds of molecular properties, with regard to subtypes including the defects of their molecular structure. In order to achieve the above goals, it was necessary to develop new research techniques and technologies. This degree of progress was possible after microarray technologies were implemented in laboratories (Pawliczak and Shelhamer, 2003; Maciejewski et al., 2005).

Introducing microarray technologies to laboratory practice have made it possible to accelerate work progress and to reduce time-consuming while not always unambiguous procedures to leave a limited number of simple experiments. With technology development, not only has the rate of discovering new genes increased, but it has also become possible to recognize metabolic pathways which they encode and to determine their significance in disease pathogenesis. In spite of high costs of equipment and software, as well as time-consuming procedures applied in the preparation and analysis of experiment results, practical use of microarray is becoming increasingly common. In particular, it is believed that popularizing microarray in clinical practice, especially in diagnosing and treating asthma, allergy and immune system conditions is particularly promising.

Microarray tests make it possible to simultaneously determine expression level of a number (hundreds of hundreds) of genes in a given system and to capture their activity in a given systemic or tissue condition. The test is performed in order to reveal the relationship between gene activity and conditions or diseases of genetic origin, also while the disease is progressing.

DNA oligonucleotide microarray (developed by Affymetrix) is a set of oligonucleotides (25-bases long probe) with sequences corresponding to various genes, with a number of copies (11 in Affymetrix arrays) in a given feature of glass slide, which makes it possible to study the activity of various genes. The measure of activity is the mRNA amount which has matched complementary probes on the array. Quantitative assessment is performed by means of washing fluorescent stain over the products of reaction. Then the array is scanned and the intensity of fluorescence of particular probes is evaluated. The activity of particular genes is calculated, not directly measured, because for each gene there is a group of copies of each probe, besides— apart from probes measuring mRNA concentration—there are also probes measuring background, i.e., nonspecific hybridization, which is also taken into account in determining gene expression.

Apart from oligonucleotide arrays, also older types of arrays are applied, so-called cDNA arrays. cDNA array (also referred to as a spotted array) is based on mRNA reverse transcription, PCR amplification, and cDNA cloning of a selected gene. cDNA probes are then machine printed on glass slides. This enables obtaining repeatable multispotted (up to 100,000 spots) arrays. Each spot corresponds to one gene. Gene expression tests conducted by means of cDNA array are comparative studies, which assess the level of sample expression against a reference sample.

The basic feature differentiating the two types of arrays is density of probes on the array glass, which is larger in the case of oligonucleotide arrays. Thanks to current technologies, it is possible to generate microarrays which contain $10^5$ probes per glass slide. The difference stems from differences in technologies applied in producing arrays (in the case of oligonucleotide ones, the probes are produced with the use of photolithographic techniques, while in the case of cDNA arrays, they are placed with an automatic pipette.

Experiments with the use of microarrays result in the collection of large data sets, which can serve as the basis for research into genetic functions, searching for relationships between gene activity and particular diseases, as well as building models to enable predicting the treatment response. Searching for this type of relationship is possible thanks to advanced data mining methods, which utilize both statistical techniques and pattern recognition techniques, as well as specialized computing tools. Methods of data analysis are now aggressively developing, and the target is the development of standard algorithms. Today the following suites are used in collecting and processing microarray data: Microarray suite (Affymetrix), GeneSpring (Silicon Genetics), Partek Pro (Partek Inc.), JMP and SAS software (SAS Institute Inc.), SAS (SAS Institute Inc.), SPSS (SPSS Inc.), or standard MS Excel packages (Maciejewski et al., 2005).

Numerous examples of efficacious application of functional genomics in research relating to allergology can be found in recent scientific papers (Pawliczak and Shelhamer, 2003; Saito et al., 2003).

Therefore, it is assumed that in near future it will become possible to diagnose the probability of asthma or other diseases of allergic origin, e.g., food allergies, in appropriately equipped clinical laboratories, also by means of screening all SNP and transcriptome information related to the diseases. Nowadays, however, despite extensive research, even the most risky SNP combination related to asthma has only a twofold odds ratio with controls and most SNP research papers deal only with statistical probability (Saito et al., 2003).

### 1.3.3 Functional Proteomics in Allergology and Clinical Immunology

The molecular mechanism of the effect of most allergens remains unknown. It also remains an open question what the reasons are for the allergizing properties of antigens. One strategy adopted in recognizing the mechanism of allergen effects is testing their relationship between their bioactivity and their 3D structure. It has been found that the 3D structure of some allergens is compliant with the 3D structure of endogenous proteins (albumins, lipocalins, topomyosins), which may be used in identifying epitopes involved in allergy processes. The most important reason for research into allergen activity at a molecular level, however, is the finding which indicates that allergen capacity to induce immunological response is to a significant extent independent of allergen metabolic (enzymatic) activity. It rather seems that the factors which determine the response development are allergen dose, history of exposure, and host's genetic predispositions. It particularly relates to the cases involving allergen processing mechanisms (so far unknown) concluding with Th2 response. Pomes et al. (2001) have analyzed a group of known allergens—proteins sampled from dust, cats, dogs, and cockroaches—and determined a close relationship between allergen immunological activity and enzymatic activity (previously suggested by other authors). They thus redefined the molecular mechanism of allergen effect to structural effects. If this is the case, allergen 3D structure analysis may become the basis for determining the reasons for allergenic cross-reactivity, at the same time providing more evidence for the already widely accepted 3D structure–function relationship.

Nowadays, computing methods are utilized in defining biological properties of proteins and peptides. Allergen vulnerability prediction can be tested on the basis of information on antigen (allergen) 1D structure, which, when combined with *in silico* methods of structural modeling, may serve as the grounds for recognizing the 3D structure of the tested molecule followed by determining the risk of allergy (Aalberse and Stadler, 2006). It is widely recognized that in predicting the possibility of allergy occurrence, several issues are taken into consideration: (1) IgE immunogenicity, (2) IgE cross-reactivity, and (3) T-cell cross-reactivity. As already mentioned, IgE immunogenicity above all depends on the factors determining response development (dose, exposure history, genetic predispositions) rather than protein structure, therefore *in silico* predictability of allergic reaction is not possible at this stage. However, it is fully efficacious to conduct *in silico* searches for the structural homology of

IgE antigens combined with *in vitro* tests of cross-reactions of IgE and sequenced antigens, as it has been found that the basic condition for positive cross-reactivity is the high structural compatibility (homology) of reagents. Compared to B-cells, T-cell cross-reactivity is far more difficult to assess because the mechanism of T-cell effects is more diverse and involves both the phase of immunological response and the effect phase of the allergic reaction.

Year by year, protein *in silico* structural analysis attracts more supporters. It has a set of increasingly improved biocomputing tools easily accessible on servers all over the world. The created databases such as GenBank (Benson et al., 1997), PIR (Barker et al., 1999), or Swiss-prot (Bairoch et al., 2004), which collect information in the form of nucleotide sequences of the structural genes or amino acid sequences, are an attractive source of information on the structure and functions of genes, and consequently proteins. Due to the increasing amount of information collected in the databases, it has become necessary to create searching tools. The most popular programs today are based on FASTA (Pearson, 1990) or BLAST (Basic Local Alignment Search Tool) (Altschul et al., 1997) algorithm types. The sequences from search results can then be compared against each other, in pairs or full sets, by the use of such programs as MUSCLE (Edgar, 2004), CLUSTAL_W (Higgins et al., 1994), and T-COFFIE (Notredame et al., 2000). Data in the form of multiple alignments may be utilized in phylogenetic analysis, etc. What is also becoming attractive is the possibility to predict protein folding for proteins which are now structurally undetermined, based merely on information of their 1D structure. Yet another possibility is creating structural models of the proteins whose spatial structure has not yet been determined. Due to the methodological complexity of this process and the necessity to obtain the largest possible set of information from other analyses, predicting secondary structure, determining folding type, and selecting appropriate patterns, Internet meta servers have become popular. Currently, the best ones include Bioinfobank.pl (Ginalski et al., 2003) and Genesilico (Kurowski and Bujnicki, 2003). These services enable gathering several analyses at one site in the form of a clear interface enabling the compilation of analyses by the user, depending on their knowledge and needs.

This, however, leads to certain consequences which are in essence related to the very method of creating virtual models followed by testing them with virtual tools. In case of incorrect initial assumptions and assessment criteria, which may be the result of poor knowledge of biological nature of the tested object, it may lead to incorrect conclusions. It seems that the best solution to the problem would be *in vivo* and/or *in vitro* experimental validation of *in silico* analysis. In this case *in silico* analysis would enable keeping the number of experiments down to a necessary minimum. Another benefit resulting from applying *in silico* analysis is the possibility of recognizing global features of molecules, such as the total electrostatic field of a molecule or detailed topography of its surface, which is virtually impossible with *in vitro* testing.

A recent example of such research was an effective experiment in January 2008 presented by Gosh and Gupta-Bhattacharya (2008). The researchers presented the results of an *in silico* study whose aim was to determine the molecular background of cross-reactivity and activity of Bet v1 allergens present in pollen and plant foods.

Bet vl proteins are a large family with high structural homology and proper-ties correlating with their cross-reactivity. The strategy of the study was based on the observation that one representative of the family—T1 protein, which is found naturally—does not have allergizing properties and does not exhibit the tendency to cross-react in spite of structural compatibility. The assumption made was that differ-ences in T1 bioactivity derive from differences in 3D structure. Next, by means of homological modeling, T1 modeling was performed which was then compared against Bet vl structure, particularly for the loci of conservative areas, solvent availability, and electrostatic effects of surface amino acid radicals. It was shown that the T1 folding type does not significantly differ from folding types of other Bet vl representatives, and that the differences in bioactivity among Bet vl representatives should be linked with differences in the surface organization of their molecules—the occurrence of conservative areas, and consequently, arrangement of electrostatic potentials.

Apart from modeling applications, protein sequence banks (data bases) and some biocomputing tools: BIOPEP (Dziuba et al., 1999), BLAST (http://www.ncbi.nlm.nih.gov/blast/Blast.cgi), CLUSTAL_W (Higgins et al., 1994), Peptide Search (http://www.narrador.embl-heidelberg.de/GroupPages/PageLink/peptidesearchpage.html), Swiss-prot (Bairoch et al., 2004), may be of use in recognizing biological properties of peptides and proteins on the level of 1D/2D structure, for example, searching for toxic sequences in proteins, which may be followed by eliminating the proteins from the diet for patients with coeliac disease (Darewicz and Dziuba, 2007). Bioactive peptides released from food proteins by proteolytic enzymes may present toxic activity. Coeliac disease is gluten-sensitive enteropathy of autoimmunological back-ground, induced by the presence of wheat proteins in the diet; the disease involves changes in the jejunal mucous membrane. α-Gliadin (an ethanol-soluble gluten frac-tion) is considered as the most toxic in coeliac disease. Ethanol-soluble protein frac-tions have been obtained in the process of ethanol extraction of other grains as well, i.e., rye (secalin), barley (hordein), and oats (avenin). Due to the significant content of proline (~15%) and glutamic acid (up to 60%), these proteins have been included in the category of prolamines. In the studies of peptides obtained from gliadin as a result of digestion with enzymes, it was shown that the harmfulness of grain pro-lamines depends on the activity of bioactive peptides released from the prolamine 1D structure. Peptides from α-gliadin, whose toxicity has been confirmed in *in vivo* tests, contain one of four amino acid sequences: PSQQ, QQQP, QQPY, or QPYP (P—proline, S—serine, Q—glutamine, Y—tyrozine). By means of utilizing syn-thetic peptides in the studies, it was proved that the application of peptides with 8–12 amino acid radicals can induce toxic reactions in coeliac disease. Although there are potentially toxic sequences in the structures of a number of food proteins, the proteins are not classified as coeliac etiological factors. In this situation, application of computing methods to assess the potential connection between food protein and coeliac disease may prove helpful in clinical practice.

In practical allergology, SuperHapten database (Günther et al., 2007) may also be useful; the recently developed database contains information on 2D and 3D struc-tures, as well as bioactive haptens (http://bioinformatics.charite.de/superhapten). The most researched haptens include not only xenobiotics but also numerous substances of natural origin which have the capacity to induce autoimmunological conditions, such as contact dermatitis or asthma. Haptens are linked with allergies which occur as side effects of certain drugs. However, knowledge of their role in allergy pathogenesis and mechanism of action is still poor. Haptens are also used in generating biosensors, immunomodulators, and new vaccines. SuperHapten compound classification is based on their origin: pesticides, herbicides, insecticides, drugs, natural compounds, etc. To date 7257 haptens, 453 commercially available related antibodies, and 24 carriers have been described in the database, which opens the opportunity for experimental approaches to cross-reactivity.

## REFERENCES

Aalberse, R. C. and Stadler, B. M. 2006. In silico predictability of allergenicity: From amino acid sequence via 3-D structure to allergenicity. *Mol Nutr Food Res* 50(7): 625–627.

Akdis, M., Blaser, K., and Akdis, C. A. 2005. T regulatory cells in allergy: Novel concepts in pathogenesis, prevention, and treatment of allergic diseases. *J Allergy Clin Immunol* 116: 961–968.

Altschul, S. F., Madden, T. L., Schaffer, A. A. et al. 1997. Gapped BLAST and PSI-BLAST: A new generation of protein database search programs. *Nucleic Acids Res* 25(17): 3389–3402.

Amoli, M. M., Hand, S., Hajeer, A. H., Jones, K. P., Rolf, S., and Sting, C. 2002. Polymorphism the STAT6 gene encodes risk for nut allergy. *Genes Immun* 3: 220–224.

Andre, C., Vatrinet, C., Galvain, S., Carat, F., and Sicard, H. 2000. Safety of sublingual-swallow immunotherapy in children and adults. *Int Arch Allergy Immunol* 121(3): 229–234.

Arentz-Hansen, H., Korner, R., Molberg, O. et al. 2000. The intestinal T cell response to α-gliadyn in adult celiac disease is focused on a single deamidated glutamine targeted by tissue transglutaminase. *J Exp Med* 191: 603–612.

Bahceciler, N. N., Arikan, C., Taylor, A. et al. 2005. Impact of sublingual immunotherapy on specific antibody levels in asthmatic children allergic to house dust mites. *Int Arch Allergy Immunol* 136: 287–294.

Bairoch, A., Boeckmann, B., Ferro, S., and Gasteiger, E. 2004. Swiss-Prot: Juggling between evolution and stability. *Brief Bioinform* 5: 39–55.

Barker, W. C., Garavelli, J. S., McGarvey, P. B. et al. 1999. The PIR-international protein sequence database. *Nucleic Acids Res.* 27: 39–43.

Barr, M., Kraepelien, S., and Zetterström, R. 1958. Hemolytic episodes as the cause of jaundice in children with allergic disease-allergic jaundice. *Acta Paediatr* 47: 113–119.

Benson, D. A., Boguski, M. S., Lipman, D. J., and Ostell, J. 1997. GenBank. *Nucleic Acids Res* 25(1): 1–6.

Bird, J. J., Brown, D. R., Mullen, A. C. et al. 1998. Helper T cell differentiation is controlled by the cell cycle. *Immunity* 9: 229–237.

Bischoff, S. and Crowe, S. 2005. Gastrointestinal food allergy: New insight into pathophysiology and clinical perspectives. *Gastroenterology* 128(4): 1089–1113.

Bjorksten, B., Sepp, E., Julge, K., Voor, T., and Mikelseaa, M. 2001. Allergy development and the intestinal microflora during the first year of life. *J Allergy Clin Immunol* 108: 516–520.

Bland, P. W. and Warren, L. G. 1986. Antigen presentation by epithelial cells of the rat small intestine. II. Selective induction of suppressor T-cells. *Immunology* 58: 9–14.

Bohle, B. 2004. T lymphocytes and food allergy. *Mol Nutr Food Res* 48: 424–433.

Böhme, M., Lannerö, E., Wickman, M., Nordyall, S. L., and Wahlgren, C. F. 2002. Atopic dermatitis and concomitant disease patterns in children up to two years of age. *Acta Derm Venerol* 82: 98–103.

Braga-Neto, U. M. and Marques, E. T. A. Jr. 2006. From functional genomics to functional immunomics: New challenges, old problems, big rewards. *PLoS Comput Biol* 2(7): 651–662.

Brand, U., Bellinghausen, I., Enk, A. H. et al. 1999. Allergen specific immune deviation from a Th2 to a Th1 response induced by dendritic cells and collagen type. *J Allergy Clin Immunol* 104: 1052–1059.

Brandtzaeg, P. 2001. Nature and function of gastrointestinal antigen-presenting cells. *Allergy* 56: 16–20.

Brandzeg, P. 2002. Current understanding of gastrointestinal immunoregulation and its relation to food allergy. *Ann N Y Acad Sci* 964: 13–45.

Braun-Fahrlander, C. 2000. Allergic diseases in farmers' children. *Pediatr Allergy Immunol* 11(13): 19–22.

Camponeschi, B., Lucarelli, S., Frediani, T., Barbato, M., and Quinteri, F. 1997. Association HLA DQ7 antigen with cow milk protein allergy in Italian children. *Pediatr Allergy Immunol* 8: 106–109.

Cella, M., Scheidegger, D., Palmer-Lehmann, K., Lane, P., Lanzavecchia, A., and Alber, G. 1996. Ligation of CD40 on dendritic cells triggers production of high levels of interleukin-12 and enhances T cell stimulatory capacity: T-T help via APC activation. *J Exp Med* 184: 747–752.

Chen, Y., Kuchroo, V. K., Inobe, J., Hafler, D. A., and Weiner, H. L. 1994. Regulatory T cell clones induced by oral tolerance: Suppression of autoimmune encephalomyelitis. *Science* 265 (5176): 1237–1240.

Chen, Y., Rennie, D., Cormier, Y., McDuffie, H., Pahwa, P., and Dosman, J. 2007. Reduced risk of atopic sensitization among farmers: The Humboldt study. *Int Arch Allergy Immunol* 144(4): 338–342.

Cheung, P. F., Wong, C. K., Ip, W. K., and Lam, C. W. 2008. FAK-mediated activation of ERK for eosinophil migration: A novel mechanism for infection-induced allergic inflammation. *Int Immunol* 20(3): 353–363

Ciprandi, G., Fenoglio, D., Cirillo, I., Milanese, M., and Minuti, P. 2006. Sublingual immunotherapy and regulatory T cells. *Allergy* 61: 511.

Cohn, L. 2001. Food for thought. Can immunological tolerance be induced to treat asthma? *Am J Respir Cell Mol Biol* 24: 509–512.

Darewicz, M. and Dziuba, J. 2007. Dietozależny charakter enteropatii pokarmowych na przykładzie celiakii. *Żywność Nauka Technologia Jakość* 34: 5–15.

Dehlink, E., Eiwegger, T., Gerstmayr, M. et al. 2006. Absence of systemic immunologic changes during dose build-up phase and early maintenance period in effective specific sublingual immunotherapy in children. *Clin Exp Allergy* 36: 32–39.

Durkin, H. G., Smith-Norowitz, T. A., Pincus, M., Nowakowski, M., Bluth, M. H., and Joks, R. 2007. New treatments for suppression of ongoing human and murine IgE responses. *J Allergy Clin Immunol* 119(1): S316–S371.

Dziuba, J., Minkiewicz, P., Nałęcz, D., and Iwaniak, A. 1999. Database of biologically active peptide sequences. *Nahrung* 43: 190–195.

Edgar, R. C. 2004. MUSCLE: A multiple sequence alignment method with reduced time and space complexity. *BMC Bioinform* 5: 113.

Eggesbø, M., Botten, G., Stigum, H., Nafstad, P., and Magnus, P. 2003. Is delivery by cesarean section a risk factor for food allergy? *J Allergy Clin Immunol* 112: 420–426.

Elson, C. O., Kagnoff, M. F., Fiocchi, C., Befus, A. D., and Targan, S. 1986. Intestinal immunity and inflammation recent progress. *Gastroenterology* 91: 746–768.

Fanta, C., Bohle, B., Hirt, W. et al. 1999, Systemic immunological changes induced by administration of grass pollen allergens via the oral mucosa during sublingual immunotherapy. *Int Arch Allergy Immunol* 120: 218–224.

Fontenot, J. D. and Rudensky, A. Y. 2004. Molecular aspects of regulatory T cell development. *Semin Immunol* 16: 73–80.

Fraser, J. H., Rincon, M., McCoy, K. D., and Le Gros, G. 1999. CTLA4 ligation attenuates AP-1, NFAT and NF-kappaB activity in activated T cells. *Eur J Immunol* 29: 838–844.

Frossard, C. P., Hauser, C., and Eigenmann, P. A. 2004. Antigen-specific secretory IgA antibodies in the gut are decreased in a mouse model of food allergy. *J Allergy Clin Immunol* 114: 377–382.

Galliaerde, V., Desvignes, C., Peyron, E., and Kaiserlian, D. 1995. Oral tolerance to haptens: Intestinal epithelial cells from 2,4-dinitrochlorobenzene-fed mice inhibit hapten-specific T-cell activation *in vitro*. *Eur J Immunol* 25: 385–390.

Gehring U, Bischof, W., Schlenvoigt, G., Richter, K., Fahlbusch, B., Wichmann, H.-E., and Heinrich, J. (for the INGA study group). 2004. Exposure to house dust endotoxin and allergic sensitization in adults. *Allergy* 59: 946–952.

Gereda, J, D., Leung, Y. M., and Liu, A. H. 2000. Levels of environmental endotoxin and prevalence of atopic disease. *JAMA* 284: 1647–1653.

Ghosh, D. and Gupta-Bhattacharya, S. 2008. Structural insight into protein T1, the non-allergenic member of the Bet v1 allergen family—An in silico analysis. *Mol Immunol* 45(2): 456–462.

Ginalski, K., Elofsson, A., Fischer, D., and Rychlewski, L. 2003. 3D-Jury: A simple approach to improve protein structure predictions. *Bioinformatics* 19(8): 1015–1018.

Giustizieri, M. L., Mascia, F., and Frezzolini, A. 2001. Keratinocytes from patients with atopic dermatitis and psoriasis show a distinct chemokine production profile in response to T cell-derived cytokines. *J Allergy Clin Immunol* 107: 871–877.

Groux, H., O'Garra, A., Bigler, M. et al. 1997. A CD4+ T-cell subset inhibits antigen-specific T-cell responses and prevents colitis. *Nature* 389: 737–742.

Günther, S., Hempel, D., Dunkel, M., Rother, K., and Preissner, R. 2007. SuperHapten: A comprehensive database for small immunogenic compounds. *Nucleic Acid Res* 35: 906–910.

Hage-Hamsten, M., Johansson, E., Kronquist, M., Loughry, A., Cookson, W. C., and Moffatt, M.F. 2002. Associations of Fc epsilon R1-beta polymorphisms with immunoglobulin antibody responses to common inhalant allergens in a rural population. *Clin Exp Allergy* 32: 838–842.

Hara, M., Kingley, C.I., Niimi, M. et al. 2001. Il 10 is required for regulatory T cells to mediate tolerance to alloantigens in vivo. *J Immunol* 166: 3789–3796.

Hecker, M., Bohnert, A., Konig, I. R., Bein, G., and Hackstein, H. 2003. Novel genetic variation of human interleukin-21 receptor is associated with elevated IgE levels in females. *Genes Immun* 4: 228–233.

Hemmi, H., Takeuchi, O., and Kawai, T. 2000. A Toll-like receptor recognizes bacterial DNA. *Nature* 408: 740–745.

Hidvegi, E., Cserhati, E., Kereki, E., Savilahti, E., and Arato, A. 2002. Serum immunoglobulin E, IgA, and IgG antibodies to different cow's milk proteins in children with cow's milk allergy: Association with prognosis and clinical manifestations. *Pediatr Allergy Immunol* 13: 255–261.

Higgins, D., Thompson, J., Gibson, T. et al. 1994. Improving the sensitivity of progressive multiple sequence alignment through sequence weighting, position-specific gap penalties and weight matrix choice. *Nucleic Acids Res.* 22: 4673–4680.

Higgins, S. C., Lavelle, E. C., McCann, C. et al. 2003. Toll-like receptor 4-mediated innate IL 10 activates antigen-specific regulatory T cells and confers resistance to *Bordetella pertusis* by inhibiting inflammatory pathology. *J Immunol* 171: 3119–3127.

Hill, P. G. and Mc Millan, S. A. 2006. Anti-tissue transglutaminase antibodies and their role in the investigation of coeliac disease. *Ann Clin Biochem.* 43: 105–117.

Hobbs, K., Negri, J., Klinnert, M., Rosenwasser, L. J., and Borish, Ł. 1998. Interleukin-10 transforming growth factor-beta promoter polymorphisms in allergies and asthma. *Am J Respir Crit Care Med* 158: 1958–1962.

Howard, T. D., Meyers, D. A., and Bleecker, E. R. 2003. Mapping susceptibility genes for diseases. *Chest* 123: 363S–368S.

Howell, W. M., Turnen, S. J., Hourihane, J. O., and Warner, J. O. 1998. HLA classes DRB1., DQB1 and DPB! Genotypic associations with peanut allergy (evidence for family-based and case control study). *Clin Exp Allergy* 28: 156–162.

Illi, S., Mutius, E., Lau, S. et al. 2004. The natural course of atopic dermatitis from birth to age 7 years and the association with asthma. *J Allergy Clin Immunol* 113(5): 925–931.

Isolauri, E., Arvola, T., Sutas, Y., Moilanen, E., and Salminen, S. 2000. Probiotics in management of atopic eczema. *Clin Exp Allergy* 30: 1605–1610.

Jansen S. C., van Dusseldorp M., Bottema K. C., and Dubois A. E. 2003. Intolerance to dietary biogenic amines: A review. *Ann Allergy Asthma Immunol* 91(3): 233–240.

Johansson, S. G. O., Hourihane, J. O. B., Bousquet, J. et al. 2001. Position paper. A revised nomenclature for allergy: An EAACI position statement from the EAACI nomenclature task force. *Allergy* 9: 813–829.

Jonhsson, C. C., Ownby, D. R., and Peterson, E. L. 1996. Parental history of atopic disease and concentration of cord blood IgE. *Clin Exp Allergy* 26: 624–629.

Kabesch, M. and Mutius, E. 2000. Adverse health effects of environmental tobacco smoke exposure in childhood. *Allergy Clin Immunol Int: J World Allergy Org* 12: 146–151.

Karlsson, H., Hessle, C., and Rudin, A. 2002. Innate immune response of human neonatal cells to bacteria from the normal gastrointestinal flora. *Infect Immun* 70: 6688–6696.

Karpus, W. J., Lujacs, N. W., Kennedy, K. J., Smith, W. S., Hurst, S. D., and Barrett, T. A. 1997. Differential CC chemokine-induced enhancement of T helper cell cytokine production. *J Immunol* 158: 4129–4136.

Kim, C. Y., Quarsten, H., Bergseng, E., Khosla, C., and Sollid, L. M. 2004. Structural basis for HLA-DQ2-mediated presentation of gluten epitopes in celiac disease. *Proc Natl Acad Sci USA* 101: 4175–4179.

Knapczyk, M. and Lauterbach, R. 2001. Porównanie wartości pH soku żołądkowego u noworodków urodzonych przedwcześnie i noworodków donoszonych—badania wstępne. *Post Neonatol* 2: 75 86 (in Polish).

Koch, F., Stanzl, U., and Jennewein, P. 1996. High level IL-12 production by murine dendritic cells: Upregulation via MHC class II and CD40 molecules and downregulation by IL-4 and IL-10. *J Exp Med* 184: 741–746.

Kohno, Y., Shimojo, N., Kojima, H., and Katsuki, T. 2001. Homing receptor expression on cord blood T lymphocytes and the development of atopic egzema in infants. *Int Arch Allergy Immunol* 124: 332–335.

Kolho, K. L., Haapaniemi, A., Haahtela, T., and Rautelin, H. 2005. Helicobacter pylori and specific immunoglobulin E antibodies to food allergens in children. *J Pediatr Gastroenterol Nutr* 40: 180–183.

Kramer, M. S. and Kakuma, R. 2006. Maternal dietary antigen avoidance during pregnancy or lactation, or both, for preventing or treating atopic disease in the child. *The Cochrane Database of Systematic Reviews*, no. 3 (July).

Kurowski, M. A. and Bujnicki, J. M. 2003. GeneSilico protein structure prediction metaserver. *Nucleic Acids Res* 31: 3305–3307.

Kusunoki, T., Okafuji, I., Yoshioka, T. et al. 2005. SPINK5 polymorphism is associated with disease severity and food allergy in children with atopic dermatitis. *J Allergy Clin Immunol* 115: 636–638.

Landete J. M., Ferrer S., Polo L., and Pardo I. 2005. Biogenic amines in wines from three Spanish regions. *J Agric Food Chem* 53: 1119–1124.

Leung, D. Y. M. and Soter, N. A. 2001. Cellular and immunologic mechanism in atopic dermatitis. *J Am Acad Dermatol* 44: S1–S12.

Levings, M. K., Sangregorio, R., and Roncarolo, M. G. 2001. Human CD25(+)CD4(+) T regulatory cells suppress naive and memory T cell proliferation and can be expanded in vitro without loss of function. *J Exp Med* 193: 1295–1302.

Levings, M. K., Sangregorio, R., Sartirana, C. et al. 2002. Human CD25+ CD4 suppressor cells clones produce transforming growth factor β, but not interleukin 10, and are distinct from type 1 T regulatory cells. *J Exp Med* 196: 1335–1336.

Lider, O., Santos., L. M., Lee, C. S., Higgins, P. J., and Weiner, H. L. 1989. Suppression of experimental autoimmune encephalomyelitis by oral administration of myelin basic protein, II. Suppression of disease and in vitro immune responses is mediated by antigen-specific CD8+ T lymphocytes. *J. Immunol* 142: 748–752.

Lugovic, L., Lipozencic, J., and Jakić-Razumovic, J. 2005. Prominent involvement of activated Th1-subset of T-cells and increased expression of receptor for IFN-gamma on keratinocytes in atopic dermatitis acute skin lesions. *Int Arch Allergy Immunol* 137: 125–133.

Macdougall, C. F., Cant, A. J., and Colver, A. F. 2002. How dangerous is food allergy in childhood? The incidence of severe and fatal allergic reactions across the UK and Ireland. *Arch Dis Child* 86: 236–239.

MacGlashan, D. W. 1993. Releasability of human basophils: Cellular sensitivity and maximal histamine release are independent variables. *J Allergy Clin Immunol* 91 (2): 605–615.

MacGlashan, D. W. and Lichtenstein, L. M. 1981. The transition from specific to nonspecific desensitization in human basophils. *J Immunol* 127: 2410–2422.

Maciejewski, H., Konarski, Ł., Jasińska, A., and Drath, M. 2005. Analysis of DNA microarray data methods and tools. *Bio-Algorithms Med-Syst.* Journal edited by Medical College – Jagiellonian University. 1(1/2): 129–132.

Macpherson, A. J., Gatto, D., Sainsbury, E., Harriman, G. R., Hengartner, H., and Zinkernagel, R. M. 2000. A primitive T cell-independent mechanism of intestinal mucosal IgA responses to commensal bacteria. *Science* 288: 2222–2226.

Magalhaes, J. G., Tattoli, I., and Girardin, S. E. 2007. The intestinal epithelial barrier: How to distinguish between the microbial flora and pathogens. *Semin Immunol* 19: 106–115.

Malaviya, R. and Abraham, S. N. 2001. Mast cell modulation of immune responses to bacteria. *Immunol Rev* 164: 589–595.

Mandhane, P. J., Greene, J. M., and Sears, M. R. 2007. Interactions between breast-feeding, specific parental atopy, and sex on development of asthma and atopy. *J Allergy Clin Immunol* 119: 1359–1366.

Matricardi, P. M., Rosmini, F., Riondino, S. et al. 2000. Exposure to foodborne and orofecal microbes versus airborne viruses in relation to atopy and allergic asthma. Epidemiological study. *BMJ* 320: 412–417.

Matysiak-Budnik, T., van Niel, G., Megraud, F. et al. 2003. Gastric Helicobacter infection inhibits development of oral tolerance to food antigens in mice. *Infect Immun* 71: 5219–5224.

Mayer, L. and Shlien, R. 1987. Evidence for function of IgA molecules on gut epithelial cells in man. *J Exp Med* 166: 1471–1483.

Millichap J. G. and Yee M. M. 2003. The diet factor in pediatric and adolescent migraine. *Pediatr Neurol* 28: 9–15.

Misra, N., Bayry, J., Lacroix-Desmazes, S., Kazatchkine, M. D., and Kaveri, S. V. 2004. Cutting edge: Human CD4+ CD25+ T cells restrain the maturation and antigen-presenting function of dendritic cells. *J Immunol* 172: 4676–4680.

Miyake, Y., Arakawa, M., Tanaka, K., Sasaki, S., and Ohya, Y. 2008. Tuberculin reactivity and allergic disorders in schoolchildren, Okinawa, Japan. *Clin Exp Allergy* 38: 388–392.

Moffatt, M., Mill, M., and Cornelis, F. 1994. Genetic likeage of T cell receptors and γ/δ complex to specific IgE response. *Lancet* 343: 1997–2001.

Moffatt, M. F., Schou, C., Faux, J. A. et al. 2001. Association between quantitative traits underlying asthma and the HLA-DRB1 locus in a family-based population sample. *Eur J Hum Genet* 9: 341–346.

Moneret-Vautrin, D. A., Rance, F., Kanny, G. et al. 1998. Food allergy to peanuts in France. Evaluation of 142 observations. *Clin Exp Allergy* 28: 1113–1119.

Moss, S. F., Attia, L., Scholes, J. V., Walters, J. R. F., and Holt, P. R. 1996. Increased small intestine apoptosis in coeliac disease. *Gut* 39: 811–817.

Mowat, A. I. 2003. Anatomical basis of tolerance and immunity to intestinal antigens. *Immunology* 3: 331–341.

Murakami, H., Akbar, S. M. F., Matsui, H., Horiike, N., and Onji M. 2002. Macrophage migration inhibitory factor activates antigen-presenting dendritic cells and induces inflammatory cytokines in ulcerative colitis. *Clin Exp Immunol* 128: 504–510.

Myung, P. S., Boerthe, N. J., and Koretzky, G. A. 2000. Adapter proteins in lymphocyte antigen-receptor signaling. *Curr Opin Immunol* 12: 256–266.

Nagata, S., McKenzie, C., Pender, S. L. F. et al. 2000. Human Peyer's patch T cells are sensitized to dietary antigen and display a Th cell type 1 cytokine profile. *J Immunol* 165(9): 5315–5321.

Nakahara, T., Uchi, H., Urabe, K., Chen, Q., Furure, M., and Moroi, Y. 2004. Role of c-Jun N-terminal kinase on lipopolysaccharide induced maturation of human monocyte-derived dendritic cells. *Int Immunol* 16: 1701–1709.

Nakamura, K., Kitani, A., and Strober, W. 2001 Cell contact-dependent immunosuppression of CD4+ CD25+ regulatory T cells is mediated by cell-surface-bound transforming growth factor-β. *J Exp Med* 195: 629–644.

Nakazato, J., Kishida, M., Kuroiwa, R., Fujiwara, J., Shimoda, M., and Shinomiya, N. 2008. Serum levels of Th2 chemokines, CCL17, CCL22, and CCL27, were the important markers of severity in infantile atopic dermatitis. *Pediatr Allergy Immunol* 19(7): 605–613 http://www.blackwell-synergy.com/doi/abs/10.1111/j.1399-3038.2007.00692.

Netea, M. G., Sutmuller, R., Herman, C. et al. 2004. Toll-like receptor 2 suppress immunity against Candida albicans through induction of IL 10 and regulatory T cells. *J Immunol* 172: 3712–3718

Noble, A., Truman, J. P., Vyas, B., Vukmanovic-Stejic, M., Hirst, W. J., and Kemeny, D. M. 2000. The balance of protein kinase C and calcium signaling directs T cell subset development. *J Immunol* 164: 1807–1813.

Noirey, N., Rougier, N., Andre, C., Schmitt, D., and Vincent, C. 2000. Langerhans-like dendritic cells generated from cord blood progenitors internalize pollen allergens by macropinocytosis, and part of the molecules are processed and can activate autologous native T lymphocytes. *J Allergy Clin Immunol* 105: 1194–1201.

Notredame, C., Higgins, D. G., and Heringa, J. 2000. T-Coffee: A novel method for fast and accurate multiple sequence alignment. *J Mol Biol* 302: 205–217.

Nuhoglu, Y., Nuhoglu, C., and Ozcay, S. 2003. The association between delayed type hypersensitivity reaction to Mycobacterium tuberculosis and atopy in asthmatic children. *Allergol Immunopathol* (Madr) 31(1): 14–17.

Oddy, W. H., Peat, J. K., and de Klerk, N. H. 2002. Maternal asthma, infant feeding and the risk of childhood asthma. *J Allergy Clin Immunol* 110: 65–67.

Pasare, C. and Medzhitov, R. 2003. Toll pathway-dependent blockade of CD4+ CD25+ T cell-mediated suppression by dendritic cells. *Science* 299: 1033–1036.

Pasare, C. and Medzhitov, R. 2004. Toll-dependent control mechanisms of CD 4 T cell activation. *Immunity* 21: 733–741.

Passalacqua, G., Guerra, L., Fumagalli, F., and Canonica, G. W. 2006. Safety profile of sublingual immunotherapy. *Treat Respir Med* 5: 225–234.

Patella, V., Florio, G., Petraroli, A., and Marone, G. 2000. HIV gp 120 induces IL4 and release from human Fc epsilon RI+ cells through interaction with the VH3 region IgE. *J Immunol* 164: 589–595.

Pawliczak, R. and Shelhamer, J. H. 2003. Application of functional genomics in allergy and clinical immunology. *Allergy* 58: 973–980.

Pearson, W. R. 1990. Rapid and sensitive sequence comparison with FASTP and FASTA. *Methods in Enzymol* 183: 63–98.

Pomés, A., Smith, A. M., Grégoire, Ch., Vailes, L. D., Arruda, L. K., and Chapman, M. D. 2001. Functional properties of cloned allergens from dust mite, cockroach, and cat. *J Allergy Clin Immunol Int: J World Allergy Org* 13: 162–169.

Ramsdell, F. 2003. FoxP3 and natural regulatory T cells: Key to a cell lineage. *Immunity* 19: 165–168.

Remes, S. T., Livanainen, K., Koskela, H., and Pekkanen, J. 2003. Which factors explain the lower prevalence of atopy amongst farmers' children? *Clin Exp Allergy* 33: 427–434.

Renz-Polster, H., David, M. R., Buist, A. S. et al. 2004. Caesarean section delivery and the risk of allergic disorders in childhood. *Clin Exp Allergy* 35: 1466–1472.

Rolland, J. M. and O'Hehir, R. E. 2001. Targeting the allergen-specific CD4+ T cell-strategies for improved allergen immunotherapy. *Allergy Clin Immunol Int: J World Allergy Org* 13: 170–177.

Romagnani, S. 2000. The role of lymphocytes in allergic disease. *J Allergy Clin Immunol.* 105: 399–408.

Romagnani, S. 2004a. Immunologic influences on allergy and the Th1/Th2 balance. *J Allergy Clin Immunol* 113: 395–400.

Romagnani, S. 2004b. The increased prevalence of allergy and the hygiene hypothesis: Missing immune deviation, reduced immune suppression, or both? *Immunology* 112: 352–363.

Roszkiewicz, J., Lange, M., Szczerkowska-Dobosz, A., and Jasiel-Walikowska, E. 2007. Alergiczne lub cytoklastyczne zapalenie naczyń (vasculitis alergica/vasculitis leukocytoclastica). *Forum Medycyny Rodzinnej* 1: 272–279.

Rothenberg, M. E., Mishra, A., Brandt, E. B., and Hogan, S. P. 2001. Gastrointestinal eosinophils in health and disease. *Adv Immunol* 78: 291–328.

Ruiz, R. G., Kemeny, D. M., and Price, J. F. 1992. Higher risk of infantile atopic dermatitis from maternal atopy than from paternal atopy. *Clin Exp Allergy* 22: 762–766.

Saito, H., Kato, A., and Matsumoto, K. 2003. Application of genomic science to clinical allergy. *Allergy Clin Immunol Int: J World Allergy Org* 15: 218–222.

Salam, M. T., Margolis, H. G., Mcconnell, R., Mcgregor J. A., Avol, E. L., and Gilliland, F. D. 2006. Mode of delivery is associated with asthma and allergy occurrences in children. *Ann Epidemiol* 16: 341–346.

Samoilova, E. B., Horton, J. L., Zhang, H., Khoury S. J., Weiner, H. L., and Chen, Y. 1998. CTLA4 is required for the induction of high-dose oral tolerance. *Int Immunol* 10: 491–498.

Schröder, J. M. and Mochizuki, M. 1999. The role of chemokines in cutaneous allergic inflammation. *Biol Chem* 389: 889–896.

Schroeder, J. T., Bieneman, A. P., Xiao, H. et al. 2005. TLR9- and FcεRI-mediated responses oppose one another in plasmacytoid dendritic cells by down-regulating receptor expression, *J Immunol* 175: 5724–5731.

Schubert, L. A., Jeffery, E., Zhang, Y., Ramsdell, F., and Ziegler, S. F. 2001. Scurfin (FOXP3) acts as a repressor of transcription and regulates T cell activation. *J Biol Chem* 276: 37672–37679.

Schulze, A., van Strien, R. T., Praml, G., Nowak, D., and Radon, K. 2007. Characterization of asthma among adults with and without childhood farm contact. *Eur Respir J* 29: 1169–1173.

Schuppan, D. 2000. Current concepts of celiac disease pathogenesis. *Gastroenterology* 119: 234–242.

Senechal, H., Geny, S., Desvaux, F. X., Busson, M., Mayer, C., and Aron, Y. 1999. General and specific immune response in allergy to birch pollen and food (evidence of allergen positive association between atopy and the HLA class II allele HLA-DR7). *J Allergy Clin Immunol* 104: 395–401.

Sepp, E., Julge, K., Vasar, M., Naaber, P., Bjorksten, B., and Mikelsaar, M.1997. Intestinal microflora of Estonian and Swedish infants. *Acta Pediatr* 86: 956–961.

Shida, K., Makino, K., Morishita, A. et al. 1998. Lactobacillus casei inhibits antigen-induced IgE secretion through regulation of cytokine production in murine splenocyte cultures. *Int Arch Allergy Immunol* 115: 278–287

Shin, H. D., Kim, L. H., Park, B. L. et al. 2003. Association of eotaxin gene family with asthma and serum total IgE. *Hum Mol Genet* 12: 1279–1283.

Shin, H.D., Park, B. L., Kim, L. H. et al. 2004. Association of tumor necrosis factor polymorphisms with asthma and serum total IgE. *Hum Mol Genet* 13: 397–403.

Shirai, Y., Hashimoto, M., Kato, R. et al. 2004. Lipopolysaccharide induces CD25-positive, IL 10 producing lymphocytes without secretion of proinflammatory cytokines in the human colon: low MD-2 mRNA expression in colonic macrophages. *J Clin Immunol* 24: 42–52.

Sokal, I. 1995. Receptory Fcγ. Właściwości i udział w wiązaniu IgG i innych procesach biologicznych. *Postępy Hig Med Dośw* 49: 47–55.

Stern, D. A., Riedler, J., Nowak, D. et al. 2007. Exposure to a farming environment has allergen-specific protective effects on TH-2 dependent isotype switching in response to common inhalants. *J Allergy Clin Immunol* 119: 351–358.

Stoll, S., Jonuleit, H., Schmitt, E. et al. 1998. Production of functional IL-18 by different subtypes of murine and human dendritic cells (DC): DC-derived IL-18 enhances IL-12-dependent Th1 development. *Eur J Immunol* 28: 3231–3239.

Swinson, C. M., Slavin, G., and Coles, E. C. 1983. Coeliac disease and malignancy. *Lancet* 1: 111–115.

Szaflarska-Szczepanik, A. 1997. Etiopatogeneza glutenozależnej choroby trzewnej ze szczególnym uwzględnieniem związku choroby z antygenami zgodności tkankowej *Ann Acad Med Siles* 33: 61–67.

Taams, L.S., Smith, J., Rustin, M. H., Salmon, M., Poulter, L. W., and Akbar, A. N. 2001. Human allergic/suppressive CD4CD25+ T cells: A highly differentiated and apoptosis-prone population. *Eur J Immunol.* 31: 1122–1131.

Takabayashi, A., Ihara, K., Sasaki, Y. et al. 2000. Childhood atopic asthma: Positive association with a polymorphism of IL-4 receptor α gene but not with that of IL-4 promoter or Fc ε receptor I β gene. *Exp Clin Immunogenet* 17: 63–70.

Thomson, A.W., Drakes, M. L., Zahorchak, A. F. et al. 1999. Hepatic dendritic cells: Immunobiology and role in liver transplantation. *J Leukoc Biol* 66: 322–330.

Thorstenson, K. M. and Khoruts, A. 2001. Generation of anergic and potentially immunoregulatory CD25+ CD4 T cells in vivo after induction of peripheral tolerance with intravenous or oral antigen. *J Immunol* 167: 188.

Thorton, A. and Mshevach, E. M. 2000. Suppressor effector function of CD4+ CD25+ immunoregulatory T cells is nonspecific. *J Immunol* 164: 183–190.

Tighe, H., Corr, M., Roman, M., and Raz, E. 1998. Gene vaccination: Plasmid DNA is more than just a blueprint. *Immunology Today* 19: 89–97.

Tlaskalova-Hogenova, H., Tućková, L., Lodinova-Żadnikova, R. et al. 2002. Mucosal immunity: Its role in defense and allergy. *Int Arch Allergy Immunol* 128: 77–89.

Townley, R. G., Barlan, I. B., Patino, C. et al. 2004. The effect of BCG vaccine at birth on the development of atopy or allergic disease in young children. *Ann Allergy Asthma Immunol* 92: 350–355.

Trautmann, A., Akdis, M., Kleeman, D. et al. 2000. T-cell mediated Fas-induced keratinocyte apoptosis plays a key pathogenic role in eczematous dermatitis. *J Clin Invest* 106: 25–35.

Tuormaa TET. 1994. The adverse effects of food additives on health (Booklet). *J Orthomolec Med* 9: 225–243.

Ulevitch, R. J.1999. Toll gates for pathogen selection. *Nature* 41: 755–756.

Upham, J. W. and Holt, P. G. 2005. Environment and development of atopy. *Curr Opin Allergy Clin Immunol* 5: 167–172.

Valenta, P. 1994. The phenotype of human eosinophils, basophils and mast cells. *J Allergy Clin Immunol* 94 (6): 1177–1183.

Van Egmond, M., Damen, C. A., van Spriel, A. B., Vidarsson, G., van Garderen, E., and van de Winkel, J. G. 2001. IgA and the IgA Fc receptor. *Trends Immunol* 22: 205–211.

van Herverden, L., Harrap, S. B., Wong, Z. Y., Abramson, M. J., Kutin, J. J., and Forbes, A. 1995. Linkage of high-affinity IgE receptor gene with bronchial hyperreactivity, even absence of atopy. *Lancet* 346: 1262–1265.

van Wijk, R. G. 2008. Sublingual immunotherapy in children. *Expert Opin Biol Ther* 8(3): 291–298.

Venkatesh, Y. P. and Venkatesh, L. H. 2003. A hypothesis for the mechanism of immediate hypersensitivity to mannitol. *Allergol Int* 52 (3): 165–170.

Ventura, A., Magazzu, G., and Greco, L. 1999. Duration of exposure to gluten and risk for autoimmune disorders in celiac patients. *Gastroenterology* 117: 303–310.

von Mutius, E., Braun-Fahrländer, C., Schierl, R. et al. 2000. Exposure to endotoxin or other bacterial components might protect against the development of atopy. *Clin Exp Allergy* 30: 1230–1234.

Vulcano, M. M., Albanesi, C. A., Stoppacciaro A. et al. 2001. Dendritic cells as a major source of macrophage-derived chemokine/CCL22 in vitro and in vitro. *Eur J Immunol* 31: 812–822.

Warner, A. and Warner, J. O. 2000. Early life events in allergic sensitization. *Br Med Bull* 56: 883–893.

Watanabe, T., Yoshida, M., and Shirai, Y. 2002. Administration of an antigen at a high dose generates regulatory CD4+ T cells expressing CD95 ligand and secreting IL-4 in the liver. *J Immunol* 168: 2188–2199.

Weiner, H. L., Gonnella, P. A., Slavin, A., and Maron, R. 1997. Oral tolerance: Cytokine milieu in the gut and modulation of tolerance by cytokines. *Res Immunol* 148: 528–533.

Yamamoto, T., Hattori, M., and Yoshida, T. 2007. Induction of T-cell activation or anergy determined by combination of intensity and duration of T-cell receptor stimulation, and sequential induction in an individual cell. *Immunology* 121: 383–391.

Yoshimoto, T., Takeda, K., Tanaka, T. et al. 1998. IL-12 up-regulates IL-18 receptor expression on T cells, Th1 cells, and B cells: Synergism with IL-18 for IFN-gamma production. *J Immunol* 161: 3400–3407.

Zhang, W., Trible, R. P., and Samelson, L. E. 1998. LAT palmitoylation: Its essential role in membrane microdomain targeting and tyrosine phosphorylation during T cell activation. *Immunity* 9: 239–246.

Zheng, S. G., Wang, J. H., Gray, J. D., Soucier, H., and Horowitz, D. A. 2004. Natural and induced CD4+ CD25+ cells educate CD4+ CD25-cells to develop suppressive activity: Role of IL 2, TGF β and IL 10. *J Immunol* 172: 5213–5221.

# 2 Immunomodulating Properties of Food Components

*Lucjan Jędrychowski, Anna Halász,*
*Edina Németh, and András Nagy*

## CONTENTS

## 2.1 NUTRITION AND HYPERSENSITIVE REACTIONS TO FOOD

Lucjan Jędrychowski

Nutrition is one of the basic physiological functions of every living organism. For many years, due to its components, it has been the subject of interest of the so-called social medicine and dietetics. Dietary solutions seem to be indispensable for certain social groups such as children, hardworking people, sportspersons, convalescents, pregnant women, elderly persons, etc. A commonly known thesis in dietetics is a possibility of treating with food. The so-called nutraceutics, or the food with elevated wholesome properties resulting from its wholesome components, are more and more commonly applied. The situation described above concerns organisms correctly reacting to food, i.e., the cases of food tolerance or a situation in which the organism does not distinguish strange-antigen food components as specifically strange. Hypersensitive allergic reactions, in those caused by foodstuffs, became a serious health problem worldwide at the turn of the twentieth and twentieth centuries, especially in the highly developed countries of Western Europe and the United States. In recent years, an increasing trend in the number of allergies, including food allergies, has been observed (Haahtela et al. 2008).

The causes of steadily increasing occurrence of allergies, especially in industrially developed countries, have not been univocally recognized. It is assumed that the main factors determining the onset of hypersensitive reactions are individual genetic, environmental (food, surroundings, others), and anatomical–physiological predispositions (Table 2.1.1). In addition, there are also factors related to the ways of food processing, application of advanced technologies often resulting in deep changes of raw material antigenic properties (extensively processed foodstuffs), increasing use of genetically modified foods, as well as new kinds of packaging. Moreover, the growth in the occurrence of allergic hypersensitivity is unquestionably connected with the pollution of environment by fuel combustion products, industrial dust, and climatic changes resulting in greater than before abiotic stress (soil salinity, droughts) causing changes in raw materials already during their production (Konopka et al. 2007).

The risk of developing allergies is higher in people whose parents both have allergies, between 40% and 60%; if only one parent is affected, the offspring has a 20%–40% chance of developing an allergy, too. Other factors apparently increasing the risk of allergic hypersensitive reactions are a very hygienic living environment, which creates favorable conditions for children but prevents their immunological system from developing, or chemical environment pollution causing changes within the protective barriers of the mucosa thus permitting their penetration by allergens (Rothenberg 2001). All this is overlapped by individual predispositions such as genetic and anatomical–physiological ones (Table 2.1.1).

Some researchers claim that also other factors, such as sex or race, may be of importance for the scale of the problem, which could be attributed to genetic factors. Allergic reactions are observed everywhere, irrespective of the geographical zone or cultural preferences. Yet, they occur more often in infancy or early childhood than in adulthood, and they affect women more often than men. The data concerning the scale are divergent, which may result from various

**TABLE 2.1.1**

**Major Factors Affecting Occurrence and Development of Food Allergy**

| Genetic (Internal) | Environmental (External—Organism Exposure to Food Allergen) | Coacting (Anatomical–Physiological) |
|---|---|---|
| Atopic genetic parents' constitution | Food | Immaturity of the digestive tract |
| Individual immunological defects | Breast-feeding | Diseases of the digestive tract (inflammatory processes) |
| Child's head size (perimeter >35 cm may be the cause of thymus ischemia) | Infant's diet | Congenital diseases of the digestive tract |
| | Mother's diet during pregnancy and lactation | |
| | Milk formulas used during infancy | |
| | Time of introducing solid food into infant's diet (too early) | |
| | Kind of microflora of the digestive tract | |
| | Vitamin D deficiency | |
| | Diet rich in salt and others | |
| | Environmental | |
| | Perinatal factors | |
| | Hygienic state of environment (pollution) | |
| | Small dusty interiors | |
| | Exposure to food and inhalatory allergens | |
| | Sunshine deficiency | |
| | Others | |
| | Frequent infections | |
| | Antibiotic treatment | |

research methods. Most often studies are fragmentary, they do not cover whole populations and generally appear to be underestimated due to diagnostic reasons. It is assumed that approximately 10%–35% of the world population suffers from some allergy (Sicherer et al. 2004, European Allergy White Paper 1997), in this 0.5%–8% from food allergy (4%–8% children and 1%–2% adults) (Nowak-Wegrzyn et al. 2001, Schäfer et al. 2001).

The actual prevalence of food allergy is lower and seems to range from 1% to 4% of the general population and about 6% of the pediatric population, but it occurs in as much as 25% of children with eczema (Samson 1996, Wüthrich 2000).

According to other sources, the levels (1%–2%) and increasing severity of allergic responses to food in the adult population are well documented as is the phenomenon of even higher (3%–8%) and apparently increasing allergy incidence in children, albeit that susceptibility decreases with age (Osterballe et al. 2005, Vierk et al. 2007).

According to other available data, one-third of the European population suffers from allergies. In the last two decades the number of allergic individuals has doubled (European Allergy White Paper). Allergic reactions to food are very dangerous. In the case of anaphylactic reactions, they pose a life threat at any age. The problem is becoming one of the most significant epidemiological and economic issues (the costs of recognizing and treating allergies in the EU are approximately €30 billion and needs international-scale solutions (Bogucki 2000).

The most significant problems related to the occurrence of hypersensitive allergic reactions are

- Hypersensitive reactions to valuable staple food products (milk, eggs, meat, and cereals) which are difficult to replace.
- High allergenic threat is posed by the so-called panallergens widely occurring in the natural world, i.e., profilins occurring in many foods such as celery, bananas, apples, pollens and seeds of some grasses, herbs, and bushes, and in latex (Jędrychowski 2001); animal proteins—lipocalins (Virtanen 2001); oleosines—proteins which along with phospholipids have a fat storage function and which occur in carrots and oilseeds (soy, rapeseed, and sunflower) (Besler et al. 2001, Jędrychowski 2001, Wilson et al. 2005). Other allergens, common due to their widespread occurrence, are storage plant proteins (2S) and lipid transfer proteins (LTPs) (Pastorello et al. 2001) responsible for lipid transport as well as proteins related to pathogenic processes namely *pathogenesis-related proteins* (PR) among which 14 groups were isolated, 7 of which contain proteins with allergenic properties and 6 of which can be found in food, e.g., PR-2 protein occurs in bananas and latex; PR-3 protein in avocado, sweet chestnuts, and bananas; PR-4 protein in turnip and black elder berries; PR-5 protein (taumatin) in peppers; and PR-10 protein in apples, apricots, cherries, pears, celery, and carrots (Ebner et al. 2001).
- The threat may be caused by the so-called hidden allergens occurring in food as a result of using food additives in order to obtain desired functional properties of a product or to increase its shelf life, or by lack of information about the potential occurrence of some allergen. In this context there is a clear worldwide need for suitable labeling of food products in order to protect consumers (Taylor and Hefle 2001).
- Widespread occurrence of the mentioned proteins may, according to some authors, be the cause of polysensitization, i.e., sensitivity to many different products and it may account for some cross-reactions, for instance between latex and celery and bananas (Jędrychowski 2001), which have been observed in peaches, apricots, plums, and apples; a high structural affinity between the proteins of the fruits mentioned and respective sweet corn proteins has been documented (Pastorello et al. 2001).
- Possible sources of threat are the previously mentioned products obtained using genetically modified organisms (GMO) (Penninks et al. 2001) as well as those made with the use of microorganisms (especially mould), antibiotics (Gay 2001), anabolics, and some food additives which have the

potential or already confirmed capability to induce allergic or pseudoaller-
gic responses (Jędrychowski and Wroblewska 2002). The issue is presented
in greater detail in Chapter 14.1 and 14.4.
- Very strong and immediate reactions, including anaphylactic shock, following consumption of even the smallest amounts of peanuts or their derived
products. In extreme cases even a trace amount of peanut protein added to
other food products may bring about death of particularly sensitive individuals (Burks et al. 1999, Wüthrich 2000).

Based on the study concerning the British population, food is the most common
cause of anaphylaxis reactions (66%) compared to anaphylaxis reactions caused by
other factors such as insect venom, medicines, or latex. The most dangerous food
products comprised by the study were in the order of threat—peanuts, nuts, eggs,
sesame seeds, soy, lentils, bananas, gelatin, fish, and crustaceans (Wüthrich 2000).
Similar results were obtained in Sweden though the threat order was different (nuts,
peanuts, eggs, celery, wheat, milk, rice, poppy seeds, and sunflower seeds). In France,
the threat of anaphylaxis reactions caused by consumption of some food products
was the highest following consumption of eggs, crustaceans, fish, milk, leguminous
seeds, peanuts, and celery. In Switzerland, the threat of anaphylaxis reactions was
highest from celery, followed by nuts, molluscs, bananas, papaya, sweet chestnuts,
peanuts, sesame seeds, olives, and honey (Wüthrich 2000). From the quoted examples it follows that many food products may, even when consumed in trace amounts,
present a threat to the health or even life of sensitive individuals.

**Possibilities of limiting the potential risk of allergy onset and development**
In the context of the above-mentioned threats it seems indispensable to undertake
actions aimed at limiting the scale of allergic hypersensitivity reactions. Possibilities
of reducing the potential risk of allergy onset and development should be sought
for in

- Educational campaigns aimed at reducing the possibilities of occurrence
and development of allergies through conscious elimination of various diet
components. It is an area in which the so-called self-help groups may act,
e.g., in the United States, a wide ranging educational campaign of the Ford
Allergy and Anaphylaxis Network (www.foodallergy.org).
- Actions aimed at suitable profiling of diets depending on the age of infants/
children.
- Actions concerning targeted modifying allergenic food constituents (application of deep enzymatic hydrolysis, applying antisense recombinant technology, or thermal processes) (Davis et al. 2001, Mosseley 2001).
- Protective effect of women's milk on the child during breast-feeding.
Numerous studies seem to confirm great significance of mother's milk,
especially colostrum, during infancy as an agent preventing the onset of
food allergies (Kirjavainen et al. 2001). Women's milk contains numerous biologically active components reinforcing the defensive functions
of the immunological system, in particular a high content of secretory

immunoglobulins of A class (s-IgA) reaching 90% of total immunoglobulins, which favors exclusion of food antigens, thus supporting the still not quite developed mechanisms of producing secretory IgA of the digestive system.

- Supervisory actions and development of Hazard Analysis Critical Control Point programs to determine food manufacturers' risk and improve the accuracy of monitoring and surveillance by food industry, commercial and enforcement of laboratories with the final goal of better consumer safety.
- Informing possibly the greatest number of consumers through improvements in compliance with labeling laws with concomitant reductions in risks to atopic consumers.
- Application of genetic engineering techniques oriented toward lowering allergenicity of raw food materials (GMO).
- Use of technological and biotechnological processes lowering product allergenicity (through deep enzymatic hydrolysis or natural enzymatic processes, e.g., seed germination).

Consumption of food, in appropriate conditions and appropriate amounts should provide all the nutrients needed for good health but food, which is a large collection of antigens, can affect allergy-sensitive individuals as well as healthy ones.

## REFERENCES

Besler, M., Steinhart, H., and Paschke, A. 2001. Stability of allergens and allergenicity of processed foods. *J Chromatogr B* 756: 207–228.

Bogucki, M. 2000. The UCB Institute of Allergy. Terapia. Special issue 21. (In Polish).

Burks, W., Bannon, G.A., Sicherer, S., and Sampson, H.A. 1999. Peanut-induced anaphylactic reaction. *Int Arch Allergy Immunol* 119: 165–172.

Davis, P.J., Smales, C.M., and James, D.C. 2001. How can thermal processing modify the antigenicity of proteins? *Allergy* 56(Suppl. 67): 56–60.

Ebner, Ch., Hoffmann-Sommergruber, K., and Breitender, H. 2001. Plant food allergens homologous to pathogenesis-related proteins. *Allergy* 56(Suppl. 67): 43–44.

European Allergy White Paper. 1997. *Epidemiology: Prevalence of Allergic Diseases.* The UCB Institute of Allergy, Belgium, pp. 14–39.

Gay, P. 2001. The biosafety of antibiotic resistance markers in plant transformation and the dissemination of genes through horizontal gene flow. In: *Safety of Genetically Engineered Crops*, R. Custers, Ed. VIB Flanders Interuniversity Institute for Biotechnology, Zwijnaarde, Belgium, pp. 135–159.

Haahtela, T., von Hertzem, L., Mäkelä, M., and Hannuksela, M. 2008. Finnish Allergy Programme 2008–2018—time to act and change the course. *Allergy* 63(6): 634–645.

Jędrychowski, L. 2001. Alergeny pokarmowe jako czynniki ryzyka zdrowotnego. *Zywn Nauka Technol Jakosc* 4 (29) 8: 62–81. (In Polish)

Jędrychowski, L. and Wroblewska, B. 2002. Food and nutrition in food allergy cases. *Pol J Food Nutr Sci* 11/52(SI 2): 160–165.

Kirjavainen, P.V., Apostolo, E., Salmine, S.J., and Isolauri, E. 2001. New aspects of probiotics application in food allergy treatment. *Alergia Astma Immunologia* 6(1): 1–6. (In Polish)

Konopka, I., Tanska, M., Pszczolkowska, A., Fordonski, G., Kozirok,W., and Olszewski, J. 2007. The effect of water stress on wheat kernel size, color and protein composition. *Pol J Nat Sci* 22(2): 157–171.

Mosseley, B.E.B. 2001. How to make foods safer—genetically modified foods. *Allergy* 56(Suppl. 67): 61–63.

Nowak-Wegrzyn, A., Conover-Walker, M.K., and Wood, R.A. 2001. Food-allergic reactions in schools and preschools. *Arch Pediatr Adolesc Med* 155(7): 790–795.

Osterballe, M., Hansen, T.K., Mortz, C.G., Høst, A., and Bindslev-Jensen, C. 2005. The prevalence of food hypersensitivity in an unselected population of children and adults. *Pediatric Allergy Immunol* 16: 567–573.

Pastorello, E.A., Pompei, C., Pravettoni, V., Brenna, O., Farioli, L., Trambaioli, C., and Conti, A. 2001. Lipid transfer proteins and 2S albumins as allergens. *Allergy* 56(Suppl. 67): 45–47.

Penninks, A., Knippels, L., and Houben, G. 2001. Allergenicity of foods derived from genetically modified organisms. In: *Safety of Genetically Engineered Crops*, R. Custers, Ed. VIB Flanders Interuniversity Institute for Biotechnology, Zwijnaarde, Belgium, pp. 108–134.

Samson, H.A. 1996. Epidemiology of food allergy. *Pediatr Allergy Immunol* 7: 42–50.

Schäfer, T., Bohler, E., Ruhdorfer, S., Weigl, L., Wessner, D., Heinrich, J., Filipiak, B., Wichmann, H.E., and Ring, J. 2001. Epidemiology of food allergy/food intolerance in adults: Associations with other manifestations of atopy. *Allergy* 56(12): 1172–1179.

Sicherer, S.H., Muñoz-Furlong, A., and Sampson, H.A. 2004. Prevalence of seafood allergy in the United States determined by a random telephone survey. *J Allergy Clin Immunol* 114: 159–165.

Taylor, S.L. and Hefle, S.L. 2001. Ingredient and labeling issues associated with allergenic foods. *Allergy* 56(67): 16–20.

Vierk, K.A., Koehler, K.M., Fein, S.B., and Street, D.A. 2007. Prevalence of self-reported food allergy in American adults and use of food labels. *J Allergy Clin Immunol* 119: 1504–1510.

Virtanen, T. 2001. Lipocalin allergens. *Allergy* 56(Suppl. 67): 48–51.

Wilson, S., Blaschek, K., and de Mejia, E.G. 2005. Allergenic proteins in soybean: Processing and reduction of P34 allergenicity. *Nutr Rev* 63: 47–58.

Wüthrich, B. 2000. Lethal or life-threatening allergic reactions to food. Review article. *Invest Allergol Clin Immunol* 10(2): 59–65.

## 2.2 IMMUNOMODULATORY PROPERTIES OF FOOD

Lucjan Jędrychowski

### 2.2.1 INTRODUCTION

The immunomodulatory effect produced by food is an extremely important and a current issue, as it is associated with potentially improved immunological tolerance of a human body and, in consequence, better health of a whole society attained via dietary components. Besides, studies on food and the immune system can help to compose food rations with a view of enhancing the health condition of whole human populations.

Apart from being complex, the human immune system also changes during the body's growth and development. The defense mechanisms involved in building immunity are equally complex. Thus, it is extremely difficult to formulate definite statements on the effect of particular environmental components on the immunological tolerance of a human body, including the impact of diet on the immune system. Until now, the research on human nutrition has focused primarily on the effect of food on the cardiovascular system, for example blood pressure (quantitative and qualitative share of fat in a diet), the thyroid (salt iodization), the osseous system, and ionic balance in the context of decalcification of bones—osteoporosis (macro- and microelemental supplementation). By comparison, the effect of diet on the immune system has been studied to a lesser degree.

However, interest in the effect of food on the immune system seems justified by the fact that the alimentary system is one of the major links in the chain of immunological barriers in the human body. It is so because of the extensive surface of the digestive tract, a large amount of ingested food (about 1 t annually per adult), which varies in its antigenic properties and comes in contact with one of the defense barriers of the human body such as the mucous membrane of the digestive tract, and finally because over 80% of antibodies in the human body are produced by the immune system of the digestive system (Gut-associated lymphoid tissue—GALT). All these considerations mean that studies on the immunomodulatory effect of food on the human body remain very important.

The definition of an immunomodulator suggests that this term refers to exogenous (drug, nutrient, physical, or psychic—stress) or endogenous (hormone, mediator) factors used for their effect on the immune system. Immunostimulatory preparations affect the nonspecific (independent from antigens) defense system of an organism, although by producing influence on the whole system regulating the immune system, such preparations can, via mediators, strengthen the immunological response of the specific immune system.

## 2.2.2 Effect of Some Foodstuffs on the Immune System

Description of food, which via nutrition sustains vital functions and "wellness" of a living organism, contains physicochemical and sensory characteristics of particular foodstuffs and their nutritional and biological values. Equally important seems the specification of antigenic and immunological properties of food. This aspect becomes essential when discussing cases of food allergies in which the immunological response of the body is not a typical one but consists of very noxious, complex, and sometimes dangerous symptoms of illness. Food, which is a large collection of antigens, can affect allergy-sensitive individuals as well as healthy ones. An example of immunomodulatory influence of food (one of the major environmental factors) on the immune system consists of pharmacological plant preparations (e.g., containing biologically active fractions of acid heteroglycans), applied *per os* in a stimulation therapy, which act specifically (on the hormone system) and nonspecifically (on the cellular system) (Table 2.2.1). The use of medicinal plants has increased considerably in the past two decades in the world. Particularly three species of the genera *Echinacea* (*E. angustifolia, E. purpurea, and E. pallida*), belonging to the *Compositae* family are recognized for their immunostimulating properties.

Stimulation of the human immune system through the lymphoid tissue of the intestines can occur directly or indirectly. Such stimulation may involve the effect produced on the primary (bone marrow, thymus, and liver) and secondary organs (spleen, lymph nodes, tonsils, lymphoid tissue of bronchi, intestines, and skin) and

**TABLE 2.2.1**

**Influence of Food Antigens (Immunostimulators) on the Immune System**

| Specific Tolerance (Humoral Response) | Nonspecific Tolerance (Cellular Response) |
|---|---|
| B lymphocytes (production of antibodies) | Granulocytes |
| T lymphocytes and T suppressive cells | Macrophages |
| | Natural killer (NK) cells |
| | Complement system, reaction mediators (IFNs, chemokines, ILs), cellular membrane receptors, enzymes, free oxygen radicals |

on the neuroendocrinological system. Local responses in the lymphatic system connected with GALT can be transferred, via the lymphatic and circulatory system, to the peripheral elements of this system and play a crucial role in the formation of the systemic tolerance of an individual. Some of the defense mechanisms of the immune system (including the GALT system), due to their complex nature, have not been fully clarified yet (e.g., the phenomenon of food tolerance or non-tolerance related to anergia, clonal deletion, and cellular suppression of CD8 lymphocytes, allergenic hypersensitivity reactions) (Brandtzaeg 2001, Mayer et al. 2001, Rothenberg 2001). In the view of the above, quality of foodstuffs for human consumption or animal feeds appears to be very important, also because of an increasingly high incidence of allergenic reactions in people and animals. The definition of an immunomodulator suggests that this term refers to exogenous (drug, nutrient, physical, or psychic factors, e.g., stress) or endogenous factors (hormone, mediator) used for their effect on the immune system. Food components can act in either way: stimulating or suppressing the immune system.

In the context of an increasingly more important role of the immune system associated with the digestive tract (GALT) as well as the growing access to the so-called functional (pro-health) foodstuffs alongside the assertion, known since ancient Rome (Lucrecius, 98–53 B.C.), that food can be a medicine or a poison, the question of the immunomodulatory effect of food on living organisms is of an undying interest. Recently, the issues of antigenic (allergenic) properties of food and their immunomodulative effect on the human have been given a priority in Europe and worldwide due to their social and economical significance. Their applicable character is revealed in the practical dietetic recommendations in some diseases and convalescence.

Undernutrition during fetal and early life impacts upon the development of the immune organs and appears to diminish cellular immunity and increase the risk of atopic disorders during childhood (Langley-Evans and Carrington 2006). The references confirm that many food components have a beneficial impact on various elements of the immune system. Proteins, some fats, vitamins (A, $B_6$, E, and folic acid), macro- and microelements (zinc, iron, selenium, and copper), and certain bacteria (probiotic bacteria), for example, have a considerable effect on the immune system.

### 2.2.2.1　Effect of Proteins

The claim that proteins and peptides affect the immune system seems confirmed by the fact that proteins are the main building material of an organism. They are essential for the production of special proteins, including antibodies, and for a proper course of cellular and humoral immune responses (Feng 2007). Proteins and protein derivatives are mediators of immune responses and can perform various functions. Dietary proteins and peptides play a significant role in the developmental expression of the secretory immune system (Tables 2.2.1 and 2.2.2) (Bounous and Kongshavn 1982, Degwert and Hoppe 1996, Sullivan et al. 1993). It has been, for example, verified that sericin and sericin-related peptides interfere with cellular interactions of immune-relevant cells of the human skin immune system (Degwert and Hoppe 1996). Equally important seems to be the role of vasoactive intestinal peptides in

### TABLE 2.2.2
### Effect of Some Dietary Characteristics on the Immune System of an Organism

| Dietary Characteristics | Type of Influence Produced by Diet | References |
|---|---|---|
| Calorie-protein undernourishment | Disturbs cellular tolerance, thus increasing infectious disease incidence and mortality; increases secretion of antioxidative enzymes, IL-2, IFN-$\gamma$, TGF-$\beta$, which control proliferation and differentiation of most types of cells | Szponar and Respondek (1999) |
| Calorie-protein excess | Increased number of macrophages, T lymphocytes [producers of inflammatory cytokines (IL-1, IL-4, IL-6, TNF-$\alpha$, IL-10)], increases number of prooxidative acids and free radicals | Szponar and Respondek (1998) |
| Pycnogenol (procyanidins extracted from *Pinus maritima*) | Free radicals scavenger, anti-inflammatory properties via indirect effect on activity of antioxidative enzymes of the oxidative system, dependent on glutathione (superoxide dismutase catalase) | Bayeta and Lau (2000) |
| Probiotics | Immunological effects<br>　Supports release of cytokines<br>　Stimulates phagocytes via leucocytes<br>　Supports IgA secretion<br>　Adjuvant effect (strengthens immunological activity),<br>　Anti-mutagenic effects<br>　Stimulates activity of enzymes<br>　Source of additional enzymes | Vitini et al. (2001), Jędrychowski (2001), Shanahan (2000), He et al. (2000), Sanders (2000), Gibson and Fuller (2000) |
| Peptides/ neuropeptides | Neuropeptides are potent modulators of immunoglobulin E synthesis | Aebischer et al. (1994) |

the functioning of both the nervous and the immune systems (Aebischer et al. 1994, Goetzl et al. 2001). It has been discovered that the vasoactive intestinal peptide (VIP) prominently mediates diverse physiological functions in the neural, endocrine, and immune systems (Goetzl et al. 2001, Grinninger et al. 2001). It needs to be added that the biological functions of the above peptides are largely conditioned by their structure as the natural deletion of part of the last transmembrane domain of $VPAC_2$ receptor abrogates signaling functions without apparent alterations of expression of ligand binding (Grinninger et al. 2004). The aforementioned peptides affect migration of the T cells and T-cell secretion of the mediators (leucotriens and cytokines), which regulate functions for other immune cells, thus being able to affect the Th1/Th2 balance, essential in occurrence of inflammatory conditions or allergies (Goetzl et al. 2001, Grinninger et al. 2004). Considerable deficiencies of proteins in diet lead to depressed secretion of interleukin-1 (IL-1) by monocytes and IL-2 and TNFs by T lymphocytes. Shortage of proteins can also cause decrease in the total number of T lymphocytes and reduction in subpopulations of circulating CD4 lymphocytes, which play an important role in the process of presentation of antigens (Szponar and Respondek 1998). Prolonged shortage of proteins in diet leads to changes in mechanisms which participate in the nonspecific defense of an organism, whereas protein-calorie malnutrition weakens production of antibodies, lowers the level of immunoglobulins, depresses IgA secretion, and impairs synthesis of the complement system proteins. Such disorders eventually lead to the impairment of both cellular and humoral tolerance mechanisms (Szponar and Respondek 1998). Some peptides (particularly neuropeptides) are potent modulators of IgE synthesis (Aebischer et al. 1994) (Table 2.2.2).

The effect of glycoproteins is likewise undeniable. For example, carbohydrate components perform critical biological functions in immune and receptor recognition, inflammation, metastasis, pathogenicity, signal transduction, and many other cellular processes (Li et al. 1999). Most of the food allergens are proteins, lipoproteins, or glycoproteins, which, in the light of the way they act, may suggest that proteins have an adverse influence on the immune system in patients who suffer from allergenic hypersensitivity (Bando et al. 1996, Wijesinha-Bettoni et al. 2007).

## 2.2.2.2   Effect of Fatty Acids

Among all other nutrients, fatty acids (particularly n-6 and n-3 fatty acids) are the food constituents that can also largely affect the immune system (Calder 1998, Erickson 1998, Ikeda 2000, Kromhout 1990) (Table 2.2.3). Shortage of fatty acids leads to depression or considerable impairment of humoral and cellular tolerance response. Exposure to prolonged low-fat diet, containing very little omega-3 acids, causes elevated production of pro-inflammatory IL-1 and TNF-α cytokines. On the other hand, a low-fat diet rich in omega-3 WNTK considerably reduces the percentage of T CD4 cells while raising the percentage of T CD8 cells. Such a diet also depresses secretion of IL-1, IL-6, and TNF-α (Erickson 1998, Ikeda 2000). It turns out that a low-fat diet rich in omega-3 WNTK produces a beneficial effect on the cardiovascular system by helping to prevent atherosclerosis but is bad for the immune system, as it reduces tolerance of an organism (Table 2.2.4).

## TABLE 2.2.3
## Effect of Some Food Components on the Immune System

| Food Components | Type of Effect Produced by Food | References |
|---|---|---|
| β-Carotene, alone and conjugated with linoleic acid (CLA), octadecadienoic acid | Cytotoxic—inhibits growth of carcinoma of the urinary bladder, breasts, esophagus, thorax, and lungs. Increases secretion of cytokins, mainly IL-1 and TNF-α factor | Shultz et al. (1992), Cook and Pariza (1998), Holik et al. (2002) |
| Octadecadienoic acid | Protective factor against cancer | Pariza et al. (2001) |
| Linolenic acid | Stimulates development of breast cancer | Yang and Cook (2003) |
| Fats (high content) | Being incorporated into cellular membranes, fats modulate the activity of macrophages. They disturb proliferation of lymphocytes and depress activity of cytotoxic cells | Szponar and Respondek (1998) |
| Essential unsaturated fatty acids (EFAs) (deficiency) | They disturb the response dependent on both B and T cells | Szponar and Respondek (1998) |
| Eicosonoids (prostaglandins, thromboxanes, leukotrienes) hydroxyperoxy-eicosatetraenoic acid hydroxy-eicosatetraenoic acid | They play an important role in maturation and differentiation of B and T lymphocytes, NK cells, macrophages, and cytokines they release | Cook and Pariza (1998) |
| Omega-3 acids | Decrease amount of lymphocytes T helpers, have anti-inflammatory action, diminish allergenic responses of delayed type, depress mitogenic response of T cells, increase level of antioxidative enzymes, decrease number of free radicals | Szponar and Respondek (1998) |
| Omega-6 acids | Depress cytotoxic activity of macrophages (increase incidence of cancers) | Szponar and Respondek (1998) |

When a diet is rich in polyunsaturated fatty acids, the inflammatory response and production of free radicals appear to be strengthened. Arachidonic acid is held responsible for this reaction, as it is used by lipoxygenases of the immune system cells to produce, via biochemical transformations, leukotrienes, compounds which function as mediators and perform an important function in the immune system (Szponar and Respondek 1998, Fimmel and Zouboulis 2005).

**TABLE 2.2.4**

**Effect of Vitamins on the Immune System**

| Type and Composition of a Component | Effect | References |
|---|---|---|
| Vitamin A and related retinoids | Strengthens the immune system; enhances lactoferrin tolerance against viruses, bacteria, and fungi; regulates keratinization, hematopoiesis, production of neutrophils, erythrocytes, basophils, eosinophils, and lymphocytes, as well as influence on immunoglobulin, TNF-$\alpha$, TGF-$\beta$, INF-$\gamma$, IL-1, IL-2, IL-3, IL-4 production | Pfahl (1996), Szponar and Respondek (1998), Semba (1998) |
| Deficient vitamin A | Disturbs functions of the immune system by damaging the continuity of mucous membranes and depressing phagocytosis by neutrophils | Pfahl (1996) |
| Deficient vitamin $B_6$ | Causes disorders in maturation and activity of T lymphocytes, depresses the level of IL-2 interleukin | Szponar and Respondek (1998) |
| Vitamin $D_3$ | Modulates the immune system via cellular proliferation and differentiation | Mukhopadhyay et al. (2000), Rigby (1988) |
| Vitamin E (norm quantities) | Strengthens the immune system and tolerance to infections (limits synthesis of prostaglandins, depresses number of free radicals) | Zhao et al. (1994), Szponar and Respondek (1998), Han and Meydani (1999) |
| Deficient vitamin E | Through increased peroxidation of fats raises production of prostaglandins, but retards production of antibodies and cytokines or proliferation of lymphocytes | Zhao et al. (1994), Szponar and Respondek (1998), Han and Meydani (1999) |

## 2.2.2.3 Immunomodulatory Effect of Antioxidants in Diet

The physiological effect of antioxidative compounds is highly diverse (Pawliczak et al. 2002). Recently, it has been reported in the literature that compounds which possess antioxidative functions help to shape the immunological tolerance of living organisms. Determination of the antioxidative activity of food is an important measure of the pro-health quality of foodstuffs (Table 2.2.3). Evaluation of the blood plasma antioxidative activity under the effect of a diet with enhanced antioxidative potential can also serve as a measure of absorption or bioavailability of certain nutrients (Ghiselli et al. 2000). Modification of diet toward increased antioxidative potential or dietary supplementation with components that are characterized by such properties (vitamin A, C, E, glutation, ubiquinon, and flavonoids) is used by sportspeople in order to maintain balance between oxygen reactive forms and antioxidants in the body cells (Table 2.2.4). The purpose of such supplementation is to combat oxidative stress, which occurs, for example, after a large physical effort (Urso and Clarkson 2003). Antioxidants in diet, owing to a large cellular redox potential, can help to reduce death rate of neurons and contribute to improved functions of the nervous system (Castagne et al. 1999).

Lack of physiological equilibrium between oxygen reactive forms and antioxidants is considered to be one of the major reasons behind civilization illnesses or the aging of an individual. For sustaining the oxygen balance, significant regulatory role in the thioredoxin reductase–thioredoxin system is played by extracellular thioredoxin (Nordberg and Arner 2001).

Reactive forms of oxygen are recognized as mediators in transmitting intercellular information, thus elevated content of reactive forms of oxygen (oxygen imbalance) can lead to oxidative stress, loss or change of cell function, cell necrosis, or apoptosis. This is of extreme importance for the immune system cells, i.e., for the defense system, and for the nervous system. Reactive forms of oxygen are dangerous to life functions of cells, but they also play an important physiological role, being mediators in signal transduction. They participate in apoptosis. By modifying the permeability of the mitochondrial membrane, reactive forms of oxygen released in mitochondria favor elevated secretion of pro-apoptic mediators (procapsase, capsase-activating compounds, and capsase independent factors, such as apoptosis-inducing factor (AIF) to the cellular solution (Fleury et al. 2002).

In the etiology of aging, an important role is assigned to accumulated changes caused by oxygen reactive species within lymphocytes, including mutations within DNA, and to reduced potential of repair mechanisms. In order to activate repair mechanisms, it is necessary to interfere in the process of balance between oxidants and antioxidants and in the enzymatic system, that is, in the antioxidative defense system, for which the levels of glutationic peroxidase (EC 1.11.1.99), catalase (EC 1.11.1.6), and caeruloplasmin are good measures. These levels are largely elevated in the age group of 75–80 years (King et al. 1997).

Some authors claim that liposaccharides can depress the content of TNF-$\alpha$ and increase the activity of superoxide dismutase (SOD) and catalase, thus—via mediators—they can affect the immune system (Can et al. 2003). It has been demonstrated that the NF-p transcription factor, (highly sensitive to the redox potential in its environment), which regulates synthesis of many mediators—cytokines, associated with inflammatory condition and the phenomenon of adhesion of cells—becomes deregulated in old age. Defense functions in such cases (and primarily in arthritis and arthritis-related conditions) are said to be performed by antioxidants (including $\alpha$-lipoic acid), which can modulate the activity of monocytes and inhibit changes caused by deregulating of the transcription factor NF-$\kappa$B under the influence of redox conditions in elderly people (Lee and Hughes 2002).

Medical observations and research suggest that oxidative stress can be related to the occurrence of memory loss, implying that this adverse effect can be restricted by application of bilirubin as an antioxidant. It has been found that bilirubin possesses antioxidative activity and prevents pathological changes which appear in multiple sclerosis patients, but does not reveal any immunosuppressive effects (Liu et al. 2003). Lack of oxidative and antioxidative balance in pneumonia can activate such transcription factors as NF-$\kappa$B and activating protein-1 (AP-1), which are sensitive to the redox potential (Rahman 2000).

It has also been discovered that physiological transformations associated with oxidative stress impair functions of macrophages, especially the ones connected with chemotaxis, substrate binding, production of reactive oxygen forms, and release of a mediator such as tumor necrosis factor-$\alpha$ (TNF-$\alpha$) (Victor et al. 2003).

Flavonoids are used in treatment of many diseases, mainly because of their capability to inhibit many harmful strains of bacteria and enzymes (proteases, reverse transcriptase), to stimulate hormones and neurotransmitters, and to capture free radicals (Havsteen 2002). There are reports confirming that supplementation of diet with an antioxidant ($\alpha$-tocopherol), by increasing the concentration of the antioxidant in blood, can reduce the titer of antibodies in hypercholesterolemia (Table 2.2.4).

The immunomodulatory activity of antioxidants depends on the age of an organism. It has been determined that in elderly people—in contrast to young ones (20–30 years of age)—antioxidants fail to produce any effect on the restoration of lymphocyte proliferative response. The effect produced by antioxidants also depends on the type of compound (Table 2.2.4). Vitamin E, in old age has a stronger inhibitory effect on lymphocyte stimulation than vitamin O (a pricey health supplement). The actual immunomodulatory effect of antioxidants is associated with the content of cholesterol in cellular walls and consequent changes in intercellular information transmission (Douziech et al. 2002). The results of research conducted in Sweden have proved that free radicals damage T lymphocytes, which means that they impair the immunological response of lymphocytes (immunosenescent effect), thus contributing to DNA damage and aging (Hyland et al. 2002).

The role of cytokines and oxygen reactive species in the pathogenesis of chronic sinusitis has not been completely clarified. However, this disorder is associated with a depressed level of IL-2 and tissue antioxidants ($\alpha$-tocopherol and superoxide dimutase), which may suggest that that these compounds can possibly play a role in the development and progress of chronic sinusitis (Kassim et al. 2002). Thiol antioxidants in diet (e.g., thioproline, N-acetyl cystein) improved the immunological functions of macrophages and lymphocytes in mice (Puerto et al. 2002). Antioxidants in diet are believed to have an inhibitory effect on the formation of reactive oxygen species, tromboxan and peroxidation of fat, the role of inhibitor of nephrotoxicity of some medications as well as an active role in renaturation of damaged tissues and their function (Parra et al. 2003).

Fruit, vegetables, and other plants, including medicinal ones, are a valuable source of antioxidants. Some (*Sida cordifolia*, *Evolvulus alsinoides*, and *Cynodon dactylon*) have been successfully used for thousands of years (without precise knowledge of the mechanisms involved in their application) by Indians to treat ailments associated with degeneration of the immune and nervous system cells (Parkinson's disease, Alzheimer's disease, Rasayan's disease, and loss of memory) (Auddy et al. 2003). Such findings raise an ever growing interest in medicinal preparations (herbal plants) used in folk and natural medicine. Satisfying treatment results have been obtained in clinical research on antioxidants. Positive changes in CD3+, CD4+, and lymphocytes of the immune system coincided with the antioxidative balance regained under the influence of an antioxidant in HIV positive patients, which resulted in an elevated level of apoptosis of lymphocytes and inhibited replication of HIV (de Martino et al. 2001).

There are interesting reports on possible application of certain antioxidants (1,3-glucan, "levamisole," and vitamins C and E) in diet. For example, supplementation of a diet given to ill fish (carp) with the above components has resulted in an improved specific immunity to diseases and lowered mortality rate (Sahoo and Mukherjee 2001). It has been verified that aqueous extracts from certain plants, e.g., mistletoe (*Viscum album*), nettle (*Urtica dioica*), and ginger (*Zingiber officinale*) added to fish diets produce an immunostimulating effect. Rainbow trout (*Oncorhynchus mykiss*) fed a diet enriched with an extract from ginger (characterized by high antioxidative activity) have been found to possess a higher nonspecific immunological tolerance (much higher activity of leucocytes) (Dugenci et al. 2003).

Because food components of high antioxidative potential are good for health, new natural sources of antioxidants (including foodstuffs) are constantly being searched for. Another solution is to increase their content in food products (e.g., through certain modifications in food processing technologies, for example, products obtained from pomegranate [*Punica granatum*]) (Schubert et al. 1999).

### 2.2.2.4    Role of Microorganisms, Particularly Probiotic Ones, in Immunomodulation

The gastrointestinal system, which comprises the largest lymphoid tissue and microbial reservoir of the body, has received more attention during the last few years as a potential determiner in the development of atopic disease (Kalliomaki and Isolauri 2003).

The up-to-date advances in sciences suggest that both commensal bacteria, resident microflora, and bacteria that enter the digestive tract with ingested food or microorganisms from the broadly understood natural environment, play an important role in the modulation of the immune system (Table 2.2.2). Hooper et al. (2001) found that commensal bacteria modulate expression of genes involved in several important intestinal functions, including nutrient absorption, mucosal barrier fortification, xenobiotic metabolism, angiogenesis, and postnatal intestinal maturation. Orihara et al. (2008), who presented the current state of knowledge on the mechanism of creating an allergenic response and illustrated it with a balancing square model, in which four T-cell types (Th1, Th2, Th17, and Treg), which antagonize each other, point to an important role of reaction mediators (including the newly discovered IL-17 producing helper T cells, which may counteract Treg cells even in allergic diseases) and environmental microorganisms in the mechanism of maintaining the immunological balance. The mechanism of mutual interactions between cells and the role that mediators play in these relationships are still being studied. Among the findings is the observation that increased production of IF-$\gamma$ (a cytokine antagonistic to IL-4) implies the capability of probiotics to diminish the atopic inflammation mediated by IgE, mast cells, and eosinophils.

The release of IL-12 initiated by macrophages may be crucial for the activation of Th1 cells. Transforming growth factor-$\beta$ (TGF-$\beta$) can produce an effect consisting of differentiation of Th0 lymphocytes and increased production of IgA (Kalliomaki and Isolauri 2003, Orihara et al. 2008). These issues are discussed in more detail in the cited references and in Chapter 1.

The effect of microflora (positive and negative) is emphasized in many other publications on this subject (Cosseau et al. 2008, Dibner et al. 2008, Kirjavainen et al. 2001, Nagy et al. 2002, Orihara et al. 2008, Shanahan 2000, Wexler 2007).

Probiotic bacteria are an important group of microorganisms, as they have a beneficial effect on the digestive tract and, consequently, the immune system (GALT)

(Fuller and Perdigon 2000, Gibson 1998, Kirjavainen et al. 2001, Marteau et al. 2002, Rautava et al. 2002, Sanders 2000, Vitini et al. 2001) (Table 2.2.2). Food products that contain probiotic bacteria are labeled functional (medicinal) food, which is used, like pharmaceuticals, to evoke specific physiological reactions of an organism. The use of probiotics as parapharmaceuticals can produce a direct effect on immunocompetent cells of the lymphoid tissue or as adjuvants of bacteria, or else they can generate an indirect effect by changing the intestinal microflora, which can result in the capture and degradation of food antigens.

In addition, probiotic bacteria

- Improve the function of the digestive system defense barrier via immunological and nonimmunological mechanisms
- Normalize increased permeability of the intestinal mucosa to food antigens
- Alleviate inflammatory conditions of the intestines caused by pathogenic bacteria
- Diminish hypersensitivity responses
- Modify microecological conditions in the alimentary tract by modifying mutual quantitative ratios between the harmful microflora and the microorganisms which produce a beneficial effect on the digestive tract (Gibson 1998)
- Interact with the mucosal cells (including epithelial cells) and immune cells
- Improve the defense barriers of the immune system by increasing production of secretory immunoglobulin class A (s-IgA)
- Through changes in the precursor cells Th0 and diminished secretion of the major cytokine, i.e., IL-4, by Th2 cells, probiotic bacteria facilitate maintaining proper proportions between subgroups of Th1 and Th2 lymphocytes
- Offer broader possibilities to treat food allergies owing to their effect consisting of depressing the level of concentration of IgE
- Cause increased activity of phagocytes and lymphocytes, cause increased secretion of certain cytokines: interferon-$\gamma$ (IFN-$\gamma$), IL-2, and IL12, which are critical for differentiation of Th0 cells toward Th1 line

The above assertions have been verified by clinical studies conducted on infants who developed dermatitis or cow's milk allergy to evaluate if lactic acid bacteria (LAB) probiotic strains could prevent or reduce allergic symptoms; *in vivo* (fecal) level of TNF-$\alpha$ was strongly reduced. Additional immunological parameters that reflect the Th1/Th2 balance were measured demonstrating reduced intestinal inflammation. Kalliomaki and Isolauri found that compositional development of *Bifidobacterium* and *Lactobacillus* in gut microflora was delayed in allergic children while a prenatal administration of lactobacilli halved the later development of atopic eczema during the first 2 years of life. The same authors also demonstrated that specific strains of the healthy gut microbiota induced the production of IL-10 and TGF-$\beta$, which play an important regulative role in the development of allergic type immune response (Kalliomaki and Isolauri 2003).

This study seems to confirm that selected LAB strains can exert a healthy effect in the context of neonatal allergy. Another positive outcome of the presence of probiotic microflora is that its exogenous enzymes participate in the transformation of the antigenic (allergenic) properties of substrate (food). Research has confirmed that Gram-positive bacteria may have distinctive importance in protection against atopic sensitization (Kirjavainen et al. 2001). Besides, Ulisse et al. (2001) found that probiotic treatments led to increasing tissue levels of IL-10, an IL which performs a very important role in activating the immune system cells. Nagy et al. (2002) discovered a stimulatory effect of some probiotic bacteria (*B. longum, B. animalis,* and *L. casei*) on the immune system of rats (higher specific and total IgG concentrations). Similar tendencies have been observed for IgA content. Noteworthy is the fact that autochthonous probiotic microorganisms have a weaker stimulatory influence on the immune system (Nagy et al. 2002).

The above questions are discussed in greater detail in Sections 2.4 and 2.5. A very detailed discussion on the immunomodulation by probiotics has been extensively addressed by Fuller and Perdigon (2000) and Sanders (2000).

However, not all studies confirm beneficial influence of probiotic bacteria on the organism when an allergy appears. For instance, a study by Helin et al. (2002) shows that that *L. rhamnosus* GG is not effective in every case of allergy, as no effect was observed in adults or teenagers with birch pollen and apple allergy. Probiotic bacteria are characterized by highly varied properties and, regardless the fact that they are discussed in a great number of scientific reports and articles, probiotics need to be studied further in order to distinguish probiotic bacteria that would have the most desirable influence on human health and would reveal a positive effect on the immune system.

### 2.2.2.5  Influence of Vitamins on the Immune System

The influence produced on the immune system by vitamins, macro- and microelements may result from the fact that many of these compounds function as activators of enzymes, mediators of immunological reactions, and compounds responsible for the transfer of information between cells. Deficiency of these nutrients can weaken the humoral and cellular response and, in many cases, the nonspecific response of the immune system. The following vitamins are believed to produce particular influence on the immune system: A, $B_6$, C, D, and E (Brock 1996, Mukhopadhyay et al. 2000, Pfahl and Chytil 1996, Semba 1998, Zhao et al. 1994) (Table 2.2.4).

Vitamin A (retinol) improves the humoral and cellular tolerance of a person who suffers from an infection. By affecting the differentiation of cells and regulating the metabolism of steroids, vitamin A stimulates the activity of macrophages and T-cytotoxic lymphocytes. It also raises secretion of cytokines and production of antibodies (Hughes 1999, Pfahl and Chytil 1996).

Vitamin C, which also stimulates the immune system, can inhibit the process of neoplasia, raises the amount of CD4 and CD8 lymphocytes in blood, stimulates functions of phagocytes, activity of NK cells, and production of cytokines and antibodies (Benzie 1999, Szponar and Respondek 1998).

Vitamin E (tocopherol) possesses antioxidative properties, which means it can protect polyunsaturated fatty acids from auto-oxidation. Deficiency of vitamin E causes increased peroxidation of lipids, which consequently leads to elevated production of prostaglandins. Increased concentration of prostaglandins, in turn, retards production of antibodies and cytokines as well as proliferation of lymphocytes. As a result, tocopherol deficit affects functions of both the humoral and cellular components of the immune system (Meydani and Biharka 1996, Zhao et al. 1994).

Deficiency of vitamin $B_6$ (pyridoxine) causes gradual disappearance of the lymphatic system, depressed number of B lymphocytes in peripheral blood, and impaired activity of antibodies and IL-2 (Szponar and Respondek 1998) (Table 2.2.4). Vitamin $D_3$ can produce an immunosupressive effect. The recent literature data suggest that one of metabolites of this vitamin, 1,2,5-dihydroxy $D_3$, by affecting a specific receptor present on monocytes and lymphocytes, can inhibit their proliferation. This effect occurs via retardation of the production of mRNA for GM CSF, IL-2, and IFN-7. At the same time, it has been demonstrated that deficiency of vitamin $D_3$ in food caused impaired cellular-type tolerance (Szponar and Respondek 1998).

## 2.2.2.6 Effect of Macro- and Microelements

The critical role performed by ions stems from the fact that they typically serve as activators of enzymatic reactions. Shortage of zinc, iron, and copper is reflected by inhibited activity of NK cells, depressed secretion of cytokines, and lower number of B and T lymphocytes in peripheral blood. The typical human adult body contains approximately 100 mg Cu, which is mainly found in oxireductases and other metalloproteins, where it serves as a catalytic cofactor. Copper participates in modulating the synthesis of the cytokine IL-2, coordinating cell-mediated immunity (Failla 1999, Failla and Hopkins 1998, Huang and Failla 2000). Iron is essential for maintaining proper functions of macrophages, and especially macrophage listericidal mechanisms, which consist of producing highly toxic hydroxyl radicals via the Fenton reaction and controlling the production of NO after activation by immunological stimuli (Alford et al. 1991, Dlaska and Weiss 1999, Mulero et al. 2002) (Table 2.2.5).

Zinc deficiency in adult mice caused depletion of thymic cell numbers, apoptosis among peripheral lymphocytes, large losses among the pre-B cells developing in the marrow, and interferentation with specific immunoglobulin or T-cell receptor (TCR) gene (Fraker 2003, Fraker et al. 2000, King et al. 2002). Zinc deficit worsens chemotactic properties of neutrophils, whereas deficient concentration of copper causes a slow decline in the absolute number of neutrophils in the blood (Brock 1996) (Table 2.2.5). Recently, selenium has been implied as another mineral essential for cellular tolerance. Selenium is found in selenoproteins, which are essential for the cellular-type immunity. Selenium deficiency coincides with depressed number of T lymphocytes in peripheral blood and lowered NK cell activity. While discussing the effect of particular dietary components on the immune system, one should not only consider the concentration of a particular nutrient but also its form and the transformations it can undergo during food production technological processes. Holding in mind the immense influence produced by food antigens on the immune system, it appears that evaluation of antigenic and immunoreactive properties of food products should be a very important element of a general assessment of pro-health effect of food.

**TABLE 2.2.3**

**Effect of Macro- and Microelements on the Immune System**

| Elements | Effect | References |
|---|---|---|
| Copper Cu$^{2+}$ (deficiency) | Copper deficit causes decreased number of T lymphocytes and disorder in their functions; it disturbs processes of antigen transformations and contributes to modulating the synthesis of cytokine IL-2, thus coordinating cell-mediated immunity; causes depressed activity of antioxidative enzymes. | Huang and Failla (2000), Failla (1999), Failla and Hopkins (1998) |
| Zinc Zn$^{2+}$ (deficiency) | Zinc deficiency in adult mice caused a negative effect on primary tissues of the immune system (bone marrow, thymus), depletion of thymic cell numbers, apoptosis among peripheral lymphocytes, large losses among the pre-B cells developing in the marrow. Interferentation with specific immunoglobulin or T-cell receptor (TCR) gene. Causes disorders in cellular and humoral tolerance, depresses number of lymphocytes and phagocytic activity of macrophages. | Fraker (2003), King et al. (2002), Fraker et al. (2000), Fraker and King (1998) |
| Iron Fe$^{2+}$ (deficiency) | Depresses cell destruction by leukocytes via phagocytosis, inhibits proliferation of lymphocytes, depresses systemic tolerance of an organism, disturbs proper functions of macrophages, especially macrophage listericidal mechanisms. | Mulero et al. (2002), Dlaska and Weiss (1999), Alford et al. (1991) |
| Selenium (deficiency) | Depresses peroxidative activity of gluthatione enzymes and tolerance to viruses. | Baum (2000) |

# REFERENCES

Aebischer, I., Stampfli, M.R., Zurcher, A. et al. 1994. Neuropeptides are potent modulators of human in vitro immunoglobulin E synthesis. *Eur J Immunol* 24(8): 1908–1913.

Alford, C.E., King, T.E. Jr, and Campbell, P.A. 1991. Role of transferrin, transferrin receptors, and iron in macrophage listericidal activity. *J Exp Med* 174(2): 459–466.

Auddy, B., Ferreira, M., Blasina, F., Lafon, L., Arredondo, F., Dajas, F., Tripathi, P.C., Seal, T., and Mukherjee, B. 2003. Screening of antioxidant activity of three Indian medicinal plants, traditionally used for the management of neurodegenerative diseases. *J Ethnopharmacol* 84(2–3): 131–138.

Bando, N., Tsuji, H., Yamanishi, R., Nio, N., and Ogawa, T. 1996. Identification of the glycosylation site of a major soybean allergen, Gly m Bd 30K. *Biosci, Biotechnol, Biochem* 60(2): 347–348.

Baum, M.K., Shor-Posner, G., and Campa, A. 2000. Zinc status in human immunodeficiency virus infection. *J Nutr* 130(5S Suppl): 1421S–1423S.

Bayeta, E. and Lau, B.H.S. 2000. Pycnogenol inhibits generation of inflammatory mediators in macrophages. *Nutr Res* 20(2): 249–259.

Benzie, I.F.F. 1999. Vitamin C: Prospective functional markers for defining optimal nutritional status. *Proc Nutr Soc* 58: 469–476.

Bounous, G. and Kongshavn, P.A. 1982. Influence of dietary proteins on the immune system of mice. *J Nutr* 112(9): 1747–1755.

Brandtzaeg, P. 2001. Nature and function gastrointestinal antigen-presenting cells. *Allergy* 56(Suppl. 67): 16–20.

Brock, J.H. 1996. Iron and immunity. *J Nutr Biochem* 2: 47–106.

Calder, P.C. 1998. Dietary fatty acids and the immune system. *Nutr Rev* 56(1) Part II: S70–S83.

Can, C., Demirci, B., Uysal, A., Akcay, Y.D., and Kocay, S. 2003. Contradictory effects of chlorpromazine on endothelial cells in a rat model of endotoxic shock in association with its actions on serum TNF- levels and antioxidant enzyme activities. *Pharmacologic Res* 48(3): 223–230.

Castagne, V., Gautschi, M., Lefevre, K., Posada, A., and Clarke, P.G.H. 1999. Relationships between neuronal death and the cellular redox status. Focus on the developing nervous system. *Prog Neurobiol* 59(4): 397–423.

Cook, M.E. and Pareza, M. 1998. The role of conjugated linoleic acid (CLA) in heath. *Int Dairy J* 8: 459–462.

Cosseau, C., Devine, D.A., Dullaghan, E. et al. 2008. The commensal Streptococcus salivarius K12 downregulates the innate immune responses of human epithelial cells and promotes host-microbe homeostasis. *Infect Immun* 76: 4163–4175.

de Martino, M., Chiarelli, F., Moriondo, M., Torello, M., and Azzari, C. 2001. Restored antioxidant capacity parallels the immunologic and virologic improvement in children with perinatal human immunodeficiency virus infection receiving highly active antiretroviral therapy. *Clin Immunol* 100(1): 82–86.

Degwert, J. and Hoppe, U. 1996. Influence of the protein sericin on cellular interactions of immune relevant cells. *Parfümerie Kosmetik* 77(2): 74, 76, 94–100.

Dibner, J.J., Richards, J.D., and Knight, C.D. 2008. Microbial imprinting in gut development and health. *J Appl Poult Res* 17: 174–188.

Dlaska, M. and Weiss, G. 1999. Central role of transcription factor NF-IL6 for cytokine and iron-mediated regulation of murine inducible nitric oxide synthase expression. *J Immunol* 162: 6171–6177.

Douziech, N., Seres, I., Larbi, A. et al. 2002. Modulation of human lymphocyte proliferative response with aging. *Exp Gerontol* 37(2–3): 369–387.

Dugenci, S.K., Arda, N., and Candan, A. 2003. Some medicinal plants as immunostimulant for fish. *J Ethnopharmacol* 88(1): 99–106.

Erickson, K.L. 1998. Dietary fat, breast cancer, and nonspecific immunity. *Nutr Rev* 56(1) Part II: S99–S104.

Failla, M.L. 1999. Considerations for determining 'optimal nutrition' for copper, zinc, manganese and molybdenum. *Proc Nutr Soc* 58: 497–505.

Failla, M.L. and Hopkins, R.G. 1998. Is low copper status immunosuppressive? *Nutr Rev* 56(1 Pt 2): S59–S64.

Feng, J.M. 2007. Minireview: Expression and function of golli protein in immune system. *Neurochem Res* 32(2): 273–278.

Fimmel, S. and Zouboulis, C.C. 2005. Influence of physiological androgen levels on wound healing and immune status in men. *Aging Male* 8: 166–174.

Fleury, C., Mignotte, B., and Vayssiere, J.L. 2002. Mitochondrial reactive oxygen species in cell death signaling. *Biochimie* 84(2–3): 131–141.

Fraker, P. 2003. Letter to the editor. Response to Dr. Woodward. *J Nutr* 133: 815.

Fraker, P.J. and King, L.E. 1998. Reprogramming of the immune system during zinc deficiency. *Annu Rev Nutr* 24: 277–298.

Fraker, P., King, L., Laakko, T., and Vollmer, T. 2000. The dynamic link between the integrity of the immune system and zinc status. *J Nutr* 130: 1399S–1406S.

Fuller, R. and Perdigon, G. 2000. *Probiotics 3: Immunomodulation by the Gut Microflora and Probiotics*. R. Fuller and G. Perdigon, Eds. Kluwer Academic Publishers, Dordrecht, the Netherlands.

Ghiselli, A., Serafini, M., Natella, F., and Scaccini, C. 2000. Total antioxidant capacity as a tool to assess redox status: Critical view and experimental data. *Free Rad Biol Med* 29(11): 1106–1114.

Gibson, G.R. 1998. Dietary modulation of the human gut microflora using prebiotics. *Br J Nutr* 80(Suppl. 2): S209–S212.

Gibson, G.R. and Fuller, R. 2000. Aspects of in vitro and in vivo research approaches directed toward identifying probiotics and prebiotics for human use. *J Nutr* 130(2S Suppl): 391S–395S.

Goetzl, E.J., Voice, J.K., Shen, S. et al. 2001. Enhanced delayed-type hypersensitivity and diminished immediate-type hypersensitivity in mice lacking the inducible VPAC2 receptor for vasoactive intestinal peptide. *Proc Natl Acad Sci USA* 98: 13854–13859.

Grinninger, C., Wang, W., Bastani Oskoui, K., Voice, J.K., and Goetzl, E.J. 2004. A natural variant type ii g protein-coupled receptor for vasoactive intestinal peptide with altered function. *J Biol Chem* 279(39): 40259–40262.

Han, S.N. and Meydani, S.N. 2000. Antioxidants, cytokines, and influenza infection in aged mice and elderly humans. *J Infect Dis* 182(Suppl 1):S74–S80.

Havsteen, B.H. 2002. The biochemistry and medical significance of the flavonoids. *Pharmacol Therapeut* 96(2&3): 67–202.

He, F., Tuomoloa, E., Arvilommi, H., and Salminen, S. 2000. Modulation of humoral immune response through probiotic intake. *FEMS Immunol Med Microbiol* 29: 47–52.

Helin, T., Haahtela, S., and Haahtela, T. 2002. No effect of oral treatment with an intestinal bacterial strain, *Lactobacillus rhamnosus* (ATCC 53103), on birch-pollen allergy: A placebo-controlled double-blind study. *Allergy* 57: 243–246.

Holick, C.N., Michaud, D.S., Stolzenberg-Solomon, R., Mayne, S.T., Pietinen, P., Taylor, P.R., Virtamo, J., and Albanes, D. 2002. Dietary carotenoids, serum {beta}-carotene, and retinol and risk of lung cancer in the alpha-tocopherol, beta-carotene cohort study. *Am J Epidemiol* 156(6): 536–547.

Hooper, L.V., Wong, M.H., Thelin, A., Hansson, L., Falk, P.G., and Gordon, J.I. 2001. Molecular analysis of commensal host-microbial relationships in the intestine. *Science* 291(5505): 881–884.

Huang, Z.L. and Failla, M.L. 2000. Copper deficiency suppresses effector activities of differentiated U937 cells. *J Nutr* 130(6): 1536–1542.

Hughes, D.A. 1999. Effects of carotenoids on human immune function. *Proc Nutr Soc* 58: 713–718.

Hyland, E.M., Rezende, L.F., and Richardson, C.C. 2003. The DNA binding domain of the gene 2.5 single-stranded DNA-binding protein of bacteriophage T7. *J Biol Chem* 278(9): 7247–7256.

Ikeda, I. 2000. Immunoactive lipids. *Nutrition and Health-Milk.* IDF World Dairy Summit, Bruges, Belgium, pp. 1–2.

Jędrychowski, L. 2001. Immunomodulative properties of food. *Biuletyn Naukowy* 13: 55–69. Edit UWM Olsztyn, Poland (in Polish).

Kalliomaki, M. and Isolauri, E. 2003. Role of intestinal flora in the development of allergy. Upper airway disease. *Curr Opin Allergy Clin Immunol* 3(1): 15–20.

Kassima, S.K., Elbeigermyb, M., Nasrb, G.F., Khalilc, R., and Nassarb, M. 2002. The role of interleukin-12, and tissue antioxidants in chronic sinusitis1. *Clinical Biochemistry* 35(5): 369–375.

King, C.M., Bristow-Craig, H.E., Gillespie, E.S., and Barnett, Y.A. 1997. In vivo antioxidant status, DNA damage, mutation and DNA repair capacity in cultured lymphocytes from healthy 75- to 80-year-old humans. *Mutat Res/Fund Mol Mech Mut* 377(1): 137–147.

King, L.E., Osati-Ashtiani, F., and Fraker, P.J. 2002. Apoptosis plays a distinct role in the loss of precursor lymphocytes during zinc deficiency in mice. *J Nutr* 132: 974–979.

Kirjavainen, P.V., Apostolou, E., Arvola, T., Salminen, S.J., Gibson, G.R., and Isolauri, E. 2001. Characterizing the composition of intestinal microflora as a prospective treatment target in infant allergic disease. *FEMS Immunol Med Microbiol* 32: 1–7.

Kromhout, D. 1990. The importance of n-6 and n-3 fatty acids in carcinogenesis. *Med Oncol Tumor Pharmacother* 7: 173–176.

Langley-Evans, S.C. and Carrington, L.J. 2006. Diet and the developing immune system. *Lupus* 15(11): 746–752.

Lee, H.A. and Hughes, D.A. 2002. Alpha-lipoic acid modulates NF-κB activity in human monocytic cells by direct interaction with DNA. *Exp Gerontol* 37(2–3): 401–410.

Li, Y., Hua, F., Carraway, K.L., and Carothers Carraway, C.A. 1999. The p185$^{neu}$-containing glycoprotein complex of a microfilament-associated signal transduction particle. Purification, reconstitution, and molecular associations with p58$^{gag}$ and actin. *J Biol Chem* 274(36): 25651–25658.

Liu, Y., Zhu, B., Wang, X., Luo, L., Li, P., Paty, D.W., and Cynader, M.S. 2003. Bilirubin as a potent antioxidant suppresses experimental autoimmune encephalomyelitis: implications for the role of oxidative stress in the development of multiple sclerosis. *J Neuroimmunol* 139: 27–35.

Marteau, P., Seksik, P., and Jian, R. 2002. Probiotics and health: New facts and ideas. *Curr Opin Biotechnol* 13(5): 486–489.

Mayer, L., Sperber, K., Chan, L., Child, J., and Toy, L. 2001. Oral tolerance to protein antigens. *Allergy* 56(Suppl. 67): 12–15.

Meydani, S.N. and Biharka, A.A. 1996. Recent developments in vitamin E immune response. *Nutr Rev* 56(1) Part II: S49–S58.

Mukhopadhyay, S., Singh, M., and Chatterjee, M. 2000. Vitamin D3 as a modulator of cellular antioxidant defence in murine lymphoma. *Nutr Res* 20(1): 91–102.

Mulero, V., Wie, X., Liew, F.Y., and Brock, J.H. 2002. Regulation of phagosomal iron release from murine macrophages by nitric oxide. *Biochem J* 365: 127–132.

Nagy, A., Jędrychowski, L., Gelencsér, É., Wroblewska, B., and Szymkiewicz, A. 2002. Immunomodulative effect of *Lactobacillus Salivarius* and *Lactobacillus Casei* strains. *Pol J Food Nutr Sci* SI 2, 11/52: 122–124.

Nordberg, J. and Arner, E.S.J. 2001. Reactive oxygen species, antioxidants, and the mammalian thioredoxin system. *Free Rad Biol Med* 31(11): 1287–1312.

Orihara, K., Nakae, S., Pawankar, R., and Saito, H. 2008. Role of regulatory and proinflammatory T-cell populations in allergic diseases. *World Allergy Org J* 9: Y14.

Pariza, M.W., Park, Y., and Cook, M.E. 2001. The biologically active isomers of conjugated linoleic acid. *Prog Lipid Res* 40(4): 283–298.

Parra Cid, T., Conejo García, J.R., Carballo Álvarez, F., and de Arriba, G. 2003. Antioxidant nutrients protect against cyclosporine A nephrotoxicity. *Toxicology* 189(1–2): 99–111.

Pawliczak, R., Huang, X.-L., Nanavaty, U.B., Lawrence, M., Madara, P., and Shelhamer, J.H. 2002. Oxidative stress induces arachidonate release from human lung cells through the epithelial growth factor receptor pathway. *Am J Resp Cell Mol Biol* 27: 722–731.

Pfahl, M. and Chytil, F. 1996. Regulation of metabolism retinoic acid and its nuclear receptors. *Annu Rev Nutr* 16: 251–283.

Puerto, M., Guayerbas, N., Víctor, V.M., and De la Fuente, M. 2002. Effects of the N-acetylcysteine on macrophage and lymphocyte functions in a mouse model of premature ageing. *Pharmacol Biochem Behav* 73: 797–804.

Rahman, I., 2000. Regulation of nuclear factor-κB, activator protein-1, and glutathione levels by tumor necrosis factorand dexamethasone in alveolar epithelial cells. *Biochem Pharmacol* 60(8): 1041–1049.

Rautava, S., Kalliomaki, M., and Isolauri, E. 2002. Probiotics during pregnancy and breast-feeding might confer immunomodulatory protection against atopic disease in the infant. *J Allergy Clin Immunol* 109: 119–121.

Rigby, W.F.C. 1988. The immunobiology of vitamin D. *Immunol Today* 9: 54–58.

Rothenberg, M.E. 2001. Gastrointestinal eosinophils. *Allergy* 56(Suppl. 67): 21–22.

Sahoo, P.K. and Mukherjee, S.C. 2001. Immunosuppresssive effects of aflatoxin B1 in Indian major carp (*Labeo rohita*). *Comp Immunol Microbiol Infect Dis* 24: 143–149.

Sanders, M.E. 2000. Considerations for use of probiotic bacteria to modulate human health. *J Nutr* 130: 384S–390S.

Schubert, S.Y., Lansky, E.P., and Neeman, I. 1999. Antioxidant and eicosanoid enzyme inhibi-
    tion properties of pomegranate seed oil and fermented juice flavonoids. *J Ethnopharmacol*
    66: 11–17.
Semba, R.D. 1998. The role of vitamin A and related retinoids in immune function. *Nutr Rev*
    56(1) Part II: S38–S48.
Shanahan, F. 2000. Immunology. Therapeutic manipulation of gut flora. *Science* 289: 1311–1312.
Shultz, T.D., Chew, B.P., Seaman, W.R., and Luedecke, L.O. 1992. Inhibition effect of conju-
    gated dienoic derivatives of linoleic acid and β-carotene on the in vitro growth of human
    cancer cells. *Cancer Lett* 63: 125.
Sullivan, D.A., Vaermanj, J.-P., and Soo, C. 1993. Influence of severe protein malnutrition
    on rat lacrimal, salivary and gastrointestinal immune expression during development,
    adulthood and ageing. *Immunology* 78(2): 308–317.
Szponar, L. and Respondek, W. 1998. *Nutrition and immunological system activity. Proceedings
    of the Scientific Conference "Improvement of Health of Human Population in Poland
    through Enhanced Health Quality of Food and More Rational Nutrition"*. National
    Institute for Research on Food and Nutrition, Warsaw, Poland, pp. 49–79 (in Polish).
Ulisse, S., Gionchetti, P., D'Alo, S. et al. 2001. Expression of cytokines, inducible nitric oxide
    synthase, and matrix metalloproteinases in pouchitis: Effects of probiotic treatment. *Am
    J Gastroenterol* 96: 2691–2699.
Urso, M.L. and Clarkson, P.M. 2003. Oxidative stress, exercise, and antioxidant supplementa-
    tion. *Toxicology* 189(1–2): 41–54.
Victor, F.C., Gottlieb, A.B., and Menter, A. 2003. Changing paradigms in dermatology: Tumor
    necrosis factor alpha (TNF-alpha) blockade in psoriasis and psoriatic arthritis. *Clin
    Dermatol* 21: 392–397.
Vitini, E., Alvarez, S., Median, M., Budeguer, M., and Pewrdigon, G. 2001. Gut mucosal
    immunostimulation by lactic acid bacteria. *Biocell* 24(3): 223–232.
Wexler, H.M. 2007. Bacteroides: the Good, the bad, and the nitty-gritty. *Clin Microbiol Rev*
    20: 593–621.
Wijesinha-Bettoni, R., Gao, Ch., Jenkins, J.A. et al. 2007. Post-translational modification of
    barley LTP1b: The lipid adduct lies in the hydrophobic cavity and alters the protein
    dynamics. *FEBS Lett* 581(24): 4557–4561.
Yang, M. and Cook, M.E. 2003. Dietary conjugated linoleic acid decreased cachexia, mac-
    rophage tumor necrosis factor-alpha production, and modifies splenocyte cytokines pro-
    duction. *Exp Biol Med* 228: 51–58.
Zhao, Z., Murasko, D.M., and Ross, A.C. 1994. The role of vitamin A in natural killer cell
    cytotoxity, number and activation in the rat. *Nat Immun* 13: 29–41.

## 2.3 BRIEF INFORMATION ABOUT THE EFFECT OF STRESS ON THE IMMUNE SYSTEM AND POSSIBLE RISK OF EVOKING ALLERGENIC HYPERSENSITIVITY RESPONSE

Lucjan Jędrychowski

### 2.3.1 INTRODUCTION

The term "stress," ever since it was coined, has been somewhat ambiguous. Initially,
it referred to physical phenomena (expressed in Hooke's law), to be later extended
to people and animals. At present, stress is associated with many physical (blaring

light, deafening noise, extreme heat or cold), chemical (crop fertilization, chemical pollution, water supply), and psychological factors (perpetual frustration). Stress affects all living organisms, in which it causes, according to Hans Selye "the nonspecific response of the body to any demand for change" (Selye 1956). Currently, it is assumed that stress generally consists of environmental events of a challenging sort as well as an organism's total response to environmental demands or pressures caused by such events (Cooper 1996, Ullrich 2007).

Depending on the type of a stimulus and its intensity, the response of an organism will vary. When the stress factor is weak and causes small discomfort, it can lead to positive changes in the affected organism. However, more intense the stress, larger the discomfort, and the inconvenience can be a source of negative reactions and changes in the body; in people, such changes can also concern the sphere of psychosomatic events, nervous and hormonal responses. Due to the complex nature of events occurring under stress as well as the influence of various types of stress on the health of humans, animals, and plants, stress has long been an area of interest to researchers representing different sciences. Since plant and animal food products can cause allergic hypersensitivity reactions, changes caused in plants and animals by biotic and abiotic stress factors can indirectly affect the human body (Konopka et al. 2007).

The direct influence of various stresses on the human body, because of the complexity of effects (involving neurological, endocrinological, and immunomodulatory responses) produced by stress factors, as mentioned above, has been investigated by specialists in medicine, psychology, neurology, immunology, sports, and nutrition (Cooper 1996).

## 2.3.2 EFFECT OF BIOTIC AND ABIOTIC STRESSES ON ANTIGENIC PROPERTIES OF FOOD PRODUCTS

The relationship between yields, total protein concentration, and biochemical composition of proteins in plant seeds on the one hand, and the plant's genome (the effect of a species and cultivar), on the other hand, is a generally well-recognized fact (Sell et al. 2005, Triboi et al. 2000, Wieser and Seilmeier 1998). It is also well known that agronomic practice affects the content of proteins in plant seeds (Daniel and Triboi 2000, Sell et al. 2005, Triboi et al. 2000, Wieser and Seilmeier 1998). In contrast, there are not many reports on the effect of stress on plants (Daniel and Triboi 2000, 2002, Sung and Krieg 1979).

During their vegetative growth, crops are at risk of being affected by various adverse abiotic factors (e.g., excess or shortage of water, nutrients, type and intensity of light, $CO_2$ and $O_2$ concentrations, radiation, chemical pollutants, such as heavy metals, herbicides, crop protection chemicals, and salinity) as well as biotic factors (e.g., infestation by fungi, bacteria, viruses, viroids, mycoplasms, rickettsia, or inter- and intra-species competition). Under the influence of these factors, the basic physiological processes in plants, and photosynthesis in particular, can be altered, which may cause plants' retarded growth, depressed yields, and inferior yield quality. Such changes may lead to modifications in the antigen (allergenic) properties of food products, which means that they can affect human health.

Stress factors can occur simultaneously and interact with one another, for example, excess water can facilitate the appearance of fungi in plants, while shortage of water limits the development of some pathogenic fungi. When crops are infested by fungi, there is a risk that, as raw food products, they will be contaminated by fungal metabolites (mycotoxins, which are not only claimed to be carcinogenic and genotoxic but also held responsible for causing damage to the liver, spleen, and immune system).

The environmental stress factors are extremely important in synthesis and accumulation of proteins (enzymatic, structural, signal, metabolism-related, including proteins which protect the organism, for example, defense proteins, known as stress proteins, or pathogen-related proteins, which are allergens—see Chapter 5) (McKersie and Leshem 1994, Yagami 2000).

It has been demonstrated that both water stress and varied fertilization rates can result in increased content and greater biochemical diversity of the fraction of gliadins in wheat (Konopka et al. 2007).

Mechanism involved in plants' response to stress situations and factors are different from those seen in animals. Plants under stress activate, at the molecular level, a general adaptation syndrome (GAS). In response to stress, plants activate acclimatization mechanisms, which enable them to survive difficult conditions with minimum damage. Two groups of factors are involved: syntoxic (expressed passively or indirectly) and catatoxic ones (active defense, expressed as production of defense metabolites, such as enzymes, antioxidants, and specific proteins) (McKersie and Leshem 1994). Among the results of plants responding to stress are lower yields and certain biochemical changes, which in turn have an impact on the biological quality of yields, technological suitability of plant raw products, and, eventually, biological properties of food products (including their antigen, allergenic characteristics). Such changes can be negative (by contributing to increased allergenic potential) or positive, when they make it possible to employ agronomic and technical means to obtain plant raw products used to make food characterized by depressed allergenicity (e.g., celiac toxicity) (Daniel and Triboi 2000, 2002).

Plants are highly adaptable to stresses (Levitt 1980, 1990). Plant cells, in response to abiotic stresses, can synthesize specific proteins, which alleviate stress by eliminating or neutralizing its effects, but which can also protect basic cellular structures and metabolic processes (Levitt 1980, 1990). Protein synthesis which occurs under the effect of a stress factor has been observed in many plants. The role of such proteins has not been elucidated completely, but in all likelihood they are defense and repair proteins.

Results of some research have indicated that oats and wheat under drought stress produce more total proteins and prolamins, which build up gluten than the same cereals growing under optimum soil moisture conditions (Podolska et al. 2006, 2007). Increased synthesis of gliadins, including $\alpha$-gliadin, under drought suggests that plants growing under drought contain more proteins which cause allergenic and nonallergenic hypersensitivity reaction (Konopka et al. 2007). Buckwheat has been found to respond differently to water deficit stress (Podolska et al. 2007) as it produced less prolamins/gliadins under drought. Thus, it seems to be suitable for the production of food products containing lower amounts of proteins causing food intolerance. However, plants growing under drought conditions can synthesize new proteins, which would not appear during a normal growth of a given plant, and this could create a large potential threat of causing allergies (Podolska et al. 2006).

Similar to water stress, application of plant protection chemicals can cause metabolic changes in plants, which will affect yields, both volumes and chemical composition, including altered protein fractions. However, the research on this issue has generated contradictory results (Goodling et al. 2002, Sulek et al. 2007). It has been found, for example, that herbicides applied in oats cultivation caused a slight increase (by about 4%) in the total protein content, which was accompanied by a decrease in the fraction of albumins and globulins and the fraction of prolamins. In contrast, when growing pea cv. Ramrod, application of herbicides caused higher concentrations of albumins and globulins (Dziuba and Fornal 2009).

It is a well-known fact that mineral fertilization, and nitrogen nutrition in particular, which is one of the strongest yield-enhancing factors, may cause quantitative and qualitative modifications in proteins (increased content), mainly in cereal grains (wheat, oats, and buckwheat), but will depress protein levels in pea seeds (Dziuba and Fornal 2009, Sulek and Podolska 2006). Likewise, some other agronomic treatments, mainly regarding dates of sowing and harvest (thermal stress) may lead to modifications in the pool of proteins. Such changes, however, are not uniform in character and depend also on other factors (mainly cultivar-related ones) (Dziuba and Fornal 2009).

The above considerations lead to the conclusion that as far as production of cereal grains or leguminous seeds is concerned, it is possible to use such technologies in farming practice that would favor depressed levels of allergenic proteins. At present, however, such solutions are theoretical rather than practical. Any further modification of allergenic properties of food products is more likely to take place at the food processing stage (Leszczyńska et al. 2003). These issues are discussed in greater detail in Chapter 5.

### 2.3.3 DIRECT INFLUENCE OF STRESS ON THE IMMUNE SYSTEM OF AN ORGANISM

Ever since the 1970s more evidence has been found in psychoneuroimmunology to confirm the opinion that the highly complex immune system interacts with an equally complex nervous system in a bidirectional manner (Fleshner and Laudenslager 2004). Today, it is a proven fact that stress is associated with altered immune function (Cooper 1996, Maier et al. 1998).

The mechanism of stress affecting humans and animals is similar and in general relies on activating the noradrenergic system and promoting release of noradrenaline (the most important neurotransmitter produced by neurons). Stress also activates the neurally mediated discharge of adrenaline from the adrenal medulla and of hypothalamic hormones that initiate the neuroendocrine cascade, culminating in glucocorticoid release from the adrenal cortex.

While an organism responds to stress, a whole range of hormones is released, e.g., corticotrophin, vasopressin, oxytocin, prolactin, and thyroid hormone; including the so-called metabolic hormones (insulin, epinephrine, and glucagon); and other metabolites, such as the endogenous opiates (endorphin and enkephalin) (Cooper 1996).

Murray and coauthors (Murray et al. 2001) claim that corticotropin-releasing hormones, catecholamines, neuropeptides, and steroid hormones produced throughout the central nervous system as well as in several peripheral sites including the pituitary, testes, ovaries, heart, adrenals, and immune tissues play an important role in the immunomodulatory mechanism of stress affecting human or animal bodies.

Activation of the neuroendocrine stress pathway, which involves release of corticotropin- hormone from the hypothalamus, stimulation of adrenocorticotropic hormone secretion from the pituitary, and release of glucocorticoids from the adrenal cortex, known as the hypothalamic-pituitary-adrenal axis, plays a prominent role in the response to psychological, physical (e.g., noise), or immunological stress (Archana and Namasivayam 1999, Murray et al. 2001, Turnbull and Rivier 1997). Increases in stress levels are associated with elevations in circulating glucocorticoids and catecholamines, which may influence disease pathophysiological factors and severity through changes in the number and activity of Th-cell populations and the relative proportion between Th1 and Th2 cells (Chrousos 2000). The effect of stress can also be seen as a decrease in the total leukocyte numbers, increase in the neutrophil numbers, and depressed levels of IgG and IgM response (Murray et al. 2001).

The above information confirms that external factors, and particularly psychological stress, play a critical role in the functioning of the immune system and appearance of inflammatory reactions, mainly in the digestive system. The mutual reactions between the endocrine, nervous, and immune systems mean that stress reactions can evoke the occurrence of allergenic hypersensitivity.

A broader look on the question of direct influence of stress via the endocrine and nervous systems on the immune system has been presented by Stein et al. (1985), Collins (2001), and Cooper (1996).

Stress may trigger allergenic reactions in the gut and other organs, and depression or anxiety may worsen symptoms in inflammatory disorders of the intestine (Buret 2006, Chrousos 2000, Collins 2001, Marshall and Agarwal 2000, Yang et al. 2005). This effect occurs on the cellular level and may become systematic by affecting particular tissues (Dunlop et al. 2003).

Stress contributes to the development of food allergies by increasing transepithelial permeability in a corticotropin-releasing hormone (CRH)-dependent fashion (Yang et al. 2005).

According to Berkes et al. (2003) and Corrado et al. (1998) paracellular permeability of the gastrointestinal epithelium may be increased by dephosphorylation degradation of transmembrane tight-junctional proteins or presence of gastrointestinal pathogens (e.g., *Helicobacter pylori*) has the ability to increase the passage of food antigens across the gastric epithelium, and infection with this gastric pathogen may be associated with the development of food allergies. In the light of a study carried out by Cao et al. (2005), it seems obvious that mast cells binding to CRH secrete vascular endothelial growth factor (VEGF), and express CRH receptors.

Human can be stressed out by many factors. Some are widely recognized, such as lack of light, temperature, both high and low, type of light (e.g., UV light), turbulences, and physical effort. Some can be classified as social or psychosocial factors, for example, risk of contracting a disease, lack of work, stress before and after an examination or public speech, etc. All stressful situations, as they cause disorders in the neurohormonal homeostasis of an organism, may contribute to the development of several ailments (stress can be indicated in hypertension, chronic fatigue syndrome, coronary artery disease, mental disorders, and a range of other illnesses). The influence of stress on the immune system, and particularly the suppression of immune responses by stress-related hormones, may provide chemical explanation of links between environmental and emotional pressures and susceptibility of diseases (Cooper 1996).

Allergenic hypersensitivity reactions have been observed as a result of physical effort or a sudden change in ambient temperature (particularly exposure to low temperatures), which is due to a sudden change in the levels of hormones or response mediators, e.g., histamine. Although moderate physical effort can strengthen the immune system (Smith et al. 1992), excessive exertion, which is also a stress factor, or cold stress, due to released compounds, can cause significant changes in the immune system, e.g., via suppression of macrophages (Kizaki et al. 1996, Ortega et al. 1996, Smith et al. 1992). Another mechanism of response is associated with such stress factors as UV light or radioactive light. All such cases of allergenic reactions to stress factors confirm the mutual relationships between the nervous, endocrine, and immune systems.

Also exposure of an organism to a pheromone as a stress factor can cause, via release of glucocorticoids, alterations in IL-4 and antibody production (Moynihan et al. 1994).

Another serious environmental threat to people in the modern world is noise. Around 80 million EU citizens (20%) are exposed to unacceptably high noise levels. High noise levels as a negative physical factor can cause such adverse health responses as sleep disturbance, mental stress, absentmindedness, heart attacks, hearing damages, and other negative consequences, including allergenic hypersensitivity, although the latter hypothesis still lacks documented research data. Other bad effects of noise on human health, which may also influence the immune system, include deregulation of physiological systems—in particular, an increase in the release of stress hormones, concentration problems, psychosomatic diseases, or neuroses.

Oxidative stress is another type of environmental stress which can negatively (either directly or indirectly) affect the immune system. Oxidative stress is thought to be a factor influencing many inflammatory responses, including arachidonic acid (AA) release and prostaglandin E2 release (Pawliczak et al. 2002) (see also Section 2.2).

Various types of stresses and the metabolites or hormones released under their influence, for instance glucocorticoids, have been shown to evoke specific changes in lymphocyte subpopulations and to increase the phagocytic activity of neutrophils and macrophages (Fleshner et al. 1992, Murray et al. 2001, Ortega et al. 1996, Smith et al. 1992).

Preventing illnesses which are basically caused by stress, including allergenic hypersensitivity response, should consist of trying to avoid or minimize exposure to stress factors. Certain legal regulations, which aim at reducing stress levels (e.g., noise) seem important in this matter, for example, European Noise Policy: Strategy Paper 2002, European Union: Green Paper 1996.

## REFERENCES

Archana, R. and Namasivayam, A. 1999. The effect of acute noise stress on neutrophil functions. *Indian J Physiol Pharmacol* 43: 491–495.

Berkes, J., Visvanathan, V.K., Savkovic, S.D., and Hecht, G. 2003. Intestinal epithelial responses to enteric pathogens: Effects on the tight junction barrier, ion transport, and inflammation. *Gut* 52: 439–451.

Buret, A.G. 2006. How stress induces intestinal hypersensitivity. *Am J Pathol* 168(1): 3–5.

Cao, J., Papadopoulou, N., Kempuraj, D., Boucher, W.S., Sugimoto, K., Cetrulo, C.L., and Theoharides, T.C. 2005. Human mast cells express corticotropin-releasing hormone (CRH) receptors and CRH leads to selective secretion of vascular endothelial growth factor. *J Immunol* 174: 7665–7675.

Chrousos, G.P. 2000. III. Therapeutic and clinical implications of systemic allergic inflammation. Stress, chronic inflammation, and emotional and physical well-being: Concurrent effects and chronic sequelae. *J Allergy Clin Immunol* 106: S275–S291.

Collins, S.M. 2001. Stress and the gastrointestinal tract IV. Modulation of intestinal inflammation by stress: basic mechanisms and clinical relevance. *Am J Physiol* 280: G315–G318.

Cooper, C. (Ed.). 1996. *Handbook of Stress, Medicine and Health.* CRC Press, Boca Raton, FL.

Corrado, G., Luzzi, I., Lucarelli, S., Frediani, T., Pacchiarotti, C., Cavaliere, M., Rea, P., and Cardi, E. 1998. Positive association between *Helicobacter pylori* infection and food allergy in children. *Scand J Gastroenterol* 33: 1135–1139.

Daniel, C. and Triboi, E. 2000. Effects of temperature and nitrogen nutrition on the grain composition of winter wheat: Effects of gliadin content and composition. *J Cereal Sci* 32(1): 45–56.

Daniel, C. and Triboi, E. 2002. Changes in wheat protein aggregation during grain development: Effects of temperatures and weather stress. *Eur J Agron* 16(1): 1–12.

Dunlop, S.P., Jenkins, D., Neal, K.R., and Spiller, R.C. 2003. Relative importance of enterochromaffin cell hyperplasia, anxiety, and depression in postinfectious IBS. *Gastroenterology* 125: 1651–1659.

Dziuba, J. and Fornal, L. 2008. *Food Biological Active Peptides and Protein—Nutrition and Healthy aspects.* Dziuba, J. (Ed.). WNT Warsaw, Poland. (in press, in Polish).

European Noise Policy: Strategy Paper of the CALM Network—DG Research of the European Commission—July 2002.

European Union: Green Paper on Future Noise Policy. 1996.

Fleshner, M., Watkins, L.R., Bellgrau, D., Laudenslager, M.L., and Maier, S.F. 1992. Specific changes in lymphocyte subpopulations: A potential mechanism for stress-induced immunosuppression. *J Neuroimmunol* 41: 131–142.

Fleshner, M. and Laudenslager, M.L. 2004. Psychoneuroimmunology: Then and now. *Behav Cognitive Neurosci Rev* 3(2): 114–130.

Goodling, M.J., Dimmock, J.P.R.E., Ruske, R., Pepler, S., Ford, K.E., and Gregory, P.J. 2002. The effect of fungicides on the yield and quality of wheat grain. VII Congress ESA Book of Proceedings. Cordoba, Spain, July 15–16, 2002, pp. 441–443.

He, F., Tuomoloa, E., Arvilommi, H., and Salminen, S. 2000. Modulation of humoral immune response through probiotic intake. *FEMS Immunol Med Microbiol* 29: 47–52.

Kizaki, T., Oh-ishi, S., Ookawara, T., Yamamoto, M., Izawa, T., and Ohno, H. 1996. Glucocorticoid-mediated generation of suppressor macrophages with high density Fc γRII during acute cold stress. *Endocrinology* 137: 4260–4267.

Konopka, I., Tanska, M., Pszczolkowska, A., Fordonski, G., Kozirok,W., and Olszewski, J. 2007. The effect of water stress on wheat kernel size, color and protein composition. *Pol J Nat Sci* 22(2): 157–171.

Leszczyńska, J., Łącka, A., Szemraj, J., Lukamowicz, J., and Zegota, H. 2003. The influence of gamma irradiation on the immunoreactivity of gliadin and wheat flour. *Eur Food Res Technol* 217(2): 143–147.

Levitt, J. 1980. *Response of Plants to Environmental Stresses.* New York, Acad. Press.

Levitt, J. 1990. Stress interactions-back to the future. *Hort Sci* 25(11): 1363–1365.

Maier, S.F., Fleshner, M., and Watkins, L.R. 1998. Neural, endocrine, and immune mechanisms of stress-induced immunomodulation. In: *New Frontiers in Stress Research: Modulation of Brain Function*, Levy A, Grauer E, Ben-Nathan D, and de Kloet E. R. (Ed.). Chur, Switzerland, Harwood Academic, pp. 117–126.

Marshall, G.D. and Agarwal, S.K. 2000. Stress, immune regulation, and immunity: Applications for asthma. *Allergy Asthma Proc* 21: 241–246.

McKersie, B.D. and Leshem, Y.Y. 1994. *Stress and Stress Coping in Cultivated Plants.* Dordrecht, the Netherlands, Kluwer Acad. Publ.

Moynihan, J.A., Karp, J.D., Cohen, N., and Cocke, R. 1994. Alterations in interleukin-4 and antibody production following pheromone exposure: Role of glucocorticoids. *J Neuroimmunol* 54: 51–58.

Murray, S.E., Lallman, H.R., Heard, A.D., Rittenberg, M.B., and Stenzel-Poore, M.P. 2001. A genetic model of stress displays decreased lymphocytes and impaired antibody responses without altered susceptibility to *Streptococcus pneumoniae. The Journal of Immunology* 167: 691–698.

Ortega, E., Rodriguez, M.J., Barriga, C., and Forner, M.A. 1996. Corticosterone, prolactin and thyroid hormones as hormonal mediators of the stimulated phagocytic capacity of peritoneal macrophages after high-intensity exercise. *Int J Sports Med* 17: 149–155.

Pawliczak, R., Huang, X.-L., Nanavaty, U.B., Lawrence, M., Madara, P., and Shelhamer, J.H. 2002. Oxidative stress induces arachidonate release from human lung cells through the epithelial growth factor receptor pathway. *Am J Resp Cell Mol Biol* 27: 722–731.

Podolska, G., Konopka, I., and Dziuba, J. 2007. Response of grain yield, yield components and allergic protein content of buckwheat to drought stress. Advances in buckwheat research. Proceedings of the 10th International Symposium on Buckwheat. Northwest A and F University. China, August 14–18, 2007, 323–328.

Podolska, G., Konopka, I., and Dziuba, J. 2006. Response of grain yield, yield components and allergic protein content of winter wheat to drought stress. Proceedings of the 9th European Society of Agronomy Congress. Warsaw, Poland, September 4–11, 2006. 11(Pt 2), 473–474.

Sell, M., Steinhart, H., and Paschke, A. 2005. Influence of maturation on the alteration of allergenicity of green pea (*Pisum sativum L.*). *J Agric Food Chem* 53(5): 1717–1722.

Selye, H. 1956. *The Stress of Life.* New York, Toronto, and London, McGraw-Hill Book Company.

Smith, J.A., McKenzie, S.J., Telford, R.D., and Weidemann, M.J. 1992. Why does moderate exercise enhance, but intense training depress, immunity? *Behav Immun* 11: 155–168.

Söderholm, J.D. and Perdue, M.H. 2001. Stress and the gastrointestinal tract. II. Stress and intestinal barrier function. *Am J Physiol Gastrintest Liver Physiol* 280: G7–G13.

Stein, M., Keller, S.E., and Schleifer, S.J. 1985. Stress and immunomodulation: The role of depression and neuroendocrine function. *J Immunol* 135: 827S–833S.

Sułek, A. and Podolska, G. 2006. The effect of selected herbicides on quality of wheat grains. *Prog Plant Protection/Post Plant Protection* 46(2): 300–304 (in polish).

Sułek, A., Noworolnik, K., Podolska, G., Dziuba, J., and Konopka, I. 2007. The effect of plant protection substances on toxic and allergenic compounds in seeds of selected plants. In: *Allergens and Compounds of Plant Raw Materials and Foods Inducing Food Intolerance. Proceedings of II Scientific National Conference*, Olsztyn, September 19, 2007, 41 (in polish).

Sung, F.J. and Krieg, D.R. 1979. Relative sensitivity of photosynthetic assimilation and translocation of 14 C-carbon to water stress. *Plant Physiol* 64(5): 852 856.

Triboi, E., Abdad, A., Michelena, A., Lloveras, J., Ollier, J.L., and Daniel, C. 2000. Environmental effect on the quality of two wheat genotypes: 1. Quantitative and qualitative variation of storage proteins. *Eur J Agron* 13(1): 47–64.

Turnbull, A.V. and Rivier, C. 1997. Corticotropin-releasing factor (CRF) and endocrine responses to stress: CRF receptors, binding protein, and related peptides. *Proc Soc Exp Biol Med* 215: 1.

Ullrich, O. 2007. Endothelial cells in microgravity. One more step to solve the "immune problem" in space. *Bioforum Eur. Trend Techniq Life Sci Res* 12: 38–39.

Wieser, H. and Seilmeier, W. 1998. The influence of nitrogen fertilization on quantities and proportions of different protein types in wheat flour. *J Sci Food Agric* 76(1): 49–55.

Yagami, T. 2000. Defense-related proteins as families of cross-reactive plant allergens. *Recent Res Dev Allergy Clin Immunol* 1: 41–64.

Yang, P.C., Jury, J., Soderholm, J.D., Sherman, P.M., McKay, D.M., and Perdue, M.H. 2005. Chronic psychological stress in rats induces intestinal sensitization to luminal antigens. *Am J Pathol* 168: 104–114.

## 2.4   INFLUENCE OF FOOD MATRIX AND GUT MICROFLORA ON IMMUNE RESPONSE AND ABSORPTION OF FOOD ALLERGENS

Anna Halász and András Nagy

The intestinal epithelium with optimal intestinal flora serves as first line of defense against the invading pathogenic microorganisms, antigens, and harmful components from the gut lumen.

The immune system secretes immunoglobulins as first-line defense and evolves specific immune protection. Oral tolerance, hyporesponsiveness to dietary antigens, and gut microbiota results purposeful immune regulation. Oral tolerance is a state of systemic specific immunologic hyporesponsiveness to specific innocuous antigen (food, commensal microbiota) challenge. It is an actively regulated state that is maintained by multiple and probably non-mutually exclusive immunoregulatory mechanism. The site of antigen-specific antigen sampling and especially the nature of the local antigen-presenting cells are critical to the development of oral tolerance or immunity to intestinal antigens. Oral tolerance does not prevent efficient immune functions against harmful antigens (Shanahan 2000). The gut prevents excessive inflammation and tissue injury by several mechanisms reviewed by Isolauri (Isolauri 1995).

In addition, the mucosal surface of the intestine is essential for the assimilation of antigens. Proteases of the intestinal bacteria degrade the antigenic structure, an important step in the introduction of unresponsiveness to dietary antigens. Specialized antigen transport mechanisms take place in different lymphoid compartments: mesenteric lymph nodes, Peyer's patches, isolated lymph follicles, isolated T lymphocytes in the epithelium and the lamina propria, as well as at the secretory sites (Heyman et al. 1982). The secretory IgA antibodies in the gut are part of the common mucosal immune system, which includes the respiratory tract and the salivary and mammary glands.

The hallmark of an inflammatory response is the generation of pro-inflammatory cytokines including IL-1, interleukin-2, TNF-$\alpha$, and IFN-$\gamma$. There are several reports indicating that pro-inflammatory cytokines may be primary mediators of inflammation in clinical conditions characterized by impaired gut barrier function (Ebert 1998, O'Farelly 1998). Ebert (1998) demonstrated that in intestinal inflammation, TNF-$\alpha$ disrupts the epithelial cells leading to shortening of the villi while being also mitogenic to the crypt cells. Thus immature cells replace those disrupted, allowing aberrant antigen uptake, immune response, and further impairment of the barrier function. Inflammation and infection are frequently accompanied by imbalance in the intestinal microflora. In unbalanced microflora, pathogenic bacteria are abundantly present. This leads to abrogation of interaction maintained in health between the microfloral bacteria and the immune system.

Probiotic bacteria may counteract the inflammatory process by stabilizing the microbial environment of gut and permeability barrier of intestine, but the underlying mechanisms are still not completely discovered. It has in fact been demonstrated by Salminen et al. (1998) that probiotics participate in the exclusion of pathogens thereby preventing the generation of inflammatory mediators by intraluminal bacteria.

Many studies showed that peptidoglycan in the cell wall stimulates macrophages, antibody formation, and T lymphocyte activity entering the intestine (Dziarski 1991). Certain strains of LAB induce pro-Th1 responses, promoted through the receptor-mediated cytokine pathway, and the ability of individual cell wall compounds to induce pro-IFN cytokines (especially IL-12) at a sub-inflammatory level. However, it should be realized that other indirect LAB-induced modulatory mechanisms may also be operative in combating atopy, such as their ability to liberate de novo immunoregulatory peptides from major food proteins via enzymatic hydrolysis. This mechanism has been demonstrated experimentally for some LAB (Matar et al. 1996, Rokka et al. 1997).

Based on several experiments that have demonstrated the beneficial effects of probiotics in the decrease of symptoms of allergic patients, probiotics appear to be one innovative mode of prevention and therapy of food allergy through hypoallergenic formula. Probiotics such as *L. lactis*, other LAB or *B. lactis* Bb 12 have been shown to significantly reduce the severity of the atopic eczema. In fact, these probiotics likely participate in the mucosal degradation of macromolecules leading to the reduction in the antigen load. Thanks to their peptidases, that hydrolyze tryptic chymotryptic peptides from $\beta$-lactoglobulin, they release numerous small peptides with immunomodulating properties, which repress the lymphocyte stimulation (Pessi et al. 2001, Sütas et al. 1996), upregulate IL-10 production, and downregulate IFN-$\gamma$ secretion (Prioult et al. 2004).

Attachment of probiotic lactobacilli to cell surface receptors of enterocytes also initiates signaling events that result in the synthesis of cytokines (Kaur et al. 2002). The effects in immune regulation are of utmost importance, because in reducing the generation of local pro-inflammatory cytokines, the anti-inflammatory effects of probiotics may extend beyond the gut. Certain strains of LAB (*Lb plantarum* VTT, *Lb rhamnosus* ATCC 53103) in viable form are potent producers of IL-6 from human peripheral blood mononuclear cells. Some strains are able to stimulate IL-10, but not in all subjects.

Modification of intestinal flora for increasing the predominance of specific nonpathogenic bacteria, and thereby alter the milieu in intestine, can have alternative therapeutic effects in intestinal inflammation and infections (Isolauri et al. 2002).

Probiotic bacteria may counteract the inflammatory process by

- Enhancing the degradation of enteral antigens and altering their immunogenicity
- Reducing the secretion of inflammatory mediators
- Promoting exclusion of antigens in the gut by enhancing mucosal IgA response to enteral antigens
- Normalizing the composition of intestinal microflora
- Normalizing of the increased intestinal permeability associated with intestinal inflammation

However, in many cases definitive proof of LAB immunoregulatory activity is still required from well-designed appropriately controlled human clinical studies.

The ability of dietary consumption of foods containing LAB to modulate immune responses has been thoroughly studied in animal models. Dietary consumption of LAB and Bifidobacteria strains have been shown to enhance protection against intracellular bacterial pathogens. Physiological responses have been shown to correspond with the cell-mediated immune responses that have the Th1 cell bias.

Furthermore, oral or systemic delivery of LAB has been show to be a potent signal for the induction of Type-I and Type-II IFNs (Kato et al. 1983, Matsuzaki 1998).

The ability of LAB diet enhanced IFN production to regulate the Th1/Th2 responses has been thoroughly studied in animal models. Feeding OVA-primed mice with *L. casei* has been shown to reduce antigen-specific IgE responses *in vivo* (Yasui et al. 1999). A murine model of food allergy has also demonstrated that intraperitoneal administration of *L. plantarum* can downregulate casein-specific IgE antibody levels *in vivo* and IL-4 secretion as well (Murosaki et al. 1998).

It is presumed that dietary consumption of fermented milk products facilitates the interaction of immunoregulatory LAB with cells of the GALT system and there is plenty of evidence for the direct interaction of LAB with intra-intestinal lymphoid foci (De Simone et al. 1987, Yasui and Ohwaki 1991). Recent studies have shown that LAB can potentiate the expression of cytokine receptors on IFN-activated human intestinal cells and can regulate immune phenotype and cytokine expression at intestinal sites following oral delivery in mice (Herias et al. 1999, Maassen et al. 2000).

Earlier studies have shown that probiotics can over regulate the Th2-type immune responses toward Th1 with improved TGT-$\beta$ secretion, which play an efficient role in maintaining an increased secretion of gut IgA (Polgár 2004). Matsuzaki and Chin (2000) demonstrated that while antigen feeding alone appears to prime for an immune response, co-feeding the antigen with probiotic bacteria was able to suppress both cellular and humoral responses. Nagy et al. (2002, 2005a) confirmed that oral administration of native or heat-denatured LAB strains together with a T-cell dependent marker antigen, for example, OVA, successfully induced gut IgA.

It has been proved in animal feeding trials that co-feeding LAB + OVA resulted in significant reduction of OVA-specific IgG$_1$, which is due to restoration of tolerance and the Th2 regulation (Nagy et al. 2005b).

However, in many cases definitive proof of LAB immunoregulatory activity is still required from well-designed appropriately controlled human clinical studies.

## REFERENCES

De Simone, C., Vesely, R., Negri, R., Bianchi Salvadori, B., Zanzoglu, S., and Cilli, A. 1987. Enhancement of immune response of murine Peyer's patches by a diet supplemented with yoghurt. *Immunopharmacol Immunotoxicol* 9: 87–100.

Dziarski, R. 1991. Demonstration of peptidoglycan-binding sites on lymphocytes and macrophages by photoaffinity cross-linking. *J Biol Chem* 266: 4713–4718.

Ebert, E.C. 1998. Tumour necrosis factor-$\alpha$ enhances intraepithelial lymphocyte proliferation and migration. *Gut* 42: 650–655.

Herias, M.V., Hessle, C., Telemo, E., Midtvedt, T., Hanson, L.A., and Wold, A.E. 1999. Immunomodulatory effects of *Lactobacillus plantarum* colonizing the intestine of gnotobiotic rats. *Clin Exp Immunol* 116: 283–290.

Heyman, M., Ducroc, R., Desjeux, J.F., and Morgat, J.L. 1982. Horseradish peroxidase transport across adult rabbit jejunum in vitro. *Am J Physiol* 242: G558–G564.

Isolauri, E. 1995. *Intestinal Integrity and IBD*. Kluwer Academic Publisher, Lancaster, UK, 85, pp. 553–555.

Isolauri, E., Kirjavainen, P.V., and Salminen, S. 2002. Probiotics: A role in the treatment of intestinal infection and inflammation? *Gut* 50: 54–59.

Kato, I., Yokokura, T., and Mutai, M. 1983. Macrophage activation by *Lactobacillus casei* in mice. *Microbiol Immunol* 27: 611–618.

Kaur, I.P., Chopra, K., and Saini, A. 2002. Probiotics: Potential pharmaceutical applications. *Eur J Pharm Sci* 15: 1–9.

Maassen, C.B., van Holten-Neelen, C., Balk, F., Heijne den Bak-Glashouwer, M., Leer, R.J., and Laman, J.D. 2000. Strain-dependent induction of cytokine profiles in the gut by orally-administered *Lactobacillus* strains. *Vaccine* 18: 2613–2623.

Matar, C., Amiot, J., Savoie, L., and Goulet, J. 1996. The effect of milk fermentation by *Lactobacillus helveticus* on the release of peptides during in vitro digestion. *J Dairy Sci* 79: 971–979.

Matsuzaki, T. 1998. Immunomodulation by treatment with *Lactobacillus casei* strain Shirota. *Int J Food Microbiol* 41: 133–140.

Matsuzaki, T. and Chin, J. 2000. Modulating immune responses with probiotic bacteria. *Immunol Cell Biol* 78: 67–73.

Murosaki, S., Yamomoto, Y., Ito, K., Inokuchi, T., Kusaka, H., and Ikeda, H. 1998. Heat-killed *Lactobacillus plantarum* L-137 suppresses naturally fed antigen-specific IgE production by stimulation of IL-12 production in mice. *J Allergy Clin Immunol* 102: 57–64.

Nagy, A., Baráth, Á., Halász, A., and Gelencsér, É. 2005a. Modulating of the immune responses to a co-administered marker antigen by selected *Lactobacillus* strains used as oral adjuvant. Inform All Plenary Meeting 6, Athens, Greece, October 24–26, 2005.

Nagy, A., Jędrychowski, L., Gelencsér, É., Wróblewska, B., and Szymkiewicz, A. 2002. Immunomodulative effect of *Lactobacillus salivarius* and *Lactobacillus casei* strains. *Pol J Food Nutr Sci* 11/52: 122–124.

Nagy, A., Jędrychowski, L., Gelencsér, É., Wróblewska, B., Szymkiewicz, A. 2005b. Induction of specific mucosal immune responses by viable or heat denatured probiotic bacteria of *Lactobacillus* strains. *Acta Alimentaria* 34: 33–39.

O'Farelly, C. 1998. Just how inflamed is the normal gut? *Gut* 42: 613–616.

Pessi, T., Isolauri, E., Sütas, Y., Kankaanranta, H., Moilanen, E., and Hurme, M. 2001. Suppression of T-cell activation by *Lactobacillus rhamnosus* GG-degraded bovine casein. *Int Immunopharmacol* 1: 211–218.

Polgár, M. 2004. A bélflóra kialakulása újszülöttekben, alakulásának és alakításának jelentösége csecsemö- és gyermekkorban. (Development of intestinal flora in new-born, importance of formation and modulation in infancy and childhood.). In: Szakály, S. (Ed) *Probiotikumok és humánegészség*. (Probiotics and human health.), Magyar Tejgazdasági Kísérleti Intézet, Mosonmagyaróvár, pp. 18–28.

Prioult, G., Pecquet, S., and Fliss, I. 2004. Stimulation of interleukin-10 production by acidic β-lactoglobulin-derived peptides hydrolyzed with *Lactobacillus paracasei* NCC2461 peptidases. *Clin Diagn Lab Immunol* 11: 266–271.

Rokka, T., Syvaoja, E.L., Tuominen, J., and Korhonen, H. 1997. Release of bioactive peptides by enzymatic proteolysis of *Lactobacillus* GG fermented UHT milk. *Milch wissenschaft* 52: 675–678.

Salminen, S., Bouley, C., Boutron-Ruault, M.C., Contor, L., Cummings, J.H., and Franck, A. 1998. Functional food science and gastrointestinal physiology and function. *Br J Nutr* 80: S147–S171.

Shanahan, F. 2000. Probiotics and inflammatory bowel disease: Is there a scientific rationale? *Inflamm Bowel Dis* 6: 107–115.

Sütas, Y., Soppi, E., Korhonen, H., Syväoja, E.L., Saxelin, M., Rokka, T., and Isolauri, E. 1996. Suppression of lymphocyte proliferation in vitro by bovine caseins hydrolyzed with *Lactobacillus casei* GG-derived enzymes. *J Allergy Clin Immunol* 98: 216–224.

Yasui, H., Shida, K., Matsuzaki, T., and Yokokura, T. 1999. Immunomodulatory function of lactic acid bacteria. *Antonie van Leeuwenhoek* 76: 383–389.

Yasui, Y. and Ohwaki, M. 1991. IgA production and intestinal microflora: Augmentation of IgA production by *Bifidobacterium breve*. *Jpn Clin Microsc* 24: 426–430.

## 2.5 ROLE OF PROBIOTIC BACTERIA IN THE PREVENTION OF FOOD ALLERGY

Edina Németh and Anna Halász

The gastrointestinal (GI) microflora plays an important role in the health status of people and animals. The GI tract represents a much larger contact area with the environment, compared to the $2\,m^2$ skin surface of our body (van Dijk 1997). The mucosal surface of the small intestine is increased by forming folds, intestinal villi, and the formation of microvilli in the enterocyte resorptive luminal membrane. The resulting surface of GI system is calculated to be $150–200\,m^2$, therefore it provides enough space for the interactions related to digestion and for the adhesion to the mucosal wall.

It is estimated that about 300–400 different cultivable species belonging to more than 190 genera are present in the colon of healthy adults. Among the colonic microbial flora only a few major groups dominate at levels around $10^{10}–10^{11}$/g, all of which are strict anaerobes such as *Bacteroides, Eubacterium, Bifidobacterium,* and *Peptostreptococcus*. Facultative aerobes are considered to belong to the subdominant flora, constituting *Enterobacteriaceae*, lactobacilli and streptococci. Minor groups of pathogenic and opportunistic organisms, the so-called residual flora according to Gedek (1993) are always present in low number.

Bacteria present in the "normal" flora may exert beneficial effect and are able to degrade certain food components, produce certain B vitamins, stimulate the immune system, and produce digestive and protective enzymes. The normal flora also takes part in the metabolism of some potentially carcinogenic substances and may play a role in drug efficacy. In the last few decades there is an increasing interest for influencing the composition of the gut flora by foods or food ingredients. The goal of these attempts is to induce the number and activities of those microorganisms which possess health-promoting properties, such as *Lactobacillus* and *Bifidobacterium* species (Szakály 2004).

The health-promoting effect of lactobacilli was first hypothesized by Metchnikoff at the beginning of the last century (Metchnikoff 1905). In the last four decades there have been growing attempts to improve the health status of the indigenous intestinal flora by living microbial adjuncts, "probiotics." Salminen and coworkers (1999) proposed that "probiotics are microbial cell preparations or components of microbial cells that have beneficial effect on the health and well-being of the host." The probiotics do not have to be viable as nonviable forms of probiotics have also been shown to exert health-promoting effect.

Over the last decade there has been accumulating evidence that consumption of fermented foods can alleviate some symptoms of atopy, and may limit allergy development. Dietary studies have suggested that long-term consumption of yoghurt can reduce some of the clinical symptoms of allergy in adults with atopic rhinitis or nasal allergies and can lower serum levels of IgE particularly among the elderly (Halpern et al. 1991, Trapp et al. 1993). Wheeler and coworkers reported that asthmatic patients who consumed Lactobacillus-supplemented yoghurt demonstrated longitudinal trend toward eosinophilia and increased production of IFN-$\gamma$ (Wheeler et al. 1997a,b).

Atopic dermatitis is a common complex, chronically relapsing skin disorder of infancy and childhood. The prevalence of atopic diseases has been progressively increasing in Western societies. The regulatory role of probiotics in human allergic disease was first emphasized in the demonstration of suppressive effect on lymphocyte proliferation and IL-4 generation *in vitro* (Sütas et al. 1996). The preventive potential of probiotics in atopic disease has been shown in a double blind placebo-controlled study (Kalliomaki et al. 2001). Administration of probiotics to pregnant women and postnatally to infants at high risk of atopic diseases for 6 months succeeded in reducing the prevalence of atopic eczema to half compared to that in infants receiving placebo.

There are observations that milk whey formula supplemented with *L. rhamnosus* (strain GG) could alleviate some aspects of atopy and intestinal inflammation among infants with atopic eczema or food allergy. Furthermore, clinical scores of the eczema were reduced in breast-fed infants whose mothers consumed Lb-GG.

Most allergic disease reflect imbalance in lymphocyte-governed immunity, with immune responses to allergenic molecules becoming overly biased toward Th2 phenotype. Secretion of the cytokines IL-4, IL-5, and IL-13 by allergen-sensitized Th2 cells recruits granular effector cells such as eosinophils, basophils, and mast cells to the site of allergenic inflammation (Djukanovic et al. 1990, Leung 1995). These effector cells alone or in combination with cytophilic/reaginic IgE class antibodies promote the clinical manifestation of allergy and atopy (Durham 1998, Wills-Karp 1999). In addition, IL-4 and IL-13 promote B lymphocyte immunoglobulin isotype switching to IgE and serves to increase circulating levels of total and allergen-specific IgE (Brown et al. 1997, Pene et al. 1988). However, during the early stages of T lymphocyte differentiation it is possible that overexpression of Th2 phenotype can be arrested by cross-regulating cytokines. IFN, particularly IFN-γ, can downregulate IL-4 expression and reduce B cell immunoglobulin switching (Brown and Hural 1997, Pene et al. 1988). Type-I INF, TNF-α, can act as an augmentative signal for INF-γ production, can promote Th1-type immune response, and reduce IgE production.

Significantly, it has been well documented that LAB can enhance IgE expression and secretion of both Type-I and Type-II.

The IL-8 production is an instant local defensive inflammatory response against various potentially harmful intestinal pathogens. IL-8 is pivotal to and governs the progress of most local intestinal inflammations. It attracts and activates neutrophils at the site of infection to combat pathogens. Persistent secretion of IL-8 that leads to neutrophil infiltration often causes chronic inflammation and may subsequently culminate into epithelial cell damage (McCafferty and Zeitlin 1989). These effects can be avoided by down-regulation of IL-8 synthesis at some stages when the inflammation is resolved. In fact, chronic inflammations characterized by high levels of IL-8 such as inflammatory bowel diseases are cured by interventions that decrease the levels of IL-8. The actual mechanism of *Lactobacillus* probiotics used in the treatment of such disorders is enigmatic.

Németh and coworkers showed that exposure of enterocyte-like Caco-2 cells to non-starter LAB induce a modest IL-8 synthesis. The levels of IL-8 induced by lactobacilli were significantly lower when compared to those induced by pathogenic *Salmonella enteritidis* 857 (*Se*. 857) (Németh et al. 2006). Indeed, the highest levels induced after 24 h were just slightly higher than those of control cells, alluding that they might be within the range of constitutive expression responsible for the normal immune surveillance *in vivo*.

Exposure of Caco-2 cells to *Se*. 857 pretreated with the spent culture supernatant (SCS) of LAB strains resulted in a marked inhibition of IL-8 synthesis. Pretreatment of *Se*. 857 with lactobacilli SCS (pH 4.5) most likely dissociates the flagella. Since flagellin is an important stimulus for epithelial IL-8 secretion because of its ability to activate Toll-like receptor 5 (Huang et al. 2004), these partly aflagellated bacteria do not equally, effectively synthesize IL-8 as the flagellated ones.

Recently, several strains of *L. rhamnosus* and *L. delbrueckii* were also observed to downregulate IL-8 production in HT-29 cells, an intestinal epithelial cell line (Wallace et al. 2003). Together with these findings, it appears that inhibition of IL-8 production may be part of the mechanism by which lactobacilli impart their welfare to the gut. This could explain their ability to treat intestinal disorders associated with high levels of IL-8.

The expression of Hsp70 by intestinal epithelial cells exposed to *Lactobacillus* spp. or their cultivation products had not been studied extensively. An experimental investigation conducted in the animal models showed that *Lactobacillus* cultivation products exerted a marked long-term protection against ischemized rat heart. This effect was attributed to an activation of the cellular defense system manifested by overexpression of Hsp70 (Oxman et al. 2000). The ability of enterocyte-like Caco-2 cells to produce the protective Hsp70 under various conditions was previously demonstrated (Malago et al. 2003, Ovelgönne et al. 2000). Németh et al. (2006) found that non-starter lactobacilli and their SCS are capable of inducing Hsp70 expression in the Caco-2 cells. Because the production of Hsp70 is a protective response (Malago et al. 2002, Ovelgönne et al. 2000), it is suggested that one mechanism for the beneficial attributes of the non-starter lactobacilli is the ability to induce the expression of Hsp70 by the bacteria and their SCS. The induced Hsp70 could function in the stabilization of the cytoskeleton of intestinal epithelial cells after being distorted during adhesion and invasion by *Salmonella* (Jepson et al. 1995, 1996). In turn, this could impede further *Salmonella* invasion. Furthermore, since SCS of *L. casei* GG hampered invasion of Caco-2 cells by *S. typhimurium* C5 without altering their viability (Hadult et al. 1997), expression of Hsp70 could protect cells against the viable intracellular bacteria and/or the pro-inflammatory cytokines they produce. It has been suggested that the beneficial effects of probiotics in host defense against infection include anti-inflammatory properties. These properties involve signaling with the gastrointestinal epithelium and with mucosal regulatory T cells (Shanahan 2000). Probiotics may also counterbalance epithelial responses to invasive bacteria by regulating the cytokine transcription factors (Neish et al. 2000). In the latter mechanism of action, Hsps might play an essential role through their ability to interfere with cytokine production in intestinal epithelial cells (Malago et al. 2002).

## REFERENCES

Brown, M.A. and Hural, J. 1997. Functions of IL-4 and control of its expression. *Crit Rev Immunol* 17: 1–32.

Djukanovic, R., Wilson, J.W., Britten, K.M. et al. 1990. Quantitation of mast cells and eosinophils in the bronchial mucosa of symptomatic atopic asthmatics and healthy control subjects using immunohistochemistry. *Annu Res Respir Dis* 142: 863–871.

Durham, S.R. 1998. Mechanisms of mucosal inflammation in the nose and lungs. *Clin Exp Allergy* 28: 11–16.

Gedek, B. 1993. Darmflora-physiologie und okologie. *J Chemotherapy* S1: 2–6.

Hadult, S., Lievin, V., Bernet-Camard, M.F., and Servin, A. 1997. Antagonistic activity exerted in vitro and in vivo by *Lactobacillus casei* (strain GG) against *Salmonella typhimurium* C5 infection. *Appl Environ Microb* 63: 513–518.

Halpern, G.M., Vruwink, K.G., van de Water, J., Keen, C.L., and Gershwin, M.E. 1991. Influence of long-term yoghurt consumption in young adults. *Int J Immunother* 7: 205–210.

Huang, F.C., Werne, A., Li, Q., Galyov, E.E., Walker, W.A., and Cherayil, B.J. 2004. Cooperative interactions between flagellin and SopE2 in the epithelial interleukin-8 response to *Salmonella enterica* serovar Typhimurium infection. *Infect Immun* 72: 5052–5062.

Jepson, M.A., Colares-Buzato, C.B., Clark, M.A., Hirst, B.H., and Simmons, N.L. 1995. Rapid disruption of epithelial barrier function by *Salmonella typhimurium* is associated with structural modification of intercellular junctions. *Infect Immun* 63: 356–359.

Jepson, M.A., Lang, T.F., Reed, K.A., and Simmons, N.L. 1996. Evidence for a rapid, direct effect on epithelial monolayer integrity and transepithelial transport in response to *Salmonella* invasion. *Eur J Physiol* 432: 225–233.

Kalliomaki, M., Salminen, S., and Kero, P. 2001. Probiotics in primary prevention of atopic disease: A randomised placebo-controlled trial. *Lancet* 357: 1076–1079.

Leung, D.Y. 1995. Atopic dermatitis: The skin as a window into the pathogenesis of chronic allergic diseases. *J Allergy Clin Immunol* 96: 302–318.

Malago, J.J., Koninkx, J.F.J.G., and van Dijk, J.E. 2002. The heat shock response and cytoprotection of the intestinal epithelium. *Cell Stress Chaperon* 7: 191–199.

Malago, J.J., Koninkx, J.F.J.G., Ovelgönne, H.H., van Asten, F.J.A.M., Swennenhuis, J.F., and van Dijk, J.E. 2003. Expression levels of heat shock proteins in enterocyte-like Caco-2 cells after exposure to *Salmonella enteritidis. Cell Stress Chaperon* 8: 194–203.

McCafferty, D.M., and Zeitlin, I.J. 1989. Short chain fatty acid-induced colitis in mice. *Int J Tissue React* 11: 165–168.

Metchnikoff, E. 1905. *Immunity in the Infectious Diseases*, Binnie, F.G. (transl.), Cambridge University Press, Cambridge.

Neish, A.S., Gewirtz, A.T., Zeng, H. et al. 2000. Prokaryotic regulation of epithelial responses by inhibition of I kappa B-alpha ubiquitination. *Science* 289: 1560–1563.

Németh, E., Fajdiga, S., Malago, J., Koninkx, J., Tooten, P., and van Dijk, J. 2006. Inhibition of Salmonella-induced IL-8 synthesis and expression of Hsp 70 in enterocyte-like Caco-2 cells after exposure to non-starter lactobacilli. *Int J Food Microbiol* 112: 266–274.

Ovelgönne, J.H., Koninkx, J.F.J.G., Pusztai, A. et al. 2000. Decreased level of heat shock proteins in gut epithelial cells after exposure to plant lectins. *Gut* 46: 679–687.

Oxman, T., Shapira, M., Diver, A., Klein, R., Avazov, N., and Rabinowitz, B. 2000. A new method of long-term preventive cardioprotection using *Lactobacillus. Am J Physiol— Heart C* 278: H1717–H1724.

Pene, J., Rousset, F., Briere, F., Chretien, I., Bonnefoy, J.Y., and Spits, H. 1988. IgE production by normal human lymphocytes is induced by interleukin 4 and suppressed by interleukins gamma and alpha and prostaglandin E2. *Proc Natl Acad Sci USA* 85: 6880–6885.

Salminen, S., Ouwehand, A., Benno, Y., and Lee, Y.K. 1999. Probiotics: How should they be defined? *Trends Food Sci Technol* 10: 107–110.

Shanahan, F. 2000. Probiotics and inflammatory bowel disease: Is there a scientific rationale? *Inflamm Bowel Dis* 6: 107–115.

Sütas, Y., Hurme, M., and Isolauri, E. 1996. Downregulation of antiCD3 antibody-induced IL-4 production by bovine caseins hydrolysed with *Lactobacillus GG*-derived enzymes. *Scand J Immunol* 43: 687–689.

Szakály, S. 2004. *Probiotikumok és humánegészség (Probiotics and human health.)*, Magyar Tejgazdasági Kísérleti Intézet, Mosonmagyaróvár.

Trapp, C.L., Chang, C.C., Halpern, G.M., Keen, C.L., and Gershwin, M.E. 1993. The influence of chronic yogurt consumption on populations of young and elderly adults. *Int J Immunother* 9: 53–64.

van Dijk, J.E. 1997. Morphology of the gut barrier. *Eur J Comparative Gastroenterol* 2: 23–27.

Wallace, T.D., Bradley, S., Buckley, N.D., and Green-Johnson, J.M. 2003. Interactions of lactic acid bacteria with human intestinal epithelial cells: Effects on cytokine production. *J Food Protect* 66: 466–472.

Wheeler, J.G., Bogle, M.L., Shema, S.J. et al. 1997a. Impact of dietary yogurt on immune function. *Am J Med Sci* 313: 120–123.

Wheeler, J.G., Shema, S., Bogle, M.L. et al. 1997b. Immune and clinical impact of *Lactobacillus acidophilus* on asthma. *Ann Allergy Asthma Immunol* 79: 229–233.

Wills-Karp, M. 1999. Immunologic basis of antigen-induced airway hyperresponsiveness. *Annu Rev Immunol* 17: 255–282.

# 3 Methods for Detection of Food Allergens

*Lucjan Jędrychowski, André H. Penninks,*
*Maciej Kaczmarski, Beata Cudowska,*
*Elżbieta Korotkiewicz-Kaczmarska, Andrea Harrer,*
*Anja Maria Erler, Gabriele Gadermaier,*
*Michael Faltlhansl, Fátima Ferreira,*
*and Martin Himly*

## CONTENTS

Allergenic hypersensitivity is a multi-organ response, which involves the occurrence of various clinical manifestations causing discomfort (see Chapter 1) and can be mistaken for other illnesses. Thus, correct diagnosis is of utmost importance. Avoiding allergenic hypersensitivity largely depends on the patient, who should assess health hazards, i.e., recognize potential allergens in his or her diet.

The most suitable method for diagnosing allergies is a double-blind, placebo-controlled (DBPC) challenge: first, because allergenic responses are highly individual in character and second, because food allergens administered *per os* undergo extensive modification while being digested. This method can be supported by open food test challenges, *in vivo* tests (skin prick tests), or *ex vivo* tests with pure, natural, or recombinant allergen molecules as well as panels of synthetic peptides as components of particular tests, or sera of allergenic patients (FAO/ WHO, 2001; Lidholm et al., 2006). (These are discussed in greater detail in Section 3.4.)

All other assays related to *in vivo* tests on allergens can only serve as a cognitive tool and assist the diagnostic process. The ultimate verification of allergenic properties of a diet or a dietary component should always be performed by an allergist.

The health hazard caused by the presence of allergens in food, alongside the legal regulations concerning food product labeling and inclusion of information on potential allergy-related risks, means that the food industry needs good, inexpensive, replicable, and precise analytic methods. The primary aim of detection of food allergens is to discover their characteristics and to specify the health risk caused by their presence in food. Improved description of allergens and better understanding of mechanisms behind the allergies can help to work out more suitable, safer diets for breastfeeding women or neonates at risk of atopy. It can also serve as a basis for elaboration of new therapeutic methods to treat food allergies (Bindslev-Jensen, 2001; Burks et al., 2001).

European law requires that the following allergen-containing food products

1. Cereals containing gluten (i.e., wheat, rye, barley, oats, spelt, kamut or their hybridized strains) and products thereof, except cereals used for making distillates or ethyl alcohol, wheat-based maltodextrins, and dextrose and glucose syrups
2. Crustaceans and products thereof
3. Eggs and products thereof
4. Fish and products thereof, except fish gelatin used as fining agent in beer and wine

5. Peanuts and products thereof
6. Soybeans and products thereof, except fully refined soybean oil and natural tocopherols, soybean oils derived phytosterols and phytosterol esters, and stanol ester
7. Milk and products thereof (including lactose), except lactitol, and whey used for making distillates or ethyl alcohol
8. Nuts, i.e., almonds (*Amygdalus communis* L.), hazelnuts (*Corylus avellana*), walnuts (*Juglans regia*), cashews (*Anacardium occidentale*), pecan nuts (*Carya illinoinensis (Wangenh.) K. Koch*), Brazil nuts (*Bertholletia excelsa*), pistachio nuts (*Pistacia vera*), macadamia nuts and Queensland nuts (*Macadamia ternifolia*), and products thereof, except nuts used for making distillates or ethyl alcohol
9. Celery and products thereof
10. Mustard and products thereof
11. Sesame seeds and products thereof
12. Sulfur dioxide and sulfites at concentrations of more than 10 mg/kg or 10 mg/L expressed as $SO_2$
13. Lupin and products thereof
14. Molluscs and products thereof

be under control (Directive 2003/89/EC, 2003; Directive 2007/68/EC, 2007).

In the USA, only the first eight food allergens is legally regulated. In Australia and New Zealand, the first nine allergens are under legal control, whereas the presence of $SO_2/SO_3$ is controlled only when in excess of 10 mg/kg. The law in Japan requires that food products be controlled for the presence of components such as gluten and buckwheat, eggs, peanuts, and milk (FALCPA, 2004; Food Standards Agency, 2006).

Detection of allergens as health risk factors can take place at several levels:

- *In vitro* determination of specific antigens in products using classical physicochemical and biochemical methods, which rely on the determination of amino acid sequences in proteins and their tertiary structure (see Section 3.4) as well as immunodetection methods using commercially available analytical tests
- *In vitro* determination of the content of general and specific IgE class antibodies, using sera of allergic people and tests based on histamine release from basophils (see Section 3.3)
- Determination of allergenic responses using *in vivo* methods on animal models (see Section 3.2)
- Determination of allergenic properties using clinical methods while diagnosing patients, e.g., using skin prick tests; patch tests (PRICK); challenge tests which involve placing antigens on mucosa of the nasal cavity, oral cavity, labia, or the stomach; open food challenge tests; and DBPC challenge tests (see Section 3.3)

## 3.1 DESCRIPTION OF PHYSICOCHEMICAL AND BIOCHEMICAL METHODS USED FOR ASSAYS ON ALLERGENIC COMPONENTS IN FOOD PRODUCTS

Lucjan Jędrychowski

Qualitative and the quantitative analyses of food allergens are essential because of the health risk they pose to food consumers (particularly to those who suffer from allergenic hypersensitivity). As most allergens are proteins, glyco- or lipoproteins, traditional protein determination assays can help examine their biochemical properties. Classical methods used for studying proteins include

Physicochemical methods

- Kjeldahl nitrogen assay
- Nephelometry
- Colorimetry
- Chromatography (SEC, ion-exchange chromatography, affinity chromatography, HPLC, FPLC)
- Electrophoresis (SDS-PAGE, capillary electrophoresis, 2D-electrophoresis)
- Spectrophotometry
- Mass spectrometry
- PCR (specific DNA for allergen)

Immunological methods

- Counterelectrophoresis
- Immunoblotting
- Immunodiffusion
- Enzyme-linked immunosorbent assay (ELISA)
- Enzyme-linked immunospot assay (ELISPOT)
- Radioimmunoassay

The classical approach to preliminary protein purification (including allergens) includes its desalting from previously prepared crude extracts using $(NH_4)_2SO_4$. This is followed by dialysis and subsequent purification.

Enhanced analytical methods contribute to improved quality control processes and better quality of food products. In short, they contribute to health safety of consumers. Immunochemical methods enable determination of micro-quantities down to trace amounts of various food components (including allergens which can be a threat to health or, in extreme cases, life of consumers).

However, we need to emphasize that although the *in vitro* determination methods used for detection of food allergens are highly sensitive and precise, their role is mainly auxiliary—they help us learn more about food allergens.

To this day, numerous groups of allergens have been defined, including complex proteins, their derivatives, and haptens—a type of food additives.

The diversity of biological material (matrix) that contains allergens and allergenic compounds means that detection methods and analytical tests need to be equally diverse. Current assays on allergens should account for the fact that allergens are now defined more completely. Previously, a factor causing allergenic response was defined as a food product which caused such a reaction (e.g., allergy to milk, eggs, fish, or nuts, etc.). Later, the factors responsible for unwanted reactions were specified more precisely (e.g., by referring to the proteins present in these food products: $\alpha$-lactalbumin, $\beta$-lactoglobulin, $\alpha_s$-casein, $\alpha_{s1}$-casein, $\beta$-casein, and ovomucoid). Today, allergens are defined as particular epitopes of proteins (e.g., 15 IgE and 10 IgG epitopes have been defined in $\beta$-casein, 4 IgE epitopes in $\alpha$-lactoalbumin-Bos d 4, 14 IgE and 5 IgG epitopes in lactoglobulin—Bos d 5, and 1 IgE epitope in bovine blood serum albumin—Bos d 6) (Sharma et al., 2001).

In order to correctly design analytical procedures used for the detection of food allergens, it is necessary to have basic knowledge of food product chemistry; to know how to collect, prepare, and store food samples; to be able to fragment, mix, disintegrate, and extract samples; to know (or be able to find quickly) relevant food quality standards and admissible contents of particular food ingredients; and finally to understand precision of determinations, their sensitivity, and detection threshold levels, reproducibility, and errors of determination methods. In addition, it is essential to be able to gather the results of assays, process them with the aid of a computer and statistical methods, and to present the analytically derived data.

### 3.1.1 PRELIMINARY SEPARATION AND INITIAL PURIFICATION OF SAMPLES

Preliminary separation and purification of samples can considerably modify the properties of products thus obtained. Therefore, these two stages should be limited to the necessary minimum, in compliance with good laboratory practice.

Obtaining and purifying an allergen is extremely important but can sometimes be difficult due to the nature of allergens (solubility, stability, resistance to enzymes) and because allergens, which are natural food components, occur in very complex combinations (proteins, fats, carbohydrates, minerals) and in complex spatial structures (storage, structural, enzymatic proteins, etc.). This is compounded by the potentially destructive nature of some food ingredients (e.g., acidity, salinity) and processing conditions (i.e., heat and pressure), which make detection of allergens a real challenge to the analyst. For quantitative determination of allergens (which is essential for establishing their threshold amounts or the lowest adverse effect level), solubility and extractability are important. Detection of a range of food allergen residues in food products can be difficult, as most of the current methods detect them individually. Besides, residues in food products appear in various physical forms, for example, some are readily soluble (eggs, milk), easily dispersed (fish, crustaceans), or come in the form of flours (wheat, buckwheat), and as such are less of a sampling concern than food fragments (nuts, sesame seeds), which require larger samples and more homogenization.

Nonsoluble allergens are highly difficult to assay. Any attempt at achieving increased solubility of a particular allergen can lead to some modification in its allergenic properties. On the other hand, when determining soluble allergens, we need to take into account all physicochemical and technological parameters which can affect the extent to which we can separate the allergenic factor (degree of fragmentation, type of a solvent, its pH, ionic strength, temperature, mixing, mutual quantitative ratios of the solvent and substrate, number of times the solvent has been used, extraction methods, stability of proteins while being desalted using dialysis).

The preliminary protein extraction stage (extracting allergens from a matrix in which they are present) is crucial for the validity of a given test, a fact which can be supported by the results on determination of immunoreactivity of gluten proteins, especially in foodstuff modified with physicochemical methods and subjected to hydrothermal processes (Wieser, 1998; Rumbo et al., 2001; Hoebler et al., 2002; Partridge et al., 2003). The solvents traditionally employed for extraction of gliadins with Osborn method (Osborne, 1907) (aqueous solutions of 40%–70% of ethanol or methanol) have proved to be less effective on samples of thermally processed foods. In such cases, and in all other assays, selecting proper extraction solvent is absolutely essential. At present, a mixture of guanidine hydrochloride (a chaotrop) with 2-mercaptoethanol (a reductor) is a recommended solvent for quantitative extraction of gluten proteins from samples of thermal processed food (Hischenhuber et al., 2006).

Improved extractability of gluten proteins from thermally processed food products, due to the formation of carbohydrate–protein bonds, can be attained by using preliminary digestion of samples with glucoamylase or α-amylase (Partridge et al., 2003). However, such modification of analytical tests can cause a change in the properties of allergenic proteins.

The analytical problem becomes more complicated when complex proteins, glyco- or lipoproteins are a cause of allergenic response. As most of allergens are proteins, which are subject to different posttranslational modifications, of which glycosylation and phosphorylation are the most common ones, conventional biochemical methods used in research on glyco- and lipoproteins comprise the most suitable analytical techniques for description of these allergens.

Analysis of glycoproteins (e.g., a major soybean allergen, Gly m Bd 30 K, which is an N-linked glycoprotein) (Bando et al., 1996) is rather difficult and involves specific methods (Gates et al., 2004). Most often, analysis of the glycan structure of glycoproteins and the peptide portion of glycoproteins normally requires enzymatic or chemical methods of deglycosylation. In studies on the allergenic characteristics of glycoproteins, removal of the carbohydrate residue can either cause a change in the specificity of the epitope or lead to the removal of carbohydrate epitopes from antigens (Gates et al., 2004).

The use of ConA affinity chromatography in SDS has proved to be very useful for glycoprotein analysis because it combines complete dissociation of the glycoproteins from associated components with a rapid, specific, and high yield method of isolation. Most importantly, the glycoproteins reform the complex after displacement of SDS by nonionic detergent (Bando et al., 1996; Li et al., 1999).

Similar problems occur when analyzing lipoproteins.

The difficulties mentioned above, along with an increasing importance of precise determination of allergens in food products stimulated by legal regulations, mean that specific application procedures are needed for each stage of extraction, purification, and analysis of allergens, which will guarantee the required reproducibility and repeatability (within and between, for example, operators, days, laboratories, food industry plants) and robustness of sample preparation and immonoassay processes, thus improving food safety to consumers. (Goodwin, 2004; Poms et al., 2004). Identification and control of hazards posed by food allergens should be an ongoing process, integrated into the existing food quality management systems and critical control points (HACCP) system.

Currently available reagent kits, which help to remove impurities (such as nucleic acids, lipids, and carbohydrates) but which do not modify properties of proteins while detecting even trace amounts of proteins in samples, enable analysts to obtain pure proteins. Such kits are often used to prepare proteins for their separation using 2D electrophoresis, which is typically a preliminary step in the proteomics research methods.

### 3.1.1.1  General Description of Methods Used for Purification of Allergens

Nearly all physical methods of analysis are applicable to examine allergenic compounds, which are predominantly proteins, polypeptides, their lipid or carbohydrate derivatives, and, less often, hapten compounds (e.g., food additives or plant ingredients responsible for contact type allergies). When assessing allergenic properties of new food and biotechnical products, including the ones produced via genetic modifications, many analytical methods are applied simultaneously (Metcalfe et al., 1996; Konig et al., 2004; Goodman and Helfe, 2005). Because of the dynamic progress in analytical techniques, it is recommendable to continually update analytical procedures according to the guidelines proposed by international organizations (FAO/WHO, 2001; Codex Alimentarius Commission, 2003).

Light, fluorometric, electronic emission, and confocal absorption microscopy techniques or their combinations with immunometric techniques are applicable to analysis of allergenic compounds regarding the structure of a product—its matrix). Cells and metabolites produced by the immune system cells involved in the allergenic response (specific types of lymphocytes) can be examined by flow cytometry techniques in addition to traditional microscopic techniques.

Chromatography, and especially solid–liquid chromatographic techniques, can be broadly used for analysis of food allergens, mainly as a tool for preparatory separation of food ingredients. High performance liquid chromatography (HPLC) and fast protein liquid chromatography (FPLC) which take advantage of gel carriers, ion-exchange carriers, and chemical affinity with an application of isocratic and gradient elution are particularly useful as they enable analysts to examine compounds in a state closer to the native one, which is quite an important analytical factor for evaluation of immunoreactive or allergenic properties. The preparatory character of the chromatographic methods ensures good purification of an allergen, which means that once it has been standardized, the allergen can serve as a standard in diagnostic kits, although the use of pure allergen molecules has led to a clearly higher sensitivity of the immunoglobulin E immunoassay compared to conventional allergen extracts (Lidholm et al., 2006). Other useful methods, which have provided much information on analyzed proteins, are isoelectrofocusing, electrophoresis under native and denaturing conditions (SDS-PAGE), and two-direction capillary electrophoresis.

When taking into account the nature of effects produced by allergens during assays, it seems recommendable to use a combination of the above methods with blotting (DOT-blotting, Western blotting), affinity chromatography, SDS-PAGE electrophoresis, two-direction (2D) electrophoresis with immunoblotting (Beyer et al., 2002; Szabo et al., 2002).

At present, there are advanced difference gel electrophoresis (DOGE) Systems and 2-D fluorescence difference gel electrophoresis (2-D DIGE) which enable the analyst to use simultaneously modern (more precise) methods of fluorescent analysis with 2-D electrophoresis (using internal patterns), aided by a fully integrated bioinformatics system. Such systems allow more complete differential protein analysis, while the application of internal standards eliminates differentiation between the intervals, thus ensuring that even the smallest differences will be detected irrespective of the multitude of components. This guarantees reproducibility of results and their statistical reliability. Such assays are one of the platforms employed in the research based on the proteomics method.

### 3.1.1.2  Characteristic of the Methods Used for the Determination of Allergens *In Vitro*

Assays performed with proteomics methods combined with immunoblotting are believed to play an important role in recognition of epitopes responsible for causing allergenic reactions (Beyer et al., 2002).

Determination of a linear sequence of amino acids, especially in the area of epitopes, is an important part in characterization of allergens (FAO/WHO, 2001). Although the reactions between an antibody and an antigen (allergen) are largely affected by conformation epitopes, i.e., spatial structures of proteins, the linear sequence of amino acids should not be neglected as it enables preliminary identification of similarities between this sequence and potential allergenicity of products obtained via biotechnological processes or genetic modification (GMO) (Metcalfe et al., 1996; FAO/WHO, 2001; Codex Alimentarius Commission, 2003; Goodman and Hefle, 2005; Goodman et al., 2005).

Studies on linear epitopes can be facilitated by using amino acids analyzers and sequentators, e.g., an Edman sequentator. Progress in analytical methods has brought about a situation in which mass spectrometry is used for determination of the properties of proteins, including allergens, which are initially separated using 2D electrophoresis or chromatography.

Combination of mass spectrophotometry with other analytical methods, e.g., 2-D electrophoresis, SDS-PAGE, capillary zone electrophoresis (CZE), HPCL, and FPLC or a combination of spectrophotometers into the so-called MS-MS tandems, provides additional information and enables us to identify compounds at even much lower concentrations.

Mass spectrophotometry competes with Edman degradation method as a protein sequencing method which enables researchers to identify posttranslational modifications or analysis of endogenous compounds which occur in very low concentrations. For amino acid sequencing, the initial step most often consists of electrophoretic separation of proteins. Spot assays on material obtained through enzymatic hydrolysis of allergens using sera of allergy patients are used to study structures of linear epitopes. An example of how this method can be applied is characterization of eight food allergens which possess the highest allergy-causing potential (e.g., eggs) and its application for the determination of the smallest fragments that are able to cause an allergenic response, i.e., informative epitopes (Mine and Rupa, 2003; Jarvinen et al., 2007) (Section 3.4 discusses this problem in more detail).

One example of practical application of the above solution involves determination of allergens in sesame seeds, for which 2-D electrophoresis and Edman degradation methods have been employed (Beyer et al., 2002) (Section 3.4 contains more information on this issue).

The up-to-date methods for protein and peptide assays, including the ones which guarantee easy protein sequencing, have enabled researchers, aided by bioinformatics techniques, to use the data collected as described above in order to assess potential allergenicity on the basis of comprehensive allergen databases (Doolittle, 1990; Gendel, 1998; Gendel, 2002; Hileman et al., 2002; Zorzet et al. 2002; Goodman, 2006). Besides, determination of the sequence of amino acids in an allergen is necessary if we want to obtain it using genetic recombination techniques, which is becoming as one of the prerequisites in the process of registration of a new allergen in a database (Section 3.4 and Chapter 4 focuses on this problem in more detail).

At present, in many parts of the world there are integrated protein assay systems, which are very useful, both in studies on amino acid sequences in peptides and in genetic engineering—in investigations on genes and genetic expression products, and in biopharmaceutical research (designing and manufacturing new pharmaceuticals). Such systems rely on well-developed bioinformatics systems. Examples include a mass spectrophotometer matrix-assisted laser desorption (MALD), mass spectrophotometer—matrix-assisted laser desorption ionization-time of flight (Ettan MALDI-ToF Pro) with a fully integrated and automatic search engine of the database, both in the area of "peptide mass fingerprint" (PMF) and "Post-source decay" (PSD), for identification of proteins. The whole set of equipment is additionally perfected by a range of innovative reagents (e.g., chemically assisted fragmentation kit, CAF, or Ettan CAF-MALDI sequencing kit, which are helpful while analyzing samples in proteomics studies. Introduction of these reagent kits prevents the occurrence of interface residues and provides quick (available in a few minutes) and precise (down to one amino acid residue) information on a protein sequence. Proteins obtained with this method undergo trypsin hydrolysis, and the hydrolysates are analyzed as ions using a MALDI-ToF mass spectrophotometer. A combination of a CAF unit with relatively inexpensive pieces of equipments, such as a MALDI PSD, can possibly replace (and in the future, owing to much lower costs, completely eliminate) such complex and expensive tools as an MS/MS (Q-ToF type) tandem or a MALDO ToF.

The possibilities of application of far-UV circular dichroism (CD) and Fourier transform infrared (FTIR) spectroscopy in analysis of thermal stability of proteins and structural changes within protein molecules as well in explanation of cross reactivity between food allergens have been described in more detail in Section 3.4. Likewise nuclear magnetic resonance (NMR), especially 2D and multidimensional NMR as well as the method based on diffraction of monochromatic x-rays widely used in examination of tertiary structures of allergens have been described in Section 3.4 and by Neudecker et al. (2001) and Schirmer et al. (2005).

Methods such as size-exclusion chromatography (SEC), differential scanning calorimetry (DSC), atomic force microscopy (AFM), or analytical ultracentrifugation (AUC) with a density gradient can be very useful in the determination of homogeneity and aggregation of food allergens, e.g., of potato (Koppelman et al., 2002). Apart from studies on allergens and their epitopes, the above methods are applicable to examinations of structures of lymphatic cell receptors and spatial structures of the product's matrix (Koppelman et al., 2002). Recently, for determination of protein structure, attention has been paid to their changeability in a dynamic pattern.

Protein structures and protein structural models are very useful tools for grasping functional properties of proteins, understanding their biological functions, and providing the information that is very useful for recognition of the mechanisms of interaction between an antigen (an allergen) and its antibody (Aalberse, 2000; Aalberse and Stapel, 2001; Bornot et al., 2007) (Section 3.4 contains more details on allergenic protein structures and methods of analyzing the physical structures of allergens).

It has been found out that the structure of proteins is flexible and there are many differences between the static spatial image of a protein and a dynamic view of its structure. This divergence is caused by the fact that the repetitive part of α-helices and β-strands of protein folds, often described as a succession of secondary structures, can assume different local spatial orientation. Two experimental methods can be used to measure "the flexibility" in precise regions of protein structures (the anatomic mean square displacement, B-factor, measured during crystallographic experiments, and indirectly by NMR experiments which show different local conformation that could correspond directly to different stages of protein structures) (Bornot et al., 2007).

Cutting-edge bioinformatics methods and several bioinformatics tools (e.g., MED.-SuMo software package) as well as other bioinformatics programs which rely on databases (Bornot et al., 2007) can help to clarify complex issues related with the flexibility of protein structures. All the above factors, including the role of external environment, which affect the spatial structure of proteins should be taken into consideration when studying allergens. Analysis of allergenic compounds and product matrix structures can be aided by light microscopy techniques, using fluorescent markers, and electron emission, absorption, or confocal microscopy, or other solutions which combine any of the above techniques with immunodetection methods, including the ones which involve colloidal silver or gold markers (e.g., studies on cereal grain proteins).

Beside conventional microscopic techniques, flow cytometry methods, including intracellular staining, can be applied to assays of lymphocytes and other immune system cells engaged in producing allergenic reactions as well as their metabolites. The current technical solutions guarantee rapid analysis and enable the analyst to sort multiple subpopulations of lymphocytes using 8–12 colors along with two scatter parameters (Schmid and Giorgi, 1995; Baumgarth and Roederer, 2000; Herzenberg et al., 2002; Roederer et al., 2004).

The major weakness of traditional analytical chemistry and biochemistry techniques, such as spectroscopy and chromatography, is that they can be labor intense, costly, and time consuming.

### 3.1.2   General Characteristics of Immunometric Methods

Stricter food quality requirements as well as the obligation to inform food consumers about possible allergy risk (in order to ensure health safety) have made immunodetection methods (applied next to PCR and real-time PCR methods) more commonplace in food research.

Immunodetection (immunochemical) methods take into advantage the naturally occurring bond between an antigen and the antibody produced to combat this antigen. Immunoassay plays an important role in food analysis, clinical observation, or serum diagnosis, and is well known (Hage et al., 1999; Hirsch et al., 2003; Nichkova et al., 2005). The effectiveness of any immunoassay depends on many factors, such as the type of an antigen and how it was obtained (the way it was separated and purified), the method applied, and the quality of the antibodies used for capture and detection of a given allergen. A proper bank of specific antibodies is needed to carry out studies on allergens and allergies based on immunoassays. Polyclonal antibodies (characterized by affinity to several epitopes) and more specific monoclonal antibodies as well as recombined antibodies are helpful in studies on allergens (Lee and Morgan, 1993). It is also possible to use specific products of biodegradation of antibodies with appropriate enzymes (Ishikawa et al., 1983), hybridoma antibodies, next generation of monoclonal antibodies with high efficiency (Tomita, 2008) or, in place of antibodies, aptamers, or aptazymes (Alexander, 2007).

Progress in biotechnology and immunology has made it possible to use such tools for immunoassays as fragments of antibodies as (Ishikawa et al., 1983; Pierce Chemical Company, 1994)

- Hydrolysis products of IgG antibodies (150 kDa) using ficin
  - F(ab´)$_2$ (110 kDa) using immobilized Ficin at 1 mM cysteine or immobilized pepsin
  - 2 Fab (50 kDa) and Fc fragment (50 kDa) at 10 mM cysteine or immobilized papain

By hydrolyzing class M immunoglobulin (Pierce Chemical Company, 1994), it is possible to obtain such products as

- F (ab´)$_2$ (150 kDa)
- Fab (45 kDa)
- Fv (25 kDa) with immobilized pepsin
- IgG type (200 kDa)
- rIgG (110 kDa)
- Inverted IgG (mouse)

with 2-MEA-HCl

- F(ab´)$_2$ IgG (150 kDa)
- Fc5µ- H (340 kDa)
- IgG type M (200 kDa)
- Fab-H (45 kDa)

with immobilized trypsin.

Each of these products has specific properties and thus is applicable to specific assays (Pierce Chemical Company, 1994).

With biotechnological modifications (which use genetic engineering techniques), it is possible to obtain antibodies which are characterized by different ratios of proteins from different animal species. Evolution of the humanization process in mouse mAb production enables us to obtain antibodies of

- Ordinary mouse—100% of mouse protein
- Chimeric—34% of mouse protein and 66% of human protein
- Humanized—10% of mouse protein and 90% of human protein
- Xenomouse—100% of human protein

These antibodies are of greater importance in clinical studies than in the analysis of antigenic properties of food products.

Sensitivity of immunoassays is largely conditioned by markers applied for conjugation with the antibody. Traditional immunodetection methods ELISA with radioactive markers (radioimmunoassay—RIA), enzymatic markers (enzyme immunoassays—EIA), or fluorescent markers (fluoroenzyme immunoassays FEIA) are currently the most widely used techniques in laboratory analysis of allergens as well as in clinical studies for determination of general and specific IgE and other subclasses of immunoglobulines, e.g., IgG4 in the Immuno-CAP system (Samson, 2001; Duran-Tauleria et al., 2004; Lidholm et al., 2006).

Because radionuclides used as markers have many drawbacks, they are more and more often replaced by enzymatic markers (horseradish peroxidase, alkaline phosphatase, glucose oxidase, $\beta$-galactosidase). In order to enhance the sensitivity of determinations, fluorescent markers have been introduced. Another solution relies on avidin—biotin bonds.

Advances in production and characterization of new compounds which can serve as protein (antibody) markers have provided us with much wider applications.

Newer immunodetection applications, and particularly the so-called microarrays, employ new fluorescent probes such as europium chelates (Scorilas et al., 2000), lanthanide oxide nanoparticles (Dosev et al., 2005; Nichkova et al., 2006), fluorophore loaded latex beads (Orth et al., 2003), dye-doped silica nanoparticles (Zhou and Zhou, 2004; Yao et al., 2006), and inorganic nanocrystals (Gerion et al., 2003; Geho et al., 2005).

Among the fluorescent materials (fluorophores or fluorochromes) which can be detected through spectrofluorimeter methods and have become the main labels for generating fluorescent signals, the most common are such fluorescent dyes as Fluoroscein, Rhodamin RITC, Rhodamin XRITC, Texas Red, R-Phycoerythrin, Phyocyanin, Allophycocyanin, or the newer ones, characterized by better properties: PromoFluor, Alexa Fluor®, or Cy™ dyes which can be covalently coupled to amino acids, proteins, antibodies, affinity tags (e.g., biotin or streptavidin) as well as to hormones, sugars, dNTPs, oligonucleotides (Hilderbrand et al., 2005). It is also possible to use chemically modified fluorescent dyes, e.g., fluorescein (5-carboxyfluorescein, 6-carboxyfluorescein, 5(6)-carboxyfluorescein, 5-carboxyfluorescein, succinimidyl ester, 6-carboxyfluorescein, succinimidyl ester,

5(6)-carboxyfluorescein, succinimidyl ester) czy rhodamine (5-carboxytetramethyl-rhodamine, 6-carboxytetramethylrhodamine, 5(6)-Carboxytetramethylrhodamine). When selecting fluorescent markers, the analyst should take into consideration their properties.

Nanoparticles, e.g., silicon, gold, silver (Dequaire et al., 2000), are often used as materials for protein labeling in immunoassays, especially in lateral flow device (LFD), where they are responsible for visualization of the results. Their advantage lies in the fact that they enhance the optical signal, and reduce the background interference (Schneider et al., 2000; Lochner et al., 2003; Matveeva et al., 2005; Chumbimuni-Torres et al., 2006; Li et al., 1999; Peng et al., 2007a).

Colloidal gold or silver marking can also be used on a microscale in protein assays by electron scanning microcopy.

At present, there are many methodological solutions available in the field of immu-noassay (Rittenburg, 1990; Stepaniak et al., 1998; Stepaniak et al., 2002; Nichkova et al., 2007).

The most frequently applied methods are

- Direct competitive ELISA
- Indirect competitive ELISA
- Antibody class capture ELISA
- Two- or three-step methods employing secondary antibodies conjugated with appropriate markers
- Double antibody sandwich ELISA along with their modifications (Hefle et al., 1994) (Figure 3.1.1)
- Multiplexed (micro-immunoassays) (Blais et al., 2003; Nichkova et al., 2007)

Immuno-enzymatic methods make a large group of analytical methods with high sensitivity, specificity, and multitude of applications. Immunometric methods are simple to carry out. ELISA can be divided into two types of assays: noncompetitive and competitive ones. Last mentioned method may be direct or indirect depending on the kind of antibodies used in assay. Using competitive ELISA, reference labeled antibody and/or antigen are incubated with the sample. During incubation, they compete for limited quantity of the antigen or antibody bound to the solid phase of the microplate. The main steps in this assay are

- Coating the solid phase with an antigen
- Incubation with the test sample and reference antibody
- Incubation with an antiglobulin conjugate
- Incubation with an enzyme substrate
- Absorbance reading (Rittenburg, 1990)

High absorbance values indicate low antigen concentration in the test sample. Using a direct immunometric method usually comprises the following stages (Rittenburg, 1990):

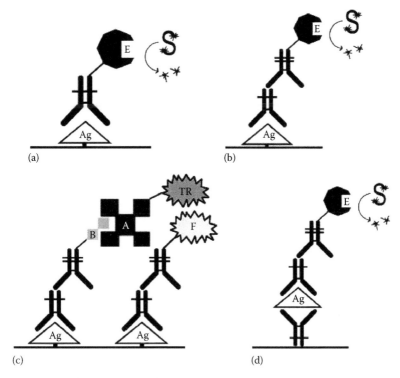

**FIGURE 3.1.1** (a) The principle of antigen determination by direct method; (b) two-stage indirect method; (c) double labeling with fluorometric markers; and (d) sandwich ELISA method. (From Jędrychowski, L., *Food Biotechnology*, 2nd edn., Bednarski, W. and Reps, A. (eds.), WNT, Warsaw, 464, 2003a (in Polish); Jędrychowski, L., *Pol. J. Food Nutr. Sci.*, 12/53(SI 2), 32, 2003b. With permission.)

- Combining antibodies with sample containing antigen and enzyme-conjugated antigen. In this operation, the antigen studied competes with the added conjugated antigen for binding with antibody
- Possible multiple washing with buffer solution (in heterogeneous methods).
- Adding substrate suitable for the marker–enzyme used in the reaction mixture (the amount of color product formed is proportional to the amount of antigen in sample)
- Absorbance reading

In an indirect two-step ELISA, major steps include

- Coating solid phase of microplate with serial dilutions of the reference antigen or with the test sample
- Incubation with primary antibodies
- Incubation with enzyme labeled secondary antibodies which attach to primary antibodies

- Incubation with enzyme substrate
- Absorbance reading

In an indirect double antibody sandwich ELISA, the major steps include (Figure 3.1.1)

- Coating solid phase with specific primary (from species first) antibodies
- Incubation with serial dilutions of reference antigen or sample antigen
- Incubation with constant amount of specific secondary antibodies (from species second)
- Incubation with enzyme labeled anti-secondary antibodies (conjugate)
- Incubation with the enzyme substrate
- Absorbance reading

Between each step of the assay, careful washing is done using PBS-T buffer.

Among the immunological methods which use amplifying markers with high mutual affinity, i.e., avidin–biotin and streptavidin–biotin, the ones most often applied methods are

- Labeled avidin–biotin (LAB)
- Bridged avidin–biotin (BRAB)
- Avidin–biotin complex (ABC)—the most sensitive of all avidin–biotin methods (Figure 3.1.2)

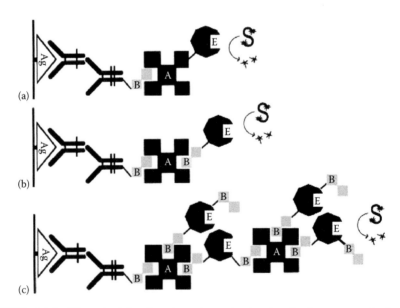

**FIGURE 3.1.2** The principle of antigen determination by the immune methods with avidin–biotin signal amplification. (a) Labeled avidin–biotin assay (LAB assay); (b) Bridged avidin–biotin assay (BRAB assay); and (c) Avidin–biotin complex method (ABC assay). (From Jędrychowski, L., *Pol. J. Food Nutr. Sci.*, 12/53(SI 2), 32, 2003b. With permission.)

Application of avidin–biotin amplification, and especially fluorescent markers, together with appropriate antibodies, makes it possible to determine simultaneously two antibodies occurring in a concentration of $10^{-21}$ M.

Such methods are used, for example, in detection of antibodies present in low concentrations (allergenic ingredients, various mediators generated by the immune system cells, interleukins, cytokines, IgE, IgG, IgA, IgG4) (Jędrychowski and Wróblewska, 1999; Hourihane et al., 2000; Davis et al., 2001; Szymkiewicz and Jędrychowski, 2002; Wróblewska and Jędrychowski, 2002a,b; Jędrychowski, 2003b), and enzymes (Forman, 1977).

Immunodetection methods find broad applications, but mainly when interactions between the antibody and the antigen (the allergen) are important, that is when assessing the possibilities of changing antigenic, immunoreactive properties, and either eliminating or drastically reducing the allergenicity of food products, mainly through various physical, enzymatic, technological, and biotechnological processes (Szymkiewicz and Jędrychowski, 2002; Wróblewska and Jędrychowski, 2002a,b; Szymkiewicz et al., 2003; Jędrychowski et al., 2005; Szymkiewicz and Jędrychowski, 2005; Wróblewska et al., 2005).

Using the ELISA (with avidin–biotin bridges) and ELISPOT methods a stimulating effect of selected probiotic bacteria (*Bifidobacterium longum, B animalis, Lactobacillus casei, L. salivarius*) on the immune system of the rat and mouse has been demonstrated (higher level of specific as well as total IgGa and IgA content) (Nagy et al., 2002).

A number of emerging methods such as fluorescence polarization immunoassays, dipsticks, or even newer methods such as biosensors have been used for rapid screening of mycotoxin (ochratoxin A and Fusarium toxins—fumonisins (FBs), moniliformin (MON), zearalenone (ZON), and type-A and -B trichothecenes in foods, fodders, blood, urea, and tissues of pigs after slaughter) (Curtui et al. 2001; Krska et al., 2007).

Immunoassays are extremely important in determination of the content of particular allergens in food, for example, Ara h 1 and Ara h 2 allergens in peanuts (Hefle, 2006), tree nuts and seeds in food (Koppelman, 2006), dairy and egg allergens as residues in food (Demeulemester and Giovannacci, 2006), soy, fish, and crustaceans in food (Koppelman, 2006), wheat gluten in food (Janssen, 2006).

The ELISA method (in its various modifications), employing radionuclide markers (radioimmunoassay RIA), enzymatic markers (enzyme immunoassay EIA) (Dill et al., 2006), or fluorescent dyes (fluorophores or fluorochromes) (Hildebrand et al., 2005) (FEIA—fluoroenzyme immunoassay, Immuno-CAP-system) or nanoparticles (Dequaire et al., 2000) are commonly used as materials for protein labeling in an immunoassay.

Enzyme immunoassay and fluoroenzyme immunoassay are often used in clinical studies to determine general and specific IgE and, owing to flow cytometry, in analyzing subpopulations such as T and B lymphocytes, the immune system cells participate in the immunological reaction of the organism to food antigens (including allergens) (Fest, 2008).

The immunoassays (Dot-blot, immunoblotting, ELISA) are often applied in combinations, for example, to characterize immunoreactive (allergenic) properties of fractions obtained via mechanical, electrophoretic (SDS-PAGE, 2-D), or chromatographic separations of proteins (Jędrychowski and Wróblewska, 1999; Hourihane et al., 2000; Davis et al., 2001, Deyer et al., 2002; Szabo et al., 2002; Szymkiewicz and Jędrychowski, 2002; Wróblewska and Jędrychowski, 2002a,b; Jędrychowski, 2003b). Under specific circumstances, it is recommendable to support immunoassays by methods which enable us to broaden our knowledge or to accelerate the results, for example, by employing surface plasmon resonance (SPR) methods, used in multichannel microprocessor analysators (SPR-BIACORE, 2000), the circular dichroism method (CD) or using a mass spectrometer MALDI-ToF, or else by additional studies on protein structures or their fragments.

Chemiluminescence immunoassay methods have many applications (Weeks, 1992). Highly sensitive chemiluminescent immunoassays were developed by Tsuji et al. (1989) for determination of enzymes (oxidases, peroxidase, glucose oxidase, $\beta$-D-galactosidase) as well as various hormones and drugs in biological fluids (Tsuji et al., 1989).

The above analytical solutions are used in the ELISPOT method, dot-bolt, and immunoblotting (Masseyeff et al., 1993; Bednarski and Reps, 2003; Jędrychowski, 2003) and in analytical systems used for clinical diagnostic purposes (Clinical Laboratory International, 2005).

The ELISPOT method can be commonly applied to determination of metabolites (e.g., cytokines) produced by cells in minute quantities.

One more interesting immune method applied in food allergens analysis is immunoblotting. It comprises the following stages: electrophoresis, transfer of separated protein onto the nitrocellulose membrane, and determination of immunoreactive proteins with the use antibodies and conjugates using some kind of immunometric method (Figures 3.1.1 and 3.1.2). The dot-blot and immunoblotting are most often employed for rapid tests of the interaction between allergenic proteins (most frequently, separated by electrophoresis) and sera of persons suffering from allergenic hypersensitivity.

Immunometric methods find increasingly wide applications owing to their superiority and continuous improvements. One of the major advantages of immunometric methods is that they provide consumers with early information (prior to food consumption) on possible health hazards (allergenic characteristics) of specific food products. The sensitivity of immunoassays is largely dependent on the type of a compound subject to analysis (up to 10 pg/mL of the analyte).

Possible obstacles to using immunoassays are created by environmental factors, such as pH, temperature, or other food product ingredients, e.g., endogenous enzymes whose specificity is similar to the specificity of the enzyme present in the conjugate, colorings present in a given samples can interfere with the color obtained from the enzyme–substrate reaction, phenolic compounds which can adsorb proteins.

Currently, the methods based on immunoassays are improved by introducing new analytical solutions (Dequaire et al., 2000; Dequaire et al., 2002; Blais et al., 2003; Hildebrandt et al., 2005; Dill et al., 2006; Nichkova et al., 2007) and miniaturizing analytical elements (Bannon et al., 2008; Wolbers et al., 2006a,b). The underlying objectives are to increase the sensitivity of the assays, to broaden the range of applications, and to simplify the analytical protocols. An attempt to replace radioactive or enzymatic markers by a method of direct measurement of intermolecular interactions using a system of biomolecular interaction detection (BIND) which involves photonic crystalline biosensors could be a good example here (Cunningham and Laing, 2008).

Extensive progress has been attained in determination techniques. Noteworthy is the broad applicability of a homogenic method known as the TRACE method (time-resolved amplified cryptate emission). Another interesting solution, TSA (tyramide signal amplification), employs a technique which amplifies the tyramide signal (Bednarski and Reps, 2003).

Today's analytical procedures are much easier to conduct owing to a broad range of commercially available test kits for analysis of food allergens. Point of care (POC) tests are at present widely used in clinical analysis, for example, to determine allergens. Precise diagnosis of atopic illnesses can be achieved with FastCheckPOC® tests, which rely on identification of allergen-specific IgE antibodies in the patient's blood. POC assays enable rapid and simultaneous qualitative or half-quantitative determination of 12 food allergens (or 12 inhalatory allergens with another kit of POC tests).

POC assays can be done quickly. Another advantage is that they can be performed on very small amounts of blood (2–3 drops of blood collected from a finger pulp), serum, or a blood sample taken earlier for EDTA or heparin tests.

The filtering membrane in the FastCheckPOC system is a carrier of allergenic extracts. After 15 min incubation, the blood dilution is rinsed off and the specific IgE bound to the membrane is detected using a half-quantitative method and chromogenic substrate. The whole analytical procedure takes about 30 min. A positive result, seen as a + sign on the membrane, means that the titer of the specific IgE antibodies in the patient's blood is above class 2. When the results obtained with FastCheckPOC tests were compared with the ones produced by the Pharmacia UniCAP system, the correlation between positive results reached 96% and that of negative results was as high as 98% in 313 cases analyzed (Runge et al., 2005).

The comparison of the sIgE titers revealed a good concordance between other methods—the Centaur and the UniCAP tests, for example—for egg (f1), cod (f3), and peanut (f13) (94%, 91%, and 96% respectively). However, the concordance was lower for cow milk (f2), wheat (f4), and soy bean (f14) (76%, 77%, and 77% respectively) because of discrepancies between the two techniques (Contin-Bordes et al., 2007).

A special POC food intolerance test (antigen-specific IgG test) has been prepared to account for an increasing incidence of food intolerance implied in different disease states. It can detect a total of 57 different antibodies. There are possibilities to analyze more than 150 different components or antigens from about 20 μL of sample using a biochip-based allergy test (ImmunoCAP ISAC) (Samson, 2001; Duran-Tauleria et al., 2004; Lidholm et al., 2006).

Observing recent advances in applying immunometrical methods in medical science and their increasing role in food industry and quality control, we have to take into account equally dynamic application of immunometric methods in food analysis.

### 3.1.3   NEW TENDENCIES IN ANALYSIS OF ALLERGENS: BIOSENSORS IN PROTEIN AND ALLERGEN ANALYSIS

In the recent years, analytical techniques used for detection of proteins, peptides, and their derivatives have relied more and more heavily on methods employing biosensors and atomic force microscopy, which rely on the determination of changes in electrochemical or spectral parameters occurring under the influence of incorporate biological probes coupled to an appropriate transducer (Wasowicz et al., 2008). Biosensors, according to Sharma et al. (2003), are analytical devices incorporating biological materials such as enzymes, tissues, microorganisms, antibodies, cell receptors or biologically derived materials, or a biomimic component intimately associated with or integrated within a physicochemical transducer or transducing microsystem, which may be either optical, electrochemical, thermometric, piezoelectric, or magnetic. The electronic signals produced are proportional to the concentration of specific analyte (biomolecules).

An essential component of a molecular sensor consists of reagent layers. Creation of these layers requires the immobilization of recognition elements for the detection method (Sharma et al., 2003).

Immunosensors, a group of biosensors, similarly to immunodetection methods, are analytical devices based on the antigen–antibody binding reaction providing a concentration-dependent response to the analyte (antigen) of interest. The application of nanotechnology to immunosensors design and fabrication, which makes it possible to immobilize the biomolecules without losing their biological activities, opens up a promising vista for revolutionary diagnostics and therapeutic solutions at the molecular and cellular levels (Gu et al., 2001; Szymanska et al., 2007).

The most critical issue in preparing an immunosensor is the immobilization of an antibody on the support surface. Therefore, preparing an underlying layer that prevents loss of the antibody activity is of great importance (Wasowicz et al., 2008). The above methods is extensively applicable to clinical studies, including tests on allergens.

An example of the application of immunodetection methods and biosensors in SPR. SPR is an optical technique based on the excitation of plasmons (a cloud of free electrons) in a dielectric (antigen–antibody or biolayer–analyte set) close to a gold surface. Excitation takes place by light from laser under different incident angles (Figure 3.1.3). At a specific angle (depending, among other factors, on the refractive index and, therefore, on the mass of bound proteins, biomolecules, on or close to the metal surface), all the energy from the photons is transferred to the free electrons in the metal surface, which leads to total attenuation of the light. The SPR method can also measure changes in the refractive index upon antigen–antibody binding. Having prepared binding curves, we can analyze parameters of the sensograms obtained with the SPR method, which enables us to determine the content of a given component or thermodynamic biding constants (de Mol et al., 2006). A sandwich format can be used to enhance the signal and increase the specificity of an assay. Currently, in order to improve the efficiency of determinations and scope of analytical procedures, two- (de Mol et al., 2006) or four-channel (Jonsson et al., 2006) systems are used. Such systems are most often used for series determinations because, having

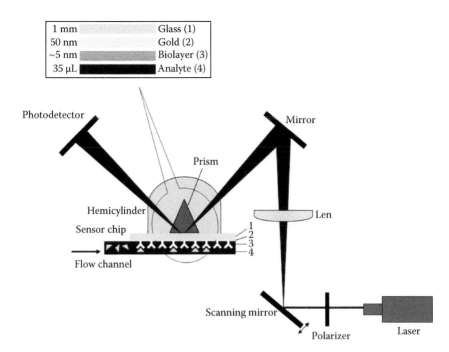

**FIGURE 3.1.3**   Principles of SPR method.

been regenerated, they can be reused many times. The SPR method has been broadly used in the food production industry (Mello and Kubota, 2002), for example, to test contamination of milk with antibiotics (Baxter et al., 2001), to determine veterinary residues in food products or presence of a staphylococcal enterotoxin B and vitamin $B_{12}$ (Medina, 2003).

Other applications involve detection of adulteration of dairy products with soy, pea, and wheat proteins (Haasnoot et al., 2001), presence of $\alpha_{S1}$-casein in milk (the detection threshold for this protein was 0.87 µg/mL) (Muller-Renaud et al., 2005), β-casein in milk and cheese (Muller-Renard et al., 2004), and detection of peanut allergenic proteins (the detection threshold for this protein was 0.7 µg/mL) (Mohammed et al., 2001).

Current advanced instrumentation and automation enable food processors to reduce the testing time and cost (Greg Cheng and Merchant, 1995), which means that new and numerous applications of the above methods that employ biosensors can be expected.

The applicability of biosensors in the food industry has been exhaustively discussed by Mello and Kubota (2002).

### 3.1.4   Applicability of Other Analytical Methods

A new type of label-free optical biosensor and the BIND system, similar to SPR, are described in detail by Cunningham and Laing (2008). These optical biosensors are based on unique properties of optical device structures known as "photonic crystals" (a patented solution). A surface photonic crystal is composed of a periodic arrangement of dielectric material, in which a low refractive index periodic surface structure made of plastic is overcoated with a high refractive index film of $TiO_2$. With proper choice of periodicity, symmetry, and material dielectric constants, the photonic crystal (sensor) will selectively couple energy at only one wavelength, which will be strongly reflected (Cunningham and Laing, 2008). The sensor, incorporated into standard 96, 384, and 1536-well microplate formats, operates by measuring changes in the peak wavelength value (PWV) of reflected light as biochemical binding events take place on the surface. The detection system is fast—operating in parallel, eight illumination/detection heads measure all the 96 wells in a microplate in ~15 s. Besides, it does not require markers. The system, compatible with standard liquid handling systems used in screening applications, utilizes single-use disposable biosensor labware and a simple, robust microplate reader instrument, which is configured for compatibility with robotic microplate handlers (Cunningham and Laing, 2008).

The system greatly reduces the assay development costs and offers simplicity and quantitative benefits of multistep monitoring. As such, it finds an increasingly broader use, for example, for label-free applications in drug discovery, to measure the effect of a small molecule interaction with the primary protein target, and to draw down cells specifically expressing cognate surface binding proteins, thus determining the functionality of an immunoprotein in complex media. In addition, because each step in the experiment provides quantitative information, an assessment of affinity for the immunoprotein can be made (Cunningham and Laing, 2008).

As we need to understand better, the molecular mechanisms responsible for allergenic reactions, we search for more precise analytical methods, which will enable us to define fragments of proteins, epitopes, which cause such reactions, as well as some lines of lymphocytes (mainly TH1, TH2, Treg, Th17) and metabolites these lymphocytes produce (these issues are discussed in greater detail in Chapter 1). As a result, methods used in molecular biology are becoming more useful. Introduction of some techniques of molecular biology in the field of allergen characterization has influenced both the methodology and the rate of identification of new allergens.

### 3.1.4.1 Microarray-Based Proteomics

Proteomic studies have been gaining importance over the past few years. The broad applicability of proteomics in large-scale analysis of proteins is stimulated by the advantages proteomic techniques create, including the possibility of rapid and thorough recognition of properties of polypeptides corresponding to spots obtained via 2-D electrophoretic protein separation. The development in proteomics and its increasing popularity in research have been achieved owing to such solutions as miniaturization, rapid determination techniques, automation, introduction of new tools such as monoclonal antibodies, and recombinant antibody microarray techniques (Borrebaeck and Wingren, 2007; Wingren and Borrebaeck, 2007). At present, proteomics can become very important in studies on allergens, especially on proteins obtained via expression of certain genes using genetic engineering techniques and protein posttranslational modification.

Proteomics and its possible applications for assessment of allergenicity of food products are described by Bannon et al. (2008), who draw attention to the fact that reproducibility of results obtained though proteomic techniques need to be improved by introducing more precise definitions of the parameters of technical determinations. Nonetheless, proteomics provides high-throughput methods for detection and characterization of proteins.

The broad use of proteomic studies and microarrays seems to prove that such diagnostic tests are useful in medicine and research on allergens, allergies, and other human diseases (Ellmark et al., 2008; Person et al., 2008). Likewise, miniaturization of analytical instruments, which profoundly enhances research potential, stimulates the development of these methods.

### 3.1.4.2   Miniaturization of Protein Arrays

In the 1970s, this tendency to produce more miniature tests led to the creation of new analytical systems—micro total analysis systems (uTAS), also known as lab-on-a-chip (LOC). Complete microsystems incorporated procedures of sample handling, analysis, and detection into a single device (Wolbers et al., 2006b). Capillary electrophoresis on the chip is an example of such a solution. Today, we witness the development of another miniature system, called the lab in a cell (LIC), which is mainly used for analysis of apoptosis (programmed cell death) in real time at a single-cell level (Wolbers et al., 2006a). The LIC technology uses the cell as a laboratory, in which complex biological operations can be performed. LIC requires appropriate micro- and even nanotechnological tools. It can greatly help to explain mechanisms involved in the occurrence of an allergenic reaction.

As such downscaling offers many advantages (such as smaller samples, less reagent use and less waste, faster analysis, lower cost, and integration of many analytical processes into one device), such solutions have found wide use in the life science research (in medical and biotechnical sciences, in proteomics, and in biotechnology). It can be expected, with large probability, that they will also be used for analysis of allergens and explanation of mechanisms involved in allergenic hypersensitivity reaction (in which the immunological mechanism is defined or strongly suspected).

Miniaturization of protein arrays (a carrier is often less than $1\,cm^2$ in size, and the diameter of spots of antibodies or antigens, carrying the desired specificity/biological function around $300\,\mu m$, whereas the density could be $<2000$ probes/$cm^2$, and the amount of the analyzed proteins is up to $1000/cm^2$; in addition, the quantities of reagents needed for the tests are very small, measured in pL or μL, and the assay sensitivity is expressed in pM to fM) makes them a very attractive research tool in proteomics.

The next step in miniaturization within proteomics is the development of protein nanoarrays. In nanoarrays of proteins, the size is within an $mm^2$ range, spot size (feature) is $3$–$1000\,nm$, and the array density (probes/$mm^2$) is $<1 \times 10^6/mm^2$. There are also some initial studies on attovial arrays, in which the miniaturization of the array components is beyond our imagination (e.g., attovial arrays use 6 (Ø 200 nm) to 4000 aL (Ø 5 μm) sized vials, at a density of 225 vials/$mm^2$ (tentative densities of 90,000–225,000 vials/$mm^2$) (Wolbers et al. 2006b).

Because protein microarrays (antibody microarrays) have been successfully used for a variety of applications, such as antibody response profiling, identification and detection of bacterial and protein analytes, as well as disease proteomics with a clear focus toward oncoproteomics, it can be assumed that they will also prove to be a useful tool in studies on allergens (Wingren and Borrebaeck, 2007).

It is estimated that by 2015, many *in vitro* diagnostic products (IVD) analyses for both the lab and point-of-care will be based on miniaturized and multiplexed technologies, for example, "chip" technologies (Kalorama, 2008; Matsson, 2008).

### 3.1.4.3   Aptamers and Aptazymes in Molecular Diagnostics and Biosensors

Aptamers—RNA or DNA oligomers that have been selected *in vitro* as sensitive detectors for defined target molecules—have recently emerged as an attractive method for the rapid development of highly specific and flexible diagnostic platforms. They are now well-established as an alternative to protein-based monoclonal antibodies detection techniques and will continue to facilitate a variety of novel biosensor technologies (Alexander, 2007).This technology has many advantages as aptamers and other functional nucleic acids (including aptazymes, which are aptamers linked to RNA enzymes, or ribozymes) are superior in many ways to antibodies in diagnostic applications (Alexander, 2007; Peng et al., 2007b).

Aptamers, as biosensors, find many applications. Possible aptamer ligands are proteins, other biological macromolecules, as well as the biological context in which these occur (i.e., viruses, bacteria, and eukaryotic cells). Aptamers can interact with small molecules such as metal ions and drugs, as well as primary and secondary metabolites (amino acids, nucleotides, sugars, peptides).

The *in vitro* procedure to select general aptamers includes choosing an appropriate target, a complex of aptamers, from the available (preferably the largest possible) nucleic acid library, using a suitable selection method (most often, affinity chromatography). The next stage consists of the regeneration of bound nucleic acid, PCR amplification, selection, and application (mainly as analytical microchips).

Another advantage of aptamers as biosensors is that they can be easily modified chemically, which offers ever broader applicability of assays based on these oligomers.

Future development of novel aptazyme technologies, in particular, those involving nanomaterials, will continue to drive the fields of diagnostics and biosensing toward more high-throughput platforms, as well as powerful new LOC devices (Alexander, 2007).

It is possible to apply SPR techniques to direct monitoring of intermolecular interactions in aptamer-target binding events, analogously to its use in studies on monoclonal antibodies (Misono and Kumar, 2005; Hwang and Nishikawa, 2006).

### 3.1.4.4   Atomic Force Microscopy

Also, atomic force microscopy (AFM) is used to characterize the binding of antigen/antibody on a molecular level (e.g., to select suitable materials for antigen immobilization), to characterize individual antigen/antibody complexes, and to investigate the mechanisms of specific antigen/antibody interactions, all of which are fundamentally important in the life sciences (Peng et al., 2007b, Browning-Kelley et al., 1997). In AFM studies, it has been demonstrated that a COOH-terminated surface can effectively immobilize proteins without sacrificing the bioreactivity and that it is possible to monitor antigen/antibody binding process *in situ* in real time via the AFM. Stable antigen/antibody complexes were observed in less than 4 min after the injection of an antibody, and such reactions cannot occur in the absence of a buffer (Browning-Kelley et al., 1997).

### 3.1.5 Conclusions

The knowledge originating from characterization of allergens is essential for constructing suitable databases on allergies and allergens. The development of such databases is mutually related to the progress in bioinformatics (which makes it possible to gather, store, retrieve, analyze, and utilize such data) as well as advances in analytical technologies (microarrays, large-scale screening technologies as well as development of genomics and proteomics), which generate a vast supply of increasingly complex allergy information (Brusic, 2006).

In the future, we can expect to witness further development of all these fields of research and science, which will certainly contribute to our better understanding of allergen as well as mechanisms of forming allergenic reactions. We should also be able to assess better cases of allergenicity, identify allergenic cross-reactivity, and offer more effective therapies (Brusic, 2006).

## REFERENCES

Aalberse, R.C. 2000. Structural biology of allergens. *J Allergy Clin Immunol.* 106:228–238.

Aalberse, R.C. and Stapel, S.O. 2001. Structure of food allergens in relation to allergenicity. *Pediatr Allergy Immunol* 12:10–14.

Alexander, C. 2007. Aptamers and aptazymes: An apt technology for molecular diagnostics and biosensors. *Clin Lab Int* 31, 7:40–41.

Bando, N., Tsuji, H., Yamanishi, R., Nio, N., and Ogawa, T. 1996. Identification of the glycosylation site of a major soybean allergen, Gly m Bd 30K. *Biosci, Biotechnol, Biochem* 60(2):347–348.

Bannon, G.A., Astwood, J.D., Dobert, R.C., and Fuchs, R.L. 2008. Biotechnology and genetic engineering. In: *Food Allergy Adverse Reactions to Foods and Food Additives*, 4th ed., D.D. Metcalfe, H.A. Sampson, and R.A. Simon, Eds., pp. 62–81. Blackwell Publishing, New York.

Baumgarth, N. and Roederer, M. 2000. A practical approach to multicolor flow cytometry for immunophenotyping. *J Immunol Methods* 243:77–97.

Baxter, G.A., Ferguson, J.P., O'Connor, M.C., and Elliot, C.T. 2001. Detection of Streptomycin residues in whole milk using an optical immunobiosensor. *J Agric Food Chem* 49(7):3204–3207.

Bednarski, W. and Reps, A. 2003. *Food Biotechnology*, W. Bednarski and A. Reps, Ed. Published by WNT (in polish).

Beyer, K., Bardina, L., Grishina, G., and Sampson, H.A. 2002. Identification of sesame seed allergens by 2-dimensional proteomics and Edman sequencing: Seed storage proteins as common food allergens. *J Allergy Clin Immunol* 110(1):154–159.

Bindslev-Jensen, C. 2001. Standardization of double-blind, placebo-controlled food challenges. *Allergy* 56(Suppl. 67):75–77.

Blais, B.W., Gaudereault, M., and Phillippe, L.M. 2003. Multiplex enzyme immunoassay system for the simultaneous detection of multiple allergens in foods. *Food Control* 14:43–47.

Bornot, A., Offmann, B., and de Brevern, A.G. 2007. How flexible are protein structure? New questions on the protein structure plasticity. *Bioforum Eur Trends Tech Life Sci Res.* 11:24–25.

Borrebaeck, C.A.K. and Wingren, C. 2007. High-throughput proteomics using antibody microarrays: An update. *Expert Rev Mol Diagn* 7:673–686.

Browning-Kelley, M.E., Wadu-Mesthrige, K., Hari, V., and Liu, G.Y. 1997. Atomic force microscopic study of specific antigen/antibody binding. *Langmuir*, 13: 343–350.

Brusic, V. 2006. Information management for the study of allergies. *Inflam Allergy—Drug Targets* 5(1):35–42.

Burks, W., Bannon, G., and Lehrer, S.B. 2001. Classic specific immunotherapy and new perspectives in specific immunotherapy for food allergy. *Allergy* 56(Suppl. 67):121–124.

Chumbimuni-Torres, K.Y., Dai, Z., Rubinova, N., Xiang, Y., Pretsch, E., Wang, J., and Bakker, E. 2006. Potentiometric biosensing of proteins with ultrasensitive ion-selective microelectrodes and nanoparticle labels. *J Am Chem Soc* 128(42):13676–13677.

Clinical Laboratory International—IgG4 ELISA to identify food intolerances. CLI. 2005. 29(2):33.

Codex Alimentarius Commission. 2003. Alinorm 03/34: Appendix III. Guideline for the conduct of food safety assessment of foods derived from recombinant DNA plants. Annex IV. Annex on the assessment for possible allergenicity, Rome, Italy.

Contin-Bordes, C., Petersen, A., Chahine, I., Boralevi, F., Chahine, H., Taïeb, A., Sarrat, A., Moreau, J.F., and Taupin, J.L. 2007. Comparison of ADVIA Centaur and Pharmacia UniCAP tests in the diagnosis of food allergy in children with atopic dermatitis. *Pediatr Allergy Immunol* 18(7):614–620.

Cunningham, B.T. Laing, L.G. 2008. Advantages and application of label-free detection assays in drug screening. *Expert Opinions in Drug Discovery* 3(8):891–901.

Curtui, V.G., Gareis, M., Usleber, E., and Artlbauer, E.M. 2001. Survey of Romanian slaughtered pigs for the occurrence of mycotoxins ochratoxins A and B, and zearalenone. *Food Addit Contaminants. Part A.* 18(8):730–738.

Davis, P.J., Smales, C.M., and James, D.C. 2001. How can thermal processing modify the antigenicity of proteins? *Allergy* 56(Suppl. 67):56–60.

de Mol, N.J., Fischer, M.J., Castrop, J., and Frelink, T. 2006. Determination by surface plasmon resonance of the binding characteristics of a kinase and its substrates. *BioTech Int Eur Mag Life Sci Industry.* 18(6):19–22.

Demeulemester, C. and Giovannacci, I. 2006. Detecting dairy and egg residues in food. In: *Detecting Allergens in Food.* S.J. Koppelman and S.L. Hefle, Eds. pp. 219–243. Woodhead Publishing Limited, Cambridge, England.

Dequaire, M., Degrand, Ch., and Limoges, B. 2000. An electrochemical metalloimmunoassay based on a colloidal gold label. *Electrosynthèse et Electroanalyse Bioorganique* UMR CNRS 6504.

Dequaire, M., Limoges, B., Moiroux, J., and Saveant, J.M. 2002. Mediated electrochemistry of horseradish peroxidase. Catalysis and inhibition. *J Am Chem Soc.* 124(2):240–253.

Dill, K., Ghindilis, A., and Schwarzkopf, K. 2006. Multiplexed analyte and oligonucleotide detection on microarrays using several redox enzymes in conjunction with electrochemical detection. *Lab on a Chip* 6(8):1052–1055.

Directive 2003/89/EC of the European Parliament and of the Council of November 10, 2003 amending Directive 2000/13/EC as regards indication of the ingredients present in foodstuffs; *Off J Eur Union* L 308/:15–18.

Directive 2007/68/EC. 2007. Amending Annex IIIa to Directive 2000/13/EC of the European Parliament and of the Council as regards certain food ingredients. Directives Commission. *Off J Eur Union* L 310/11.

Doolittle, R.F. 1990. Molecular evolution: Computer analysis of protein and nucleic acid sequences. In *Methods in Enzymology*, Vol. 183, R. F. Doolittle, Ed. Academic Press, Inc.: San Diego, Chapter 6.

Dosev, D., Nichkova, M., Mao Liu, Bing Guo, Gang-Yu Liu, Hammock, B.D., and Kennedy, I.M. 2005. Application of fluorescent Eu:Gd2O3 nanoparticles to the visualization of protein micropatterns. *J Biomed Opt* 10(6):064006.

Duran-Tauleria, E., Vignati, G., Guedan, M.J.A., and Petersson, C.J. 2004. The utility of specific immunoglobulin E measurements in primary care. *Allergy* 59:(Suppl. 78):35–41.

Ellmark, P, Woolfson, A, Belov, L., and Christopherson, R.I. 2008. The applicability of a cluster of differentiation monoclonal antibody microarrays to the diagnosis of human disease. In: *Genomic Protocols*, 2nd ed., M. Starkey and R. Elaswarapu, Eds., Humana Press, Totowa, NJ; *Meth Mol Biol* 439:199–209.

FALCPA. 2004 (Food Allergen Labeling Consumer Protection Act of 2004) at http://www.cfsan.fda.gov/~dms/alrgact.html

FAO/WHO. 2001. Joint FAO/WHO Expert Consultation on Allergenicity of Foods Derived from Biotechnology. Rome, Italy.

Fest, T. 2008. Flow cytometry—the key to automated, objective validation of abnormal samples. *Clin Lab Int* 32(3):24–26.

Food Standards Agency. 2006. Guidance on Allergen Management and Consumer Information at http://www.food.gov.uk/multimedia/pdfs/maycontainguide.pdf

Forman, D.T. 1977. Immunoassay of enzymes. *Ann Clin Lab Sci* 7(4):329–334.

Gates, R., Rathbone, E., Masterson, L., Wright, I., and Electricwala, A. 2004. *Glycoprotein Analysis Manual*, 1st ed., Sigma-Aldrich Co.: St Louis, MO.

Geho, D.H., Espina, V., Wulfkuhle, J., Petricoin, E.F., and Liotta, L.A. 2005. Biomarkers and surrogate markers. Protein pathway analysis in Clinical Proteomics using protein microarrays. *Drug Discov Today: Technol* 2(4):353–359.

Gendel, S.M. 1998. The use of amino acid sequence alignments to assess potential allergenicity of proteins used in genetically modified foods. *Adv Food Nutr Res* 42:45–62.

Gendel, S.M. 2002. Sequence analysis for assessing potential allergenicity *Ann NY Acad Sci* 964:87–98.

Gerion, D., Chen, F.Q., Kannan, B., Fu, A.H., Parak, W.J., Chen, D.J., Majumdar, A., and Alivisatos, A.P. 2003. Room-temperature single-nucleotide polymorphism and multiallele DNA detection using fluorescent nanocrystals and microarrays. *Anal Chem* 75(18): 4766–4772.

Goodman, R.E. 2006. Practical and predictive bioinformatics methods for the identification of potentially cross-reactive protein matches. *Mol Nutr Food Res* 50:655–660.

Goodman, R.E. and Hefle, S.L. 2005. Gaining perspective on the allergenicity assessment of genetically modified food crops. *Expert Rev Clin Immunol* 1(4):561–578.

Goodwin, P.R. 2004. Food allergen detection methods: A coordinated approach. *J AOAC Int* 87(6):1383–1390.

Greg Cheng, S.G. and Merchant, Z.M. 1995. Biosensors in food analysis. In *Characterization of Food. Emerging Methods* (Chapter 14), A.G. Gaonkar, Ed., pp. 329–345. Edition Elsevier B.V., London, U.K.

Gu, H.Y., Yu, A.M., and Chen, H.Y. 2001. Direct electron transfer and characterization of hemoglobin immobilized on a Au colloid–cysteamine-modified gold electrode. *J Electroanal Chem* 516:119–126.

Haasnoot, W., Olieman, K., Cazemier, G., and Verheijen, R. 2001. Direct biosensor immunoassays for the detection of nonmilk proteins in milk powder. *J Agric Food Chem* 49:5201–5206.

Hage, D.S., Thomas, D.H., Chowdhuri, A.R., and Clarke, W. 1999. Development of a theoretical model for chromatographic-based competitive binding immunoassays with simultaneous injection of sample and label. *Anal Chem* 71(15):2965–2975.

Hefle, S. 2006. Methods for detecting peanuts in food. In *Detecting Allergens In Food*, S.J. Koppelman and S.L. Hefle, Eds., pp. 183–200. Woodhead Publishing Limited, Cambridge, U.K.

Hefle, S.L., Bush, R.K., Yunginger, J.W., and Chu, F.S. 1994. A sandwich enzyme linked immunosorbent assay (ELISA) for the quantitation of selected peanut proteins in foods. *J Food Protect* 57:419–423.

Herzenberg, L.A., Parks, D., Sahaf, B., Perez, O., Roederer, M., and Herzenberg, L.A. 2002. The history and future of the fluorescence activated cell sorter and flow cytometry: A view from Stanford. *Clin Chem* 48:1819–1827.

Hilderbrand, S.A., Kelly, K.A., Weissleder, R., and Tung, Ch-H. 2005. Monofunctional near-infrared fluorochromes for imaging applications. *Bioconjugate Chem* 16(5), 1275–1281.

Hileman, R.E., Silvanovich, A., Goodman, R.E., Rice, E.A., Holleschak, G., Astwood, J.D., and Hefle, S.L. 2002. Bioinformatic methods for allergenicity assessment using a comprehensive allergen database *Int Arch Allergy Immunol* 128:280–291.

Hirsch, L.R., Jackson, J.B., Lee, A., Halas, N.J., and West, J. 2003. A whole blood immunoassay using gold nanoshells. *Anal Chem* 75(10):2377–2381.

Hischenhuber, C., Crevel, R., Jarry, B., Mäki, M., Moneret-Vautrin, D.A., Romano, A., Troncone, R., and Ward, R. 2006. Review article: Safe amounts of gluten for patients with wheat allergy or celiac disease. *Aliment Pharmacol Ther* 23(5):559–575.

Hoebler, C., Lecannu, G., Belleville, C., Devaux, M.F., Popineau, Y., and Barry, J.L. 2002. Development of an in vitro system simulating bucco-gastric digestion to assess the physical and chemical changes in food. *Int J Food Sci Nutr* 53(5):389–402.

Hourihane, J.O'B, Miemann, L.M., Hlywka, J.J., and Hefle, S.L. 2000. Immunochemical analysis of retail foods labeled as "may contain Peanut" or other similar declaration: Implication for food allergic individuals. *J Allergy Clin Immunol* 105:188.

Hwang, J. and Nishikawa, S. 2006. Novel approach to analyzing RNA aptamer-protein interactions: Toward further applications of aptamers. *J Biomol Screening* 11:599–605.

Ishikawa, E., Imagawa, M., Hashida, S., Yoshitake, S., Hamaguchi, Y., and Ueno, T. 1983. Enzyme-labeling of antibodies and their fragments for enzyme immunoassay and immunohistochemical staining. *J Immunoassay* 4(3):209–327.

Janssen, F. 2006. Detecting wheat gluten in food. In: *Detecting Allergens in Food*, S.J. Koppelman and S.L. Hefle, Eds., pp. 244–272. Woodhead Publishing Limited, Cambridge, England.

Jarvinen, K.M., Beyer, K., Vila, L., Bardina, L., Mishoe, M., and Sampson, H.A. 2007. Specificity of IgE antibodies to sequential epitopes of hen's egg ovomucoid as a marker for persistence of egg allergy. *Allergy* 62(7):758–765.

Jędrychowski, L. 2003a. Immunoenzimatical methods. In: *Food Biotechnology*, 2nd ed., W. Bednarski and A. Reps, Eds., pp. 464–479, WNT, Warsaw (in Polish).

Jędrychowski, L. 2003b. Examination of immunoreactive and immunomodulative properties of food components with the application of immunometric methods. *Pol J Food Nutr Sci* 12/53(SI 2):32–39.

Jędrychowski, L. and Wróblewska, B. 1999. Reduction of the antigenicity of whey proteins by lactic acid fermentation. *Food Agric Immunol* 11:91–99.

Jędrychowski, L., Wróblewska, B., and Szymkiewicz, A., 2005. Technological aspects of food allergen occurrence in food products. *Pol J Environ Stud* 14(Suppl. II): 171–180.

Jonsson, H., Erikson, A., and Yman, M. 2006. Detecting food allergens with a surface plasmon resonance immunoassay. In: *Detecting Allergens in Food*. S. J. Koppelman and L. Hefle, Eds., pp. 158–173. Woodhead Publishing Limited, Cambridge, England.

Kalorama. 2008. *The Worldwide Market for In Vitro Diagnostic (IVD) Tests*, 6th ed. (with 2009 economy preface). Kalorama Information, www.kaloramainformation.com

Konig, A., Cockburn, A., Crevel, R.W. et al. 2004. Assessment of the safety of foods derived from genetically modified (GM) crops *Food Chem Toxicol* 42:1047–1088.

Koppelman, S.J. 2006. Detecting soy, fish and crustaceans in food. In *Detecting Allergens in Food*, S.J. Koppelman and S.L. Hefle, Eds., pp. 273–290, Woodhead Publishing Limited, Cambridge, England.

Koppelman, S.J., van Koningsveld, G.A., Knulst, A.C., Gruppen, H., Pigmans, I.G., and de Jongh, H.H. 2002. Effect of heat-induced aggregation on the IgE binding of patatin (Sol t 1) is dominated by other potato proteins. *J Agric Food Chem* 50(6): 1562–1568.

Krska, R., Welzig, E., and Boudra, H. 2007. Analysis of Fusarium toxins in feed. *Animal Feed Sci Technol* 137(3–4):241–264.

Lee, H.A. and Morgan, M.R.A. 1993. Food immunoassay: Applications of polyclonal, monoclonal and recombinant antibodies. *Trends Food Sci Technol* 4:129–132.

Li, Y., Hua, F., Carraway, K.L., and Carothers Carraway, C.A. 1999. The p185$^{neu}$-containing glycoprotein complex of a microfilament-associated signal transduction particle. purification, reconstitution, and molecular associations with p58$^{gag}$ and actin. *J Biol Chem* 274(36):25651–25658.

Lidholm, J., Ballmer-Weber, B., Mari, A., and Vieths, S. 2006. Component-resolved diagnostics in food allergy. *Curr Opin Allergy Clin Immunol* 6:234–240.

Lochner, N., Lobmaier, C., Wirth, M., Leitner, A., Pittner, F., and Gabor, F. 2003. Silver nanoparticle enhanced immunoassays: One step real time kinetic assay for insulin in serum. *Eur Pharm Biopharm* 56(3):469–477.

Masseyeff, R.F., Albert, W.H., and Staines, N.A. 1993. *Methods of Immunological Analysis*. Vol. 1: *Fundamentals*. VCH Verlagsgesellschaft mbH, Weinheim.

Matsson, P. 2008. Allergy. The future of allergy testing: New technologies and opportunities. *Clin Lab Int* 32(6):26–28.

Matveeva, E.G., Gryczynski, Z., and Lakowicz, J.R. 2005. Myoglobin immunoassay based on metal particle-enhanced fluorescence. *J Immunol Methods* 302:26–35.

Medina, M.B. 2003. Detection of staphylococcal enterotoxin B (SEB) with surface plasmon resonance biosensor. *J Rapid Methods Autom Microbiol* 11:225–243.

Mello, L.D. and Kubota, L.T. 2002. Analytical, nutritional and clinical methods. Review of the use of biosensors as analytical tools in the food and drink industries. *Food Chem* 77(2):237–256.

Metcalfe, D.D., Astwood, J.D., Townsend, R., Sampson, H.A., Taylor, S.L., and Fuchs, R.L. 1996. Assessment of the allergenic potential of foods derived from genetically engineered crop plants *Crit Rev Food Sci Nutr* 36(Suppl):S165–S186.

Mine, Y. and Rupa, P. 2003. Fine mapping and structural analysis of immunodominant IgE allergenic epitopes in chicken egg ovalbumin. *Protein Eng* 16(10):747–752.

Misono, T.S. and Kumar, P.K.R. 2005. Selection of RNA aptamers against human influenza virus hemagglutinin using surface plasmon resonance. *Anal Biochem* 342:312–317.

Mohammed, I., Mullet, W.M., Lai, E.P.C., and Yeung, J.M. 2001. Is biosensor a viable method for food allergen detection? *Ann Chim Acta* 444:97–102.

Muller-Renaud, S.P., Dupont, D., and Delie, P. 2004. Quantification of beta-casein in milk and cheese using an optical immunosensor. *J Agric Food Chem* 52:659–664.

Muller-Renaud, S.P., Dupont, D., and Dulieu P. 2005. Development of a biosensor immunoassay for the quantification of $\alpha_{s1}$-casein in milk. *J Dairy Res* 72:57–64.

Nagy, A., Jędrychowski, L., Gelencsér, É., Wróblewska, B., and Szymkiewicz, A. 2002. Immunomodulative effect of *Lactobacillus Salivarius* and *Lactobacillus Casei* strains. *Pol J Food Nutr Sci* 11/52(SI 2):122–124.

Neudecker, P., Schweimer, K., Nerkamp, J., Scheurer, S., Vieths, S., Sticht, H., and Stricht, P. 2001. Allergic cross-reactivity made visible: Solution structure of the major cherry allergen Pru av 1. *J Biol Chem* 276(25):22756–22763.

Nichkova, M., Dosev, D., Gee, S.J., Hammock, B.D., and Kennedy, I.M. 2005. Microarray immunoassay for phenoxybenzoic acid using polymer encapsulated Eu: Gd2O3 nanoparticles as fluorescent labels. *Anal Chem* 77(21):6864–6873.

Nichkova, M., Dosev, D., Gee, S.J., Hammock, B.D., and Kennedy, I.M. 2007. Multiplexed immunoassays for proteins using magnetic luminescent nanoparticles for internal calibration. *Anal Biochem* 369(1):34–40.

Nichkova, M., Dosev, D., Perron, R., Gee, S.J., Hammock, B.D., and Kennedy, I.M. 2006. Eu3+-doped Gd2O3 nanoparticles as reporters for optical detection and visualization of antibodies patterned by microcontact printing. *Anal Bioanal Chem* 384(3):631–637.

Orth, J.H., Blöcker, D., and Aktories, K. 2003. His1205 and His1223 are essential for the activity of the mitogenic *Pasteurella multocida* toxin. *Biochemistry* 42(17): 4971–4977.

Osborne, T.B. 1907. *The Proteins of the Wheat Kernel*. Carnegie Institution, Washington DC, Publ. 84.

Partridge, M.A.K., Yiang, Y., Skerritt, J.H., and Schaich, K.M. 2003. Immunochemical and electrophoretic analysis of the modification of wheat proteins in extruded flour products. *Cereal Chem* 80(6):791–798.

Peng, H.S., Wu, C.F., Jiang, Y.F. et al. 2007a. Highly luminescent Eu3+ chelate nanoparticles prepared by a reprecipitation-encapsulation method. *Langmuir* 23(4):1591–1595.

Peng, L., Stephens, B.J., Bonin, K. et al. 2007b. A combined atomic force/fluorescence microscopy technique to select aptamers in a single cycle from a small pool of random oligonucleotides. *Microsc Res Tech* 70(4):372–381.

Person, J.L., Colas, F., Compère, C., Lehaitre, M., Anne, M., Boussard-Plédel, C., Bureau, B., Adam, J.-L., Deputier, S., and Guilloux-Viry, M. 2008. Surface plasmon resonance in chalcogenide glass-based optical system. *Sens Actuators B: Chem* 130(2):771–776.

Pierce Chemical Company. 1994. *Pierce Catalog and Handbook. Life Science and Analytical Research Products*. Pierce a Perstorp Biotec (Chemical) Company, Rockford, IL, T19–T34.

Poms, R.E., Agazzi, M., Bau, A., Brochee, M., Capelletti, C., Nordgaard, J.V., and Anklam, E. 2004. Inter-laboratory validation study of five commercially different ELISA test kits for the determination of peanut residues in cookie and dark chocolate. European Commission 2004, GE/R/FSQ/D08/05/2004.

Rittenburg, J.H. 1990. *Development and Application of Immunoassay for Food Analysis*. Elsevier Applied Science, London and New York.

Roederer, M., Darzynkiewicz, Z., and Parks, D.R. 2004. Guidelines for the presentation of flow cytometric data. *Methods Cell Biol* 75:241–256.

Rumbo, M., Chirdo, F.G., Fossati, C.A., and Anón, M.C. 2001. Analysis of the effects of heat treatment on gliadin immunochemical quantification using a panel of anti-prolamin antibodies. *J Agric Food Chem* 49(12):5719–5726.

Runge, D.M. Westpfahl-Wiesener, K.-P., and Schwertner, H. 2005. Development and performance evaluation of a visual fast test for the detection of specific IgE in capillary blood or heparin blond. *Allergologie* 28(7):263–268.

Samson, H. 2001. Utility of food-specific IgE concentrations in predicting symptomatic food allergy. *J Allergy Clin Immunol* 107:891–896.

Schirmer, T., Hoffmann-Sommergruber, K., Susani, M., Breiteneder, H., and Markovic-Housley, Z. 2005. Crystal structure of the major celery allergen Api g 1: Molecular analysis of cross-reactivity. *J Mol Biol* 351(5):1101–1109.

Schmid, I. and Giorgi, J.V. 1995. Preparations of cells and reagents for flow cytometry, Intracellular staining. In *Current Protocols in Immunology*, Vol 1, Unit 5.3. J.E. Coligan, A.M. Kruisbeek, D.H. Margulies, E.M. Shevach, and W. Strober, Eds., pp. 5.3.1–5.3.23, John Wiley & Sons, New York.

Schneider, B.H., Dickinson, E.L. Vach, M.D. Hoijer J.V., and Howard L.V. 2000. Highly sensitive optical chip immunoassays in human serum. *Biosens Bioelec* 15(1):13–22(10).

Scorilas, A., Bjartell, A., Lilja, H., Moller, C., and Diamandis, E.P. 2000. Streptavidinpolyvinylamine conjugates labeled with a europium chelate: Applications in immunoassay, immunohistochemistry, and microarrays. *Clin Chem* 46:(9):1450–1455.

Sharma, S., Kumar, P., Betzel, C., and Singh, T.P. 2001. Structure and function of proteins involved in milk allergies. *J Chromatogr* 756(1):183–187.

Sharma, S., Murphy, S.P., Wilkens, L.R., Shen, L., Hankin, J.H., and Henderson, B. 2003. Adherence to the food guide pyramid recommendations among Japanese Americans, Native Hawaiians, and whites: Results from the multiethnic cohort study. *J Am Dietetic Assoc* 103(9):1195–1198.

Stepaniak, L., Jędrychowski, L., Grabska, J., Wróblewska, B., and Sorhang F. 1998. Application of immunoassays for proteins and peptides in milk and dairy products. *Recent Res Dev Agric Food Chem.* 2:673–687.

Stepaniak, L., Jędrychowski, L., and Sorhaug, T. 2002. Analysis/immunochemical in dairy food sciences encyklopedia. *Sci Technol* 62–67.

Szabo, E., Hajós, G., and Matuz, J. 2002. Identification of major allergens of cereal proteins by electrophoretic methods. *Pol J Food Nutr Sci* 11/52(Suppl. 2):131–134.

Szymanska, I., Radecka, H., Radecki, J., and Kaliszan, R. 2007. Electrochemical impedance spectroscopy for study of amyloid β-peptide interactions with (−) nicotine ditartrate and (−) cotinine. *Biosen Bioelec* 22(9–10):1955–1960.

Szymkiewicz, A. and Jędrychowski, L. 2002. Influence of selected technological processes on immunogenic properties of pea proteins. *Pol J Food Nutr Sci* 11/52(SI 1):100–103.

Szymkiewicz, A. and Jędrychowski, L. 2005. Reduction of immunoreactive properties of pea globulins as the result of enzymatic modification. *Acta Alimentaria* 34(3):295–306.

Szymkiewicz, A., Wróblewska, B., and Jędrychowski, L. 2003. The application of immunoblotting method in the analysis of cow milk and pea protein hydrolysis. *Pol J Food Nutr Sci* 12/53(SI 1):84–88.

Tomita, M. 2008. Next generation of monoclonal antibodies shortlisting lymphocytes via B-cell targeting. *BIOforum Eur* 4:33–34.

Tsuji, A., Maeda, M., and Arakowa, H. 1989. Chemiluminescent enzyme immunoassay: A review. *Anal Sci* 5(5):497–506.

Wasowicz, M., Viswanathan, S., Dvornyk, A., Grzelak, K., Kludkiewicz, B., and Radecka, H. 2008. Comparison of electrochemical immunosensors based on gold nano materials and immunoblot techniques for detection of histidine-tagged proteins in culture medium. *Biosens Bioelec* 24:284–289.

Weeks, I. 1992. Chemiluminescence immunoassay, In *Wilson and Wilson's Comprehensive Analytical Chemistry*, Volume XXIX. G. Svehla, Ed., Elsevier, Amsterdam London New York Tokyo.

Wieser, H. 1998. Investigation of the extractability of gluten proteins from wheat bread in comparison with flour. *Z Lebensm Unters Forsch* 207(2):128–132.

Wingren, C.h. and Borrebaeck, C.A.K. 2007. Progress in miniaturization of protein arrays—a step closer to high-density nanoarrays. *Drug Discovery Today* 12(19–20):813–819.

Wolbers, F., Haanen, C., Andersson, H., van den Berg, A., Vermes, I. 2006a. Analysis of apoptosis on Chip. Why the move to chip technology? In: *Lab-on-Chips for Cellomics Micro and Nanotechnologies for Life Science*, H. Andersson and A. van den Berg, Eds., pp. 197–224, Kluwer Academic Publishers, Dordrecht, Boston, London.

Wolbers, F., Andersson, H., Vermes, I., van den Berg, A. 2006b. Miniaturisation in the biotechnology laboratory. *BioTech Int* 18(6):10–14.

Wróblewska, B. and Jędrychowski, L. 2002a. Influence of technological and biological processes on the immunoreactivity of cow milk proteins. *Pol J Food Nutr Sci* 11/52 (SI 2):156–159.

Wróblewska, B. and Jędrychowski, L. 2002b. Effect of conjugation of cow milk whey proteins with polyethylene glycol on changes in their immunoreactive and allergic properties. *Food Agric Immunol* 14:155–162.

Wróblewska, B., Jędrychowski, L., Szabó, E., and Hajós, G. 2005. The reduction of cow milk proteins immunoreactivity by two–step enzymatic hydrolysis. *Acta Alimantaria.* 34(3):307–315.

Yao, G., Wang, L., Wu, Y.R., Smith, J., Xu, J.S., Zhao, W.J., Lee, E.J., and Tan, W.H. 2006. FloDots: Luminescent nanoparticles. *Anal Bioanal Chem* 385(3):518–524.

Zhou, X.C. and Zhou, J.Z. 2004. Improving the signal sensitivity and photostability of DNA hybridizations on microarrays by using dye-doped core-shell silica nanoparticles. *Anal Chem* 76(18):5302–5312.

Zorzet, A., Gustafsson, M., and Hammerling, U. 2002. Prediction of food protein allergenicity: A bioinformatic learning systems approach. *In Silico Biol* 2:525–534.

## 3.2 ANIMAL MODELS IN FOOD ALLERGEN ANALYSIS AND INVESTIGATING THE MECHANISMS OF ALLERGY

André H. Penninks

### 3.2.1 INTRODUCTION

In concert with the increasing incidence in food allergy, the interest in animal models for food allergy research has raised in the past two decades. Most animal research models of food allergy are focused on the elucidation of immunological mechanisms that underlie the sensitization and challenge phase of food allergy, and the development of new prophylactic and therapeutic strategies. Furthermore, due to the development of new (bio)technology-derived proteins and genetically modified foods, there has been a growing interest in animal models that can predict the potential allergenicity and potency of (novel) proteins in our food. In this section, the important criteria for the development of food allergy models will be discussed. In addition, the developed mechanistic and predictive animal models for food allergy in rodents (rat, mice), swine, and dog will be reviewed.

Animal models for food allergy have been developed to expand our knowledge on food allergy and to identify new therapeutic and prophylactic strategies or for predicting the allergenicity of novel food products. The increased knowledge of the immune system and the availability of a wide variety of immunological tools allow to study certain aspects of food allergy in more detail and to obtain more insight into the mechanistic aspects of food allergy. Moreover, it will be important to study the clinical reactions (including hopefully the assessment of thresholds) elicited in animal models when they are challenged with allergenic food and that the results obtained can be extrapolated to and will be predictive for the human allergic response. Furthermore, the development and introduction of genetically engineered food crops in the market has gained a lot of interest in approaches to assess the allergenic potential of these novel gene products. It is evident that especially in animal models, which mimic as much as possible the allergic response in humans, the relative potency of sensitization of existing and new proteins can be studied as for ethical reasons this cannot be studied in human volunteers.

The first systematic attempt to develop a structured approach to assess the allergenic potential of novel food proteins was jointly developed by the International Food Biotechnology Council and the ILSI Allergy and Immunology Institute that was published in 1996 (Metcalfe et al., 1996). Attention should be given to several factors like amino acid sequence homology, various physicochemical properties such as heat and digestive stability of the protein, but the use of animal models was not yet possible as they were not existing. A revision of the IFBC/ILSI decision tree strategy, including additional testing, was proposed in 2001 by an expert consultation of the Food and Agriculture Organization (FAO) and the World Health Organization (WHO) (FAO/WHO, 2001). Among the introduction of several new tests animal testing was also proposed, despite the fact that widely accepted and validated animal models were not yet available. However, the Codex Alimentarius Commission guidelines (Codex, 2003) emphasized subsequently that only scientifically validated testing should be used. This resulted among others in the removal of the demand for non-validated animal models in the weight of evidence approach of the Codex Alimentarius Commission to predict the potential allergenicity of novel proteins. These different recommendations may have led to some confusion and different request of regulatory authorities in respect to tests needed for evaluation of the potential allergenicity of novel proteins or genetically engineered crops.

An important advantage of the availability of animal models will be the possibility to obtain information on the sensitizing potential of the new protein(s) or genetically engineered crops in relation to its potency, relative to well-known allergens. As it is clear that both specific characteristics of the protein itself and specific conditions of the human individual will play an important role in the sensitization process, this also explains the difficulty of finding the right animal model if ever possible. However, it is evident that only in animal models, which mimic as much as possible the allergic response in humans, the relative sensitization of existing and new proteins can be studied as for ethical reasons this cannot be studied in human volunteers. In food allergy research, three animal species have been most frequently used, viz., guinea pigs, rats, and mice although in recent years attention is also being given to allergy research in other species like dogs and pigs. In this section, the special problems related to the development of animal models for food allergy research are discussed, and furthermore the progress is summarized that comprises of promisful animal models for predictive and more mechanistic research in food allergy.

### 3.2.2 IMPORTANT CRITERIA FOR ANIMAL MODELS FOR FOOD ALLERGY

It has become clear that important criteria for animal models of food allergy may differ somewhat depending on the specific use of the model to either study the immunological mechanisms that underlie the development of food allergy, and the development of new immunoprophylactic and therapeutic strategies or to predict the potential allergenicity of novel proteins. As in the human situation, allergic patients often have a predisposed atopic genetic background, it is also desirable for animal models to use a strain of animal that is more susceptible to develop allergic disorders. Examples are, for instance, the Balb/c mouse (Hilton et al., 1997; Kimber et al., 2003; Dearman and Kimber, 2005) and the BN rat (Atkinson and Miller, 1994;

Knippels et al., 1998a), which both have a propensity toward a Th2 type phenotype, which will result in relatively high immunoglobulin production, in particular IgE. To mimic the normal conditions as closely as possible, one of the first important criteria to study the sensitizing potential of a novel protein would be the oral administration of the protein or food. The oral route is the preferred route for sensitization and challenge studies as it is evident that natural barriers such as the gastrointestinal tract (acid denaturation and enzymatic digestion of proteins) and the mucosal/epithelial layers (e.g., uptake), are all known to influence the allergenicity of proteins and should be taken into account (Pauwels et al., 1979; Strobel and Ferguson, 1984; Turner et al., 1990; Atkinson et al., 1996). However, from human experience and various rodent studies it has become clear that oral administration of proteins will, in general, not result in immunological sensitization, but rather in tolerance induction, in particular high-dose protein exposure (Strobel and Ferguson, 1984; Turner et al., 1990). The unscheduled dietary pre-exposure of the test animals or their parental generations to the protein under investigation, or a cross-reacting allergen, is also of great importance as this may have resulted already in tolerance induction (Knippels et al., 1998b). Only in case this active state of immune suppression is abrogated adverse reactions like IgE-mediated food allergy may develop, which can be achieved using adjuvants such as cholera toxin (Li et al., 1999; Kroghsbo et al., 2003). The limitation of not using adjuvants is that despite the choice of a good responder strain, only a limited number of animals might become allergic. Still, this condition of not using adjuvants is preferred in studies to determine the potential allergenicity of novel proteins, as their use may not mimic a natural response of the immune system and result in allergic sensitization which might not be the case in the absence of adjuvants. In models studying the mechanism of food allergy and/or immunotherapeutic strategies, adjuvants are frequently used, in order to increase the number of allergic animals.

Important key factors, in particular, for animal models to distinguish between allergic (from weak to strong sensitizers) and nonallergic proteins are summarized in Table 3.2.1. To ultimately validate such model(s), the test animal should tolerate most food proteins, so well-known non-allergenic food proteins should be negative, and a differentiated response would be preferred when using a wide range of known weak to strong allergenic food proteins. In this context also, in case whole allergenic foods are used, allergic responses should be directed against the known allergenic proteins in the food, based on human experience, and not to other proteins in the food.

### 3.2.3 Animal Models to Predict the Potential Allergenicity of Proteins

#### 3.2.3.1 Predictive Food Allergy Models in Brown Norway Rats

As the BN rat has an atopic-like phenotype, which might result in relatively high IgE antibody production, the BN was considered to be a promising species for the development of an oral feeding protocol. Various approaches with BN rats have been described using different routes and duration of exposure and in the presence or absence of adjuvants (Atkinson and Miller, 1994; Atkinson et al., 1996; Miller et al., 1999). The oral sensitization to food proteins was studied in Brown Norway (BN)

**TABLE 3.2.1**

**Key Factors for Predictive Animal Models for Food Allergy**

- Genetic predisposition (species/strain-high/low responder/atopic prevalence)
- Prior exposure of test animals to test protein/food (diet, parents)
- Sensitization conditions:
- Age of the animals—neonate, adolescent, adult
  - ○ Route of exposure—oral/gavage/i.p./others
  - ○ Use of adjuvant—cholera toxin/alum
  - ○ Test material—whole foods/purified proteins
  - ○ Dose frequency—e.g., daily, twice weekly, weekly
  - ○ Dose amount—high dose (tolerance!)/low dose(sensitization)
- Comparable allergenicity—strong/week/nonallergic proteins
- Comparable IgE responses to allergenic proteins in foods as found in patients
- Clinical reactions upon challenges

rats by administration through the diet or by gavage-dosing either in the presence (Atkinson and Miller, 1994) or absence of an adjuvant (Knippels et al., 1998a,b, 1999a,b, 2000). Daily intra-gastric administration of 1 mg ovalbumin (OVA) for 42 days, without the use of adjuvants, resulted in antigen-specific IgG as well as IgE responses as measured by both ELISA and PCA (Knippels et al., 1998a). In a subsequent study in this OVA-induced allergy model in BN rats, clinical reactions upon an oral challenge with OVA were studied, like increased gut permeability, changes in respiratory functions and blood pressure (Knippels et al., 1999b). From a comparative sensitization study with Wistar-, PVG-, Hooded Lister-, and BN rats, it was evident that upon oral exposure to OVA, only the BN rats developed OVA-specific IgE antibodies confirming the choice of the BN rat for oral sensitization studies (Knippels et al., 1999a). Also the sensitizing potential of hen's egg white and cow's milk (Knippels et al., 2000) and in addition a peanut protein extract (Knippels and Penninks, 2005) were studied in this BN rat model. From the results obtained with these different food products, it was clear that the number of responding animals differed with the various food products tested and that it also is necessary to test different dose levels of the food protein to obtain a good range order (Knippels and Penninks, 2005). It was also clear from these studies with hen's egg white and cow's milk that the IgG- and IgE-antibodies raised in the BN rat were raised to the same allergenic proteins as are recognized in sera of patients allergic to these food products (Knippels et al., 2000).

In this BN rat model also various purified weak-, strong- or nonallergenic proteins, based on human experience, have been tested in order to study the relative allergenicity of the selected proteins. In these BN rat studies, 2S albumin purified from Brazil nut (Ber e1), a peanut allergen (Ara h 1) purified from peanut, shrimp tropomyosin (Pen a1), beef tropomyosin (nonallergenic), and patatin (Sol t1) purified from potatoes were used. These purified proteins were tested in the BN rat model as it was done for OVA using daily gavage with 1 mg of each of the test proteins for 42 days. Although most of the animals developed specific IgG antibodies to the proteins tested, not all animals developed protein-specific IgE antibodies. The order of the oral sensitization potential observed in these separate tests was found to be OVA > Ber e1 > Ara h 1 > Pen a1 > Sol t1 (Knippels and Penninks, 2005).

Experiences with the BN rat model in different laboratories has indicated that by using almost comparable experimental regimes some laboratories were able to demonstrate the allergic sensitization to OVA upon oral application (Akiyama et al., 2001; Pilegaard and Madsen, 2004; Xu-Dong et al., 2005;) whereas others could not stimulate IgE antibody responses to OVA (Dearman et al., 2001). A possible explanation for these discrepancies might be minor differences in study protocols or the naivety of animals for the tested protein, as it is clear that unscheduled dietary pre-exposure of test animals or their parental generation to the test protein under investigation, or a cross-reacting allergen, will be of importance as this may result in tolerance induction as was demonstrated with soy (Knippels et al., 1998b).

In conclusion, the results obtained with the BN rat model up to date at different laboratories indicate that the BN rat might be a useful model to study the potential oral allergenicity of "novel" food proteins. However, further testing with either more allergenic and nonallergenic whole foods or with purified allergenic and nonallergenic proteins will be needed to further evaluate and validate this Brown Norway rat model.

### 3.2.3.2 Predictive Food Allergy Models in Mice

As the Balb/c inbred mice strain has an atopic-like phenotype, it was considered to be a promising species to evaluate the potential predictivity for human allergenicity of novel protein. Exploring studies of Hilton et al. (1994, 1997), which focused on the nature of immunological responses in Balb/c mice upon intraperitoneal (i.p.) application of proteins, were followed by more detailed studies by Dearman et al. (2000, 2001), Kimber et al. (2000), and Dearman and Kimber (2001). They examined upon repeated i.p. exposure, without using adjuvants, the intrinsic ability of various food proteins to stimulate IgG (immunogenicity) and IgE (allergenicity) antibody responses. The i.p. route of exposure was selected as this will avoid the development of oral tolerance and was considered to better predict the inherent ability of proteins to induce IgE antibody responses. In their standard protocol, mice are injected i.p. with different concentrations of the test proteins in phosphate buffered saline at days 0 and 7. Blood is collected at days 14, 28, or 42 and serum is prepared for analysis of antibody production. In the first studies (Dearman et al., 2000), bovine serum albumin (BSA, a protein with limited potential to induce sensitization) and ovalbumin (OVA, a major egg-white allergen) were compared for the strength of the immune response that they can elicit. Apart from vigorous IgG antibody responses elicited by both proteins, relatively high IgE levels were only observed for OVA whereas no or only low IgE titers were detected against BSA. In a subsequent study (Dearman and Kimber, 2001), three proteins were compared, viz., peanut agglutinin (a minor peanut allergen), OVA, and a crude extract of type II acid phosphatase (PAP, no or limited potential to induce sensitization) from potato. IgG responses were induced by all proteins, whereas IgE production was protein- and dose-dependent with good responses for peanut agglutinin and OVA and no IgE response with PAP. In other studies, OVA and potato protein extract (PPE) were compared upon i.p administration (Dearman et al., 2001) as well as several allergens and nonallergens (Dearman et al., 2003a). Moreover, in an inter-laboratory study with various allergens it was demonstrated that this assay was transferable between various laboratories (Dearman et al., 2003b). From all these studies, it can be concluded that with the i.p. administration it was possible with the selected proteins to distinguish between allergenic and nonallergenic proteins, which despite being immunogenic fail to provoke IgE antibody production. These data suggest that this Balb/c model could be of importance in the identification and characterization of the immunogenic/allergenic potential of novel proteins. However, there is still a need for further research in order to elucidate whether this systemic (i.p.) exposure will be representative for the more relevant oral route of exposure, as false-positive and false-negative identification may occur. Further testing with a larger panel of allergenic and nonallergenic proteins will still be needed to evaluate if this test approach in mice will be feasible as a stand alone test or that combinations with other oral tests will be needed.

In literature also, several other mice models using, e.g., Balb/c mice and different routes of exposure are available dealing with predictive aspects of allergenicity upon oral/gavage treatment (Akiyama et al., 2001; Prescott et al., 2005; Gizzarelli et al., 2006), or combinations of oral and i.p. application (Strid et al., 2004). In Balb/c mice also the allergenicity of some whole foods (milk and peanut) was studied by Adelpatient et al. (2005) upon oral application with an adjuvant. All these models lack sufficient testing with a range of allergenic and nonallergenic proteins.

### 3.2.3.3 Predictive Food Allergy Models in Guinea Pigs

Guinea pigs are infrequently used for regulatory allergenicity testing of different type of products (industrial chemicals, cosmetics, pharmaceuticals, infant formula's) but are less commonly used in models for food allergy research. As guinea pigs can be easily sensitized by the oral route without adjuvants, they are still used in a model for testing the hypoallergenicity of cow's milk-derived infant formulas or other formulas based on modified (hypoallergenic) proteins (Piacentini et al., 1994; Kitagawa et al., 1995; Devey et al., 1976; Fritsché, 2003). Ad libitum administration of cow's milk in the drinking water for about 5 weeks will result in an allergic sensitization and upon an i.v. challenge with cow's milk proteins, after a resting period of about 2 weeks, severe clinical reactions such as anaphylaxis will occur. Drawbacks for the further use of the guinea pig in the prediction of the potential allergenicity of novel proteins and in more mechanistic food allergy research are the significant differences in immunophysiology when compared with other species, the limited knowledge of its immune system (e.g., the reagenic antibody is of the IgG1a subtype instead of IgE), the lack of tools to study its immune system, and its questionable specificity in allergic sensitization.

### 3.2.3.4 Predictive Food Allergy Models in Dogs

Occasionally also the dog is used for food allergy research (Paterson, 1995; Jeffers et al., 1996; Buchanan et al., 1997; Ermel et al., 1997; Buchanan and Frick, 2002; Teuber et al., 2002; Jackson et al., 2003). In these studies, a colony of spaniel/basenji-type dogs with a genetic predisposition to allergy that had histories of sensitivity to pollen and foods is used. These dogs resemble the high IgE responsiveness of allergic patients, and after oral challenges they develop clinical manifestations of food allergy observed in humans such as skin effects and gastrointestinal effects such as vomiting and diarrhea. In the studies of Ermel et al. (1997) and Buchanan et al. (1997, 2002), newborn pups are sensitized by subcutaneous (s.c.) injection of very low doses (1 µg) of the different allergens, e.g., cow's milk, ragweed, beef, or wheat extracts using alum as an adjuvant. The pups received several additional s.c. immunizations over a course of weeks following the same regime as used for the first immunization. The allergic sensitization was further maintained by daily feeding of a diet containing small amounts of the same allergen and by s.c. boost immunizations at bimonthly intervals. In these sensitized dogs, allergic responses are measured in particular by skin reactions upon intradermal injection of the offending allergens or by gastrointestinal reactions upon oral challenges. In this dog allergy model, various allergenic food extracts have been tested such as extracts from cow's milk, beef, ragweed, and wheat (Buchanan and Frick, 2002), of barley, brazil nut, peanut, soy, and walnut (Teuber et al., 2002), and of cornstarch, corn, soy, and a soy hydrolysate (Jackson et al., 2003). In the study of Teuber et al. (2002), the hierarchy of skin reactivity in dogs sensitized with the multiple allergenic food extracts was found to be similar as observed in humans resulting in the following order of response; peanut > walnut > wheat > soy > barley.

Although the atopic dog model might not be the first choice to evaluate the relative allergenic potency of new proteins, it still might be a useful model to study novel proteins or genetically modified foods, in particular because of the low protein levels needed for sensitization and the similarity in typical human symptoms of food allergy upon oral challenges. In addition, the model might be attractive for further mechanistic studies underlying the development of food allergy and the clinical manifestations upon skin and oral challenges.

### 3.2.4 Mechanistic and Therapeutic Animal Models for Food Allergy Research

#### 3.2.4.1 Mechanistic and Therapeutic Models in Mice

Several mice models have been published which are especially designed to study the potency to elicit clinical reactions such as anaphylaxis upon oral challenges with the offending food to which the animals are sensitized (Ito et al., 1997; Li et al., 1999, 2000; Brandt et al., 2003; Finkelman et al., 2005; Finkelman, 2007), to study the mechanism of sensitization (van Wijk et al., 2004, 2005), or to study the development of prophylactic and therapeutic approaches (Li et al., 2003a,b). In order to obtain optimal IgE responses in the animal models used to study challenge reactions the mice are sensitized by different routes (e.g., i.p. or intragastric) and mostly in the presence of adjuvants. In the model of Li et al. (1999), sensitization of 3 week old C3H/HeJ mice was achieved by an intragastric immunization of different concentrations of cow's milk in the presence of cholera toxin as adjuvant, which was boosted five times at weekly intervals. Six weeks after the initial intragastric sensitization, the mice were challenged. Clinical reactions were assessed based on skin testing, symptom scores of systemic anaphylaxis which was accompanied by vascular leakage and significantly increased plasma histamine levels and increased intestinal permeability. Histopathology of the intestinal tissue also revealed marked signs of vascular congestion, edema, and enterocyte pathology. The kinetics of serum IgE production was followed and its reactivity was confirmed by passive cutaneous anaphylaxis. In addition, cytokine production was followed after *ex vivo* stimulation of spleen cells that resulted in increased levels of IL-4 and IL-5 which is indicative for a Th2 cell-mediated reactivity.

Li et al. (2000) also developed a mice model of IgE-mediated peanut allergy that closely mimics human peanut allergy. In this model C3H/HeJ, mice were sensitized by an intragastric administration of freshly ground whole peanut in the presence of cholera toxin as adjuvant. After intragastric challenges, anaphylactic reactions were determined and found to be fatal or near fatal for part of the animals. Apart from the anaphylactic symptom scores, hypersensitivity responses were assessed by vascular leakage, plasma histamine release, serum IgE titers, passive cutaneous anaphylaxis, histopathological examination, and *ex vivo* splenocyte proliferation against the purified major peanut allergens Ara h 1 and Ara h 2. Both the cow's milk allergy and peanut allergy models were regarded to be useful models for the evaluation of the immunopathogenic mechanisms that involved cow's milk allergy and peanut allergy and for exploring new therapeutic approaches for food allergy.

Therefore this peanut-allergy model in C3H/HeJ mice was further used in many studies that focused on more mechanistic-, prophylactic-, or therapeutic aspects. In studies of van Wijk et al. (2004), it was observed that both Th1 and Th2 phenomena were involved in the development of peanut allergy in the C3H/HeJ mice model. In a subsequent study in this peanut allergy C3H/HeJ mice model, it was shown by van Wijk et al. (2005) that the co-stimulatory molecule CTLA-4, predominantly expressed on activated T cells, is not the crucial factor in preventing sensitization to food allergens, but rather plays a pivotal role in regulating the intensity of a food allergic sensitization response.

The peanut-allergy model in C3H/HeJ mice is also used in studies focused on therapeutic strategies. Possibilities for specific immunotherapy with modified antigens/epitopes, regulatory cytokines, immunomodulatory microorganisms, anti-IgE antibodies, DNA vaccination, and alternative medicine has been reviewed by Li and Sampson (2002). Antigen-specific immunotherapy has been used in patients to generate tolerance to their offending allergens. As this strategy has a high level of serious side effects, there is a need to improve this treatment using animal models. To reduce IgE binding of allergens used for therapy (responsible for the observed clinical side effects), modified recombinant peanut allergens were produced to reduce the risk of severe systemic reactions in combination with different bacterial strains that also produce peanut allergens just to potentiate the desensitization (Li et al., 2003a,b). In these studies, a shift to a more Th1-driven response was observed, which is a promisful result for the further development of antigen-specific immunotherapy.

In literature also, several other mice models using different stains of mice or routes of exposure are available that were considered to be helpful to elucidate the pathogenesis of food allergy. Also these last models lack sufficient testing with a range of allergenic and nonallergenic proteins. Ito et al. (1997) studied the development of a relevant mice model by using different mice strains. They used DBA/2,

Balb/c, and B10A mice, and oral exposure to either casein or ovalbumin without the use of adjuvant. The mice were maintained on a diet that contained bovine casein or ovalbumin as the only protein source from 6 weeks of age and continued for 9 weeks. It was shown that only in the DBA/2 mice and only in case of casein feeding, casein-specific IgE was produced from day 28 onward. No IgE production was observed against ovalbumin in DBA/2 mice, whereas in the other two mice strains no IgE response was observed at all against both casein and ovalbumin. The authors did not really have a conclusive explanation with respect to the differences observed in sensitization by the tested allergens in the different mice models. A Balb/c mouse model mimicking both the sensitization and challenge phase against milk β-lactoglobulin was developed by Adel-Patient et al. (2003). They showed that biochemical and clinical manifestations differed depending on the structure of the β-lactoglobulin used in the challenge reactions.

### 3.2.4.2  Mechanistic Models in Pigs

Model development for food allergy research in pigs was initiated by Helm and Helm et al. (2002). Neonatal pigs have some important advantages over the other animal species discussed as they closely mimic several human physiological and immunological properties; they closely resemble humans in gastrointestinal physiology and in the development of the mucosal immunity, and they are immunocompetent at birth (Helm et al. (2003). This model was set up with peanuts as allergenic source and might be attractive to improve our knowledge of gastrointestinal hypersensitivity to peanuts. To assure naivity of the piglets for peanut the pregnant sows, during the last period of gestation, as well as the new-born piglets were fed with a soy and peanut free diet. Sensitization of the piglets was started when they were 3 days of age. Groups of piglets were sensitized intragastrically on three consecutive days with crude peanut meal and cholera toxin as adjuvant. A booster was given 1 week later with the same sensitization protocol. After a resting period of 3 weeks, the animals received an oral challenge with crude peanut meal. The allergic responses were measured by symptoms such as erythematous rashes, cyanosis around snout and ears, lethargy, vomiting, and respiratory distress. Also lymphocyte proliferation, skin prick tests, and gastrointestinal symptoms, also by histopathology, were studied. To confirm that IgE played a role in the allergic symptoms observed, passive cutaneous anaphylaxis tests were also performed. In summary, the data showed that this pig model might be of importance to study the mechanisms of IgE-mediated mechanisms, the characterization of clinical symptoms, and possibly also immunotherapeutic intervention strategies. As only peanut is tested in this model, it is still unclear if the pig model would also have the potential to predict allergenicity of novel proteins. Important disadvantages when using this model to predict the potential allergenicity of new proteins will of course be costs, handling of the pigs, and the amount of protein needed in case of oral sensitization.

### 3.2.5  Conclusions and Future Trends

In the past 10–15 years, a lot of effort has been put in the development of food allergy models by immunologists and toxicologists, either to elucidate mechanisms involved in food allergy and to study new prophylactic and therapeutic strategies, or to predict the potential allergenicity in humans of novel proteins. It can be concluded that in contrast to the slow progress made in the development of predictive animal models, more progress has been achieved in respect to animal models to study the mechanism of IgE-induced food allergy and to develop new approaches for prophylaxis and therapy of food allergy. Due to the still limited progress concerning predictive models, we have not succeeded yet in presenting an effective and validated model in rats, mice, dogs, or pigs. The current view is that especially the prediction of the sensitizing potential of a novel protein/food will likely be difficult to attain with a single model. It is even thought that because of the complexity of the immune system, the range of environmental factors that may influence the onset of allergic sensitization and the limited knowledge of specific physicochemical characteristics of the allergenic proteins, it may be extremely difficult to succeed in the development of such an animal model predictive for human food allergy (McClain and Bannon, 2006). This should, however, not restrain us from proceeding with our research, as it is a challenge to further explore the promising progress made with in particular both most studied rodent models, viz., the i.p. immunization model in Balb/c mice and the oral immunization model in BN rats, in order to refine these methods. Further improvement will especially need the integration of new knowledge and methods that is associated with the generation of more insight in the mechanisms involved in the sensitization process, what is the impact of exposure conditions on the development of food allergy, and which factors may influence inter-individual differences in susceptibility (Kimber et al., 2007). Future research should be focused therefore on the improved understanding needed on the mechanism(s) of sensitization to food proteins and the clinical symptoms on challenge reactions, and on the contribution of host and environmental factors in the presented well-studied mechanistic rodent, dog, and pig models for food allergy. Also for validation purposes of the proposed predictive rodent models, additional studies are still needed with a wider range of proteins (including well-known strong, weak, or no allergenic capacity) to study their predictability.

As it is still uncertain, whether these efforts will finally result in a conclusive animal model to predict food allergy in humans, it is anticipated that the information that finally can be obtained from animal models will have to be evaluated in concert with other parameters related to the potential allergenic activity of the protein/food, in order to assess if the protein/food might have a low or high allergenic potential in humans.

## REFERENCES

Adel-Patient, K., Nahori, M.A., Proust, B. et al. 2003. Elicitation of allergic reaction in β-lactoglobulin sensitised Balb/c mice: Biochemical and clinical manifestations differ depending on the structure of the BLG used for the challenge. *Clin Exp Allergy* 33:376–385.

Adel-Patient, K., Bernard, H., Ah-Leung, S., Créminon, C., and Wal, J.M. 2005. Peanut and cow's milk specific IgE, Th2 cells and local anaphylactic reaction are induced in Balb/c mice orally sensitised with cholera toxin. *Allergy* 60:658–664.

Akiyama, H., Teshima, R., Sakushima, J. et al. 2001. Examination of oral sensitisation with ovalbumin in Brown Norway rats and three strains of mice. *Immuno Lett* 78:1–5.

Atkinson, H.A. and Miller, K. 1994. Assessment of the Brown Norway rat as a suitable model for the investigation of food allergy. *Toxicol* 91:2 81–8.

Atkinson, H.A.C., Johnson, I.T., Gee, J.M., Grigoriadou, F., and Miller, K. 1996. Brown Norway rat model of food allergy: Effect of plant components on the development of oral sensitisation. *Food Chem Toxicol* 34:27–32.

Brandt, E.B., Strait, R.T., Hershko, D., Wang, Q., Muntel, E.E., and Schribner, T.A. 2003. Mast cells are required for experimental oral-allergen induced diarrhea. *J Clin Invest* 112:1666–1677.

Buchanan, B.B. and Frick, O.L. 2002. The dog as model for food allergy. *Ann NY Acad Sci* 964:173–183.

Buchanan, B.B., Adamidi, C., and Lozano, R.M. 1997. Thioredoxin-linked mitigation of allergic response to wheat. *Proc Acad Sci USA* 94:5372–5377.

Codex Alimentarius Commission. 2003. Alinorm 03/34: Joint FOA/WHO Food Standard Programme, Codex Alimentarius Commission, Twenty-Fifth Session, Rome, June 30–July 5, 2003. Appendix III, Guideline for the conduct of food safety assessment of foods derived from recombinant-DNA plants and Appendix IV, Annex on the assessment of possible allergenicity, 44–60.

Dearman, R.J. and Kimber, I. 2001. Determination of protein allergenicity: Studies in mice. *Toxicol Lett* 120:181–186.

Dearman, R.J. and Kimber,. 2005. Characterization of immune responses to food allergens in mice. *Proc Nutr Soc* 64:426–433.

Dearman, R.J., Caddick, H., Basketter, D.A., and Kimber, I. 2000. Divergent antibody isotope responses induced in mice by systemic exposure to proteins: A comparison of ovalbumin with bovine serum albumin. *Food Chem Toxicol* 38:351–360.

Dearman, R.J., Caddick, H., Stone, S., Basketter, D.A., and Kimber, I. 2001. Characterization of antibody responses induced in rodents by exposure to food proteins: Influence of route of exposure. *Toxicology* 167:217–231.

Dearman, R.J., Stone, S., Caddick, H.T., Basketter, D.A., and Kimber, I. 2003a. Evaluation of protein allergenic potential in mice: Dose-response analyses. *Clin Exp Allergy* 33:1586–1594.

Dearman, R.J., Skinner, R.A., Herouet, C., Labay, K., Debruyne, E., and Kimber, I. 2003b. Induction of IgE antibody responses by protein allergens: Inter-laboratory comparisons. *Food Chem Toxicol* 41:1509–1516.

Devey, M.E., Anderson, K.J., and Coombs, R.R.A. 1976. The modified anaphylaxis hypothesis for cot death. Anaphylactic sensitisation in guinea pigs fed cow's milk. *Clin Exp Immunol* 26:542–548.

Ermel, R.W., Kock, M., Griffey, S.M., Reinhart, G.A., and Frick, O.L. 1997. The atopic dog: A model for food allergy. *Lab Anim Sci* 47:40–49.

FAO/WHO. 2001. Evaluation of allergenicity of genetically modified foods. Report of a joint FAO/WHO expert consultation on allergenicity of foods derived from biotechnology. Food and Agriculture Organization of the United Nations (FAO), Rome.

Finkelman, F.D. 2007. Anaphylaxis: Lessons learned from mouse models. *J Allergy Clin Immunol* 120:506–515.

Finkelman, F.D., Rothenberg, M.E., Brandt, E.B., Morris, S.C., and Strait, R.T. 2005. Molecular mechanisms of anaphylaxis: Lessons from studies with murine models. *J Allergy Clin Immunol* 115:449–457.

Fritsché, R. 2003. Animal models in food allergy: Assessment of allergenicity and preventive activity of infant formulas. *Toxicol Lett* 140–141:303–309.

Gizzarelli, F., Corinti, S., Barletta, B. et al. 2006. Evaluation of allergenicity of genetically modified soybean protein extract in murine model of oral allergen-specific sensitization. *Clin Exp Allergy* 36:238–248.

Helm, R.M. 2002. Food allergy animal models: An overview. *Ann NY Acad Sci* 964:139–150.

Helm, R.M., Furuta, J.S., Ye, J. et al. 2002. A neonatal swine model for peanut allergy. *J Allergy Clin Immunol* 109:136–142.

Helm, R.M., R.W. Ermel, and Frick, O.L. 2003. Non-murine animal models of food allergy. *Environ Health Perspect* 111:239–244.

Hilton, J., Dearman, R.J., Basketter, D.A., and Kimber, I. 1994. Serological responses induced in mice by immunogenic proteins and by protein respiratory allergens. *Toxicol Lett* 73:43–53.

Hilton, J., Dearman, R.J., Sattar, N., Basketter, D.A., and Kimber, I. 1997. Characteristics of antibody responses induced in mice by protein allergens. *Food Chem Toxicol* 35:1209–1218.

Ito, K., Ohara, K.I., Murosaki, S. et al. 1997. Murine model of IgE production with a predominant Th2-response by feeding protein antigen without adjuvants. *Eur J Immunol* 27:3427–3437.

Jackson, H.A., Jackson, M.W., Coblenz, L., and Hammerberg, B. 2003. Evaluation of the clinical and allergen-specific serum immunoglobulin-E responses to oral challenge with cornstarch, corn, soy and a soy hydrolysate diets in dogs with spontaneous food allergy. *Vet Derm* 14:181–187.

Jeffers, J.G., Meyer, E.K., and Sosis, E.J. 1996. Responses of dogs with food allergies to single-ingredient dietary provocation. *J Am Vet Assoc* 209:608–611.

Kimber, I., Atherton, K.T., Kenna, G.J., and Dearman, R.J. 2000. Predictive methods for food allergenicity: Perspectives and current status. *Toxicology* 147:147–150.

Kimber, I., Stone, S., and Dearman, R.J. 2003. Assessment of the inherent allergenic potential of proteins in mice. *Environ Health Perspect* 111:227–231.

Kimber, I., Penninks, A.H., and Dearman, R.J. 2007. Food allergy: Immunological aspects and approaches to safety assessment. In *Immunotoxicology and Immunopharmacology*. R. Leubke, R. House, and I. Kimber, Eds., pp. 607–622. CRC Press, Boca Raton, FL.

Knippels, L.M.J. and Penninks, A.H. 2005. Recent advances using rodent models for predicting human allergenicity. *Toxicol Appl Pharmacol* 207: S157–S160.

Knippels, L.M.J., Penninks, A.H., Spanhaak, S., and Houben, G.F. 1998a. Oral sensitisation to food proteins: A Brown Norway rat model. *Clin Exp Allergy* 28:368–375.

Knippels, L.M.J., Penninks, A.H., and Houben, G. 1998b. Continued expression of anti soy-protein antibodies in rats bred on a soy-protein free diet; the importance of dietary control in oral sensitization research. *J Allergy Clin Immunol* 101:815–820.

Knippels, L.M.J., Penninks, A.H., Van Meeteren, M., and Houben, G.F. 1999a. Humoral and cellular immune responses in different rat strains upon oral exposure to ovalbumin. *Food Chem Toxicol* 37:881 888.

Knippels, L.M.J., Penninks, A.H., Smit, J.J., and Houben, G.F. 1999b. Immune-mediated effects upon oral challenge of ovalbumin sensitised Brown Norway rats; further characterization of a rat food allergy model. *Toxicol Appl Pharmacol* 156:161–169.

Knippels, L.M.J., Felius, A.A., van der Kleij, H.P.M., Penninks, A.H., Koppelman, S.J., and Houben, G.F. 2000. Comparison of antibody responses to hen's egg and cow's milk-proteins in orally sensitised rats and human patients. *Allergy* 55:251–258.

Kitagawa, S., Zhang, S., Harari, Y., and Castro, G.A. 1995. Relative allergenicity of cow's milk and cow's milk-based infant formulas in an animal model. *Am J Med Sci* 310:183–187.

Kroghsbo, S., Christensen, H.R., and Frokiar, H. 2003. Experimental parameters differentially affect the humoral response of the cholera-toxin-based murine model for food allergy. *Int Arch Allergy Immunol* 131:256–263.

Li, X.M. and Sampson, H.A. 2002. Novel approaches for the treatment of food allergy. *Curr Opin Allergy Clin Immunol* 2:213–218.

Li, X.M., Schofield, B.H., Huang, C.K., Kleiner, G.I., Sampson, H.A. 1999. A murine model for IgE-mediated cow's milk hypersensitivity. *J Allergy Clin Immunol* 103:206–214.

Li, X.M., Serebrisky, D., Lee, S.J. et al. 2000. A murine model of peanut anaphylaxis: T- and B-cell responses to a major peanut allergen mimic human responses. *J Allergy Clin Immunol* 106:150–158.

Li, X.M., Srivastava, K., Grishin, A. et al. 2003a. Persistant protective effect of heat-killed Escherichia coli producing engineered', recombinant peanut proteins in a murine model of peanut allergy. *J Allergy Clin Immunol* 112:159–167.

Li, X.M., Srivastava, K., Huleatt, J.W. et al. 2003b. Engineered recombinant peanut protein and heat-killed Listeria monocytogenes coadministration protects against peanut-induced anaphylaxis in a murine model. *J Immunol* 170:3289–3295.

McClain, S. and Bannon, G.A. 2006. Animal models of food allergy: Opportunities and barriers. *Curr Allergy Asthma Rep* 6:141–144.

Metcalfe, D.D., Astwood, J.D., Townsend, R., Sampson, H.A., Taylor, S.L., Fuchs, R.L. 1996. Assessment of the allergenic potential of foods from genetically engineered crop plants. *Crit Rev Food Sci Nutr* 36(S):165–186.

Miller, K., Meredith, C., Selo, I., Wal, J-M. 1999. Allergy to ß-lactoglobulin: Specificity of immunoglobuline E generated in the Brown Norway rat to tryptic and synthetic peptides. *Clin Exp Allergy* 29:1696–1704.

Paterson, S. 1995. Food hypersensitivity in 20 dogs with skin and gastrointestinal signs. *J Small Anim Pract* 36:529–534.

Pauwels, R., Bazin, H., Platteau, B., van der Straeten, M. 1979. The effect of age on IgE production in rats. *Immunology* 36:145–159.

Piacentini, G.L., Bertolini, A., Spezia, E., Piscione, T., Boner, A.L. 1994. Ability of a new infant formula prepared from partially hydrolyzed whey to induce anaphylactic sensitisation; evaluation in a guinea pig model. *Allergy* 49:361–364.

Pilegaard, K., Madsen, C. 2004. An oral Brown Norway rat model for food allergy: Comparison of age, sex, dosing volume, and allergen preparation. *Toxicology* 196:247–257.

Prescott, V.E., Campbell, P.M., Moore, A., Mattes, J., Rothenberg, M.E., Foster, P.S., Higgins, T.J.V., Hogan, S.P. 2005. Transgenic expression of bean α-amylase inhibitor in peas results in altered structure and immunogenicity. *J Agric Food Chem* 53:9023–9030.

Strid, J., Thomson, M., Hourihane, J. et al. 2004. A novel model of sensitization and oral tolerance to peanut protein. *Immunology* 113:293–303.

Strobel, S., Ferguson, A. 1984. Immune responses to fed protein antigens in mice. Systemic tolerance or priming is related to age at which antigen is first encountered. *Pediatr Res* 18:588–594.

Teuber, S.S., del Val, G., Morigasaki, S. et al. 2002. The atopic dog as a model of peanut and tree nut food allergy. *J Allergy Clin Immunol* 110:921–927.

Turner, M.W., Barnett, G.E., Strobel, S. 1990. Mucosal mast cell activation patterns in the rat following repeated feeding of antigen. *Clin Exp Allergy* 20:421–427.

van Wijk, F., Hartgring, S., Koppelman, S.J., Pieters, R., Knippels, L.M.J. 2004. Mixed antibody and T cell responses to peanut and peanut allergens Ara h1, Ara h2, Ara h3 and Ara h6 in an oral sensitization model. *Clin Exp Allergy* 34:1422–1428.

van Wijk, F., Hoeks, S., Nierkens, S. et al. 2005. CTLA-4 signaling regulates the intensity of hypersensitivity responses to food allergens, but is not decisive in the induction of sensitization. *J Immunol* 174:174–179.

Xu-Dong, J., Ning, L., Yong-Ning, W. 2005. Studies on BN rats model to determine the potential allergenicity of proteins from genetically modified foods. *World J Gastroenterol* 11:5381–5384.

## 3.3   CLINICAL METHODS FOR THE DIAGNOSIS OF FOOD ALLERGIES

Maciej Kaczmarski, Beata Cudowska, and
Elżbieta Korotkiewicz-Kaczmarska

> Allergy in general, and food allergy (FA) in particular, is probably the most commonly self-diagnosed health problem whereas it is overdiagnosed by public. FA is often underdiagnosed by physicians and is frequently misdiagnosed by allergists
>
> **Bahna (2003)**

Food allergy is defined as an immuno-mediated adverse reaction to foods, whereas the term nonallergic hypersensitivity has been proposed when immunological mechanisms cannot be proven (Burks and Sampson, 1992; Sampson, 1999a; Johansson et al., 2001; Sicherer, 2002; Høst et al., 2003). In humans, food allergies are often accused of causing numerous ailments. This is particularly true for the pediatric population, in which food allergy affects about 6%–8% of infants and young children and approximately 3.5%–4.0% of adults (Reibel et al., 2000; Guarderas, 2001; Sicherer, 2002; Høst et al., 2003; Nowak-Wegrzyn, 2003, 2006; Niggemann et al., 2005). Since the critical factor is that the immune system can be shown to be involved in the pathophysiology of the illness, food allergic disorders are usually classified according to the pathophysiological role of immunoglobulin E (IgE antibody), as an IgE-mediated, non-IgE-mediated (cell-mediated) or mixed reactions (IgE- and cell-mediated) (Bahna, 2002a; Sicherer, 2002; Bock, 2003; Høst et al., 2003; Nowak-Wegrzyn, 2003; Chapman et al., 2006).

Regarding these pathomechanisms, the clinical pattern of symptoms observed after ingestion of harmful food may be helpful in clinical classification to differentiate the onset of immediate (quick), semi-delayed, and delayed (late) reactions (Table 3.3.1) (Sicherer, 2002; Bock, 2003; Høst et al., 2003; Nowak-Wegrzyn, 2003; Bindslev-Jensen et al., 2004; Chapman et al., 2006).

---

**TABLE 3.3.1**

**IgE-Mediated versus Non-IgE-Mediated Reactions**

| IgE | Non-IgE |
|---|---|
| • Quick onset | • Delayed (usually) |
| • Anaphylaxis, other symptoms | • GI symptoms, eczema |
| • Well-defined mechanisms | • Unclear mechanism |
| • Easy to diagnose | • Difficult to diagnose |
| • Validated tests | • No validated test |

*Note:*   According to Fox A., Diagnosing immediate food allergy, *Food Allergy—Practical Diagnosis and Management*, Eastern Europe AAA Academy Meeting, Prague, 2008.

---

A number of laboratory tests may be useful in delineating specific foods responsible for IgE disorders, whereas laboratory techniques are of limited value in non-IgE-mediated reactions. This fact explains why until now there has been no one simple, quick, cheap, and easily accessible laboratory test for such diagnosis. This explanation must be enriched by the knowledge that allergic symptoms occur either individually or in combination and are not specific for a definite food. They usually change when the allergic child grows up (allergic marsh). Therefore, the diagnostic work-up of food allergy in patients in developmental age is a complex and time-consuming procedure, creating a great challenge for pediatricians, allergists, and other specialists including primary care providers (Kaczmarski et al., 1997; Ahlstedt et al., 2002; Bock, 2003; Høst et al., 2003; Chapman, 2006) (Table 3.3.2)

The diagnostic procedure used to evaluate suspected food allergy in infants and children includes: medical history (including family history of atopic/allergic diseases—parents, siblings, others), symptom-food diary (in some cases), *in vitro* tests (total and specific IgE measurements in serum), *in vivo* tests (prick skin tests, PST; atopy patch tests, APT), oral food challenges and other tests (Table 3.3.2). None of the above tests used alone can accurately confirm food allergy or predict the process of food tolerance (Kaczmarski et al., 1997; Burks, 2000; Bahna, 2003; Niggemann et al., 2005; Chapman et al., 2006).

Allergy testing is a very important prerequisite for specific allergy treatment. Proper diagnosis will allow the patient to receive the knowledge of the offending foods to avoid unnecessary dietary restrictions when a suspected food allergy is not present.

Who should be tested for allergy? All individuals with severe, persisting, or recurrent possible allergic symptoms and individuals with the need for permanent

---

**TABLE 3.3.2**

**Methods Used in the Evaluation of Food-Allergic Reactions**

Medical history and physical examination

Food diary

Elimination diet

Skin prick testing

RAST, ELISA—testing (specific IgE)

Double Blind Placebo Controlled Food Challenge (DBPCFC)

Other immunological and nonimmunological tests

    Basophil histamine release assay

    Intestinal mast cell histamine release

    Intragastric provocation under endoscopy

    Intestinal biopsy after allergen elimination and feeding

Others (see text below)

*Source:*   Burks, W. et al., *J. Pediatr.* 121, 64, 1992; Kaczmarski, M. et al., Sympozjum 1, 1997 (in Polish).

prophylactic treatment irrespective of the child's age (Høst et al., 2003; Niggemann et al., 2005; Chapman et al., 2006).

### 3.3.1 MEDICAL HISTORY

The general aims of diagnosis are to determine if the ingested foods cause clinical symptoms and to identify them as specific causal food products.

The diagnostic approach to suspected adverse food reactions begins with medical history and physical examination (Sampson, 1999a; Burks, 2000).

The information elicited from a detailed history helps the physician determine the clinical classification and possible pathogenetic mechanisms of food allergy. The physician attempts to establish the likelihood of a food-induced disorder on the basis of symptoms, as well as timing of the reaction and food suspected of causing the reaction (Sampson, 1999a). There are a few crucial facts in anamnesis that should be considered: family history of atopic (allergic) disease, type of signs and symptoms following food ingestion, quantity and nature of the ingested food, the timing of onset of symptoms, details of last (recent) clinical reaction, and factors interfering with allergic food reaction (Burks and Sampson, 1992; Bahna, 2003; Bock, 2003) (Table 3.3.3).

The value of the medical history depends largely on the patient's recollection of symptoms and examiner's ability to differentiate between disorders provoked by food hypersensitivity and those with other causes (Burks and Sampson, 1992; Chapman et al., 2006).

The medical history is helpful when we choose particular allergens for laboratory tests (PST or sIgE) or for food challenge. Thus, the medical history is the most important guide in diagnosing food allergy. However, it is important to recognize that the medical history is primarily subjective and has marked limitations (Guarderas, 2001; Chapman et al., 2006).

In some research series, fewer than 50% (30%–50%) of reported food allergic reactions from anamnesis could be verified by DBPCFC (Burks and Sampson, 1992; Sampson, 1999a; Burks, 2000).

---

**TABLE 3.3.3**
**History Details to be Ascertained**

Description of symptoms and signs
Timing from ingestion to the onset of symptoms
Frequency with which reactions have occurred
Time of most recent occurrence
Quantity of food required to evoke reaction
Associated factors (activity)
Medication
Reproducibility, especially for subjective symptoms (behavior, headaches)
Potential cross-contact (contamination with other food, dust mites)

*Source:* Bock, S.A., *Pediatrics*, 11, 1638, 2003.

---

Authors suggest that this is due to incorrect identification of food nonallergic causes of reactions and outgrowing allergies (Sampson, 1999a; Burks and Sampson, 1999; Sicherer, 2002; Bock, 2003).

For acute reactions, a food which is ingested, infrequently is more probably responsible for a reaction than one that has been previously tolerated. Additionally, reactions are more often caused by constant exposure to previously identified allergens than they are by a new sensitivity (Sicherer, 2002).

For chronic disorders, suspicions about particular foods are notoriously inaccurate and are only verified in about 30% of cases (Sicherer, 2002).

### 3.3.2   FOOD DIARY

This method is used to detect recognized and unrecognized associations between the foods ingested and the symptoms experienced. The parents (or patients) are advised to keep a chronologic record of all foods ingested during a specified period. Any symptoms that have occurred are recorded and reviewed by a physician later on. A dietary diary is used as the examining tool adjunct to the medical history (Burks and Sampson, 1992; Burks, 2000; Guarderas, 2001).

Accurate records of the ingested foods or beverages and any developed symptoms might focus suspicion on one or more food products. The findings are often confusing when symptoms are recorded frequently and in relation to a wide variety of foods (Bahna, 2003).

Food diary is frequently used to evaluate harmful food influence in chronic allergic disease (atopic dermatitis, allergic eosinophilic gastroenteritis, or esophagitis) (Sampson, 1999a).

Diet records and symptom diaries are helpful but rarely diagnostic. Table 3.3.4 shows the examples of nonimmunological adverse reactions to food and masquerades of food allergy (Sicherer, 2002) (Table 3.3.4).

---

**TABLE 3.3.4**

**Examples of Nonimmunological Adverse Reactions to Food and Masquerades of Food Allergy**

Intolerance (lactase deficiency)

Infection (bacterial, viral, parasitic)

Pharmacological effects (caffeine, histamine, tyramine)

Anatomical (pyloric stenosis)

Digestive (gallbladder disease, pancreatic insufficiency)

Metabolic disorders (galactosemia)

Toxins (bacterial contamination, scombroid fish poisoning)

Nonfood allergy (reactions to pollen, mould, dust mite, dander)

Neurological (gustatory rhinitis from spicy foods, facial flush from tart foods)

Factitious (Munchausen's syndrome/Munchausen's syndrome by proxy)

Psychological (panic disorder)

*Source:*   Sicherer, S.H., *Lancet*, 360, 701, 2002.

---

### 3.3.3 Physical Examination

Attention must be directed toward organs or systems involved in the allergic process, such as skin, gastrointestinal tract, respiratory tract (very common), and to other less common disorders (central nervous system—behavioral and neurologic symptoms, arthropathy, nephropathy, trombocytopenia, vasculitis, and others) (Guarderas, 2001; Bahna, 2002b; Bock, 2003). Systemic reactions due to food allergy can be observed: i.e., periodically increased temperature, regional enlargement of lymphatic nodes, "common cold-like symptoms" or failure to thrive (infants) (Kaczmarski et al., 1997; Bock, 2003; Chapman et al., 2006).

The physical examination is directed toward stigmata of atopic disease (Bock, 2003). According to Marks, in older children and adults the features include allergic shiner, allergic salute, nasal itching, transverse nasal grove, open mouth breathing, discoloration in the supraorbital area, geographic tongue, adenoid or tonsils hyperplasia, snoring, tooth grinding, allergic ticks, etc. (Marks, 1977).

The physical examination might reveal whether the presenting signs are more likely to be those of allergy or of other disorders. None of the signs of clinical manifestations are pathognomonic and the differential diagnosis needs to be established depending on the information derived from the medical history and physical examination (Bahna, 2003).

From the doctor's point of view, it is the patient who makes the diagnosis of food allergy when the mechanism is IgE-mediated, since the time interval between ingestion and allergic reaction is short.

When the symptoms are chronic and reaction to food is delayed the patient is usually unaware of the time relationship between ingestion of the food and the appearance of symptoms (Brostoff and Challacombe, 2002).

### 3.3.4 Diagnosis of IgE-Mediated Food Allergy

A wide spectrum of adverse reactions may occur after ingestion of food. Adverse food reactions can be divided on the basis of immunologic and nonimmunologic pathogenetic mechanisms (Johansson et al., 2001; Sicherer, 2002).

Two types of diagnostic tests are commonly used to detect antibodies to food allergens: prick skin tests (PST) and blood tests (CAP RAST or RAST). They both measure specific IgE (sIgE) antibodies = IgE-mediated allergic reaction (Nowak-Wegrzyn, 2003). The positive PST and sIgE show the presence of IgE specific for the food allergy tested (sensitization to susceptible allergens). Only those sensitized subjects can develop associated disease. In praxis, either test must be related and used in combination with clinical history (Nowak-Wegrzyn, 2003; Chapman et al., 2006).

Tests for food allergy, like other medical tests, are neither 100% sensitive nor 100% specific.

Sensitivity refers to the proportion of patients with an illness and with positive test results. Specificity refers to the proportion of individuals without disorder and with negative test results.

The importance of clinical question to the physician concerns the likelihood that the patient has food allergy if the test result is positive (positive predictive value).

The negative predictive value means that the test result is negative and the patient does not have food allergy (Chapman et al., 2006).

### 3.3.4.1 Prick Skin Tests

Appropriate laboratory tests can be selected for type I reaction (IgE-mediated)—serum total IgE, specific IgE, and SPT, all used as good screening tests to identify specific offending foods.

Prick skin tests are used to screen patients with suspected IgE-mediated food allergies. In Table 3.3.5, there is a list of clinical conditions in which the methods of IgE detection are indicated (Chapman et al., 2006).

PST is a bioassay in which a minuscule amount of food allergen is introduced into the skin by gently disrupting the integrity of the outer skin (scratching, puncturing, or pricking by special needle or lancet). Glycerinated food extracts of 1:10 or 1:20 dilution and appropriate positive (histamine, codeine) and negative (saline) controls are applied by the prick or puncture technique. In a sensitized individual, food allergen binds to specific IgE antibody present on the surface of mast cells in the skin and causes degranulation of mast cells. Histamine released from mast cells leads to a flare (erythema) and wheal response within 10–15 min (Burks and Sampson, 1992; Bock, 2003; Nowak-Wegrzyn and Sampson, 2006).

PST are judged positive if there is a mean wheal diameter of 3 mm or greater, after subtraction of saline control; all others are considered negative (Sampson and Ho, 1997; Høst et al., 2003; Nowak-Wegrzyn and Sampson, 2006). These diameter provides acceptable sensitivity of 75%–95% and specificity of 30%–60% (Sicherer, 2002; Chapman et al., 2006).

---

**TABLE 3.3.5**

**Diversity of Conditions Associated with IgE-Mediated Reactions to Foods**

Systemic IgE-mediated reactions (anaphylaxis)
    Immediate-onset reactions
    Late-onset reactions
IgE-mediated gastrointestinal reactions
    Oral allergy syndrome
    Immediate gastrointestinal allergy
IgE-mediated respiratory reactions
    Asthma and rhinitis secondary to ingestion of food
    Asthma and rhinitis secondary to inhalation of food (e.g., occupational asthma)
IgE-mediated cutaneous reactions
    Immediate-onset reactions
      Acute urticaria or angioedma
      Contact urticaria
    Late-onset reactions
      Atopic dermatitis

*Source:* Chapman, J.A. et al., *Ann. Allergy Asthma Immunol.* 96, 1, 2006.

---

**TABLE 3.3.6**

**The Diagnostic Value of PST in Children with Food Allergy**

| Food Allergen | Cutoff Levels |
|---|---|
| Cow's milk proteins | 5.8 mm[a] (8.0)[b] |
| Hen's egg | 4.0 mm[a] (7.0)[a] |
| Peanuts | 6.0 mm[a] (8.0)[a] |
| Wheat | 3.0 mm[a] |
| Soy | 3.0[a] |

[a] Eigenmann and Sampson (1998).
[b] Hill et al. (2004).

A positive PST indicates the presence of IgE but cannot univocally confirm that actual hypersensitivity for definite food allergy still exists. The diagnostic value of PST in children with food allergy is shown in Table 3.3.6 (Eigenmann and Sampson, 1998; Sporik et al., 2000; Hill et al., 2004) (Table 3.3.6).

A positive PST indicates the presence of IgE but cannot predict reactivity and does not always indicate food allergy (Eigenmann and Sampson, 1998; Sporik et al., 2000; Hill et al., 2004).

A negative prick test usually rules out food allergy mediated by IgE mechanisms. The PST with a commercial food allergen extract has a high negative predictive value (>95%), whereas a positive PST has only a 30%–40% positive predictive value (Burks and Sampson, 1992; Sampson, 1999a; Nowak-Wegrzyn and Sampson, 2006).

Testing with native food allergens is more sensitive than testing with commercial extracts. The responsible allergens are very unstable and disintegrate during the allergen extraction process. Prick by prick method involves puncturing the allergen product through the peel and then puncturing the skin (Nowak-Wegrzyn, 2003; Nowak-Wegrzyn and Sampson, 2006).

There is no lower age limit for performing PST. Earlier a lower age limit of 3 years has wrongly been recommended (Malinowska et al., 2002; Høst et al., 2003).

Limitation of PST include: active atopic eczema on the test side, local treatment with steroids or immunomodulator ointment, use of antihistamines (should be avoided at least 3 days prior to PST) (Høst et al., 2003).

Some authors propose to use the combination of PST, sIgE, and patch testing in the diagnosis of food allergy in infants (Isolauri and Turjanmaa, 1999; Vanto et al., 1999; Roehr et al., 2001) (Table 3.3.7).

### 3.3.4.2 Blood Tests

IgE antibody formation and allergy commence early in life, which can be reflected by specific IgE antibody determination in serum samples with the use of particular systems developed for commercial use (Ahlstedt et al., 2002). The paper technique and methods have been developed for the detection of free allergen-specific antibody

**TABLE 3.3.7**

**Combinations of APT, PST, and Specific IgE Determinations (≥0.35 kJ/L)**

| PST + sIgE + APT | Cow's Milk Proteins (n-71) | Hen's Egg (n-42) | Wheat (n-35) | Soy (n-25) |
|---|---|---|---|---|
| Sensitivity (%) | 81.0 | 94.0 | 91.0 | 100.0 |
| Specificity (%) | 100.0 | 75.0 | 86.0 | 100.0 |

*Source:* Roehr, C.C. et al., *J. Allergy Clin. Immunol.* 107, 548, 2001.

circulating in the blood stream. Test for specific IgE should be conducted with a validated method and can be performed at any age (Ahlstedt et al., 2002; Bock, 2003; Høst et al., 2003).

The determination of food-specific IgE (sIgE) may be preferred in the patients with following clinical situations (Kaczmarski et al., 1997; Sicherer and Sampson, 1999; Brostoff and Challacombe, 2002):

- Very young patients (infants)
- With severe skin diseases (e.g., atopic dermatitis) and limited surface area for testing
- Patients who have difficulty in discontinuing antihistamines
- With significant dermographism
- With suspected exquisite sensitivity to certain foods

A negative test (specific IgE) <0.35 kJ/L has a high negative predictive value (>95%) (Nowak-Wegrzyn and Sampson, 2006).

Clinical decision points indicating greater than 95% likelihood of reactions were established for the most common food allergens. The measurements are indicative of greater than 95% chance of clinical reaction (Chapman et al., 2006) (Table 3.3.8).

A patient with serum food allergy-specific IgE in excess of the 95% predictive value may be considered reactive and an oral food challenge would not be warranted. A patient with a food allergen-specific IgE levels less than 95% predictive value may be reactive but would require a food challenge to confirm the diagnosis (Sampson and Ho, 1997; Sampson, 1999a, 2001; Bock, 2003) (Table 3.3.9).

### 3.3.5 DIAGNOSIS OF NON-IgE-MEDIATED FOOD ALLERGY

### 3.3.6 ATOPY PATCH TEST

Patch testing is typically used for the diagnosis of delayed contact hypersensitivity reaction in which T cells play a prominent role (Nowak-Wegrzyn, 2003). Patch testing involves prolonged contact of the allergenic extract with intact skin under occlusion for 48 h. The results are evaluated 20 min after removing the patch and again at 72 h (final assessment). Positive reactions to patch tests consist of erythema and induration. As shown in Table 3.3.10, the correct interpretation of this test allows

**TABLE 3.3.8**

**Food Allergen-Specific IgE Antibody Thresholds of Clinical Reactivity**

| Food | Serum Food-IgE (kIU/L) | PPV (%) |
|------|------------------------|---------|
| Milk | 15 | 95 |
|  | 5 if ≤1 year | >95 |
| Eggs | 7 | >95 |
|  | 2 if ≤2 years | >95 |
| Peanuts | 14 | >95 |
| Fish | 20 | >95 |
| Tree nuts | ≈15 | >95 |

*Source:* Chapman, J.A. et al., *Ann Allergy Asthma Immunol*, 96, 1, 2006.

*Note:* PPV, positive predictive value; kIU/L is a unit for measurement of the concentration of food-specific IgE.

**TABLE 3.3.9**

*In Vitro* **Test Values that may be Used to Determine whether Food Challenges Are Needed**

| Clinical Reaction | Serum Food IgE kIU/L | | | | | | PPV% |
|-------------------|-----|------|--------|------|-----|-------|------|
|  | Egg | Milk | Peanut | Fish | Soy | Wheat | |
| Reaction highly probable (no challenge needed) | >7 | >15 | >14 | >20 | >60 | >80 | 95.0 |
| Young children (reaction highly probable) | >2 (2 years) | >5 (1 year) | — | — | — | — | >95.0 |
| Reaction unlikely (home or physician challenge) | <0.35 | <0.35 | <0.35 | <0.35 | <0.35 | <0.35 | — |

*Source:* Bock, S.A., *Pediatrics* 11, 1638, 2003.

*Note:* After Sampson (2001), Garcia Ara et al. (2001) and Boyano-Martinez et al. (2001).

differentiation between positive and negative or questionable reactions in atopic dermatitis with food allergy. If the result is positive, both infiltration and at least seven papules can correlate with clinical relevance (Turnjamaa et al., 2006).

To date, the APT with foods is not well standardized and different methods in preparing the test materials are likely to cause controversial results. Most studies with foods have been performed with cow's milk, hen's egg, and wheat. The fresh foods should be preferred over commercial extracts for testing. The APT with foods like cow's milk or hen's egg has been studied in infants and children since food allergy plays a role especially in this age group, whereas aeroallergens (house dust mite) have been studied more intensively in adults (Turnjamaa et al., 2006).

**TABLE 3.3.10**

**Revised European Task Force on Atopic Dermatitis (ETFAD) Key for Atopy Patch Test (APT) Reading**

| | |
|---|---|
| – | Negative |
| ? | Only erythema, questionable |
| + | Erythema, infiltration |
| ++ | Erythema, few papules |
| +++ | Erythema, many or spreading papules |
| ++++ | Erythema, vesicles |

*Source:*   Turnjamaa, K. et al., *Allergy*, 61, 1377, 2006.

In allergic disease, in which T cells play a major role in pathogenesis (e.g., infantile atopic dermatitis), combined skin prick and patch testing may enhance identification of the offending foods (Roehr et al., 2001; Bahna, 2003). According to Turnjamaa et al. the APT with food (cow's milk, hen's egg, cereals, and peanut) may increase the identification of food allergy in patients with atopic eczema (AE) in the following cases:

- Suspicion of food allergy without predictive-specific IgE levels or a positive PST
- Severe and/or persistent AE with unknown trigger factors
- Multiple IgE sensitizations without proven clinical relevance in patients with AE

Usually the APT has been used to diagnose delayed reactions in children with cow's milk allergy, atopic dermatitis, and for identification of causative food in eosinophilic esophagitis (Turnjamaa et al., 2006).

Patch tests were positive in 89% of children with delayed-onset reactions, with challenge-proven milk allergy. In children with atopic dermatitis, the combination of positive patch tests with evidence of sIgE or positive PST had the highest positive predictive value (see Table 3.3.7) (Roehr et al., 2001).

In the diagnosis of cow's milk allergy, skin prick tests (PST) and APT yielded nearly similar mean sensitivity (0.53 and 0.51, respectively) and specificity figures (0.81 and 0.86, respectively) (Turnjamaa et al., 2006).

Lately a novel technique with milk in a commercially available test kit has been introduced in France (Diallartest). A positive APT has a high diagnostic accuracy for predicting the outcome of DBPCFC (Turnjamaa et al., 2006).

### 3.3.7    CHALLENGE TESTING

#### 3.3.7.1    Diagnostic Elimination Diet

Elimination diets are often used both in diagnosis and management of adverse food reactions. If certain foods are suspected of providing allergic symptoms or if the constellation of symptoms is thought to be caused by one or more particular foods, the foods are completely omitted in the diet (Burks and Sampson, 1992).

Cow's milk is usually the first product to be eliminated from the diet. The first criteria for the diagnosis of cow's milk protein hypersensitivity were established by Goldman and coworkers in 1963 and refer to the observation that symptoms must subside following dietary elimination of milk and become exacerbated within 48 h of its reintroduction (three challenges in all) (Goldman et al., 1963). For safety of this biological method (mainly because of risk of anaphylactic shock), the criteria have been modified and one food tested is given either in open or blinded challenging test (Lifschitz, 2005).

Elimination of milk formula in infants lasts for at least 2 weeks. In this period, the infants are given extensively hydrolyzed casein or whey-based formulas. If they refuse to drink such formulas, adverse food reactions to these are suspected. The child should receive elementary (amino-acid) formula. If a breast-fed infant is suspected of hypersensitivity to cow's milk product or other food(s) via breast milk, the mother is also requested to temporarily avoid these products (Lifschitz, 2005).

In older children, elimination of one or two suspected foods may be appropriate. Elimination of a large number of foods before evaluation can lead to unnecessarily broad restrictions and subsequent nutritional deficiencies. It is important to remember that the diet cannot be more troublesome than the allergic disease itself (Kaczmarski et al., 1997; Bock, 2003; Lifschitz, 2005).

The selection of foods to eliminate should be based on a variety of items, including history of illness, age of patient, results of diagnostic tests, epidemiological considerations, adherence to the diet, and elimination of additional triggers which may cause symptoms (Sampson, 1999a; Sicherer and Sampson, 1999).

When the food to which the patient is sensitized is removed from the diet for 2–4 weeks (depending on symptoms), reintroduction can induce the same clinical reaction (reproducibility and repeatability of symptoms) (Kaczmarski et al., 1997; Sampson, 1999a; Sicherer and Sampson, 1999; Burks, 2000).

The amelioration of symptoms during dietary elimination of suspected foods provides presumptive evidence of causality. Finally, a trial with elimination diet may be useful to determine if a disorder with frequent or chronic symptoms is responsive to dietary manipulations especially in atopic dermatitis, respiratory or gastrointestinal symptoms (Diagnostic Criteria for Food Allergy ESPGN, 1992; Kaczmarski et al., 1997; Sicherer and Sampson, 1999b; Bahna, 2002b).

Since no gold standard has been established for true diagnosis of allergy, such a diagnosis is complicated. For patients with food allergy and intolerance, DBPCFC is considered the standard diagnostic test; however, this technique does not distinguish between allergy and intolerance (Niggemann et al., 1994; Ahlstedt et al., 2002; Bindslev-Jensen et al., 2004).

The diagnostic elimination diet procedure is shown in Figure 3.3.1.

### 3.3.7.2   Oral Food Challenge

Oral food challenge (OFC) is the basis of diagnosis of food allergy or intolerance, forming the standard to which other testing methods are compared. OFC may be used to diagnose IgE-mediated as well as non-IgE-mediated food hypersensitivity. Oral food challenges are used to identify, confirm, or rule out a suspected allergy to

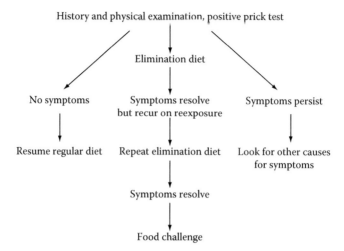

**FIGURE 3.3.1**    The diagnostic elimination diet procedure. *Note:* According to Szitányi P and Frühauf P. Food allergy—local perspectives? Food Allergy—Practical diagnosis and management, *Eastern Europe AAA Academy Meeting*, Prague, 2008.

food(s) (Nowak-Wegrzyn, 2003; Nowak-Wegrzyn and Sampson, 2006). Food challenge is recognized as the "gold standard" for confirming whether the patient has a true food allergy (Høst et al., 2003; Bindslev-Jensen et al., 2004; Niggemann et al., 2005). This is a biological response of the organism to the increasing amount of suspected food allergen, with simultaneous observation of signs and symptoms of this reaction. The results of the reaction give us three important pieces of information concerning (1) the presence or lack of food allergy, (2) pathogenetic mechanisms of induction of clinical symptoms (IgE-dependent = rapid onset, non-IgE-dependent = late onset), and (3) patient's tolerance of the ingested food (outgrowing his/her allergy).

Food challenges can be performed as follows:

Open—both the patient and the physician are aware of the challenge content

Single-blind—only the clinician, but not the patient, is aware of the challenge content

Double-blind placebo-controlled—neither the patient nor the physician is aware of the challenge content (Niggemann et al., 1994; Kaczmarski et al., 1997; Høst et al., 2003; Bindslev-Jensen et al., 2004; The Food Allergy and Anaphylaxis Network, 2005; Nowak-Wegrzyn and Sampson, 2006).

For the safety of the patient, the food challenge should be performed in hospital after receiving informed consent of the patient or his parents/caretakers in a separate room. The test is performed by a physician (supervisor) and others (nurse, dietician, and child parents). The setting must be available for emergency equipment, proper medicines (epinephrine, antihistamines, glucocorticosteroides, beta-agonists), the chart of challenge procedure as well as emergency treatment protocol should be in place (Niggemann et al., 1994; Høst et al., 2003; The Food Allergy and Anaphylaxis Network, 2005; Chapman et al., 2006).

Prior to oral food challenges, patients should avoid the suspected food(s) for at least two weeks and discontinue antihistamines or long-term asthma medications (beta-agonists) according to their elimination half-life. They should be evaluated carefully, before the challenge, for the presence of any clinical symptoms (The Food Allergy and Anaphylaxis Network, 2005; Chapman et al., 2006).

There is still debate whether oral food challenges should be performed in an open or double-blind fashion. Figure 3.3.2 offers a flow sheet for the decision-making process. Placebo challenges are indicated when, e.g., day-to-day variations (children with atopic dermatitis) or subjective symptoms play a role (abdominal discomfort, burning of the tongue, palpitations). Children under one year of age will rarely report subjective symptoms and might therefore undergo open food challenges (Niggemann et al., 1994; Høst et al., 2003; Bindslev-Jensen et al., 2004).

The food challenge is considered positive if a single symptom or a combination of objective clinical reactions is observed (i.e., urticaria, wheezing, vomiting, diarrhea, abdominal pain, exacerbation of eczema, shock) (Niggemann et al., 2005). Provocation is stopped if clinical symptoms are observed and the highest dose of harmful food is noted (Niggemann et al., 1994; Høst et al., 2003; Bindslev-Jensen et al., 2004; Niggemann et al., 2005; Nowak-Wegrzyn and Sampson, 2006) (Table 3.3.11).

In children older than 2–3 years, positive open food challenge may need a confirmatory DBFCPC in order to avoid a false positive reaction due to psychological and other mechanisms (Høst et al., 2003). Negative DPBCFC should always be followed by open food challenge up to normal daily intake of the food (Høst et al., 2003; Niggemann et al., 1994, 2005).

Upon completing the challenge, the patients are usually observed for the two subsequent hours in the absence of any symptoms. The total time for food challenge in the office setting can be as long as 4 h (The Food Allergy and Anaphylaxis Network, 2005; Nowak-Wegrzyn and Sampson, 2006).

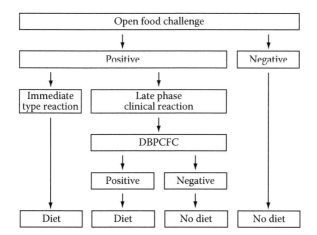

**FIGURE 3.3.2**    Flow sheet for deciding whether to perform open or double-blind oral challenges. (According to Niggemann, B. et al., *Allergy*, 60, 865, 2005.)

**TABLE 3.3.11**

**Procedure after De-Blinding of DBPCFC**

| Allergen | Placebo | Procedure |
|----------|---------|-----------|
| + | − | Elimination diet |
| + | + | Repeat challenge |
| − | − | No diet |
| − | + | No diet |

*Source:* Niggemann, B. et al., *Allergy*, 60, 865, 2005.

The practical procedure for conducting challenge tests differs from center to center and depends on the experience of authors (Sampson, 1999b; Reibel et al., 2000; Bock, 2003; Høst et al., 2003; Bindslev-Jensen et al., 2004; Niggemenn et al., 2005; The Food Allergy and Anaphylaxis Network, 2005) (Table 3.3.12).

For the IgE-mediated reactions, Sampson uses 8–10 g of dry food (double for wet food) such as meat and fish, which are mixed in the vehicle of choice and are administered gradually in three feedings over a period of 45 min (Sampson, 1999; The Food Allergy and Anaphylaxis Network, 2005; Nowak-Wegrzyn and Sampson, 2006).

For the non-IgE-mediated reactions, such as in food protein-induced enterocolitis, 0.15–0.3 gram protein/kg/body weight and no more than 8–10 g of dry food are also given in the vehicle of choice (The Food Allergy and Anaphylaxis Network, 2005; Nowak-Wegrzyn and Sampson, 2006).

**TABLE 3.3.12**

**The Practical Procedure for Conducting DBPCFC Depending on Diagnostic Centers and Experience of Authors (Own Comparison)**

| Day | Procedure of Performing Milk Challenge | | Proposal for Starting Dose for Different Foods | |
|-----|----------------------------------------|---------|----------------------------|------|
| | Australia | Germany | Food | Dose |
| 1 | 1 drop inside lip; 0.5, 2.5, 5.0, 10.0, 20.0, 30 mL at 30 min intervals | Successive doses in randomized manner (verum, placebo) are given: 0.1; 0.3; 1.0; 3.0; 10.0; 30.0; 100.0 mL fresh pasteurized milk, time interval 20 min | Milk | 0.1 mL |
| | | | Egg | 1.0 mg |
| | | | Wheat | 100 mg |
| 2 | 30, 60, 120 mL at 30 min intervals | | Peanut | mg |
| | | | Cod | mg |
| 3 | Normal volumes of milk, i.e. 7450 mL per day | | Soy | 1.0 mg |
| | | | Shrimp | 5.0 mg |
| | | | Hazelnut | 0.1 mg |
| References | Sporik R. et al. (2000) | Reibel et al. (2000) | Bindslev-Jensen et al. (2004) | |

*Source:* From Bindslev-Jensen, C. et al., *Allergy*, 59, 690, 2004; Host, A. et al., *Allergy*, 58, 559, 2003; Reibel et al., 2005.

These challenges are administered in a vehicle that completely obscures the nature of the food being challenged or at least masks it enough to render the doses difficult to identify (Bock, 2003).

For other foods (i.e., white of egg and yolk, wheat), powder is dissolved in a milk-free formula or water and given in a similar regiment (mL) as for cow's milk (The Food Allergy and Anaphylaxis Network, 2005; Nowak-Wegrzyn and Sampson, 2006).

Niggemann, Wahn, and Sampson have designed the following procedure for oral food challenges (Niggemann et al., 1994):

1. Oral food challenges have to be performed in a control manner if used for clinical studies.
2. In infants, oral food challenges may also be performed in an open manner while in older children, oral challenges should be done double-blind and placebo-controlled food challenge (DBPCFC)—especially in the case of atopic dermatitis.
3. Medication should be withdrawn according to half-life.
4. Blinding should be guaranteed by a dietician. The "blind" effect can best be achieved by using an extensively hydrolyzed formula (eHF) or an amino-acid formula (AA).
5. The relation of placebo to allergen challenges should be at least 1:2.
6. Oral challenges are performed in a titrated manner, starting with very low doses followed by increasing steps (every 30 min) up to the equivalent amount of the usual daily intake of an infant/child.
7. Observation time should be 24 h for expected early clinical reactions and 48 h for expected late-phase reactions (patients with AD).
8. Thorough documentation of the challenge results is mandatory. The responsible physician should sign the form after 24 h, after 48 h, and after the final result.
9. Challenges should be observed and supervised by professionals capable of dealing with anaphylaxis.

Precautions: if there is any doubt about the safety of giving food to a patient, everything should be done under the physician supervision with possible appropriate emergency medications (The Food Allergy and Anaphylaxis Network, 2005).

Contraindications: food challenges are contraindicated for patients with a history of past or present anaphylactic reaction to a single food or a group of food products ingested and with a simultaneous positive test for specific food (sIgE) (The Food Allergy and Anaphylaxis Network, 2005).

### 3.3.8   OTHER TESTS: NON-IGE AND NONIMMUNOLOGICAL ADVERSE FOOD REACTIONS

These tests are mainly used for the research purposes. Atopic dermatitis and allergic eosinophilic gastroenteritis are examples for disorders with mixed mechanisms, in which both IgE antibody and cell immunity may play a role (Sampson, 2004).

1. Determination of IgE in serum (total IgE)—normal values of total IgE increase gradually since infancy till puberty reaching adult level. Normal total IgE does not rule out specific allergy (Høst et al., 2003).
2. Peripheral blood eosinophil count > 450/mm$^3$.
3. Histamine released test (HRtest)—measurement of histamine release from basophile granulocytes. HR is more complicated for daily clinical practice but may be a helpful tool in certain cases of infrequent food or drug allergy (Burks and Sampson, 1992; Burks, 2000).
4. Low IgA and reduced fraction of $C_3$ complement (Lifschitz, 2005).
5. IgG subclass antibodies to food antigens (IgG$_4$ antibodies). The appearance of the IgG type of antibodies to food antigens is a sign of contact with the food antigen in normal or allergic patients. Cow's milk allergic individuals may show higher titres of IgG$_4$ subclass antibodies as compared to those tolerating cow's milk. Circulating IgA antibodies behave in a similar way as IgG antibodies. The predicted value of this test in delayed onset of clinical symptoms is poor (Lifschitz, 2005).
6. Test on cellular immunity: *in vitro* assays for lymphocyte and eosinophil activation; it is performed for distinguishing between children with and without food allergy, based on determination of Th2 type cytokines (Il-4), as compared to nonallergic children producing predominately Th1 cytokines (interferon-$\gamma$) (Nowak-Wegrzyn, 2003).
7. Lymphoblast transformation test, the leukocyte migration inhibition test with specific allergen (Kaczmarski et al. 1997).
   Lymphocyte stimulation test shows that the lymphocytes from patients with food allergy are more often stimulated by the food antigen than the lymphocytes of control subjects, although both sensitivity and specificity of the test have been low in most patients.
   The leukocyte migration inhibition test has been suggested to be a reliable test in cow's milk allergy but has been shown to be quite unspecific in other conditions (Kaczmarski et al. 1997).
8. Cytokine release upon food stimulation in serum and stool (IL-4, TNF-$\alpha$).
9. Markers of eosinophil activation in stool (ECP, TNF-$\alpha$) (Nowak-Wegrzyn, 2003).
10. Functional tests: intestinal permeability, tests of malabsorption (Lifschitz, 2005).
11. In some cases, invasive tests such as endoscopy are needed. For most gastroenterological allergies, small bowel biopsy shows a patchy enteropathy with nonspecific inflammatory infiltrate (lymphocytes, monocytes, eosinophils). If the diagnosis is positive, the mucosa improves when the offending proteins are removed from the diet. Histology of the biopsy samples often confirms the diagnosis but does not indicate which foods are responsible for the reaction (Sampson, 2004).
12. Intragastric provocation under endoscopy:
    Small quantities of food extracts (1:10 solution of food in 0.9 saline solution) are applied to the mucosa of the stomach by a gastroscope. The clinical

reaction is observed and scored (Reiman and Levin, 1988; Burks and Sampson, 1992; Romański and Bartuzi, 2004).

### 3.3.9 FUTURE DIAGNOSTIC PERSPECTIVES

New methods of diagnosing the IgE-mediated reaction are:

1. Recombinant allergens of high purity offer superior safety and specificity in allergy testing. There is an opinion that diagnostic sensitivity is generally lower than that of allergen extracts. Recombinant allergens may be of special value in diagnosing allergy to plant foods in subjects who are allergic to pollens (Nowak-Wegrzyn, 2003).
2. Immunoblotting (Pawliczak and Shelhamer, 2003).
3. Microarrays can be used for identifying the genes responsible for the allergic process. Microarray technologies can be classified into two types. One consists of oligonucleotide microarrays that use synthesized oligonucleotide as probes, whereas the other involves cDNA microarrays that use whole cDNA molecules with irregular lengths as probes. Two technologies (oligonucleotide array and cDNA microarray) have been developed in parallel and may be used in a parallel or sequential fashion (Pawliczak and Shelhamer, 2003; Saito et al., 2005).
4. Possibility of enhanced development of allergy to genetically modified foods (Bernstein et al., 2003; Chapman et al., 2006) (Table 3.3.13).

The diagnosis of food sensitivity leads to removal of the offending food from the patient's diet with concomitant improvement in the patient's symptoms which reappear when the food is added back preferably in a double-blind manner (Brostoff and Challacombe, 2002).

The rational selection and interpretation of diagnostic tests require an appreciation for the utility of the tests themselves and evaluation of the level of certainty required for the diagnosis of food allergy (Chapman et al., 2006).

---

**TABLE 3.3.13**
**Patients Who Are Likely to Develop Allergy to Genetically Modified Foods**

- Atopic patients with single or multiple IgE-mediated allergy to foods
- Patients with atopic dermatitis and confirmed allergy to one or more foods
- Workers previously sensitized by inhalant exposure to related food proteins
- Atopic patients previously sensitized by inhalant exposure to consumer products containing food-related proteins
- Atopic neonates being breast-fed

*Source:* Bernstein, J.A. et al., *Environ. Health Perspect.* 11, 1114, 2003.

---

## REFERENCES

The Food Allergy & Anaphylaxis Network and Shindeh Mofidi, Eds., 2004. *A Health Professional's Guide to Food Challenges*. S. Alan Bock (Medical Editor). The Food Allergy & Anaphylaxis Network, Fairfax, VA.

Ahlstedt, S., Holmquist, I., Koner, A. et al. 2002. Accuracy of specific IgE antibody assay for diagnosis of cow's milk allergy. *Ann Allergy Asthma Immunol* 89:21–25.

Bahna, S.L. 2002a. Cow's milk allergy versus cow milk intolerance. *Ann Allergy Asthma Immunol* 89:56–60.

Bahna, S.L. 2002b. Unusual presentation of food allergy. *Ann Allergy Asthma Immunol* 86:414–420.

Bahna, S.L. 2003. Diagnosis of food allergy. *Ann Allergy Asthma Immunol* 90:77–80.

Bernstein, J.A., Bernstein, I.L., Miller, M. et al. 2003. Clinical and laboratory investigation of allergy to genetically modified foods. *Environ Health Perspect* 11:1114–1121.

Bindslev-Jensen, C., Ballmer-Weber, B.K., Bengtsson, U. et al. 2004. Standardization of food challenges with immediate reactions to foods—position paper from the European Academy of Allergology and Clinical Immunology. *Allergy* 59:690–697.

Bock, S.A. 2003. Diagnostic evaluation. *Pediatrics* 11:1638–1644.

Brostoff, J. and Challacombe, S.J. 2002. Food Allergy and Intolerance. Part IV: Clinical Diagnosis of Food Allergy and Intolerance. Saunders, London.

Burks, W. 2000. Diagnosis of allergic reactions to food. *Pediatr Ann* 29:744–755.

Burks, W. and Sampson, H.A. 1992. Diagnostic approaches to the patient with suspected food allergies. *J Pediatr* 121:64–71.

Chapman, J.A., Bernstein, I.L., Lee, R.E. et al. 2006. Food allergy: a practice parameter. The American Academy of Allergy, Asthma and Immunology (AAAAI) and American College of Allergy, Asthma and Immunology document. *Ann Allergy Asthma Immunol* 96:1–68.

Diagnostic criteria for food allergy with predominantly intestinal symptoms. 1992. The European Society for Paediatrics Gastroenterology and Nutrition Working Group for the Diagnostic Criteria for Food Allergy. *J Ped Gastroenterol Nutr* 14:108–112.

Eigenmann, P. and Sampson, H.A. 1998. Interpreting skin prick tests in the evaluation of food allergy in children. *Pediatr Allergy Immunol* 9:186–191.

Goldman, A.S., Anderson, D.W., Sellers, W.A. et al. 1963. Milk Allergy. I. Oral challenge with milk and isolated milk proteins in allergic children. *Pediatrics* 32:425–443.

Guarderas, J.C. 2001. Is it food? Differentiating the cause of adverse food reactions to food. *Postgrad Med* 109:125–127, 131–134.

Hill, D.J., Heine, R.G., and Hosking, C.S. 2004. The diagnostic value of SPT in children with food allergy. *Pediatr Allergy Immunol* 15:435–444.

Høst, A., Andrae, S., and Charkin, S. 2003. Allergy testing in children: why, who, when and how? *Allergy* 58:559–569.

Isolauri, E. and Turnjamaa, K. 1999. Combined skin prick and patch testing enhances identification of food allergy in infants with atopic dermatitis. *J Allergy Clin Immunol* 97:9–15.

Johansson, S.B.O., Hourihane, J.O.B., Bousquet, J. et al. 2001. A revised nomenclature for allergy: An EAACI position statement from the EAACI nomenclature task force. *Allergy* 56:813–824.

Kaczmarski, M., Kruszewski, J., Czerwionka-Szaflarska, M., Socha, J., Wąsowska-Królikowska, K., Siwińska-Gołębiowska, M., Romański, B., Chmielewska-Szewczyk, D., Piotrowska-Jastrzębska, J., Buczyłko, K., Silny, W., Korzon, M. 1997. Alergia i nietolerancja pokarmowa. Stanowisko Polskiej Grupy Ekspertów. Sympozjum 1. *Oficyna Wydawnicza UNIMED, Jaworzno, Poland*.

Lifschitz, C. 2005. Allergy to cow milk. *J Ped Neonatal* 2:1–7.

Malinowska, E., Kaczmarski, M., and Wasilewska, J. 2002. Total IgE levels and skin test results in children under three years of age with food hypersensitivity. *Med Sci Monit* 8:280–287.

Marks, M.B. 1977. Recognizing the allergic person. *Am Fam Physician* 16:72–79.

Niggemann, B., Rolinck-Werninghaus, C., Mehl, A. et al. 2005. Controlled oral food challenges in children—when indicated, when superfluous? *Allergy*. 60:865–870.

Niggemann, B., Wahn, U., and Sampson, H.A. 1994. Proposals for standardization of oral food challenges in infants and children. Diagnosis of cow's milk and food allergy. *Pediatr Allergy Immunol* 5:11–13.

Nowak-Wegrzyn, A. 2003. Future approaches to food allergy. *Pediatrics* 111:1672–1680.

Nowak-Wegrzyn, A. and Sampson, H.A. 2006. Adverse reactions to foods. *Med Clin N Am* 90:97–127.

Pawliczak, R. and Shelhamer, J.H. 2003. Application of functional genomics in allergy and clinical immunology. *Allergy* 58:973–980.

Reibel, S., Röhr, M., Ziegert, M. et al. 2000. What safety measures need be taken in oral food challenges in children? *Allergy* 55:940–944.

Reiman, H.J. and Levin, J. 1988. Gastric mucosal reactions in patients with food allergy. *Am J Gastroenterol* 83:1212–1219.

Roehr, C.C., Reibel, S., Ziegert, M. et al. 2001. Atopy patch tests, together with determination of specific IgE levels, reduce the need for oral food challenges in children with atopic dermatitis. *J Allergy Clin Immunol* 107:548–553.

Romański, B. and Bartuzi, Z. 2004. Alergia i nietolerancja pokarmów. Problem społeczny i lekarski współczesnej cywilizacji. Wydawnictwo Naukowe Sląsk. (in Polish).

Saito, H., Abe, J., and Matsumoto, K. 2005. Allergy-related genes in micro array: An update review. *J Allergy Clin Immunol* 116:56–59.

Sampson, H.A. 1999a. Food allergy. Part 2: Diagnosis and management. *J Allergy Clin Immunol* 103:981–989.

Sampson, H.A. 1999b. Food allergy; When and how to perform oral food challenges. *Pediatric Allergy Immunol* 10:226–234.

Sampson, H.A. 2001. Utility of food-specific IgE concentrations in predicting symptomatic food allergy. *J Allergy Clin Immunol* 107:891–896.

Sampson, H.A. 2004. Update of food allergy. *J Allergy Clin Immunol* 113:805–809.

Sampson, H.A. and Ho, D.G. 1997. Relationship between food-specific IgE concentrations and the risk of positive food challenges in children and adolescents. *J Allergy Clin Immunol* 100:444–451.

Sicherer, S.H. 2002. Food allergy. *Lancet* 360:701–710.

Sicherer, S.H. and Sampson, H.A. 1999. Food hypersensitivity and atopic dermatitis: pathophysiology, epidemiology, diagnosis and management. *J Allergy Clin Immunol* 104:114–122.

Sporik, R., Hill, D.J., and Hosking, C.S. 2000. Specificity of allergen skin testing in predicting positive open food challenges to milk, egg and peanut in children. *Clin Exp Allergy* 30:1541–1546.

Turnjamaa, K., Darsow, U., Niggemann, B. et al. 2006. EAACI/GA$^2$ LEN Position Paper: Present status of the atopy patch tests. Position paper of the Section on Dermatology and the section on Pediatrics of the European Academy of Allergy and Clinical Immunology. *Allergy* 61:1377–1384.

Vanto, T., Juntunen-Backman, K., Kalimo, K. et al. 1999. The patch test, skin prick test, and serum milk-specific IgE as diagnostic tools in cows' milk allergy in infants. *Allergy* 54:837–842.

## 3.4 METHODS FOR STRUCTURAL DETERMINATION AND EPITOPE MAPPING OF FOOD ALLERGENS

Andrea Harrer, Anja Maria Erler, Gabriele Gadermaier, Michael Faltlhansl, Fátima Ferreira, and Martin Himly

### 3.4.1 INTRODUCTION

Epidemiologic data suggest rising prevalence of food allergy, which affects 2%–4% of adults and up to 6% of young children (Breiteneder and Mills, 2005). Thus, the detailed characterization of the molecular properties of food allergens represents a common endeavor within the scientific community targeting at development of molecule-based diagnosis and immunotherapy. Structural data obtained by an array of physicochemical methods need to be linked to results from immunological characterization at the level of IgE antibody binding and T cell reactivity. An overview of techniques addressing these questions in food allergy research will be given in this section. Furthermore, sophisticated computational algorithms have been developed to allow prediction of allergenicity, as regulatory authorities are highly interested in estimating the allergenic potential of a given protein for safety assessment of novel foods being introduced by biotechnological industry.

### 3.4.2 PHYSICOCHEMICAL CHARACTERIZATION OF FOOD ALLERGENS

At the stage a new allergen has been purified from its natural source or a recombinant protein has been produced in a heterologous expression system, several physicochemical techniques are applicable for characterizing the allergen at the molecular level. Classically, gel electrophoresis, IgE immunoblotting, and N-terminal sequencing are well-established methods in molecular allergology and will therefore not be covered in this section. As reviewed recently (Breiteneder and Mills, 2005), molecular characteristics can influence the immunological behavior of the molecule. These characteristics include identity of the recombinant product with its amino acid sequence, the presence of potential modifications, e.g., disulfide bonds or N/O-glycosylation, conformation, thermal and/or proteolytic stability, homogeneity, and aggregation. A wide array of physicochemical methods has been developed that are capable of answering questions on the nature of food allergens.

### 3.4.2.1 Mass Spectrometry

Mass spectrometry (MS)-based methods applied for characterizing food allergens include intact mass determination using MALDI or ESI mass spectrometers and peptide mapping with prior separation by reversed phase-HPLC and tandem MS-based sequencing. For proteolytic digestion, the most widely used protease is trypsin. Additionally, either V8 protease or CNBr is applicable to improve the sequence coverage. A typical proteomic workflow is depicted in Figure 3.4.1. Moreover, MS-based methods have been used for disulfide bridge mapping, as shown for peanut 2S albumin (Clement et al., 2005).

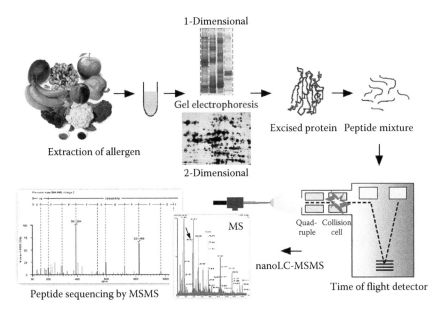

**FIGURE 3.4.1 (See color insert following page 234.)** Proteomic-based approach for identification of food allergens from natural source.

Determination of molecular mass by MS can be conducted for intact proteins as well as for peptides derived from proteolytic digestion. Since ionization can be affected by the presence of salts or ionic detergents, it is advisable to pretreat purified proteins by solid-phase extraction ($C_4$ or $C_{18}$ reversed phase beads). In matrix-assisted laser desorption ionization (MALDI), a gentle transition of sample from solid to gaseous phase is facilitated by co-crystallization with low molecular weight compounds like gentisic acid, sinapic acid, or α-cyano-4-hydroxycinnamic acid, which enables energy transfer from light to primarily singly charged protein/peptide ions. Alternatively, series of multiply charged protein ions with mass-to-charge (*m/z*) ratios of few hundreds to several thousands for intact proteins are measured in electrospray ionization (ESI) mode. Using ESI, online coupling of MS to preceding reversed phase chromatography is possible. In the usual miniaturized setup operating at flow rates <1 μL/min, this procedure is referred to as nano-liquid chromatography-tandem MS (nanoLC-MSMS). At present, an array of high-resolution hybrid MS instruments are available, which combine either a linear/three-dimensional ion trap or a quadrupole with a time-of-flight or Fourier Transform ion cyclotron resonance mass analyzer operating at mass accuracies down to 1 ppm. Thus, peptide sequencing based on collision with helium or argon atoms is performed. The resulting fragments (b/y-ion series) can be searched in databanks and the corresponding peptides identified unequivocally. For data validity, at least four consecutive ions of a y-ion series should be present for positive peptide assignment. Furthermore, tandem MS technology enables *de novo* sequencing (without databank search) of new protein stretches or characterization of protein modifications. In this context, detailed structural analyses on ion traps having the potential of sequentially fragmenting sugars shall be mentioned ($MS^n$ mode).

### 3.4.2.2 Secondary Structure Determination

Secondary structure content and conformation of food allergens has been studied in many cases applying far-UV circular dichroism (CD) measurements or Fourier Transform infrared (FTIR) spectroscopy. This was of utmost importance for food allergens as the effect of heat-denaturation and its impact on allergenicity was investigated. Notably, IgE cross-reactivity of food allergens is rather defined by conformational epitopes than by sequential epitopes. Just recently, important conclusions on the influence of secondary structure content of the major carrot allergen Dau c 1 on its allergenicity and antigenicity were drawn using this method (Reese et al., 2007).

The phenomenon of CD depends on the presence of a chiral center in close proximity to UV-absorbing groups, which in proteins is represented by the chiral $C_\alpha$ atom (except for glycine) located between two adjacent peptide bonds absorbing UV light at 214 nm. Experiments are usually conducted between 190–260 nm and have to be temperature controlled. Heating the sample in small increments to 95°C while recording the ellipticity signal at fixed wavelength (e.g., 222 nm) can be performed to determine the denaturation temperature of the allergen, which is equal to the inflection point of the sigmoidal heating curve. In order to assess the reversibility of protein denaturation, a CD spectrum at 25°C can be compared with the one recorded prior to heat denaturation. The heat resistance has been investigated for many food allergens including members of the nonspecific lipid-transfer proteins (nsLTPs) (Pastorello et al., 2003). Often, the secondary structure content of food allergens has been predicted from normalized CD spectra by nonlinear least-squares regression procedures (SELCON3 as part of the CDPro package) (Sreerama and Woody, 2000); however, results can easily be compromised by the method used for determination of protein concentration. Increments of five typical secondary structure elements ($\alpha$-helix, $\beta$-sheet, $\beta$-turn, random coil, and poly-L-proline) on the CD spectrum are shown in Figure 3.4.2. CD-based determination of secondary structure content of proteins relies on the availability of reference datasets of CD spectra of proteins whose structures have been solved experimentally. A new reference database has been introduced recently encompassing CD data of 74 proteins with known crystal structure (Lees et al., 2006).

Determination of secondary structure content can also be performed by FTIR spectroscopy, as shown for the major peanut allergen, Ara h 1 (Koppelman et al., 1999). In principle, a frequency and intensity shift of the amide I (longitudinal C=O) and partly also the amide II (combination of longitudinal C=O and N-H deformation) vibration can be observed when secondary structure changes in proteins occur. In comparative studies on stabilizing/destabilizing effects of hydrogen bonds in $\beta$-sheets, transitions from $\alpha$-helices (absorption at 1652 cm$^{-1}$) and from parallel to antiparallel $\beta$-sheets (absorption at 1633 cm$^{-1}$) leading to protein aggregation can be visualized and denaturation temperatures can be obtained. Notably, FTIR spectroscopy can be performed on both liquid and solid samples using the transmission or attenuated total reflection (ATR) modes, respectively. Thus, the influence of formulation (e.g., lyophilization) on protein stability can be physicochemically investigated by ATR-FTIR.

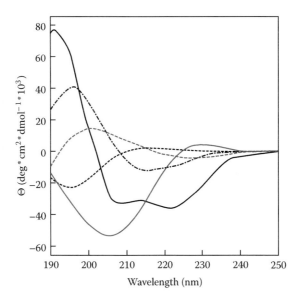

**FIGURE 3.4.2** Increments on circular dichroism spectra of secondary structure elements α-helix (black solid line), β-sheet (black dashed-dotted line), β-turn (gray dashed line), poly-L-proline (gray solid line), and random coil (black dashed line).

### 3.4.2.3 Investigation of Protein Aggregation

The question of homogeneity and aggregation behavior of food allergens has been addressed by size-exclusion chromatography (SEC), differential scanning calorimetry (DSC), atomic force microscopy (AFM), tryptophan fluorescence, and analytical ultracentrifugation (AUC). Applying these methods, heat-induced aggregation and its effect on IgE binding of the major potato allergen, Sol t 1 has been investigated extensively (Koppelman et al., 2002).

Given that aggregates formed by food allergens are not reversible by diluting effects or shear forces appearing during the chromatography process, SEC represents a suitable method capable of quantifying the separated subsets of protein. However, assumptions on the size and moreover, the molecular weight by simply comparing retention times of sample with standard proteins can be incorrect, as aggregates have been shown to adopt irregular shapes (Mills et al., 2001). As AFM allows the visualization of structures at the molecular level, the soybean 7S globulin β-conglycinin has been shown to adopt fibers and cylinders of 8–11 nm diameter during heat-set gel formation. This transition was preceded by small changes in secondary structure at 75°C determined by CD and DSC. In principle, DSC measures the heat required to increase the temperature of a sample compared to reference as a function of temperature. Thus, the thermodynamic behavior of food allergens during endothermic phase transitions like denaturation or aggregation can be determined.

To get structural insight at the tertiary and quaternary folding level, fluorescence spectroscopy can be used to monitor the local environment of tryptophan residues.

Upon excitation at 295 nm, free tryptophan in aqueous environment shows a fluorescence maximum at 353 nm, whereas solvent-buried tryptophan residues have maxima at 330–335 nm. Therefore, the extent of solvent exposure of tryptophan residues can be estimated from the wavelength of the fluorescence maximum indicating the formation of aggregates. Accordingly, the quenching susceptibility using iodide has been used as indicator for compactness of aggregation of Sol t 1 (Koppelman et al., 2002).

As AUC has been used widely for protein characterization, the sedimentation coefficient (S) has firmly manifested in nomenclature of food allergens. In principle, AUC can be operated in equilibrium mode, where the molecular weight and thus, the aggregation/oligomerization state of a protein can be estimated in a manner unaffected by molecular shape, and in velocity mode, for which modern analytical ultracentrifuges are equipped with absorbance and interference optics. For estimation of the aggregation state of Ara h 1, samples were run in a linear 5%–20% sucrose gradient at >180.000 g until equilibrium was reached (>20 h), and the S values were estimated by comparison to protein standards. In the case of Ara h 1, AUC and SEC gave comparable results. However, performing AUC is very time consuming and cannot be standardized due to the necessity of comparison to protein standards. It is not possible to determine the absolute molecular weight by AUC.

More sophisticated methods that have been used for investigating the aggregation state of allergens include x-ray and various types of light scattering techniques (Ferreira et al., 2005). Multi-angle or right-angle light scattering (LS) detectors operating in flow are available and can be coupled online to SEC or field flow fractionation instruments, which are claimed to expose sample to less shear forces than SEC. In combination with refractive index or UV detection for concentration determination, the molecular weight of the eluting protein fraction can be determined from the LS signal, thus, unequivocally resulting in the aggregation state. For investigation of the aggregation behavior in solution (without chromatographic separation), dynamic light scattering (DLS) and small-angle x-ray scattering (SAXS) can be used. While DLS determines the hydrodynamic radius of molecules from their diffusion constants, the scattering curve determined by SAXS is subjected to an indirect Fourier Transform algorithm, which gives the pair distance distribution function (PDDF). The PDDF represents the frequency of intramolecular distances between electrons and reaches a maximum at the hydrodynamic radius. The maximal dimension of the molecule results from where the PDDF meets the $x$-axis again and allows an estimation of the molecular weight. As larger particles scatter to lower angles an observation window of 0.5–25 nm can be set rendering SAXS insusceptible to particles eventually present from sample preparation (chromatography media). However, for molecules <20 kDa protein concentrations >1 mg/mL have to be used for SAXS, whereas DLS measurements can still give reliable results at 0.3 mg/mL. Notably, both methods are very sensitive to high molecular weight aggregates, but can be compromised by highly polydisperse (i.e., heterogeneous in size) solutions.

### 3.4.2.4   Nuclear Magnetic Resonance

Advanced structural analyses of food allergens have been performed by Nuclear Magnetic Resonance (NMR), which can be carried out in aqueous solution. Other advantages are the possibility to examine structural flexibilities and conformational changes during protein–ligand interaction. Moreover, problems arising with crystallization are avoided. However, structure determination by NMR is limited by size constraints and long data collection/analysis times. At present, more than 6300 structures solved by NMR are deposited in the RCSB Protein Data Bank™.

The fundamentals of NMR spectroscopy are based on nuclear spin of $^1$H, $^{13}$C, $^{15}$N, and $^{31}$P atoms. For more complex NMR applications of proteins >10 kDa, isotopic labeling using $^{13}$C- and/or $^{15}$N-enriched media for protein expression has to be performed, and milligram amounts of recombinant food allergen dissolved at high concentration are required. Under influence of the magnetic field, the nuclei align along the magnetic axis. Upon perturbation from equilibrium by radio frequency pulses, the nuclei start to "relax" in dependence of their chemical environment and spin–spin coupling with other active nuclei. The process of relaxation to equilibrium can be described by the longitudinal and transversal relaxation times, $T_1$ and $T_2$, being measured by 2D-NMR spectroscopy. Crucial is the sequential NMR assignment including the resonance frequencies of all nuclei, which is achieved by homo- and hetero-nuclear multidimensional NMR experiments. Most importantly for tertiary structure determination, cross-relaxation from one spin population to another takes place through space and can be measured by nuclear Overhauser enhancement (NOE) spectroscopy. The NOEs between nuclei can be quantified and the corresponding inter-proton distances determined. These distances can be used as constraints for predicting the three-dimensional structure. Recent developments of computational methods for structure determination have been reviewed (Liu and Hsu, 2005).

For long time, two major problems have hindered NMR spectroscopy on proteins >25 kDa. First, the larger number of resonances cause signal overlaps and second, larger molecules tend to relax faster leading to line broadening and poor spectral sensitivity. Upon development of transverse relaxation-optimized spectroscopy (TROSY) on strategically labeled molecules, the former size limit of investigated proteins could be increased significantly (Fernandez and Wider, 2003). In TROSY, the labeling strategy is based on $^2$D/$^{13}$C/$^{15}$N-triple labeling and subsequent protonation of amide in $H_2O$ enabling efficient backbone assignments.

The three-dimensional structure of the major cherry allergen, Pru av 1, has been calculated by 2438 restraints from five different NOESY experiments on $^{15}$N, $^{13}$C, and $^1$H nuclei (Neudecker et al., 2001). Pru av 1 is a member of the pathogenesis-related (PR-10) protein family, which has high sequence and structural homology to Bet v 1, the major birch pollen allergen. PR-10 proteins present in foodstuff are implicated in the pollen-food syndrome (PFS). Typically, individuals sensitized by birch pollen display clinical reactions to certain fruits and vegetables due to cross-reacting IgE-antibodies. As shown in Figure 3.4.3, Pru av 1 has a folded seven-stranded antiparallel β-sheet and two short α-helices arranged in a V-shaped manner wrapped around a long C-terminal α-helix forming a large hydrophobic cavity.

### 3.4.2.5 X-Ray Crystallography

X-ray crystallography can be regarded as the ultimate workhorse for structure determination. Presently, more than 37,000 three-dimensional structures are available in

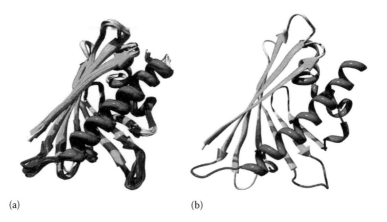

(a)                                                           (b)

**FIGURE 3.4.3 (See color insert following page 234.)** Cartoon representation of the three-dimensional structures of (a) Pru av 1 determined by NMR and (b) Api g 1 determined by x-ray crystallography. Pru av 1 represents an overlay of 22 chains retrieved from RCSB Protein Data Bank (accession number: 1e09), Api g 1 (2bk0). Highly flexible loops between β3-β4 and β7-α3 structures are depicted in blue, β-sheets in green, and α-helices in red.

the RCSB Protein Data Bank. The method is based on diffraction of monochromatic x-rays by well-ordered protein crystals. Based on the diffraction pattern, the electron density map of the macromolecule is converted by Fourier Transform and the protein sequence can be fitted into the atomic coordinates.

Two major bottlenecks arise in x-ray crystallography: crystallization and the "phase problem." In regard to the first, a homogeneous well-scattering crystal of the protein is needed. When growing such a crystal, a saturated protein solution becomes slightly dehydrated. If the process goes too fast, the protein would just precipitate in amorphous configurations. This growth is divided in two steps: nucleation of a microcrystal and subsequent growth for several days or weeks, to reach a size of 50–100 μm (Carter 1997). The process of crystallization is still not fully understood. Homologous proteins of different species grow sometimes under totally different conditions in variable forms (Georgieva et al., 2007).

When subjecting the obtained crystal to the x-ray beam, the scattered radiation leaves spots on a screen behind. Subsequently, the crystal is rotated three-dimensionally degree-by-degree to achieve enough data for clarification. Next, the generated diffraction pattern undergoes data reduction and processing. This gives a list of reflections with the corresponding intensities and errors, but no phase information (phase problem). Thus, the phases have to be obtained from a structural model with significant similarity to the target protein, or heavy atoms have to be incorporated into the protein. Measuring data sets at different wavelengths and differences caused by the heavy atoms can then be exploited to give first estimates of phases. Resulting electron density maps undergo several rounds of refinement. Although those calculation algorithms have become more and more potent, knowledge of the amino acid sequence is still required. New developments reducing measurement time and thereby, increasing crystal life-time during beaming have been reviewed comprehensively (Beauchamp and Isaacs, 1999). Although protein crystals contain 40%–70% of solvent, the comparison of NMR structures in solution and crystal structures by x-ray diffraction remains a highly discussed topic. However, only in few cases differences have been found. Unlike NMR spectroscopy, x-ray crystallography cannot give information about dynamics of the molecule, and the positions of the hydrogen atoms remain unresolved.

The crystal structure of the major celery allergen Api g 1, a PR-10 family member showing 42% sequence identity to Pru av 1, was determined at a resolution of 2.9 Å (Schirmer et al., 2005). Api g 1 consists of a seven-stranded antiparallel β-sheet, which curves around a long C-terminal helix surrounded by two short α-helices. Thus, Api g 1 adopts a similar structure as Pru av 1 (Figure 3.4.3). However, major differences occur in the two loops β7-α3 and β3-β4.

### 3.4.3   B Cell Epitope Mapping of Food Allergens

From the various existing B cell epitopes IgE-binding epitopes are the ones responsible for allergenicity. These epitopes either induce IgE antibodies themselves—class

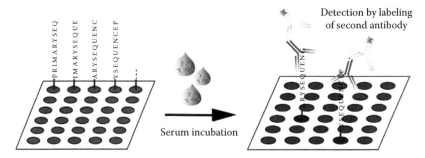

Identification of relevant epitopes using overlapping peptides spotted onto membranes

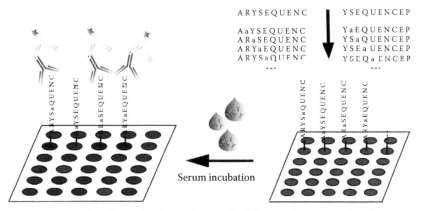

Fine-mapping of crucial amino acids for antibody binding by mutational analysis

**FIGURE 3.4.4**   Mapping of linear B cell epitopes and determination of crucial IgE-binding amino acids by SPOTs technology.

1 (complete) food allergens—or they react with IgE antibodies induced by other proteins as in case of class 2 (pollen-related) food allergens (Aalberse and Stadler, 2006). The difference between IgE immunogenicity and cross-reactivity appears to rely on the route of sensitization. While IgE immunogenicity of heat- and acid-stable glycoproteins encompassed by class 1 food allergens seems to be associated with sensitization upon ingestion, IgE cross-reactivity has been linked to respiratory sensitization by pollen allergens and clinically manifests as PFS after ingestion of certain foods (Lidholm et al., 2006). With the exception of cross-reactive carbohydrate determinants (CCD) (van der Veen et al., 1997), IgE-binding epitopes are described to be either linear or conformational with conformational IgE-binding epitopes being prevalent in pollen-related food allergy. As allergens usually lose conformational integrity during uptake in the gastrointestinal tract, linear epitopes seem to be more important in class 1 food allergy (Bannon and Ogawa, 2006).

### 3.4.3.1  Linear IgE-Binding Epitopes

There is increasing evidence that linear IgE-binding epitopes play a functional role in a large spectrum of food allergies. From these, the eliciting allergens derived from egg, milk, peanut, tree nuts, soybean, wheat, fish, and crustaceans have been described as the most prominent. Methods for mapping linear B cell epitopes include enzymatic and chemical cleavage, generation of synthetic peptides in various formats, and the use of predictive algorithms.

The advantage of the enzymatic and chemical cleavage methods has been exploited in the past as amino acid sequence information of food allergens was scarce. Peptide fragments obtained by protease digestion of food allergens were screened with sera from allergic individuals for eventual IgE-binding epitopes and subsequently sequenced. Limitations of this procedure included the positions of protease cleavage sites, the size of peptides as they were subjected to gel electrophoresis, and the quantity of peptide required for amino acid analysis (Bannon and Ogawa, 2006). Further methodological refinement has been achieved by molecular biology techniques, which facilitated expression of small protein fragments resulting in more precise maps of IgE-binding epitopes independent of proteolytic cleavage sites. However, knowledge of the amino acid sequence represented a prerequisite. Ultimately, advances in peptide chemistry led to the development of the SPOTs technology (Frank, 1992), which has been widely used for B cell epitope mapping (Reineke et al., 2001). As depicted in Figure 3.4.4, short peptides covering the entire sequence of an allergen with a two or three amino acids offset are synthesized on derivatized membranes by repeated cycles of coupling, blocking, and deprotection reactions. These membranes are then incubated with a pool of human sera and IgE-binding peptides are identified by immunoenzymatic or radioactive detection. Adapting SPOTs technology to the protein microarray format facilitated IgE epitope mapping using sera (in microliter quantities) of individual patients. Thus, a large panel of sera and allergens may be tested at once and the limitations of serum pools can be overcome.

Mapping the IgE epitopes of Gal d 2, the major hen egg white ovalbumin causing allergic reactions particularly in children, was performed by SPOTs technology

(Mine and Rupa, 2003). In a second step, the five immunodominant epitopes were fine mapped by mutational analysis to define amino acid positions critical for allergenicity of ovalbumin. Therefore, peptides with sequential single amino acid exchanges to alanine, glycine, or glutamine were synthesized on a membrane and subjected to IgE-binding analysis. Accordingly, the IgE-binding epitopes of Gal d 1, the hen egg white ovomucoid, were mapped (Jarvinen et al., 2007) and striking differences in IgE specificity were found between patients with transient versus persistent egg allergy. Four IgE epitopes were not recognized by any of the transient patients, but by all children with persistent hypersensitivity. Thus, these epitopes were termed "informative" epitopes and detectable levels of specific IgE against a combination of them might serve as a valuable tool for the prognosis of persistent egg allergy in children.

A similar approach was used for the investigation of cow's milk allergy, which also mainly affects children. IgG- and IgE-binding epitopes of all six major milk proteins, $\alpha$S1-, $\alpha$S2-, $\beta$-, and $\kappa$-caseins, $\alpha$-lactalbumin and $\beta$-lactoglobulin, were mapped using SPOTs technology and immunodominant B cell epitopes were identified (Chatchatee et al., 2001a,b; Jarvinen et al., 2001; Busse et al., 2002). Furthermore, differences in epitope recognition of major and minor IgE-binding epitopes between serumpools of patients with persistent and transient cow's milk allergy were observed (Jarvinen et al., 2002). Mutational analysis of the major IgE-binding epitopes of $\alpha$S1-casein was performed by substituting single or multiple amino acids (Cocco et al., 2003), aiming at the detection of variants with reduced IgE-binding for future immunotherapeutic interventions.

Applying SPOTs technology in the microarray format, complete sets of overlapping peptides of three major peanut allergens, Ara h 1, Ara h 2, and Ara h 3, were spotted onto activated glass slides, and the corresponding IgE epitopes were identified using sera of 77 patients (Shreffler et al., 2004). As signal intensity in microarray-based immunoassays is more dependent on affinity and tolerant to low concentration, this technology has been exploited for correlating specific IgE and $IgG_4$ responses to Ara h 2 with clinical severity and effector function (Shreffler et al., 2005). Forty-five peanut-allergic sera were assayed on six complete sets (10, 15, and 20-mers) of overlapping (2 and 3 amino acids offset) peptides covering the sequence of Ara h 2. Nine putative epitopes were found with significant inter-patient heterogeneity. Hierarchical cluster analysis of $IgE/IgG_4$ signal ratio to peptide arrays supported the hypothesis that IgG may act to block IgE access to the allergen. These findings supported earlier experimental results on differences in the IgE-recognition patterns between patients with persistent allergy and individuals who outgrew food allergy. Thus, evidence for the prognostic potential of such an analysis is increasing.

Severe allergic reactions have been described upon ingestion of tree nuts including almond, Brazil nut, hazelnut, pecan nut, English walnut, cashew, pine nut, pistachios, and macadamia nut. However, little is known about the IgE-binding epitopes being responsible for allergenicity. One immunodominant epitope was identified in Jug r 1, a 2S albumin seed storage protein of the English walnut, and the critical amino acid positions were mapped by mutational analysis (Robotham et al., 2002). Mapping for linear IgE-binding epitopes was also performed with Ana o 1, a major allergen of the vicilin seed storage protein family in cashew (Wang et al., 2002).

From the 11 epitopes tested, 3 appeared to be immunodominant. Hazelnut is known to cross-react with tree pollen and only little data exist on pollen unrelated allergens causing hazelnut allergy. As one example, the cDNA of Cor a 9, an 11S globulin seed storage protein has been cloned, but no experimental data on sequential IgE-binding epitopes have been obtained (Beyer et al., 2002).

Soybean, a member of the legume family, represents an important source of food allergens. More than 20% of seed dry weight is composed of glycinin, which consists of hexamers of G1 and G2 subunits linked by interchain disulfide bridges. Both proteins have been identified as food allergens that belong to the group of 11S storage proteins. From the 22 kD G2 glycinin, 11 linear IgE-binding epitopes were found by SPOTs technology (Helm et al., 2000). By molecular modeling, these epitopes were predicted to be distributed asymmetrically on the surface of trimeric G2 glycinin. The IgE-binding epitopes of G1 glycinin have also been characterized (Xiang et al., 2002). One epitope has been described as conserved among the two glycinins and Ara h 3 possibly accounting for severe reactions to soybean in patients with known or latent peanut allergy based on IgE cross-reactivity between the corresponding peanut and soybean allergens.

Allergy to wheat flour clinically manifests as atopic eczema/dermatitis syndrome (AEDS) affecting primarily children in the context of multiple food allergies. More severe reactions, as wheat-dependent exercise-induced anaphylaxis (WDEIA), affect mainly adults. The major wheat allergens have been characterized as α-amylase inhibitor, nsLTP, glutenins, or gliadins. Early studies using hexapeptides in ELISA format identified an IgE-epitope of the water-soluble α-amylase inhibitor (Walsh and Howden, 1989). Applying SPOTs technology and mutational analysis an IgE-binding epitope of glutenin was identified consisting of five amino acids in length. However, this epitope alone failed to release histamine from autologous basophils (Tanabe et al., 1996). Mapping of the IgE-binding epitopes of gliadins revealed ω-gliadin as the most prominent allergen with a few immunodominant sequential IgE epitopes from the repetitive domain recognized by WDEIA patients (Battais et al., 2005). Furthermore, it was hypothesized that conformational epitopes were responsible for allergenicity in children suffering from AEDS. However, a definite connection between the type of IgE epitopes recognized by patients and persistence of wheat allergy, as demonstrated for egg and milk allergies, still remains to be shown.

Tropomyosins are ubiquitous eukaryotic proteins involved in allergic reactions to shellfish, and are thus referred as invertebrate panallergens (Reese et al., 1999) eliciting allergic reactions to shellfish. The IgE-binding epitopes of Pen a 1, a shrimp tropomyosin, have been identified by SPOTs analysis (Reese et al., 2005). Based on these data, a hypoallergenic Pen a 1 mutant was generated by combinatorial substitution analysis and site-directed mutagenesis. In detail, the amino acid sequences of the shrimp IgE epitopes were aligned to the nonallergenic vertebrate homologue to compare amino acid substitutions. For each individual epitope, a set of modified peptides was synthesized containing all possible combinations of substitutions and screened for reduced IgE-binding. Twelve substitutions were selected for insertion into the Pen a 1 sequence by site-directed mutagenesis resulting in a correctly folded Pen a 1 mutant. The allergenic potency of this mutant was reduced by 90%–98%, as measured by allergen-specific mediator release from humanized rat basophil leukemia cells.

Severe allergic reactions after the consumption of fish are a worldwide medical problem. However, limited data is available concerning IgE-binding epitopes of major fish allergens, as most experimental setups made use of crude fish extracts. With the exception of the calcium-binding protein parvalbumin, mapping of IgE-binding epitopes has not been described. The relevant IgE-binding epitopes of this major fish allergen are considered to be conformational (Untersmayr et al., 2006).

### 3.4.3.2  Conformational IgE Epitopes

As many B cell epitopes are described to be conformational (Aalberse, 2000), peptides identified by sequential approaches may render limited information and might exhibit reduced antibody-binding affinity. In a very stringent definition, conformational epitopes are composed of amino acids from different loci in the allergen sequence brought into proximity by the tertiary structure of the protein. Systematic characterization of conformational epitopes is much more difficult compared to linear epitopes, because it requires knowledge of the 3D structure, which is often limited.

In the past, the issue of conformational IgE epitopes has been addressed by investigating the influence on IgE binding upon heat denaturation and reduction of disulfide bonds. However, using these approaches the exact localization of IgE epitopes remains obscure, as the loss of allergenic activity simply relies on destruction of conformational epitopes. Examples represent Mal d 3 (Sancho et al., 2005) and Ara h 2 (Sen et al., 2002). By mutational analysis and using IgE-inhibiting monoclonal antibodies (mAbs), the IgE cross-reactivity within the PR-10 family members Pru av 1 (cherry) and Api g 1 (celery) has been partially linked to a conformational epitope located in the P-loop motif (Neudecker et al., 2003). In another study involving IgE-inhibiting mAbs and CD spectropolarimetry, a second epitope of Pru av 1 has been mapped (Wiche et al., 2005). However, the involvement of a conformational epitope remains unclear.

A combinatorial approach for precise localization of conformational IgE-binding epitopes of the major fish allergen parvalbumin was performed using the phage display methodology (Untersmayr et al., 2006). In general, phage display can be used for identification of both, linear and conformational antibody-binding sites. In the case of parvalbumin, a phage library displaying a large number of random peptides was screened for high binding affinity to parvalbumin-specific IgE. Five affinity-selected peptides were sequenced and aligned to the allergen sequence providing information about epitope localization. Due to conformational mimicry by phage display the epitopes were termed mimotopes. Moreover, computational matching of the selected peptides onto the solvent-exposed surface of carp parvalbumin revealed the shape of three IgE-binding epitopes. Two of them were located at the axes joining the AB and CD domains and the CD domain and EF-hand motif, respectively, whereas the third was part of the EF-hand motif. Similarly, this approach has been used to compare the patterns of specific and cross-reactive IgE epitopes between individual patients of the PR-10 family allergens Pru av 1, Gly m 4, Ara h 8, and Bet v 1 (Mittag et al., 2006). Three antigenic areas likely to be IgE-binding epitopes were identified and mapped on the surface of the three-dimensional structures of the allergens using a computer-based algorithm. They consisted of regions mimicked by combinations of different peptides and showed heterogeneous IgE recognition among the tested patients.

### 3.4.3.3 Future Approaches by Hydrogen and Deuterium Exchange

As the characterization of conformational B cell epitopes depends on knowledge of tertiary structure of the respective allergen, NMR-based methods have been introduced for mapping antibody-binding sites. Using hydrogen exchange NMR, a reduction of the exchange rate of the amide hydrogens (from deuterium) as a result of the allergen–antibody complex formation was measured, and thus, the interacting amino acid positions in the sequence of Der p 2, a major allergen of house dust mite, were mapped (Mueller et al., 2001). So far, this technique has not been applied to food allergens, but still it should be mentioned as it represents a promising tool for IgE epitope mapping. Likewise, this phenomenon has been employed for amide deuterium exchange mass spectrometry (DXMS) described for the mapping of protein–protein interfaces and studying structural dynamics (Woods and Hamuro, 2001). As depicted in Figure 3.4.5, deuterium on the labeled allergen can be exchanged with $H_2O$, while this process is prevented in the IgE-binding epitope. By adjusting low pH and +4°C, a shift toward slow exchange conditions is achieved, and the amides within the interface remain deuterated. Subsequently, localization of deuterated amino acids is elucidated by progressive proteolysis with pepsin (acidic pH) followed by nanoLC-MSMS-based peptide mapping. As an advantage to NMR, MS-based proteomic technology is more readily accessible.

### 3.4.3.4  *In Silico*-Based IgE Epitope Prediction

Within the last years many food allergens have been mapped, and the majority of sequential IgE-binding epitopes were found. These data have been feeding evergrowing databases (Korber et al., 2006) and can be used in bioinformatic approaches

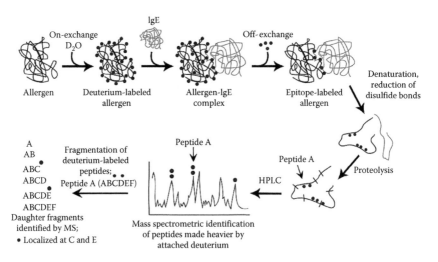

**FIGURE 3.4.5** Mapping of conformational IgE-binding epitopes by deuterium exchange mass spectrometry.

performing *in silico* predictions of allergenicity (Aalberse and Stadler, 2006). However, linear IgE-binding epitopes of minor food allergens have not been determined yet, and conformational epitopes are not included. These limitations compromise the predictability of allergenic potential or cross-reactivity with known food allergens.

An *in silico*-based approach was pursued investigating potential IgE cross-reactivity within the 2S albumin seed storage proteins. Linear IgE-binding epitopes mapped on the surface of Ara h 2 showed no structural homology with the corresponding regions of the walnut Jug r 1, Brazil nut Ber e 1, and pecan nut Car i 1 allergens (Barre et al., 2005). For homology modeling of Ara h 2, the NMR structure of Ric c 3 was used.

Conversely, cross-reactive IgE epitopes were predicted for Api g 4 (celery) and Cap a 2 (bell pepper) based on structural homology of food allergens within the profilin family (Radauer et al., 2006). The structures of these two food allergens were modeled using the crystal structures of profilins from birch and arabidopsis pollen and latex as templates. Thus, two highly cross-reactive conformational epitopes were predicted based on calculation of solvent accessible surface areas, and good correlation with inhibition data was found. However, no strong connection to clinical cross-reactivity could be established.

### 3.4.4 MAPPING T CELL EPITOPES OF FOOD ALLERGENS

Up to now, many cDNA sequences and thus, recombinant food allergens are readily available. Based on that, T cell responses to single allergens and mapping of distinct T cell proliferation regions within a sequence can be examined in allergic and non-allergic individuals. A comprehensive overview on the topic was reviewed recently (Bohle et al., 2006).

### 3.4.4.1 Technical Approach

For identification of T cell epitopes on allergenic molecules, specific T lymphocytes from the peripheral blood need to be enriched, as their frequency in the blood is quite low. As depicted in Figure 3.4.6, peripheral blood mononuclear cells (PBMCs) are incubated with optimal amounts of allergen. Thereafter, dendritic cells, monocytes, and B lymphocytes present in the peripheral blood can be used to activate allergen-specific T cells. By adding suboptimal concentrations of IL-2, the proliferation of allergen-specific T cells is supported, as they express IL-2 receptor (CD25) on their surface. Such an oligoclonal T cell line (TCL) contains a mixture of T lymphocytes with enriched specificity for the allergen, but still recognizes different epitopes. Monoclonal cultures can be obtained from these TCLs by limiting dilutions. Then, T cell blasts are enriched and seeded in the presence of irradiated PBMCs and growth factors in various concentrations. After 2 weeks, single T cell clones (TCC) are further expanded by the addition of IL-2 and in presence of irradiated PBMCs fed with allergen. Monoclonal TCCs are specific for one single epitope. For determination of specificity, TCLs or TCCs are stimulated with allergen, and the proliferative response is measured by the uptake of [$^3$H]-thymidine.

For mapping of allergen-specific T cell epitopes, either specific TCLs or TCCs can be used. T cell epitopes represent short, linear peptides in the primary

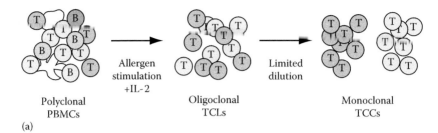

(a)

PRIMARYSEQUENCEPRIMARYSEQUENCEPRIMARYSEQUENCE

Peptide 1–12        PRIMARYSEQUE
Peptide 4–15        MARYSEQUENCE
Peptide 7–18          YSEQUENCEPRI

Peptide 27–38                                    NCEPRIMARYSE
Peptide 30–41                                    PRIMARYSEQUE
Peptide 33–44                                        MARYSEQUENCE

(b)

**FIGURE 3.4.6**  Production of oligoclonal T cell lines (TCLs) from peripheral blood mono-nuclear cells (PBMCs) by stimulation with allergen and IL-2 promoting the proliferation of allergen-specific T cells, which recognize different epitopes. By limited dilution, T cell clones (TCCs) specific for a single epitope are obtained (a). B, B cell. T cell epitope mapping using a primary sequence is performed with 12-mer peptides with overlaps of nine amino acids for stimulation of TCLs and TCCs (b).

sequence of a protein, which are, in case of allergens, presented on MHC class II molecules. To determine the exact position of the T cell epitope(s) on a protein, synthetic peptides covering the whole primary sequence are routinely used. MHC class II molecules predominately bind peptides of length 12–15 amino acids, and therefore, synthetic peptides for most studies were designed in a favorable length (10–20 residues). Peptides should furthermore contain broad overlaps of the primary sequence to ensure that epitopes are not excluded by experimental design. In addition, fragments with single amino acid exchanges can be exploited to identify critical residues necessary for T cell receptor (TCR) or MHC class II binding. Ideally, these fragments should maintain stable biochemical and biophysical properties, e.g., solubility, stability, and avoidance of oligomerization. TCLs with oligoclonal specificity obtained from a large amount of individuals can be used to identify immunodominant T cell epitopes, which are defined as being recognized by more than 50% of allergic individuals. Furthermore, T cells can be assessed for specific surface markers and cytokine production.

### 3.4.4.2   T Cell Epitopes of Class 1 Food Allergens

Class 1 food allergens are mostly found in milk, egg, peanut, tree nuts, soybean, wheat, fish, and crustaceans, and one of their characteristics is resistance to heating and enzymatic degradation. T cell epitope mapping with synthetic peptides revealed that food allergens contain multiple T cell-activating regions distributed over the whole sequence and that the patterns differ inter- and intra-individually. T cell epitopes of allergens derived from Brazil nut, halzelnut, celery, peanut, milk, beef, and egg were identified, and are described here in more detail.

Ber e 1 is a 2S storage protein from Brazil nut consisting of a heavy and light chain. For epitope mapping, 27 overlapping synthetic peptides (15-mers) were used (Stickler et al., 2003). Ninety-two community blood bank donors were included in the study and one epitope corresponding to amino acids 10–24 was found to be an immunodominant epitope located within the light chain. Three other prominent regions were found within the heavy chain (16–30, 28–42, and 40–55), although these values were not significant.

Cor a 1.04, the major allergen of hazelnut is homologous to Bet v 1, the major birch pollen allergen, and belongs to the PR-10 protein family. Allergen-specific TCLs and TCCs were established using recombinant Cor a 1.04 (Bohle et al., 2005). Peptide mapping was performed with TCLs from 17 different allergic individuals and tested with fifty 12-mer peptides covering the complete sequence. Identified epitopes were distributed over the entire hazelnut molecule, and epitopes were found that corresponded to T cell-activating regions of Bet v 1. In 8 of 17 TCLs, peptide 142–153 was recognized, and thus, it represents the most prominent T cell epitope of the hazelnut allergen. Cross-reactivity of this hazelnut allergen at the T cell level was demonstrated with recombinant Bet v 1 and Cor a 1, the major allergen of hazel pollen, although the T cell-proliferative responses to Cor a 1.04 were shown to be stronger. At a clonal level (18 TCCs), the majority of the TCCs specific for Cor a 1.04 did not react with the pollen protein, but rather with the homologous allergen in carrot. Thus, it was concluded that peptide 142–153 represented a food-specific T cell epitope found in hazelnut and carrot.

Api g 1, the major allergen of celery tuber, is another member of the PR-10 family. Using 48 overlapping 12-mers, seven distinct T cell epitopes of Api g 1 derived from 8 TCLs were identified (Bohle et al., 2003). Epitope 109–126 represented the major T cell-activating region of this molecule showing 72% sequence identity with the corresponding region of Bet v 1.

The major allergen of peanut, Ara h 2, was investigated using eight peanut-specific TCLs, and proliferative responses were assessed with overlapping 20-meric peptides representing the entire molecule (Glaspole et al., 2005). Eight out of 17 peptides showed significant proliferation, and T cell reactivity was shown to be clustered in two regions (19–47 and 73–119). Interestingly, a major IgE binding epitope was located in region 27–36, which overlapped with one prominent T cell epitope. A potential use for T cell peptides in treatment of peanut allergy was proposed, but further clarification of the precise localization regarding this epitope is needed.

The major allergen of beef, Bos d 6, is also known as bovine serum albumin and belongs to the most abundant proteins in the circulatory system. The immunological and allergological properties of Bos d 6 were investigated (Tanabe et al., 2002). Nineteen peptides consisting of 7- to 20-mers corresponding to regions not homologous to human serum albumin were used with PBMCs from 4 Bos d 6-allergic individuals. Three regions (107–123, 364–382, and 451–459) were identified to induce T cell proliferation, and all these peptides were also able to bind the patients' IgE.

α-S1-casein, a major allergen in cow's milk was mapped using TCLs from 2 allergic patients, and thus, 5 T cell activating regions have been identified (Nakajima-Adachi et al., 1998). Further clarification regarding the T cell pattern was achieved using 13 overlapping peptides with 17–20 residues length (Elsayed et al., 2004). Seven peptides did specifically stimulate α–S1-casein-specific TCLs, with peptide 1–8 and 136–155 showing the best response. β-Lactoglobulin, another allergen found in cow's milk, was mapped using TCLs and TCCs of four cow's milk allergic individuals. Peptides of 12–21 residues length were used, and seven T cell epitopes were identified (Inoue et al., 2001).

T cell reactivity of Gal d 1, a chicken ovomucoid was first studied with peptides of 55–65 residues length using PBMCs, TCLs, and TCCs (Eigenmann et al., 1996; Cooke and Sampson, 1997). Based on that, more detailed studies using shorter peptides were performed with TCLs derived from 6 hen egg-allergic patients (Holen et al., 2001). Eighteen overlapping peptides (14- to 18-mers) were investigated and 10 peptides were recognized by specific TCLs. Six of these peptides were also recognized by patients' IgE, and only four of them were exclusive T cell epitopes with no affinity to specific antibodies. Further studies corroborated the previously identified T cell epitopes (Suzuki et al., 2002). In this study, TCLs and TCCs from 4 hen egg white-allergic patients were mapped with synthetic fragments of 14–22 residues length. In total, 6 peptides were identified and 3 of them corresponded to the previously identified ones. Therefore, it was suggested that T cell epitopes specific to ovomucoid were identical regardless of species under investigation. Besides ovomucoid, an ovalbumin termed Gal d 2 causes allergic reactions in atopic individuals. Using TCLs, two T cell epitopes were identified at positions 105–122 and 323–339 of ovalbumin (Shimojo et al., 1994; Holen and Elsayed, 1996). Further studies revealed that peptide 323–339 also possessed allergenic capacity, as it reacted with a serum pool of patients allergic to hen egg (Johnsen and Elsayed, 1990).

### 3.4.4.3 T Cell Epitopes of Class 2 Food Allergens

In addition to class 1 (complete) food allergens, numerous class 2 (pollen-related) food allergens were identified that do not act as primary sensitizers, but elicit IgE-mediated reactions due to the cross-reactivity to homologous proteins. Accordingly, these reactions were termed pollen-fruit syndrome, and a prominent example for this pollen-related food allergy is the "birch-fruit syndrome."

Detailed investigations of the cross-reactivity of Mal d 1 (apple), Api g 1 (celery), and Cor a 1 (hazelnut) on the T cell level were carried out in comparison to Bet v 1 (Fritsch et al., 1998; Bohle et al., 2003; Bohle et al., 2005). Bet v 1 and food-specific TCLs and TCCs were stimulated with 12-mer peptides representing the sequence of each allergen. T cell epitopes identified in food allergens corresponded to T cell-activating regions previously found in Bet v 1. Interestingly, T cell cultures induced with Mal d 1 and Api g 1 proliferated more pronouncedly in response to Bet v 1 than to the food proteins, suggesting that these food allergens were pollen-specific and the primary sensitizer was the inhalant allergen Bet v 1 (Jahn-Schmid et al., 2005). Though members of the PR-10 family undergo rapid gastric digestion, which leads to total loss of IgE-binding activity, small peptides representing T cell epitopes may survive gastrointestinal degradation. In fact, fragments of Mal d 1, Api g 1, and Cor a 1 obtained after treatment with pepsin and trypsin were still able to activate Bet v 1-specific TCLs and TCCs (Schimek et al., 2005). A clinical impact of these pollen-related foods for patients without symptoms was proposed, as they might provide important stimuli for pollen-specific T cells throughout the whole year (Bohle, 2007).

#### 3.4.4.4  *In Silico* Analysis of T Cell Epitopes

In recent years, several Web-based tools were created in order to circumvent experimental work for epitope mapping using TCLs and TCCs. As T cell epitopes and some B cell epitopes in food allergens represent short linear peptides, prediction of these epitopes was made feasible. A summary of immunoinformatic resources including *in silico* T cell prediction was recently published (Korber et al., 2006).

### 3.4.5  CONCLUDING REMARKS

The structural and immunological properties of many food allergens have been investigated so far applying the above-mentioned methods for protein characterization. However, the question "what makes food an allergen?" has not been answered yet. Differentiation in the etiology can be made between complete and pollen-related food allergens, as prediction of IgE cross-reactivity within class 2 food allergens appears to be a feasible objective of future research. In contrast, sensitization to class 1 food allergens seems to be determined rather by the environment in which the protein is introduced to the immune system than the protein itself. Furthermore, the techniques within the scope of this section represent valuable tools for quality control and standardization of allergen products to be used for molecule-based diagnosis and immunotherapy of food allergens.

### REFERENCES

Aalberse, R.C. 2000. Structural biology of allergens. *J Allergy Clin Immunol* 106(2):228–238.
Aalberse, R.C. and Stadler, B.M. 2006. In silico predictability of allergenicity: From amino acid sequence via 3-D structure to allergenicity. *Mol Nutr Food Res* 50(7):625–627.
Bannon, G.A. and Ogawa, T. 2006. Evaluation of available IgE-binding data and its utility in bioinformatics. *Mol Nutr Food Res* 50(7):638–644.
Barre, A., Borges, J.P., Culerrier, R., and Rouge, P. 2005. Homology modelling of the major peanut allergen Ara h 2 and surface mapping of IgE-binding epitopes. *Immunol Lett* 100(2):153–158.
Battais, F., Mothes, T., Moneret-Vautrin, D.A., Pineau, F., Kanny, G., Popineau, Y. et al. 2005. Identification of IgE-binding epitopes on gliadins for patients with food allergy to wheat. *Allergy* 60(6):815–821.
Beauchamp, J.C. and Isaacs, N.W. 1999. Methods for x-ray diffraction analysis of macromolecular structures. *Curr Opin Chem Biol* 3(5):525–529.
Beyer, K., Grishina, G., Bardina, L., Grishin, A., and Sampson, H.A. 2002. Identification of an 11S globulin as a major hazelnut food allergen in hazelnut-induced systemic reactions. *J Allergy Clin Immunol* 110(3):517–523.
Bohle, B. 2007. The impact of pollen-related food allergens on pollen allergy. *Allergy* 62(1):3–10.
Bohle, B., Radakovics, A., Jahn-Schmid, B., Hoffmann-Sommergruber, K., Fischer, G.F., and Ebner, C. 2003. Bet v 1, the major birch pollen allergen, initiates sensitization to Api g 1, the major allergen in celery: Evidence at the T cell level. *Eur J Immunol* 33(12):3303–3310.

Bohle, B., Radakovics, A., Luttkopf, D., Jahn-Schmid, B., Vieths, S., and Ebner, C. 2005. Characterization of the T cell response to the major hazelnut allergen, Cor a 1.04: Evidence for a relevant T cell epitope not cross-reactive with homologous pollen allergens. *Clin Exp Allergy* 35(10):1392–1399.

Bohle, B., Zwolfer, B., Heratizadeh, A., Jahn-Schmid, B., Antonia, Y.D., Alter, M. et al. 2006. Cooking birch pollen-related food: Divergent consequences for IgE- and T cell-mediated reactivity in vitro and in vivo. *J Allergy Clin Immunol* 118(1):242–249.

Breiteneder, H. and Mills, E.N. 2005. Molecular properties of food allergens. *J Allergy Clin Immunol* 115(1):14–23; quiz 24.

Busse, P.J., Jarvinen, K.M., Vila, L., Beyer, K., and Sampson, H.A. 2002. Identification of sequential IgE-binding epitopes on bovine alpha(s2)-casein in cow's milk allergic patients. *Int Arch Allergy Immunol* 129(1):93–96.

Carter, C.W.J. 1997. Response surface methods for optimizing and improving reproducibility of crystal growth. *Methods Enzymol* 276:74–99.

Chatchatee, P., Jarvinen, K.M., Bardina, L., Beyer, K., and Sampson, H.A. 2001a. Identification of IgE- and IgG-binding epitopes on alpha(s1)-casein: Differences in patients with persistent and transient cow's milk allergy. *J Allergy Clin Immunol* 107(2):379–383.

Chatchatee, P., Jarvinen, K.M., Bardina, L., Vila, L., Beyer, K., and Sampson, H.A. 2001b. Identification of IgE and IgG binding epitopes on beta- and kappa-casein in cow's milk allergic patients. *Clin Exp Allergy* 31(8):1256–1262.

Clement, G., Boquet, D., Mondoulet, L., Lamourette, P., Bernard, H, and Wal. J.M. 2005. Expression in Escherichia coli and disulfide bridge mapping of PSC33, an allergenic 2S albumin from peanut. *Protein Expr Purif* 44(2):110–120.

Cocco, R.R., Jarvinen, K.M., Sampson, H.A., and Beyer, K. 2003. Mutational analysis of major, sequential IgE-binding epitopes in alpha s1-casein, a major cow's milk allergen. *J Allergy Clin Immunol* 112(2):433–437.

Cooke, S.K. and Sampson, H.A. 1997. Allergenic properties of ovomucoid in man. *J Immunol* 159(4):2026–2032.

Eigenmann, P.A., Huang, S.K., and Sampson, H.A. 1996. Characterization of ovomucoid-specific T-cell lines and clones from egg-allergic subjects. *Pediatr Allergy Immunol* 7(1):12–21.

Elsayed, S., Eriksen, J., Oysaed, L.K., Idsoe, R., and Hill, D.J. 2004. T cell recognition pattern of bovine milk alphaS1-casein and its peptides. *Mol Immunol* 41(12):1225–1234.

Fernandez, C. and Wider, G. 2003. TROSY in NMR studies of the structure and function of large biological macromolecules. *Curr Opin Struct Biol* 13(5):570–580.

Ferreira, F., Wallner, M., Gademaier, G., Erler, A., Fritz, G., Glatter, O. et al. 2005. *Physicochemical Characterization of Candidate Reference Materials*. Verlag Chmielorz, Wiesbaden.

Frank, R. 1992. Spot-synthesis: An easy technique for the positionally addressable, parallel chemical synthesis on a membrane support. *Tetrahedron* 84(9217–9232).

Fritsch, R., Bohle, B., Vollmann, U., Wiedermann, U., Jahn-Schmid, B., Krebitz, M. et al. 1998. Bet v 1, the major birch pollen allergen, and Mal d 1, the major apple allergen, cross-react at the level of allergen-specific T helper cells. *J Allergy Clin Immunol* 102(4 Pt 1):679–686.

Georgieva, D.G., Kuil, M.E., Oosterkamp, T.H., Zandbergen, H.W., and Abrahams, JP. 2007. Heterogeneous nucleation of three-dimensional protein nanocrystals. *Acta Crystallogr D Biol Crystallogr* 63(Pt 5):564–570.

Glaspole, I.N., de Leon, M.P., Rolland, J.M., and O'Hehir, R.E. 2005. Characterization of the T-cell epitopes of a major peanut allergen, Ara h 2. *Allergy* 60(1):35–40.

Helm, R.M., Cockrell, G., Connaughton, C., Sampson, H.A., Bannon, G.A., Beilinson, V. et al. 2000. A soybean G2 glycinin allergen. 2. Epitope mapping and three-dimensional modeling. *Int Arch Allergy Immunol* 123(3):213–219.

Holen, E. and Elsayed, S. 1996. Specific T cell lines for ovalbumin, ovomucoid, lysozyme and two OA synthetic epitopes, generated from egg allergic patients' PBMC. *Clin Exp Allergy* 26(9):1080–1088.

Holen, E., Bolann, B., and Elsayed, S. 2001. Novel B and T cell epitopes of chicken ovomucoid (Gal d 1) induce T cell secretion of IL-6, IL-13, and IFN-gamma. *Clin Exp Allergy* 31(6):952–964.

Inoue, R., Matsushita, S., Kaneko, H., Shinoda, S., Sakaguchi, H., Nishimura, Y. et al. 2001. Identification of beta-lactoglobulin-derived peptides and class II HLA molecules recognized by T cells from patients with milk allergy. *Clin Exp Allergy* 31(7):1126–1134.

Jahn-Schmid, B., Radakovics, A., Luttkopf, D., Scheurer, S., Vieths, S., Ebner, C. et al. 2005. Bet v 1142–156 is the dominant T-cell epitope of the major birch pollen allergen and important for cross-reactivity with Bet v 1-related food allergens. *J Allergy Clin Immunol* 116(1):213–219.

Jarvinen, K.M., Chatchatee, P., Bardina, L., Beyer, K., and Sampson, H.A. 2001. IgE and IgG binding epitopes on alpha-lactalbumin and beta-lactoglobulin in cow's milk allergy. *Int Arch Allergy Immunol* 126(2):111–118.

Jarvinen, K.M., Beyer, K., Vila, L., Chatchatee, P., Busse, P.J., and Sampson, H.A. 2002. B-cell epitopes as a screening instrument for persistent cow's milk allergy. *J Allergy Clin Immunol* 110(2):293–297.

Jarvinen, K.M., Beyer, K., Vila, L., Bardina, L., Mishoe, M., and Sampson, H.A. 2007. Specificity of IgE antibodies to sequential epitopes of hen's egg ovomucoid as a marker for persistence of egg allergy. *Allergy* 62(7):758–765.

Johnsen, G. and Elsayed, S. 1990. Antigenic and allergenic determinants of ovalbumin-III. MHC Ia-binding peptide (OA 323–339) interacts with human and rabbit specific antibodies. *Mol Immunol* 27(9):821–827.

Koppelman, S.J., Bruijnzeel-Koomen, C.A., Hessing, M., and de Jongh, H.H. 1999. Heat-induced conformational changes of Ara h 1, a major peanut allergen, do not affect its allergenic properties. *J Biol Chem* 274(8):4770–4777.

Koppelman, S.J., van Koningsveld, G.A., Knulst, A.C., Gruppen, H., Pigmans, I.G., and de Jongh, HH. 2002. Effect of heat-induced aggregation on the IgE binding of patatin (Sol t 1) is dominated by other potato proteins. *J Agric Food Chem* 50(6):1562–1568.

Korber, B., LaBute, M., and Yusim, K. 2006. Immunoinformatics comes of age. *PLoS Comput Biol* 2(6):e71.

Lees, J.G., Miles, A.J., Wien, F., and Wallace, B.A. 2006. A reference database for circular dichroism spectroscopy covering fold and secondary structure space. *Bioinformatics* 22(16):1955–1962.

Lidholm, J., Ballmer-Weber, B.K., Mari, A., and Vieths, S. 2006. Component-resolved diagnostics in food allergy. *Curr Opin Allergy Clin Immunol* 6(3):234–240.

Liu, H.L. and Hsu, J.P. 2005. Recent developments in structural proteomics for protein structure determination. *Proteomics* 5(8):2056–2068.

Mills, E.N., Huang, L., Noel, T.R., Gunning, A.P., and Morris, V.J. 2001. Formation of thermally induced aggregates of the soya globulin beta-conglycinin. *Biochim Biophys Acta* 1547(2):339–350.

Mine, Y. and Rupa, P. 2003. Fine mapping and structural analysis of immunodominant IgE allergenic epitopes in chicken egg ovalbumin. *Protein Eng* 16(10):747–752.

Mittag, D., Batori, V., Neudecker, P., Wiche, R., Friis, E.P., Ballmer-Weber, B.K. et al. 2006. A novel approach for investigation of specific and cross-reactive IgE epitopes on Bet v 1 and homologous food allergens in individual patients. *Mol Immunol* 43(3):268–278.

Mueller, G.A., Smith, A.M., Chapman, M.D., Rule, G.S., and Benjamin, D.C. 2001. Hydrogen exchange nuclear magnetic resonance spectroscopy mapping of antibody epitopes on the house dust mite allergen Der p 2. *J Biol Chem* 276(12):9359–9365.

Nakajima-Adachi, H., Hachimura, S., Ise, W., Honma, K., Nishiwaki, S., Hirota, M. et al. 1998. Determinant analysis of IgE and IgG4 antibodies and T cells specific for bovine alpha(s)1-casein from the same patients allergic to cow's milk: existence of alpha(s)1-casein-specific B cells and T cells characteristic in cow's-milk allergy. *J Allergy Clin Immunol* 101(5):660–671.

Neudecker, P., Schweimer, K., Nerkamp, J., Scheurer, S., Vieths, S., Sticht, H. et al. 2001. Allergic cross-reactivity made visible: Solution structure of the major cherry allergen Pru av 1. *J Biol Chem* 276(25):22756–22763.

Neudecker, P., Lehmann, K., Nerkamp, J., Haase, T., Wangorsch, A., Fotisch, K. et al. 2003. Mutational epitope analysis of Pru av 1 and Api g 1, the major allergens of cherry (Prunus avium) and celery (Apium graveolens): correlating IgE reactivity with three-dimensional structure. *Biochem J* 376(Pt 1):97–107.

Pastorello, E.A., Pompei, C., Pravettoni, V., Farioli, L., Calamari, A.M., Scibilia, J. et al. 2003. Lipid-transfer protein is the major maize allergen maintaining IgE-binding activity after cooking at 100 degrees C, as demonstrated in anaphylactic patients and patients with positive double-blind, placebo-controlled food challenge results. *J Allergy Clin Immunol* 112(4):775–783.

Radauer, C., Willerroider, M., Fuchs, H., Hoffmann-Sommergruber, K., Thalhamer, J., Ferreira, F. et al. 2006. Cross-reactive and species-specific immunoglobulin E epitopes of plant profilins: an Experimental and structure-based analysis. *Clin Exp Allergy* 36(7):920–9.

Reese, G., Ayuso, R., and Lehrer, SB. 1999. Tropomyosin: An invertebrate pan-allergen. *Int Arch Allergy Immunol* 119(4):247–258.

Reese, G., Viebranz, J., Leong-Kee, S.M., Plante, M., Lauer, I., Randow, S. et al. 2005. Reduced allergenic potency of VR9-1, a mutant of the major shrimp allergen Pen a 1 (tropomyosin). *J Immunol* 175(12):8354–8364.

Reese, G., Ballmer-Weber, B.K., Wangorsch, A., Randow, S., and Vieths, S. 2007. Allergenicity and antigenicity of wild-type and mutant, monomeric, and dimeric carrot major allergen Dau c 1: Destruction of conformation, not oligomerization, is the roadmap to save allergen vaccines. *J Allergy Clin Immunol* 119(4):944–951.

Reineke, U., Volkmer-Engert, R., and Schneider-Mergener, J. 2001. Applications of peptide arrays prepared by the SPOT-technology. *Curr Opin Biotechnol* 12(1):59–64.

Robotham, J.M., Teuber, S.S., Sathe, S.K., and Roux, K.H. 2002. Linear IgE epitope mapping of the English walnut (Juglans regia) major food allergen, Jug r 1. *J Allergy Clin Immunol* 109(1):143–149.

Sancho, A.I., Rigby, N.M., Zuidmeer, L., Asero, R., Mistrello, G., Amato, S. et al. 2005. The effect of thermal processing on the IgE reactivity of the non-specific lipid transfer protein from apple, Mal d 3. *Allergy* 60(10):1262–1268.

Schimek, E.M., Zwolfer, B., Briza, P., Jahn-Schmid, B., Vogel, L., Vieths, S. et al. 2005. Gastrointestinal digestion of Bet v 1-homologous food allergens destroys their mediator-releasing, but not T cell-activating, capacity. *J Allergy Clin Immunol* 116(6):1327–1333.

Schirmer, T., Hoffimann-Sommergrube, K., Susani, M., Breiteneder, H., and Markovic-Housley, Z. 2005. Crystal structure of the major celery allergen Api g 1: Molecular analysis of cross-reactivity. *J Mol Biol* 351(5):1101–1109.

Sen, M., Kopper, R., Pons, L., Abraham, E.C., Burks, A.W., and Bannon, G.A. 2002. Protein structure plays a critical role in peanut allergen stability and may determine immunodominant IgE-binding epitopes. *J Immunol* 169(2):882–887.

Shimojo, N., Katsuki, T., Coligan, J.E., Nishimura, Y., Sasazuki, T., Tsunoo, H. et al. 1994. Identification of the disease-related T cell epitope of ovalbumin and epitope-targeted T cell inactivation in egg allergy. *Int Arch Allergy Immunol* 105(2):155–161.

Shreffler, W.G., Beyer, K., Chu, T.H., Burks, A.W., and Sampson, H.A. 2004. Microarray immunoassay: association of clinical history, in vitro IgE function, and heterogeneity of allergenic peanut epitopes. *J Allergy Clin Immunol* 113(4):776–782.

Shreffler, W.G., Lencer, D.A., Bardina, L., Sampson, H.A. 2005. IgE and IgG4 epitope mapping by microarray immunoassay reveals the diversity of immune response to the peanut allergen, Ara h 2. *J Allergy Clin Immunol* 116(4):893–899.

Sreerama, N. and Woody, R.W. 2000. Estimation of protein secondary structure from circular dichroism spectra: Comparison of CONTIN, SELCON, and CDSSTR methods with an expanded reference set. *Anal Biochem* 287(2):252–260.

Stickler, M., Mucha, J., Estell, D., Power, S., and Harding, F. 2003. A human dendritic cell-based method to identify CD4+ T-cell epitopes in potential protein allergens. *Environ Health Perspect* 111(2):251–254.

Suzuki, K., Inoue, R., Sakaguchi, H., Aoki, M., Kato, Z., Kaneko, H. et al. 2002. The correlation between ovomucoid-derived peptides, human leucocyte antigen class II molecules and T cell receptor-complementarity determining region 3 compositions in patients with egg-white allergy. *Clin Exp Allergy* 32(8):1223–1230.

Tanabe, S., Arai, S., Yanagihara, Y., Mita, H., Takahashi, K., and Watanabe, M. 1996. A major wheat allergen has a Gln-Gln-Gln-Pro-Pro motif identified as an IgE-binding epitope. *Biochem Biophys Res Commun* 219(2):290–293.

Tanabe, S., Kobayashi, Y., Takahata, Y., Morimatsu, F., Shibata, R., and Nishimura, T. 2002. Some human B and T cell epitopes of bovine serum albumin, the major beef allergen. *Biochem Biophys Res Commun* 293(5):1348–1353.

Untersmayr, E., Szalai, K., Riemer, A.B., Hemmer, W., Swoboda, I., Hantusch, B. et al. 2006. Mimotopes identify conformational epitopes on parvalbumin, the major fish allergen. *Mol Immunol* 43(9):1454–1461.

van der Veen, M.J., van Ree, R., Aalberse, R.C., Akkerdaas, J., Koppelman, S.J., Jansen, H.M. et al. 1997. Poor biologic activity of cross-reactive IgE directed to carbohydrate determinants of glycoproteins. *J Allergy Clin Immunol* 100(3):327–334.

Walsh, B.J. and Howden, M.E. 1989. A method for the detection of IgE binding sequences of allergens based on a modification of epitope mapping. *J Immunol Methods* 121(2):275–280.

Wang, F., Robotham, J.M., Teuber, S.S., Tawde, P., Sathe, S.K., and Roux, K.H. 2002. Ana o 1, a cashew (Anacardium occidental) allergen of the vicilin seed storage protein family. *J Allergy Clin Immunol* 110(1):160–166.

Wiche, R., Gubesch, M., Konig, H., Fotisch, K., Hoffmann, A., Wangorsch, A. et al. 2005. Molecular basis of pollen-related food allergy: identification of a second cross-reactive IgE epitope on Pru av 1, the major cherry (Prunus avium) allergen. *Biochem J* 385(Pt 1):319–327.

Woods, V.L. Jr. and Hamuro, Y. 2001. High resolution, high-throughput amide deuterium exchange-mass spectrometry (DXMS) determination of protein binding site structure and dynamics: Utility in pharmaceutical design. *J Cell Biochem* Suppl 37:89–98.

Xiang, P., Beardslee, T.A., Zeece, M.G., Markwell, J., and Sarath, G. 2002. Identification and analysis of a conserved immunoglobulin E-binding epitope in soybean G1a and G2a and peanut Ara h 3 glycinins. *Arch Biochem Biophys* 408(1):51–57.

# 4 Recombinant Food Allergens and Their Role in Immunoassay and Immunotherapy

*Karin Hoffmann-Sommergruber,*
*Christina Oberhuber, and Merima Bublin*

## CONTENTS

In the recent years, standardization and characterization of allergen extracts from natural source have been improved, but extracts are often heterogeneous and may contain a mixture of nonallergenic molecules and relevant allergens which can vary in composition and quantity (Chapman et al. 2002). Molecular biology could be the solution for these problems. Many recombinant food allergens have been expressed using various systems, both prokaryotic and eukaryotic. The large-scale production of such defined molecules facilitates the proper molecular and immunological characterization of allergens, and offers new perspectives in allergy diagnosis, research, and therapy.

## 4.1   PRODUCTION, PURIFICATION, AND AUTHENTICATION OF RECOMBINANT FOOD ALLERGENS

To identify relevant IgE binding components from natural source extracts, various techniques like IgE immunoscreening of expression cDNA libraries, reverse transcriptase polymerase chain reaction (PCR), or phage-display technology combined with immunoscreening are used (Wallner et al. 2004).

For the expression of recombinant food allergens, the genomic- or cDNA-derived clone is ligated into a vector and introduced into the host organism. Bacteria, yeast, plants, and mammalian cells can be host systems.

Numerous recombinant allergens were successfully expressed in *Escherichia coli*, the most frequently used expression system for recombinant food allergens (Lorenz et al. 2001). *E. coli* cells are easy to handle and usually a high yield can be achieved. Many different *E. coli* strains that can solve some shortcomings of this expression system are commercially available.

Specialized strains can overcome the difficulties of translation for eukaryotic codons, and vectors for cytoplasmic and periplasmic expression (enable correct folding of disulfide bridges containing allergens) are available.

However, *E. coli* strains are unable to perform posttranslational modifications such as glycosylations, comparable to the glycosylation pattern of eukaryotic cells. Such lack of glycosylations may end up in reduced IgE binding capacity, caused by an altered tertiary structure or because of lacking carbohydrate IgE binding epitopes (Smith et al. 1996; Petersen et al. 1997). As mentioned above, plant-derived food allergens often posses posttranslational modifications (e.g., glycosylations, disulfide bridges), so the chosen expression model for the production of the desired recombinant food allergen should be able to produce such posttranslational modifications, important for IgE binding capacity and enzymatic activity. Transient plant expression systems, e.g., tobacco mosaic virus (TMV)-based plant viral expression vector, offer these opportunities, but due to the difficult handling, variable expression levels, and the instability of the viral vector, the only food allergen expressed in plants was a thaumatin-like protein from apple (Krebitz et al. 2003).

Yeast cells provide advanced protein folding pathways and thus process and fold recombinant proteins correctly. Especially when producing food allergens with enzymatic activity (e.g., endochitinase), the cleavage of the signal (leader) peptide is an essential requirement for the potential expression system. Food allergens possess numerous diverse properties and important functional and physicochemical characteristics, which should be considered when choosing the most suitable expression system for each allergen.

When using common *E. coli* expression system, recombinant allergens are present, either soluble in the supernatant of the cell lysate, or the proteins aggregate and form poorly soluble inclusion bodies. Inclusion bodies have to be solubilized under denaturing conditions (e.g., urea, guanidine-HCl treatment) and the protein has to be carefully refolded (Rea et al. 2004). One advantage of a eukaryotic yeast expression system is that yeast cells can segregate the expressed protein into the culture medium and thus can easily be purified.

For easier purification of the recombinant protein from cell lysate, many proteins are expressed with a fusion peptide. Arg-tag, His-tag, maltose-binding protein, FLAG-tag, and many others are used frequently when expressing recombinant proteins. After the purification step, the tag may either remain at the recombinant protein, or can be removed after purification, using appropriate techniques for the respective tag. In the recent years, many recombinant allergens were expressed carrying a fusion peptide without influencing the immunological properties of the allergen (Lorenz et al. 2001; Terpe 2003). For protein purification, either from *E. coli* or from natural source, many different chromatographic approaches can be followed. Commonly used techniques are ion exchange chromatography, size exclusion chromatography, hydrophobic interaction chromatography, and affinity chromatography—e.g., poly-L-proline, mainly used for the purification of profilins (Ma et al. 2006).

### 4.1.1 Analysis of the Purified Allergens

After successful purification, recombinant produced allergens have to undergo several investigations to ensure that the product has biophysical, biochemical, biological, and immunological properties equivalent to the natural counterpart.

There are several methods to detect possible impurities, influencing the recombinant proteins' quality: SDS-PAGE followed either by Coomassie staining or silver staining, ES-MS (electrospray-ionization), or high-performance liquid chromatography (HPLC)-size exclusion chromatography can identify co-migrating proteins.

Correct mass of purified proteins is determined using matrix-assisted laser desorption ionization-time of flight (MALDI-TOF). N-terminal sequencing and/or LC-ES-MS can verify correct amino acid sequence. Folding of the recombinant protein should be compared to the natural counterpart by measuring CD-spectra. Furthermore, nuclear magnetic resonance (NMR) analysis can be performed to ensure the presence of tertiary structure, important for IgE binding activity (Neudecker et al. 2003).

Only well-characterized recombinant allergens of constant quality, purity, and stability offer tools to replace extracts in diagnosis and therapy (Bublin et al. 2008; Gaier et al. 2008; Ma et al. 2008).

## 4.2  RECOMBINANT FOOD ALLERGENS AND DIAGNOSTIC TESTS

### 4.2.1  IgE-Dependent Assays

Diagnosis of food allergy consists of careful anamnesis, *in vitro* diagnosis, and skin prick tests (SPTs). The golden standard is still the double blind placebo controlled food challenge (DBPCFC). *In vitro* diagnosis is based on the identification of specific IgE antibodies present in human serum. All these data together have to be taken into account for diagnosing Type 1 food allergies (Asero et al. 2007). Up-to-date total crude protein extracts are used for SPTs as well as for *in vitro* diagnosis. Since these extracts display batch-to-batch variation and may lack relevant food allergens due to intrinsic enzymatic activities, the concept of component resolved diagnosis has gained more attraction in the recent past. Once the relevant allergens of a given food source have been identified, the allergen-specific *in vitro* diagnosis may not only offer improved patient tailored diagnosis—it can additionally provide information about cross-reactivity patterns.

Production of recombinant well-defined allergens seems to be the method of choice in most cases (Bohle and Vieths 2004).

### 4.2.1.1 *In Vitro* Assays

Today various routinely used clinical assays are available (Bousquet et al. 1990; Kleine-Tebbe et al. 1992). They are based on different types of solid phases bearing the immobilized allergen preparations. The patients' serum sample is incubated, and bound IgE antibodies are detected by labeled specific anti-IgE antibodies in the allergosorbent-type of assay (Figure 4.1, Panel A). Another type of assay first isolates IgE antibodies out of the serum and detection is performed with labeled specific allergen preparations (Figure 4.1, Panel B). A third format allows the binding of the serum IgE antibodies to bind to tagged allergens, and these complexes are captured out of fluid phase via the allergen tag and the read out is performed by labeled anti-IgE reagent (Figure 4.1, Panel C). For the read out, a standard curve with purified IgE calibrators is used in parallel and the signals are converted to mass units of allergen-specific IgE in international unit (IU) per milliliter of serum (plasma).

Quality criteria that need to be addressed comprise issues such as antibody isotype specificity, no unspecific antibody binding to the solid phase, level of background signals, and known level of interference of IgG antibodies with the IgE-based assay. Needless to say, that the quality of the allergen preparation plays a crucial role for the reliability of the test.

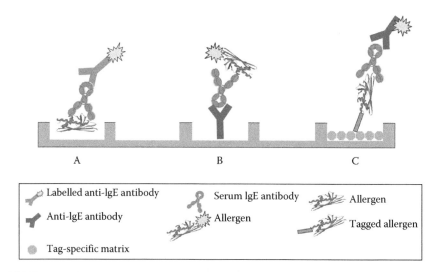

A                              B                              C

| 🔅 Labelled anti-IgE antibody | Serum IgE antibody | Allergen |
| Anti-IgE antibody | Allergen | Tagged allergen |
| Tag-specific matrix | | |

**FIGURE 4.1** *In vitro* allergy diagnostic assays used in clinical routine. Specific IgE antibodies can be quantified from human serum by labeled anti-IgE antibodies (Panel A, Panel C) or by labeled allergen (Panel B).

Until recently, the routine allergy tests were based on total protein extracts of plant and animal food as mentioned above. In the recent past, purified individual allergen preparations either of recombinant or natural origin have started to replace these extracts—in order to overcome some shortcomings such as batch-to-batch variability, considerable variation in concentration ranges of individual allergens, and even lack of some allergens in the total composition. In the recent past the protein chip technology has been applied to develop a new and smaller diagnostic format which allows to rapidly screen as minute volumes as 20 µL of serum samples for allergen-specific IgE antibodies using a large panel of purified allergens. Since the first prototype of diagnostic chip (Hiller et al. 2002) the panel of analytes has continuously expanded and includes recombinant inhalant allergens as well as recombinant food allergens (Harwanegg et al. 2003; Deinhofer et al. 2004; Harwanegg and Hiller 2006). Regardless the format—allergosorbent or microarray based—the list of recombinant food allergens used expands continuously and comprises animal-derived food allergens from fish (rCyp c 1, parvalbumin) and shrimp (rPen a 1, tropomyosin). Just to mention some examples from plant food allergens: seed storage proteins from peanut, hazelnut, and Brazil nut are available in recombinant form (e.g., rAra h 1, peanut vicilin, rAra h 2, peanut 2S albumin, rAra h 3, 11S globulin from peanut) and are offered in a diagnostic test format. In addition, a range of pollen-related food allergens such as the Bet v 1 homologous food allergens (e.g., Pru p 1 from peach, Mal d 1 from apple, Api g 1 from celery, Gly m 4 from soy) or the profilins (e.g., Pru p 4 from peach) are present on these test formats. Specific IgE binding to lipid transfer proteins can be tested with peach LTP (rPru p 3) and also wheat gliadins are available.

Dipstick-based IgE testing allows rapid testing for positive IgE present in serum samples. In most cases these assays use total protein extracts (Straumann and Wuthrich 2000). However the proof of concept has also been performed with a recombinant protein, Bet v 1, the birch pollen allergen. Crystalline bacterial cell-surface layers were used as immobilization matrices. Covalently bound monoclonal anti-Bet v 1 antibody served as a monolayer onto the recombinant allergen was bound. Quantitative determination of Bet v 1-specific IgE from human serum samples was possible within 90 min (Breitwieser et al. 1996, 1998).

Regardless the test format used, it is evident that the specificity and sensitivity of the diagnostic tests depends on the quality of the allergen preparation. With the use of well-characterized single allergens several shortcomings of the extract approach can be overcome. That is the underrepresentation of individual allergenic components as well as the batch-to-batch variation as mentioned above. However, it is mandatory to interpret IgE reactivity to allergens, that is sensitization in relation to clinically relevant food allergic symptoms. Based on sequence similarity of proteins cross-reactivity can frequently occur accompanied with or without clinical significance. For example, cross-reactive carbohydrates (CCDs) have been reported to frequently induce production of specific IgE antibodies without food allergic symptoms. For profilins cross-reactivity among these proteins even from distantly related plant species has been reported. However, in certain cases this seropositivity can be clinically relevant as shown for food allergies to melon, tomato, citrus fruits, and Rosaceae fruits (van Ree et al. 1995; Asero et al. 2003).

In the recent past serological tests of IgG4 against foods have been persistently promoted for the diagnosis of food-induced hypersensitivity. However, the presence of food-specific IgG4 points at a physiological response of the immune system after exposure to food components and does not represent a meaningful diagnostic readout for IgE-mediated food allergies. Therefore, food-specific IgG4 testing is considered irrelevant for diagnosis of food allergy as stated from the European Academy of Allergology and Clinical Immunology (EAACI) Task force group (Stapel et al. 2008).

### 4.2.1.2 *In Vivo* Assays

#### 4.2.1.2.1 SPTs

For detection of food-specific IgE, SPTs are regarded as a safe and cheap method. These tests are easily performed within 20 min. However, the diagnostic outcome depends on the quality of the food extracts used. Recently the predictive value of SPTs in relation to oral food challenges has been determined for certain foods and patients' groups (Hill et al. 2004; Verstege et al. 2005). It is commonly accepted that certain food extracts are of poor reliability, especially fruit derived extracts, resulting in false negative tests. These extract seem to lack one or more relevant allergens due to intrinsic enzymatic activity. In those cases prick-to-prick tests using the fresh fruit are currently performed. However, standardization in those cases is impossible.

In the recent past, purified recombinant and natural allergens have been used for SPTs in order to improve this method regarding reproducibility (Schmid-Grendelmeier and Crameri 2001). Indeed, increased sensitivity could be shown when using purified recombinant Api g 1, from celery, recombinant apple profilin, Mal d 4, and recombinant cherry allergens (Hoffmann-Sommergruber et al. 1999; Ballmer-Weber et al. 2002; Ma et al. 2006).

Recently, Astier and coworkers used purified recombinant peanut allergens rAra h 1, rAra h 2, and rAra h 3 in SPTs and compared the performance of single recombinant allergens to the natural total extract (Astier et al. 2006). The application of these recombinant peanut allergens proved to be a safe method, and reactivity toward individual allergens could be correlated with symptom severity. Either cosensitization to rAra h 1 and rAra h 2 or sensitization to rAra h 3 was predictive of more severe reactions (Astier et al. 2006).

Nevertheless, cross-reactive IgE antibodies may cause positive SPTs without clinical symptoms, e.g., in the pollen-fruit syndrome, and thus reduce specificity. Nowadays, only recombinant food allergens of pharmaceutical grade can be applied for SPTs which means reproducible production criteria under Good Manufacturing Practice (GMP) guidelines.

#### 4.2.1.2.2 Histamine Release Assays

In addition to *in vivo* tests, cell-based assays mimicking the *in vivo* situation can be performed. Upon addition of individual allergens, sensitized basophils can be activated via cross-linking of specific IgE which induces mediator release (Reese et al. 2006; Kaul et al. 2007). Different types of assays have been established. Either basophils are used from allergic patients, or human basophils are stripped off from their surface-bound IgE and allergen-specific IgE is added. In both cases release of histamine is recorded. Alternatively, sulfidoleukotriene release (Ballmer-Weber et al. 2008) can be measured as well as tryptase (Peterson et al. 2007). Recently, Fluorescent Activated Cell Sorting (FACS) analysis of surface markers such as CD63 or CD203c has been proved to be an adequate system for analysis of allergenic activity of allergens as well as a useful cell-based assay for diagnosis of food allergy (Erdmann et al. 2003, 2005).

### 4.2.2 FOOD ALLERGEN DETECTION IN RAW AND PROCESSED FOODS

Detection of known allergens present in food is an important issue for the production either to label the product accordingly or to exclude any unintended contamination of allergen, e.g., by a carryover effect during production. Several enzyme-linked immunosorbent assay (ELISA)-based assays and lateral flow devices are available for detection of the most important food allergens as listed by the allergen labeling directive valid for Europe (EU directive 2003/89/EG). A detailed description of the allergen detection tests is presented in Chapter 3 of this book and in the book edited by Koppelman and Hefle (Koppelman and Hefle 2006).

However, new and highly sensitive methods are still needed for rapid and reliable screening for the presence of food allergens. In those assays recombinant allergens are used as standards and/or antigens to develop the test. Besides the well-established ELISA formats new techniques have also been used for tracing allergens in diverse food matrices. Real-time PCR for detection of trace amounts of Ara h 2, a major peanut allergen was established and a detection limit of <10ppm was found, which was in agreement with the ELISA (Stephan and Vieths 2004). Another assay, developed for Cor a 1.0104, the major hazelnut allergen, biotinylated the PCR products and via Fluoresceinisothiocyanate (FITC) hybridization-specific antibodies detected the hazelnut positive probes (Holzhauser et al. 2002). Mass spectrometry is a highly sensitive method to identify the presence of individual proteins in picomolar level. For example, by Q-TOF mass spectrometry individual isoforms of Mal d 1, the major apple allergen, could be identified with this method (Helsper et al. 2002). Similarly, Shefcheck and colleagues detected Ara h 1 in a model food matrix in a ration of 10mg/kg (Shefcheck and Musser 2004). Once, the most relevant food allergens for a given food source have been identified and their primary sequence determined, *in silico* analysis of allergen sequences is also an option (Jenkins et al. 2005; Radauer et al. 2008). By screening of either sequence similarities between new proteins and already known allergens or structural determinants, possible new food allergens could be identified.

## 4.3  RECOMBINANT ALLERGENS AND IMMUNOTHERAPY OF FOOD ALLERGY

Specific immunotherapy (SIT) to inhalant allergens has proven to be successful (Moller et al. 2002; Wilson et al. 2005). This immunotherapeutic approach involves subcutaneous injection or sublingual application of progressively higher doses of allergen to induce immune tolerance. Immune tolerance is defined as redirecting the T-cell immune response from a Th2- to a Th1-type response (Durham and Till 1998). However, SIT against food allergy in humans, is currently not viable because of the high risk of the adverse reactions including anaphylaxis with lethal outcome and limited efficacy (Nelson et al. 1997; Bock et al. 2001). Nevertheless, isolated reports suggested that such approaches appear to be effective in inducing short-term desensitization for egg, milk (Staden et al. 2007), and hazelnut (Enrique et al. 2005). Several trials suggest that birch pollen immunotherapy also decreased allergy to oral allergy syndrome-related foods containing Bet v 1-homologous allergens (Bolhaar et al. 2004; Niederberger et al. 2007). In contrast, Kinaciyan reported that the successful sublingual immunotherapy with birch pollen extract may have no clinical effect on associated apple allergy (Kinaciyan et al. 2007).

Currently, inhalant allergies SIT relies on traditional allergen extracts prepared from natural allergen sources that contain undefined nonallergenic and allergenic proteins, increasing the risk of unwanted side effects such as priming of Th2 responses (Traidl-Hoffmann et al. 2005) or developing of new IgE reactivity (Moverare et al. 2002; Pajno et al. 2002). In many cases, important allergens are present in small amounts or lacking due to low abundance or the lack of stability of several allergens to endogenous enzymatic processes in plant food extracts. The use of recombinant allergens with high purity and defined molecular, immunological, and biological characteristics would resolve these issues (Valenta and Niederberger 2007). Current theory hypothesizes that allergens should be administered in high doses to shift the T-cell cytokine production from a proallergic, Th2 profile to an antiallergic Th1-type profile of allergen-specific responses (Secrist et al. 1995). The use of recombinant wild-type allergens retains the risk of adverse allergic reactions as a consequence of reactivity with IgE. Therefore, recombinant food allergens need to display a reduced capacity to bind IgE bound to mast cells or basophils, ensuring a lower risk of IgE-mediated side effects, while retaining their T-cell epitopes. Retention of the allergen's ability to interact with T-cells allows the modulation of the immune response (Ferreira et al. 1998). Consequently, future therapeutic options, currently under investigation in murine models include the use of mutated recombinant proteins, T- or B-cell-based peptide immunotherapy, or plasmid DNA-based immunotherapy.

### 4.3.1 MUTATED RECOMBINANT ALLERGENS

Recombinant allergens have been modified to hypoallergenic molecules that have reduced IgE reactivity. The IgE binding sites can be converted *in vitro* to non-IgE binding sites by altering as little as a single amino acid within the epitope (preferably a hydrophobic residue) to eliminate or reduce IgE binding (Stanley et al. 1997). For example, the three engineered peanut allergens (modified Ara h 1, Ara h 2, and Ara h 3) in which sequential IgE epitopes have been modified by site-directed mutagenesis bind minimal IgE from peanut allergic patients, but induced T-cell proliferation comparable to that of peanut native allergens (Bannon et al. 2001). Furthermore, bacterial adjuvants, as potent stimulants of Th1 immune responses were used to increase efficacy of modified peanut vaccines. The subcutaneous coadministration of heat-killed *Listera monocytogenes* and modified peanut allergens in a murine model of peanut anaphylaxis was shown to reduce plasma histamine levels, peanut-specific IgE synthesis, as well as anaphylactic responses after intragastric peanut challenge compared with sham-treated mice (Li et al. 2003b). Similarly, peanut-sensitized mice treated with heat-killed *E. coli* expressing modified Ara h 1–3 (HKE-mAra h 1–3) delivered by the rectal route had lowest symptoms scores, reduced production of IL-4, IL-5, and IL-13 by splenocytes, and long-term "down regulation" of peanut hypersensitivity compared to the mAra h 1–3 alone and placebo-treated mice (Li et al. 2003a). Currently, the HKE-mAra h 1–3 produced in a GMP facility for use in human beings is undergoing final toxicological studies before an investigational new drug application is submitted to the U.S. Food and Drug Administration for approval (Sicherer and Sampson 2007).

Major apple allergen, Mal d 1, was mutated introducing five point mutations into IgE binding critical positions. Bolhaar et al. confirmed by *in vitro* methods, i.e., radio-allergosorbent test (RAST) inhibitions, immunoblotting and basophile histamine release, and *in vivo* by DBPCFC and skin test, the hypo-allergenicity of the mutated apple allergen. In contrast to wild-type Mal d 1, an oral dose of 100 μg of the hypoallergenic Mal d 1 (rMal d 1mut) was well tolerated, and 1 mg caused only mild symptoms (Bolhaar et al. 2005).

In murine models and histamine release experiments, stimulating the human basophils from patients with carrot allergy, Reese et al. demonstrated that destruction of the native conformation of major carrot allergen Dau c 1 rather than oligomerization of the wild-type allergens increased antigenicity and reduced allergenicity. Further the authors suggested that immunotherapy with the food allergen, rather than homologous pollen proteins might be more successful (Reese et al. 2007).

Also, destruction of native conformation by mutation of calcium-binding domains of major carp allergen resulted in reduced IgE reactivity confirmed by skin prick testing. Immunization of mice with the mutated parvalbumin induced IgG antibodies, which inhibited the binding of allergic patient's IgE to wild-type parvalbumin (Swoboda et al. 2007).

### 4.3.2  T- OR B-CELL-BASED PEPTIDE IMMUNOTHERAPY

Peptides that present allergen-specific T-cell epitopes retain the ability to immunomodulate T-cells, but less an ability to cross-link IgE and activate effectors cells. For example, synthetic peptides-based vaccine derived from major peanut allergen, Ara h 2 composed of thirty 20-mers that overlapped by 15 amino acids (Sicherer and Sampson 2007). Subcutaneous or intranasal administration of the vaccine reduced Ara h 2-specific IgE and plasma histamine release levels as well as anaphylactic symptoms scores in a murine model of peanut anaphylaxis.

More recently, phage-display technology has been used to isolate random peptides that are recognized by parvalbumin-specific IgE and IgG. Subsequent molecular modeling showed that the peptides correspond to IgE binding epitopes on allergen surface (Untersmayr et al. 2006). Such mimics of B-cell epitopes could partly inhibit binding of IgE to the allergen (Ganglberger 2001) and had the potential to induce the production of blocking IgG (Focke et al. 2001).

### 4.3.3  PLASMID DNA-BASED IMMUNOTHERAPY

DNA-based vaccination has proven effective in the prevention of Th2-mediated hypersensitivity in mouse models of allergic diseases (Raz et al. 1996; Li et al.

1999; Roy et al. 1999). There are four basic DNA-based immunotherapeutic approaches: Immunization with DNA gene vaccines, allergen mixed with immunostimulatory oligodeoxynucleotide (ISS-ODN), allergen–ISS-ODN conjugates, and immunomodulation with ISS-ODN alone. ISS-ODN or CpG motifs provide Th1 adjuvant activity for the immune response that developed toward the gene product (Sato et al. 1996).

DNA vaccination to induce host cell expression of allergenic protein can prevent moderate anaphylactic reactions to peanut allergen, Ara h 2, as evidenced in a mouse model of peanut allergy (Roy et al. 1999). Mice vaccinated orally with chitan particles containing plasmid encoding Ara h 2 were shown to express the food protein in their gut and inhibited the development of an allergic sensitization to Ara h 2 upon challenge with peanut. Chitosan, a widely available, mucoadhesive polymer, increases cellular permeability enhancing vaccine uptake and promoting gene expression. Also, vaccination with Ara h 2 linked to immunostimulatory sequence (ISS) had preventive effect on peanut-induced allergic symptoms in an antigen-specific manner (Sicherer and Sampson 2007).

However, there are no published reports of successful plasmid DNA-based immunotherapy reversing established food allergy.

Although the current standard to care for patients with food allergy is based on avoidance of the triggering food, these novel therapeutic approaches in murine models provide insights toward more definitive future therapies.

## 4.4   FUTURE TRENDS IN APPLYING RECOMBINANT FOOD ALLERGENS

In the recent past great efforts to improve food allergy diagnosis have been undertaken. By the use of DNA technology more than 50 food allergens have been produced in the recombinant form.

As a proof of concept these recombinant food allergens can be used for *in vitro* diagnosis as well as for *in vivo* diagnostic approaches. Once, their equivalence to the respective natural counterpart is established, these proteins are available in unlimited quantity and can be produced in standardized quality. This offers a great improvement in setting up reliable diagnostic tools as well as allergen detection assays.

In the recent past, a rigorous European legislative has come into force which aims at protecting the food allergic consumer. However, labeling the allergenic compounds in food products challenges the food producers to set up adequate quality criteria for production. In this respect highly sensitive allergen detection tests together with reliable standards are required. Hopefully, standardized allergen tests for the most important food allergen sources will be available in the near future.

Nevertheless, another aspect should not be neglected: It has become evident that the food matrix does play an important role on the allergenic activity of the individual allergenic protein. It may either down regulate the allergenic activity or increase the unwanted activity. How to address these aspects of this complex issue remains to be the scientific challenge for the coming years. For sure, the recombinant food allergens will be a key player in that research area.

## ACKNOWLEDGMENT

This study was supported by EC grant Europrevall 514000 and grant SFB-F01802 (financing Merima Bublin) from the Austrian Science Fund.

## REFERENCES

Asero, R., B. K. Ballmer-Weber, K. Beyer, A. Conti, R. Dubakiene, M. Fernandez-Rivas, K. Hoffmann-Sommergruber, J. Lidholm, T. Mustakov, J. N. Oude Elberink, R. S. Pumphrey, P. Stahl Skov, R. van Ree, B. J. Vlieg-Boerstra, R. Hiller, J. O. Hourihane, M. Kowalski, N. G. Papadopoulos, J. M. Wal, E. N. Mills, and S. Vieths. 2007. IgE-mediated food allergy diagnosis: Current status and new perspectives. *Mol Nutr Food Res* 51 (1):135–147.

Asero, R., G. Mistrello, D. Roncarolo, S. Amato, D. Zanoni, F. Barocci, and G. Caldironi. 2003. Detection of clinical markers of sensitization to profilin in patients allergic to plant-derived foods. *J Allergy Clin Immunol* 112 (2):427–432.

Astier, C., M. Morisset, O. Roitel, F. Codreanu, S. Jacquenet, P. Franck, V. Ogier, N. Petit, B. Proust, D. A. Moneret-Vautrin, A. W. Burks, A. Bihain, H. A. Sampson, and G. Kanny. 2006. Predictive value of skin prick tests using recombinant allergens for diagnosis of peanut allergy. *J Allergy Clin Immunol* 118 (1):250–256.

Ballmer-Weber, B. K., S. Scheurer, P. Fritsche, E. Enrique, A. Cistero-Bahima, T. Haase, and B. Wuthrich. 2002. Component-resolved diagnosis with recombinant allergens in patients with cherry allergy. *J Allergy Clin Immunol* 110 (1):167–173.

Ballmer-Weber, B. K., J. M. Weber, S. Vieths, and B. Wuthrich. 2008. Predictive value of the sulfidoleukotriene release assay in oral allergy syndrome to celery, hazelnut, and carrot. *J Investig Allergol Clin Immunol* 18 (2):93–99.

Bannon, G. A., G. Cockrell, C. Connaughton, C. M. West, R. Helm, J. S. Stanley, N. King, P. Rabjohn, H. A. Sampson, and A. W. Burks. 2001. Engineering, characterization and in vitro efficacy of the major peanut allergens for use in immunotherapy. *Int Arch Allergy Immunol* 124 (1–3):70–72.

Bock, S. A., A. Munoz-Furlong, and H. A. Sampson. 2001. Fatalities due to anaphylactic reactions to foods. *J Allergy Clin Immunol* 107 (1):191–193.

Bohle, B. and S. Vieths. 2004. Improving diagnostic tests for food allergy with recombinant allergens. *Methods* 32 (3):292–299.

Bolhaar, S. T., M. M. Tiemessen, L. Zuidmeer, A. van Leeuwen, K. Hoffmann-Sommergruber, C. A. Bruijnzeel-Koomen, L. S. Taams, E. F. Knol, E. van Hoffen, R. van Ree, and A. C. Knulst. 2004. Efficacy of birch-pollen immunotherapy on cross-reactive food allergy confirmed by skin tests and double-blind food challenges. *Clin Exp Allergy* 34 (5):761–769.

Bolhaar, S. T., L. Zuidmeer, Y. Ma, F. Ferreira, C. A. Bruijnzeel-Koomen, K. Hoffmann-Sommergruber, R. van Ree, and A. C. Knulst. 2005. A mutant of the major apple allergen, Mal d 1, demonstrating hypo-allergenicity in the target organ by double-blind placebo-controlled food challenge. *Clin Exp Allergy* 35 (12):1638–1644.

Bousquet, J., P. Chanez, I. Chanal, and F. B. Michel. 1990. Comparison between RAST and Pharmacia CAP system: A new automated specific IgE assay. *J Allergy Clin Immunol* 85 (6):1039–1043.

Breitwieser, A., S. Kupcu, S. Howorka, S. Weigert, C. Langer, K. Hoffmann-Sommergruber, O. Scheiner, U. B. Sleytr, and M. Sara. 1996. 2-D protein crystals as an immobilization matrix for producing reaction zones in dipstick-style immunoassays. *Biotechniques* 21 (5):918–925.

Breitwieser, A., C. Mader, I. Schocher, K. Hoffmann-Sommergruber, W. Aberer, O. Scheiner, U. B. Sleytr, and M. Sara. 1998. A novel dipstick developed for rapid Bet v 1-specific IgE detection: recombinant allergen immobilized via a monoclonal antibody to crystalline bacterial cell-surface layers. *Allergy* 53 (8):786–793.

Bublin, M., I. Lauer, C. Oberhuber, S. Alessandri, P. Briza, C. Radauer, M. Himly, H. Breiteneder, G. Vieths, and K. Hoffmann-Sommergruber. 2008. Production and characterization of an allergen panel for component-resolved diagnosis of celery allergy. *Mol Nutr Food Res* 52 (2):241–250.

Chapman, M. D., A. M. Smith, L. D. Vailes, and A. Pomes. 2002. Recombinant allergens for immunotherapy. *Allergy Asthma Proc* 23 (1):5–8.

Deinhofer, K., H. Sevcik, N. Balic, C. Harwanegg, R. Hiller, H. Rumpold, M. W. Mueller, and S. Spitzauer. 2004. Microarrayed allergens for IgE profiling. *Methods* 32 (3):249–254.

Durham, S. R. and S. J. Till. 1998. Immunologic changes associated with allergen immuno-therapy. *J Allergy Clin Immunol* 102 (2):157–164.

Enrique, E., F. Pineda, T. Malek, J. Bartra, M. Basagana, R. Tella, J. V. Castello, R. Alonso, J. A. de Mateo, T. Cerda-Trias, M. San Miguel-Moncin Mdel, S. Monzon, M. Garcia, R. Palacios, and A. Cistero-Bahima. 2005. Sublingual immunotherapy for hazelnut food allergy: A randomized, double-blind, placebo-controlled study with a standardized hazelnut extract. *J Allergy Clin Immunol* 116 (5):1073–1079.

Erdmann, S. M., N. Heussen, S. Moll-Slodowy, H. F. Merk, and B. Sachs. 2003. CD63 expres-sion on basophils as a tool for the diagnosis of pollen-associated food allergy: sensitivity and specificity. *Clin Exp Allergy* 33 (5):607–614.

Erdmann, S. M., B. Sachs, A. Schmidt, H. F. Merk, O. Scheiner, S. Moll-Slodowy, I. Sauer, R. Kwiecien, B. Maderegger, and K. Hoffmann-Sommergruber. 2005. *In vitro* analysis of birch-pollen-associated food allergy by use of recombinant allergens in the basophil activation test. *Int Arch Allergy Immunol* 136 (3):230–238.

Ferreira, F., C. Ebner, B. Kramer, G. Casari, P. Briza, A. J. Kungl, R. Grimm, B. Jahn-Schmid, H. Breiteneder, D. Kraft, M. Breitenbach, H. J. Rheinberger, and O. Scheiner. 1998. Modulation of IgE reactivity of allergens by site-directed mutagenesis: Potential use of hypoallergenic variants for immunotherapy. *FASEB J* 12 (2):231–242.

Focke, M., V. Mahler, T. Ball, W. R. Sperr, Y. Majlesi, P. Valent, D. Kraft, and R. Valenta. 2001. Nonanaphylactic synthetic peptides derived from B cell epitopes of the major grass pollen allergen, Phl p 1, for allergy vaccination. *FASEB J* 15 (11):2042–2044.

Gaier, S., J. Marsh, C. Oberhuber, N. M. Rigby, A. Lovegrove, S. Alessandri, P. Briza, C. Radauer, L. Zuidmeer, R. van Ree, W. Hemmer, A. I. Sancho, C. Mills, K. Hoffmann-Sommergruber, and P. R. Shewry. 2008. Purification and structural stability of the peach allergens Pru p 1 and Pru p 3. *Mol Nutr Food Res* 52 (2):220–229.

Ganglberger, E., B. Sponer, I. Schöll, U. Wiedermann, S. Baumann, C. Hafner, H. Breiteneder, M. Suter, G. Boltz-Nitulescu, O. Scheiner, and E. Jensen-Jarolim. Monovalent fusion proteins of IgE mimotopes are safe for therapy of type I allergy. *FASEB J* 2001, 15(13):2524–2526.

Harwanegg, C., S. Laffer, R. Hiller, M. W. Mueller, D. Kraft, S. Spitzauer, and R. Valenta. 2003. Microarrayed recombinant allergens for diagnosis of allergy. *Clin Exp Allergy* 33 (1):7–13.

Harwanegg, Ch. and R. Hiller. 2006. Protein microarrays for the diagnosis of allergic diseases: State-of-the-art and future development. *Eur Ann Allergy Clin Immunol* 38 (7):232–236.

Helsper, J. P., L. J. Gilissen, R. van Ree, A. H. America, J. H. Cordewener, and D. Bosch. 2002. Quadrupole time-of-flight mass spectrometry: A method to study the actual expression of allergen isoforms identified by PCR cloning. *J Allergy Clin Immunol* 110 (1):131–138.

Hill, D. J., R. G. Heine, and C. S. Hosking. 2004. The diagnostic value of skin prick testing in children with food allergy. *Pediatr Allergy Immunol* 15 (5):435–441.

Hiller, R., S. Laffer, C. Harwanegg, M. Huber, W. M. Schmidt, A. Twardosz, B. Barletta, W. M. Becker, K. Blaser, H. Breiteneder, M. Chapman, R. Crameri, M. Duchene, F. Ferreira, H. Fiebig, K. Hoffmann-Sommergruber, T. P. King, T. Kleber-Janke, V. P. Kurup, S. B. Lehrer, J. Lidholm, U. Muller, C. Pini, G. Reese, O. Scheiner, A. Scheynius, H. D. Shen, S. Spitzauer, R. Suck, I. Swoboda, W. Thomas, R. Tinghino, M. Van Hage-Hamsten, T. Virtanen, D. Kraft, M. W. Muller, and R. Valenta. 2002. Microarrayed allergen mol-ecules: Diagnostic gatekeepers for allergy treatment. *FASEB J* 16 (3):414–416.

Hoffmann-Sommergruber, K., P. Demoly, R. Crameri, H. Breiteneder, C. Ebner, M. Laimer Da Camara Machado, K. Blaser, C. Ismail, O. Scheiner, J. Bousquet, and G. Menz. 1999. IgE reactivity to Api g 1, a major celery allergen, in a Central European population is based on primary sensitization by Bet v 1. *J Allergy Clin Immunol* 104 (2 Pt 1):478–484.

Holzhauser, T., O. Stephan, and S. Vieths. 2002. Detection of potentially allergenic hazelnut (*Corylus avellana*) residues in food: A comparative study with DNA PCR-ELISA and protein sandwich-ELISA. *J Agric Food Chem* 50 (21):5808–5815.

Jenkins, J. A., S. Griffiths-Jones, P. R. Shewry, H. Breiteneder, and E. N. Mills. 2005. Structural relatedness of plant food allergens with specific reference to cross-reactive allergens: An in silico analysis. *J Allergy Clin Immunol* 115 (1):163–170.

Kaul, S., D. Luttkopf, B. Kastner, L. Vogel, G. Holtz, S. Vieths, and A. Hoffmann. 2007. Mediator release assays based on human or murine immunoglobulin E in allergen standardization. *Clin Exp Allergy* 37 (1):141–150.

Kinaciyan, T., B. Jahn-Schmid, A. Radakovics, B. Zwolfer, C. Schreiber, J. N. Francis, C. Ebner, and B. Bohle. 2007. Successful sublingual immunotherapy with birch pollen has limited effects on concomitant food allergy to apple and the immune response to the Bet v 1 homolog Mal d 1. *J Allergy Clin Immunol* 119 (4):937–943.

Kleine-Tebbe, J., M. Eickholt, M. Gatjen, T. Brunnee, A. O'Connor, and G. Kunkel. 1992. Comparison between MAGIC LITE- and CAP-system: Two automated specific IgE antibody assays. *Clin Exp Allergy* 22 (4):475–484.

Koppelman, S.J. and S.L. Hefle. In *Detecting Allergens in Food*, S.J. Koppelman and S.L. Hefle (eds.). Woodhead Publishing Limited, Cambridge, U.K., 2006.

Krebitz, M., B. Wagner, F. Ferreira, C. Peterbauer, N. Campillo, M. Witty, D. Kolarich, H. Steinkellner, O. Scheiner, and H. Breiteneder. 2003. Plant-based heterologous expression of Mal d 2, a thaumatin-like protein and allergen of apple (*Malus domestica*), and its characterization as an antifungal protein. *J Mol Biol* 329 (4):721–730.

Li, X., C. K. Huang, B. H. Schofield, A. W. Burks, G. A. Bannon, K. H. Kim, S. K. Huang, and H. A. Sampson. 1999. Strain-dependent induction of allergic sensitization caused by peanut allergen DNA immunization in mice. *J Immunol* 162 (5):3045–3052.

Li, X. M., K. Srivastava, A. Grishin, C. K. Huang, B. Schofield, W. Burks, and H. A. Sampson. 2003a. Persistent protective effect of heat-killed *Escherichia coli* producing "engineered," recombinant peanut proteins in a murine model of peanut allergy. *J Allergy Clin Immunol* 112 (1):159–167.

Li, X. M., K. Srivastava, J. W. Huleatt, K. Bottomly, A. W. Burks, and H. A. Sampson. 2003b. Engineered recombinant peanut protein and heat-killed Listeria monocytogenes coadministration protects against peanut-induced anaphylaxis in a murine model. *J Immunol* 170 (6):3289–3295.

Lorenz, A. R., S. Scheurer, D. Haustein, and S. Vieths. 2001. Recombinant food allergens. *J Chromatogr B Biomed Sci Appl* 756 (1–2):255–279.

Ma, Y., U. Griesmeier, M. Susani, C. Radauer, P. Briza, A. Erler, M. Bublin, S. Alessandri, M. Himly, S. Vazquez-Cortes, I. R. Rincon de Arellano, E. Vassilopoulou, P. Saxoni-Papageorgiou, A. C. Knulst, M. Fernandez-Rivas, K. Hoffmann-Sommergruber, and H. Breiteneder. 2008. Comparison of natural and recombinant forms of the major fish allergen parvalbumin from cod and carp. *Mol Nutr Food Res* 52 (2):S196–S207.

Ma, Y., L. Zuidmeer, B. Bohle, S. T. Bolhaar, G. Gadermaier, E. Gonzalez-Mancebo, M. Fernandez-Rivas, A. C. Knulst, M. Himly, R. Asero, C. Ebner, R. van Ree, F. Ferreira, H. Breiteneder, and K. Hoffmann-Sommergruber. 2006. Characterization of recombinant Mal d 4 and its application for component-resolved diagnosis of apple allergy. *Clin Exp Allergy* 36 (8):1087–1096.

Moller, C., S. Dreborg, H. A. Ferdousi, S. Halken, A. Host, L. Jacobsen, A. Koivikko, D. Y. Koller, B. Niggemann, L. A. Norberg, R. Urbanek, E. Valovirta, and U. Wahn. 2002. Pollen immunotherapy reduces the development of asthma in children with seasonal rhinoconjunctivitis (the PAT-study). *J Allergy Clin Immunol* 109 (2):251–256.

Moverare, R., L. Elfman, E. Vesterinen, T. Metso, and T. Haahtela. 2002. Development of new IgE specificities to allergenic components in birch pollen extract during specific immunotherapy studied with immunoblotting and Pharmacia CAP System. *Allergy* 57 (5):423–430.

Nelson, H. S., J. Lahr, R. Rule, A. Bock, and D. Leung. 1997. Treatment of anaphylactic sensitivity to peanuts by immunotherapy with injections of aqueous peanut extract. *J Allergy Clin Immunol* 99 (6 Pt 1):744–751.

Neudecker, P., K. Lehmann, J. Nerkamp, T. Haase, A. Wangorsch, K. Fotisch, S. Hoffmann, P. Rosch, S. Vieths, and S. Scheurer. 2003. Mutational epitope analysis of Pru av 1 and Api g 1, the major allergens of cherry (*Prunus avium*) and celery (*Apium graveolens*): Correlating IgE reactivity with three-dimensional structure. *Biochem J* 376 (Pt 1):97–107.

Niederberger, V., J. Reisinger, P. Valent, M. T. Krauth, G. Pauli, M. van Hage, O. Cromwell, F. Horak, and R. Valenta. 2007. Vaccination with genetically modified birch pollen allergens: Immune and clinical effects on oral allergy syndrome. *J Allergy Clin Immunol* 119 (4):1013–1016.

Pajno, G. B., S. La Grutta, G. Barberio, G. W. Canonica, and G. Passalacqua. 2002. Harmful effect of immunotherapy in children with combined snail and mite allergy. *J Allergy Clin Immunol* 109 (4):627–629.

Petersen, A., K. Grobe, B. Lindner, M. Schlaak, and W. M. Becker. 1997. Comparison of natural and recombinant isoforms of grass pollen allergens. *Electrophoresis* 18 (5):819–825.

Peterson, C. G., T. Hansson, A. Skott, U. Bengtsson, S. Ahlstedt, and J. Magnussons. 2007. Detection of local mast-cell activity in patients with food hypersensitivity. *J Investig Allergol Clin Immunol* 17 (5):314–320.

Radauer, C., M. Bublin, S. Wagner, A. Mari, and H. Breiteneder. 2008. Allergens are distributed into few protein families and possess a restricted number of biochemical functions. *J Allergy Clin Immunol* 121 (4):847–852.e7.

Raz, E., H. Tighe, Y. Sato, M. Corr, J. A. Dudler, M. Roman, S. L. Swain, H. L. Spiegelberg, and D. A. Carson. 1996. Preferential induction of a Th1 immune response and inhibition of specific IgE antibody formation by plasmid DNA immunization. *Proc Natl Acad Sci USA* 93 (10):5141–5145.

Rea, G., P. Iacovacci, P. Ferrante, M. Zelli, B. Brunetto, D. Lamba, A. Boffi, C. Pini, and R. Federico. 2004. Refolding of the Cupressus arizonica major pollen allergen Cup a1.02 overexpressed in *Escherichia coli*. *Protein Expr Purif* 37 (2):419–425.

Reese, G., B. K. Ballmer-Weber, A. Wangorsch, S. Randow, and S. Vieths. 2007. Allergenicity and antigenicity of wild-type and mutant, monomeric, and dimeric carrot major allergen Dau c 1: Destruction of conformation, not oligomerization, is the roadmap to save allergen vaccines. *J Allergy Clin Immunol* 119 (4):944–951.

Reese, G., S. Schicktanz, I. Lauer, S. Randow, D. Luttkopf, L. Vogel, S. B. Lehrer, and S. Vieths. 2006. Structural, immunological and functional properties of natural recombinant Pen a 1, the major allergen of Brown Shrimp, Penaeus aztecus. *Clin Exp Allergy* 36 (4):517–524.

Roy, K., H. Q. Mao, S. K. Huang, and K. W. Leong. 1999. Oral gene delivery with chitosan—DNA nanoparticles generates immunologic protection in a murine model of peanut allergy. *Nat Med* 5 (4):387–391.

Sato, Y., M. Roman, H. Tighe, D. Lee, M. Corr, M. D. Nguyen, G. J. Silverman, M. Lotz, D. A. Carson, and E. Raz. 1996. Immunostimulatory DNA sequences necessary for effective intradermal gene immunization. *Science* 273 (5273):352–354.

Schmid-Grendelmeier, P. and R. Crameri. 2001. Recombinant allergens for skin testing. *Int Arch Allergy Immunol* 125 (2):96–111.

Secrist, H., R. H. DeKruyff, and D. T. Umetsu. 1995. Interleukin 4 production by CD4 + T cells from allergic individuals is modulated by antigen concentration and antigen-presenting cell type. *J Exp Med* 181 (3):1081–1089.

Shefcheck, K. J. and S. M. Musser. 2004. Confirmation of the allergenic peanut protein, Ara h 1, in a model food matrix using liquid chromatography/tandem mass spectrometry (LC/MS/MS). *J Agric Food Chem* 52 (10):2785–2790.

Sicherer, S. H. and H. A. Sampson. 2007. Peanut allergy: Emerging concepts and approaches for an apparent epidemic. *J Allergy Clin Immunol* 120 (3):491–503; quiz 504–505.

Smith, P. M., C. Suphioglu, I. J. Griffith, K. Theriault, R. B. Knox, and M. B. Singh. 1996. Cloning and expression in yeast Pichia pastoris of a biologically active form of Cyn d 1, the major allergen of Bermuda grass pollen. *J Allergy Clin Immunol* 98 (2):331–343.

Staden, U., C. Rolinck-Werninghaus, F. Brewe, U. Wahn, B. Niggemann, and K. Beyer. 2007. Specific oral tolerance induction in food allergy in children: Efficacy and clinical patterns of reaction. *Allergy* 62 (11):1261–1269.

Stanley, J. S., N. King, A. W. Burks, S. K. Huang, H. Sampson, G. Cockrell, R. M. Helm, C. M. West, and G. A. Bannon. 1997. Identification and mutational analysis of the immunodominant IgE binding epitopes of the major peanut allergen Ara h 2. *Arch Biochem Biophys* 342 (2):244–253.

Stapel, S. O., R. Asero, B. K. Ballmer-Weber, E. F. Knol, S. Strobel, S. Vieths, and J. Kleine-Tebbe. 2008. Testing for IgG4 against foods is not recommended as a diagnostic tool: EAACI Task Force Report. *Allergy* 63 (7):793–796.

Stephan, O. and S. Vieths. 2004. Development of a real-time PCR and a sandwich ELISA for detection of potentially allergenic trace amounts of peanut (*Arachis hypogaea*) in processed foods. *J Agric Food Chem* 52 (12):3754–3760.

Straumann, F. and B. Wuthrich. 2000. Food allergies associated with birch pollen: Comparison of Allergodip and Pharmacia CAP for detection of specific IgE antibodies to birch pollen related foods. *J Investig Allergol Clin Immunol* 10 (3):135–141.

Swoboda, I., A. Bugajska-Schretter, B. Linhart, P. Verdino, W. Keller, U. Schulmeister, W. R. Sperr, P. Valent, G. Peltre, S. Quirce, N. Douladiris, N. G. Papadopoulos, R. Valenta, and S. Spitzauer. 2007. A recombinant hypoallergenic parvalbumin mutant for immunotherapy of IgE-mediated fish allergy. *J Immunol* 178 (10):6290–6296.

Terpe, K. 2003. Overview of tag protein fusions: From molecular and biochemical fundamentals to commercial systems. *Appl Microbiol Biotechnol* 60 (5):523–533.

Traidl-Hoffmann, C., V. Mariani, H. Hochrein, K. Karg, H. Wagner, J. Ring, M. J. Mueller, T. Jakob, and H. Behrendt. 2005. Pollen-associated phytoprostanes inhibit dendritic cell interleukin-12 production and augment T helper type 2 cell polarization. *J Exp Med* 201 (4):627–636.

Untersmayr, E., K. Szalai, A. B. Riemer, W. Hemmer, I. Swoboda, B. Hantusch, I. Scholl, S. Spitzauer, O. Scheiner, R. Jarisch, G. Boltz-Nitulescu, and E. Jensen-Jarolim. 2006. Mimotopes identify conformational epitopes on parvalbumin, the major fish allergen. *Mol Immunol* 43 (9):1454–1461.

Valenta, R. and V. Niederberger. 2007. Recombinant allergens for immunotherapy. *J Allergy Clin Immunol* 119 (4):826–830.

van Ree, R., M. Fernandez-Rivas, M. Cuevas, M. van Wijngaarden, and R. C. Aalberse. 1995. Pollen-related allergy to peach and apple: An important role for profilin. *J Allergy Clin Immunol* 95 (3):726–734.

Verstege, A., A. Mehl, C. Rolinck-Werninghaus, U. Staden, M. Nocon, K. Beyer, and B. Niggemann. 2005. The predictive value of the skin prick test weal size for the outcome of oral food challenges. *Clin Exp Allergy* 35 (9):1220–1226.

Wallner, M., P. Gruber, C. Radauer, B. Maderegger, M. Susani, K. Hoffmann-Sommergruber, and F. Ferreira. 2004. Lab scale and medium scale production of recombinant allergens in *Escherichia coli*. *Methods* 32 (3):219–226.

Wilson, D. R., M. T. Lima, and S. R. Durham. 2005. Sublingual immunotherapy for allergic rhinitis: Systematic review and meta-analysis. *Allergy* 60 (1):4–12.

# 5 General Characteristics of Food Allergens

*Lucjan Jędrychowski*

## CONTENTS

## 5.1 GENERAL CHARACTERISTICS OF CAUSES OF ALLERGIC HYPERSENSITIVITY REACTIONS AND SCALE OF THE PROBLEM

All people are affected by harmless foreign antigens such as pollen, nutritional ingredients, house dust, animals, and chemicals (cosmetics, medicines, washing powder, textiles, and toys). Ever increasing numbers of people have hypersensitive reactions (allergic and nonallergic). At present, a clearly increasing tendency is observed in the occurrence of allergic and nonallergic hypersensitive reactions to mentioned antigens in foods. In the European Union and in the highly developed countries, it is estimated that approximately 35% of the population of these regions complains about different forms of hypersensitive reactions, and the figure is growing, e.g., bronchial asthma occurs twice as often as 15 years ago. Pollen allergy, coming second in the statistics, concerns 10%–20% of Europeans (European Allergy White Paper). Up to 15% of the human population is reported to have had some adverse form of food reactions (Samson, 1996; Wüthrich, 2000).

The European Allergy White Paper reports that the number of cases of atopic skin inflammation, one of the underlying allergic symptoms, increased by over 100% in the years 1960–1970. From the beginning of the 1980s to 1997, allergy prevalence increased two- to threefold in all European countries. At present, the problem concerns approximately 25%–30% of the European population (5%–8% of adults, 10%–15% of children) (European Allergy White Paper, 1997; Jahnz-Rozyk, 2007).

According to INFOSAN Information (2006), the prevalence of food allergies is estimated to be around 1%–3% in adults and 4%–6% in children, and more than 70 foods have been reported as causing food allergies (FAO/WHO Bulletin, 2006). The foods which cause the most severe reactions and most cases of food allergies are cereals containing gluten, crustaceans, eggs, fish, peanuts, soy, milk, and tree nuts.

According to Sicherer and Sampson (2006), food allergic hyperactivity affects as many as 6% of young children and 3%–4% of adults.

The above divergent data concerning the scale of the problem reflect lack of coordinated actions both in European countries and other parts of the world (Table 5.1).

The available literature data show how big the scale of food allergy occurrence in particular countries is; the differences observed concern both patients' age and kind of allergens inducing most frequent allergic symptoms in a given area (Schafer et al., 2001) (Table 5.1). Another significant factor is culinary habits. In the Scandinavian countries, among all allergy cases the dominant group is that of allergic responses to fish (39% of children); in the United States to milk (65%), chocolate and coke (45%), peanuts (33%), cereals (30%), vegetables (26%), egg white (26%), citrus fruit (25%), walnuts and hazelnuts (22.7%); in Israel to fruits and vegetables (to peaches 75%, almonds 39%, sunflower seeds 35%, and peanuts 31%); in France to egg white (46.3%), peanuts (40%), mustard (20%), cow's milk (7.5%) (Kaczmarski, 1997). In Denmark 2.2% of the total children population is allergic to cow's milk.

In Holland, 28% of all allergic reactions was caused by milk, 23% by broad beans, 22% by coffee, 18% by tomatoes, 16% by egg white, 14% by chocolate, 13% by fish, and 11% by oranges. In Asia the greatest number of allergic responses is induced by extensively consumed certain unique food allergens such as buckwheat, chestnuts, chickpeas, bird's nest, and royal jelly. In the populations of other countries these products pose less threat (Lee et al., 2008), or patients are not diagnosed in the direction of these allergens. Also crustacean shellfish is of importance in the Asian region when compared to other common food allergens. In contrast, the prevalence of peanut allergy is relatively low there. The reasons for this difference are not apparent (Lee et al., 2008) (Table 5.1).

In a large-scale study (40,246 adults were polled, yielding data on 8,825 children) carried on behalf of the REDALL study consortium by a randomized telephone survey method in 10 countries of Europe (Austria, Belgium, Denmark, Finland, Germany, Greece, Italy, Poland, Slovenia, and Switzerland), it was revealed that 4.2%–5.2% (on average 4.7%) of children population had allergic hypersensitivity to food (Steinke et al., 2007). The most affected age group of children was 2–3 year olds (7.2%); a considerable diversification of data between particular countries was observed from 1.7% in Austria to 11.7% in Finland. In the 10 European countries mentioned above, the most often implicated allergenic products were milk (38.5%), fruits (29.5%), eggs (19.0%), and vegetables (13.5%), with significant country- and age-linked variations. The most widespread allergy symptoms were skin symptoms (71.5%), followed by gastrointestinal (27.6%) and respiratory (18.5%) symptoms (Steinke et al., 2007).

In every country the scale of food allergy and epidemiological characteristics are different (Table 5.1).

The findings are confirmed by the statistical and epidemiological data of the Department of Health and Human Services, National Institutes of Health (NIH), Bethesda, (http://www.nih.gov/news/research_matters):

- The prevalence of allergic rhinitis has increased substantially over the past 15 years.
- Each year more than 50 million Americans suffer from allergic diseases.

## TABLE 5.1
## Occurrence of Food Allergies in Various Countries

| Country | Major Allergy Cause | Percent among the Allergic Population |
|---------|---------------------|---------------------------------------|
| United States | Milk | 65 |
| | Chocolate and coke | 45 |
| | Peanuts | 33 |
| | Cereals | 30 |
| | Vegetables | 26 |
| | Egg white | 26 |
| | Citrus fruits | 25 |
| | Walnuts and hazelnuts | 22.7 |
| Scandinavia | Fish | 39 (children) |
| Israel | Peaches | 75 |
| | Almonds | 39 |
| | Sunflower seeds | 35 |
| | Peanuts | 31 |
| France | Egg white | 46.3 |
| | Peanuts | 40 |
| | Mustard | 20 |
| | Cow's milk | 7.5 |
| Holland | Milk | 28 |
| | Broad beans | 23 |
| | Coffee | 22 |
| | Tomatoes | 18 |
| | Egg white | 16 |
| | Chocolate | 14 |
| | Fish | 13 |
| | Oranges | 11 |
| Denmark | Cow's milk | 2.2 (children) |
| Poland | Cow's milk | 45 |
| | Egg white and poultry | 30–37 |
| | Cereals and other plant proteins | 25 |
| | Tomatoes, potatoes, and fish | To a smaller extent |
| Far East countries | Milk, eggs, rice, buckwheat, and seafood | Not determined |
| African countries | Seafood | 14.7 |
| | Cereals | 11.4 |
| | Leguminous seeds | 11.4 |
| | Milk and dairy products | 9.8 |
| | Bulbous plants | 9.8 |
| | Fruits | 7.6 |
| | Eggs | 5.4 |
| | Alcoholic beverages | 5.4 |
| | Other beverages | 4.9 |

According to Lee et al. (2008), Commission Directive 2006/142/EC, Arbes et al. (2005), Jędrychowski (2001), Iikura et al. (1999), and Achinewu (1983).

- Allergic hypersensitivity is the sixth leading cause of chronic diseases in the United States, costing the health care system $18 billion annually.
- Estimates of allergy prevalence in the United States are 9%–16%.
- Food allergic hypersensitivity occurs in 8%–9% of children 6 years of age or under, and in 1%–2% of adults.
- Peanut or tree nut allergies affect approximately 3 million Americans and cause the most severe food-induced allergic reactions.
- Approximately 100 Americans, mostly children, die annually from food-induced anaphylaxis.
- Approximately 16.7 million office visits to health care providers each year are attributed to allergic rhinitis.

In 2007 in United States, approximately 3 million children under age 18 years (3.9%) were reported to have a food or digestive allergy in the previous 12 months. In the last decade (from 1997 to 2007), the prevalence of reported food allergic hypersensitivity increased 18% among children under age 18 years (Branym and Lukacs, 2008).

At present, the problem of food allergy becomes essential also in Europe and Poland. About 1%–2% of the adult population and 5%–8% infants/children have problems with the IgE-mediated form of food allergy (Jędrychowski, 2003). These specific reactions are directed toward several proteins present in peanuts, milk, soy, tree nuts, fish, or egg white. From the results presented it follows that food allergies in sensitive patients may be caused by the allergens contained by many food products at the same time. In Poland, allergic reactions are most often induced by the proteins of milk, eggs, fish, meat, poultry, tomatoes, and potatoes.

Recently special attention has been paid to a number of food additives, for instance of biotechnological origin, which may be responsible for causing allergic reactions. Many substances used as food additives display potential or confirmed capability to induce allergic reactions in sensitive patients (E102, E104, E110, E122, E124, E128, E129, E 129, E151, E154, E155, E180, E210, E211, E212, E213, E214, E215, E216, E218, E219, E220, E231, etc.) (The problem is presented in a more detailed way in Section 14.4.). It may be assumed that the above-mentioned additives cause pseudo-allergic reactions as they are haptens. Diagnostic differentiation between allergy and pseudoallergy is very difficult (see Chapter 1).

A significant group of food allergies are allergies to the proteins of leguminous plants, among which soy seeds take a prominent position (perhaps due to size of consumption and availability). Out of 34 proteins with antigenic properties occurring in soy flour 17 are IgE-reactive and have been suggested as allergens (Besler et al., 2001; Wilson et al., 2005). See also Table 12.1. Two of them have high structural affinity to other leguminous seed proteins and occur also in most other legumes, thus contributing to the occurrence of allergic cross-reactions within this species. It was found that individuals sensitive to soy proteins often have allergic reactions also to the proteins of sweet lupine. A similar threat is posed by food products produced with the addition of some legumes flour or proteins. The threat of potential allergic cross-reactions in individuals sensitive to soy proteins may also extend onto other foodstuffs, e.g., dairy products from cow's milk, which seems to be especially significant in the case of using soy proteins for producing hypoallergenic infant formulas for patients with allergy to cow's milk. The issue of allergens and potential cross-reactions of the allergens of particular food products are addressed in Chapters 6–14.

The increasing number of allergenic products is related to globalization processes, international trade, growth of cultivation areas, and popularization of Western habits (Iikura et al., 1999); for instance, products which bring in a significant allergenic threat are citrus fruits, lemons, kiwi, pineapples, and avocado. Recently, the cases of severe allergic reactions to many "exotic" allergens (among others—to patent blue, carmine dye, yeast, buckwheat, and macrogol) were identified in Finland (Hyry et al., 2006; Makinen-Kiljunen and Haahtela, 2008).

Wüthrich (2000) also reports a number of fatal cases caused by allergic reactions to foods pointing out particular threat posed by the so-called hidden allergens.

In Finland, from 2000 to 2007, the frequency of cases of severe allergic reactions annually was found to be 0.001%. The reaction was a life-threatening anaphylactic shock in 26% of the mentioned cases, with no deaths reported. Food was the causative agent in 53% of the cases. Out of the foodstuffs, the majority of reactions was induced by nuts and seeds: fruit and vegetables in the case of the adult population, and nuts, important allergens, for children along with milk, egg, and wheat (Makinen-Kiljunen and Haahtela, 2008).

The costs of treating patients with allergic hypersensitivity is very high (estimated to be €29 billion in Western Europe) (Bogucki, 2000).

In the view of Codex Alimentarius Commission on food labeling, all the products mentioned as well as ingredients derived from them should be listed on the product label (Codex Alimentarius Commission, 1979; Directive, 2003/89/EC 2003; Commission Directive, 2006/142/EC 2006; van Hengel, 2007).

### 5.1.1 ALLERGENS TERMINOLOGY

Over the recent years many allergens from different sources have been identified and characterized. In order to catalog and suitably describe the recognized compounds the International Union of Immunological Societies Subcommittee for Allergen Nomenclature suggested a system of terminology for purified allergens. When isolating allergenic compounds it is essential to define the source of their origin, taxonomic name of the species and genus of the organism and, if possible, a most detailed description identifying, for instance, the strain.

King et al., (1994) and Larsen and Lowenstein (1996) presented an updated version of allergens taxonomy compared to that of 1986 (Marsh et al., 1987). According to these documents, isolated and purified allergens are described as follows: the three first letters (*in italics*) determine the genus, next a single letter being the first letter of the species name (*also in italics*) and a Roman digit indicating the subsequently entered new allergen. In practice the rule is applied as follows: allergens of, for instance, hen egg white, formerly referred to as ovomucoid and ovoalbumin, are presented as *Gal d* 1 and *Gal d* 2 (*Gallus domesticus*). Apart from the traditional genus name, species name, and sequential number of allergen identification, allergen taxonomy comprises also the number of the isoallergen, genetic variant, gene responsible for polypeptide change synthesis, and the method of obtaining allergen

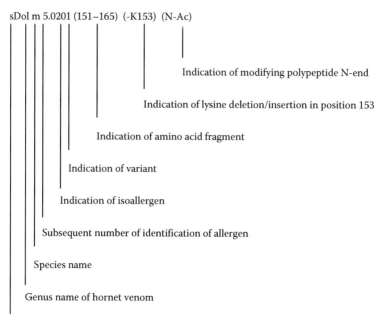

sDol m 5.0201 (151–165) (-K153) (N-Ac)

Indication of modifying polypeptide N-end

Indication of lysine deletion/insertion in position 153

Indication of amino acid fragment

Indication of variant

Indication of isoallergen

Subsequent number of identification of allergen

Species name

Genus name of hornet venom

Way of obtaining allergen fragment (s-syntetic, n-natural)

**FIGURE 5.1**    Example of the nomenclature of the hornet venom allergen.

and its modification. Below (Figure 5.1) is an example of taxonomic formula for hornet venom allergen obtained synthetically (after WHO/IUIS Allergen Nomenclature Subcommittee).

Structural and conformational affinity of epitopes from different sources, cross-reactions between different food products and airborne, food or contact allergens make an additional complication (Sharma et al., 2001; Chapman et al., 2007). Many allergens and food allergens have been characterized at a molecular level, which has increased our understanding of the immunopathogenesis of food allergy and might soon lead to novel diagnostic and therapeutic approaches (Sicherer and Sampson, 2006). A large group of food allergens and their extensive characteristics are comprised in allergen databases (e.g., Allergome database see Appendix). The most important food allergens are described in Chapters 6–14.

## REFERENCES

Achinewu, S.C. 1983. Food allergy and its clinical symptoms in Nigeria. *Food Nutr Bull* 5(3): 18–19.

Arbes, S. Jr., Gergen, P., Elliott, L., and Zeldin, D. 2005. Prevalences of positive skin test responses to 10 common allergens in the US population: Results from the Third National Health and Nutrition Examination Survey. *J Allergy Clinical Immunol* 116(2): 377–383.

Besler, M., Steinhart, H., and Paschke, A. 2001. Stability of allergens and allergenicity of processed foods. *J Chromatogr B* 756: 207–228.

Bogucki, M. 2000. The UCB Institute of Allergy. *Terapia*. Special issue 21 (in Polish).

Branym, A.M. and Lukacs, S.L. 2008. Food allergy among U.S. children: Trends in prevalence and hospitalizations. NCHS data brief no. 10. Hyattsville, MD: National Center for Health Statistics. (http://www.cdc.gov/nchs/data/databriefs/db010.pdf)

Chapman, M.D., Pomés, A., Breiteneder, H., and Ferreira, F. 2007. Nomenclature and structural biology of allergens. *J Allergy Clin Immunol* 119(2): 414–420.

Codex Alimentarius Commission (1979) Guide to the safe use of food additives. (CAC/FAL 5–1979)

Commission Directive 2006/142/EC of December 22, 2006 amending Annex IIIa of Directive 2000/13/EC of the European Parliament and of the Council listing the ingredients which must under all circumstances appear on the labeling of foodstuffs. *Official Journal of the European Union*. L 368/110 EN. 23.12.2006.

Directive 2003/89/EC of the European Parliament and of the Council of November 10, 2003 (amending Directive 2000/13/EC as regards indication of the ingredients present in foodstuffs. *Official Journal of the European Union*. L 308/15, 25.11.2003.

European Allergy White Paper. Epidemiology: Prevalence of allergic diseases. 1997. The UCB Institute of Allergy, Belgium, 14–39.

FAO/WHO Bulletin. 2006. International Food Safety Authorities Network (INFOSAN). INFOSAN Information Note No. 3/2006—Food Allergies, June 9, 2006.

Health and Human Services National Institutes of Health (NIH), Bethesda, MD (http://www.nih.gov/news/research_matters).

Hyry, H., Vuorio, A., Varjonen, E., Skyttä, J., and Mäkinen-Kiljunen, S. 2006. Two cases of anaphylaxis to macrogol 6000 after ingestion of drug tablets. *Allergy* 61(8): 1021.

Iikura, Y., Imai, Y., Imai T., Akasawa, A., Fujita, K., Hoshiyama, K., Nakura, H., Kohno, Y., Koike, K., Okudaira, H., and Iwasaki, E. 1999. Frequency of immediate-type food allergy in children in Japan. *Int Arch Allergy Immunol* 118(2–4): 251–252.

Jahnz-Rozyk, K. 2007. Choroby alergiczne na początku XXI w. *Przew Lek* 2: 155–159 (in Polish).

Jędrychowski, L. 2001. Alergeny pokarmowe jako czynniki ryzyka zdrowotnego. *Zywn Nauka Technol Jakosc* 4(29) 8: 62–81 (in Polish).

Jędrychowski, L. 2003. Examination of immunoreactive and immunomodulative properties of food components with the application of immunometric methods. *Pol J Food Nutr Sci* 12/53(SI 2): 32–39.

Kaczmarski, M. 1997. Food Allergy In Children. In Płusa T. *Allergology Progress -II*. Medpress, Warszawa, 120–129 (in Polish).

King, T.P., Hoffman, D., Lowenstein, H., Marsh, D.G., Platts-Mills, T.A., and Thomas, W. 1994. Allergen nomenclature. WHO/IUIS Allergen Nomenclature Subcommittee. *Int Arch Allergy Immunol* 105(3): 224–233.

Larsen J. N. and Lowenstein H. 1996. Allergen nomenclature. *J Allergy Clin Immunol* 97: 577–578.

Lee, B. W., Shek, L. P-Ch., Gerez, I.F.A., Soh, S.E., and Van Bever, H.P. 2008. Food allergy-Lessons from Asia. Review Article. *World Allergy Organization Journal (WAOJ)* 1(7): 129–133.

Makinen-Kiljunen, S. and Haahtela, T. 2008. Eight years of severe allergic reactions in Finland: A register-based report. *World Allergy Org J* 1(11):184–189.

Marsh, D.G., Goodfriend, L., Te Piao King, Lowenstein H., and Platts-Mills T.A.E. 1987. Allergen nomenclature. *J Allergy Clin Immunol* 5(80): 639–645.

Samson, H.A. 1996. Epidemiology of food allergy. *Pediatr Allergy Immunol* 7: 42–50.

Schäfer, T., Bohler, E., Ruhdorfer, S., Weigl, L., Wessner, D., Heinrich, J., Filipiak, B., Wichmann, H.E., and Ring, J. 2001. Epidemiology of food allergy/food intolerance in adults: Associations with other manifestations of atopy. *Allergy* 56(12): 1172–1179.

Sharma, S., Kumar, P., Betzel, Ch., and Singh, T. P. 2001. Structure and function of proteins involved in milk allergies. *J Chromatogr B: Biomed Sci Appl* 756(1–2): 183–187.

Sicherer, S.H. and Sampson, H.A. 2006. 9. Food allergy. *J Allergy Clin Immunol* 117(2 Suppl Mini-Primer). 470–475.

Steinke, M., Fiocchi, A., and Kirchlechner, V. 2007. Perceived food allergy in children in 10 European Nations. A randomised telephone survey. *Int Arch Allergy Immunol* 143(4): 290–295.

van Hengel, A.J. 2007. Declaration of allergens on the label of food products purchased on the European market. *Trends Food Sci Technol* 18(2): 96–100.

Wilson, S., Blaschek, K., and de Mejia, E.G. 2005. Allergenic proteins in soybean: Processing and reduction of P34 allergenicity. *Nutr Rev* 63: 47–58.

Wüthrich, B. 2000. Lethal or life-threatening allergic reactions to food. Review article. *Invest Allergol Clin Immunol* 10(2): 59–65.

# 6 Milk Allergens

*Barbara Wróblewska and Lucjan Jędrychowski*

## CONTENTS

## 6.1 CHARACTERIZATION OF ALLERGENS IN COW'S MILK: STRUCTURE AND FUNCTION OF MILK ALLERGENS

Barbara Wróblewska

Animal milk produced by cows (*Bos Taurus*) contains many allergenic proteins, which is why milk and milk products, including lactose, are listed in Annex IIIa of the EU Directive on the labeling of foods for human consumption. Allergy to cow's milk is the most common food allergy in childhood, especially in the third year of age, but most cases become tolerant to milk within a few years. Sometimes, but less frequently, cow allergy appears in adults. Symptoms caused by allergenic proteins in cow's milk are various and affect nearly all human systems. The easiest ones to observe and associate with Cow's Milk Allergy (CMA) are gastrointestinal symptoms such as abdominal cramps, loose stool, diarrhea, vomiting, chronic constipation, colic, eosinophilic gastroenteritis, nausea, and edema of the tongue. Cutaneous symptoms, including atopic dermatitis, angioedema, urticaria, redness, and pruritus, are embarrassing for both the sufferers and their closest circles. There can also be symptoms from the respiratory system, for example, allergic nasal blockade, cough, bronchospasm, sneezing, wheezing, and asthma. The most dangerous are systemic reactions, such as anaphylaxis and exercise-induced anaphylaxis, which can even cause death.

Cow's milk contains about 30–35 g proteins per liter, of which caseins make 80% and whey proteins 20%. One of the best list of known allergens of animal origin, with a good description of milk allergen, is InformAll (http://www.foodallergens.ifr.html).

### 6.1.1 CASEIN

Bovine casein is listed by the International Union of Immunological Societies as a single allergen, Bos d 8. However, it contains four main protein components, $\alpha$-s1-, $\alpha$-s2-, $\beta$-, and $\kappa$-Casein, in approximate proportions of 40%: 10%: 40%: 10%, respectively (Bernard et al. 1998). The fractions obtained after acid coagulation of individual caseins are cross-linked to aggregates called nanoclusters, which combine into micelles. Their central part is hydrophobic and peripheral hydrophilic parts contain sites of phosphorylation.

Caseins do not maintain a unique folded conformation (Horne 2002), which has led them to being termed as rheomorphic, and are highly sensitive to proteolysis. However, as the folded structure is limited, heating does not generally change the structure and hence its IgE binding (Kohno et al. 1994).

$\alpha$-s1-Casein, $\alpha$-s2-Casein, and $\beta$-Casein are able to chelate $Ca^{2+}$, $Zn^{2+}$, and $Fe^{3+}$. It has been proved that dephosphorylation reduces IgE binding to caseins (Bernard et al. 2000). Caseins are the major source of phosphate and calcium for the calf.

$\alpha$-s1-Casein has a molecular weight in the range of 27–32 kDa, depending on analysis conditions (Creamer and Richardson 1984). $\alpha$-s1 Casein consists of major and minor polypeptides that are built of the same amino acid (AA) sequence but differ in a phosphorylation degree (Monaci et al. 2006). Caseins form stable micellar calcium phosphate protein complexes. However, large aggregates are also reported. Allergenic epitopes were identified by Spuergin et al. (1997) in regions 19–30, 93–98, and 141–150 as immunodominant epitopes. Some sequential IgE-binding regions were recognized at AA 17–36, 39–48, 69–78, 93–102, 109–120, 123–132, 139–154, 159–174, and 173–194 using sera from nine older children (>9 years old) and the epitopes AA: 69–78 and 175–192 were recognized by 60% and 80% of sera from older children (Vila et al. 2001). Moreover, binding appeared to be predictive in the case of children who would not grow out of their allergy (Chatchatee et al. 2001a). A later study by Elsayed et al. (2004) has shown that the N- and C-terminal peptides, AA 16–35 and 136–155, have the highest human IgE-binding affinity, and AA 1–18 and 181–199 showed high binding to rabbit IgG.

$\alpha$-s2-Casein has a molecular weight in the range of 27–32 kDa and is the most hydrophilic of all the caseins because it has a cluster of anionic groups. $\alpha$-s2-Casein consists of two major and several minor components exhibiting varying levels of posttranslational phosphorylation. $\alpha$-s2-Casein is phosphorylated at multiple sites. The structure of $\alpha$-s2-Casein consists of approximately 25% $\alpha$-helix. $\alpha$-s2 Casein contains three cysteines and forms disulfide-linked dimers. Using 99 synthetic decapeptides, 10 regions binding IgE from the sera: AA: 31–44, 43–56, 83–100, 93–108,

105–114, 117–128, 143–158, 157–172, 165–188, and 191–200 were identified as aller-genic (Busse et al. 2002). Research on the presence of some α-s2-Casein epitopes has led to the identification of persistent and transient allergies. Residues AA: 33–42, 87–96, and 159–168 with weak binding to 145–154 and 171–180 originate from indi-viduals with persistent cow's milk allergy. Patients with transient allergies showed only weak binding to α-s2-Casein peptides (Järvinen et al. 2002).

Bernard et al. (2000) suggested that some of the phosphorylated regions, residues 23–31, 73–76, and 144–146, form part of the IgE epitopes and that the phosphates are involved in antibody recognition.

β-Casein has a molecular weight of 26.6 kDa. β-Casein is the most hydropho-bic component of the total casein. Sequence variants are known due to both partial proteolysis and variant genes (Farrell et al. 2004). β-Casein is less heavily phos-phorylated than α-Caseins with five potential phosphoserine sites in the N-terminal part of the sequence. The protease cleaves β-Casein into gamma 1, gamma 2, and gamma 3 fragments (Monaci et al. 2006). β-Casein also binds calcium forming "nanoclusters" (Smyth et al. 2004). One hundred overlapping synthetic decapep-tides were used to estimate the β-Casein region that binds IgE of patients and AA: 1–16, 45–54, 55–70, 83–92, 107–120, 135–144, 149–164, 167–184, and 185–208 were described as characteristic for patients with persistent cow's milk allergies. Sera from eight younger patients gave a simpler pattern with IgEs binding to residues 1–16, 45–54, 83–92, 107–120, and 135–144 with weak binding to residues 57–66 and the C-terminal region (Chatchatee et al. 2001b). It was also observed that the IgE response to dephosphorylated β-Casein was lower than that to native β-Casein, thus the N-terminal phosphorylated region, residues 30–50, probably includes important IgE epitopes (Bernard et al. 2000).

κ-Casein has a molecular weight of 21,269 Da as a precursor, and 19,023 Da as a mature form. κ-Casein consists of a major carbonate-free component and a mini-mum of six minor components. It was isolated from milk as a mixture of disulfide-bonded polymers ranging from dimers to octamers. κ-Casein plays an important role in the stability and coagulation properties of milk (Monaci et al. 2006). κ-Casein is probably more structured than α- and β-Caseins and contains specific disulfides (Rasmussen et al. 1992, 1994). These can rearrange on heating (Creamer et al. 1998). κ Casein is very sensitive to proteolysis. Its hydrolysis by chymosin in rennet pro-duces para-κ-Casein and a caseinomacropeptide that participates actively in the cheese-making process. Allergenic potential survives cooking. κ-Casein is critical to the stability of casein micelles (Creamer et al. 1998). Diagnosing patients with persistent cow's milk allergies with the use of 80 overlapping synthetic decapeptides helped to identify some regions binding to IgE from sera: AA: 15–24, 37–46, 55–80, 83–92, and 105–116 (Chatchatee et al. 2001b).

Whey proteins contain several major allergens, such as β-lg and α-la, and minor constituents, e.g., lactoferrin, bovine serum albumin (BSA), and immunoglobulins. In this fraction, proteolytic fragments of casein and fat globule membrane proteins can occur during analysis.

α-Lactalbumin, Bos d 4, α-la is a homologue of the C-type lysozymes. It is a member of glycohydrolase family 22 and Pfam family, 14,186 (mature form protein), 15,840 to 16,690 Da (glycosylated structure). α-la is stabilized by binding to calcium.

Polverino de Laureto et al. (2002) reported that α-la is cleaved by pepsin at pH 2 in the region of residues 34–57, producing large fragments. Veprintsev et al. (1997) report that differential scanning calorimetry (DSC) of α-la at pH 8.1 showed transitions at 20°C–30°C with the calcium chelator ethylene glycol tetraacetic acid (EGTA) and near 70°C with added calcium. McGuffey et al. (2005) investigated the effects of heating purified α-la and showed that the extent of irreversible aggregation varies at the temperatures between 67°C and 95°C. When milk is heated to 95°C, α-la denatures more slowly than β-lg (Chen et al. 2005). α-la folded structure is destabilized at low pH with the formation of a molten globule (Redfield 2004). The stability to denaturation is also strongly lowered by the reduction of disulfides (Chang 2004). Disulfide exchange can occur during thermal denaturation, leading to the formation of aggregates (Livney et al. 2003). Although evolved from a lysozyme (Mckenzie 1996), the function of α-la is to form a complex with galactosyltransferase, altering its substrate specificity to increase the rate of lactose formation in milk synthesis. The complex of galactosyltransferase and α-la is called lactose synthase (Ramakrishnan and Qasba 2001). α-la alone does not have any catalytic activity as a lysozyme or a synthase. Several other properties of α-la and possible additional functions have been described (Permyakov and Berliner 2000), including binding of several ligands and antimicrobial activity, both as a complete molecule (Hakansson et al. 2000) and as peptides (Pellegrini et al. 1999). The cytotoxic effects against mammalian cells have also been investigated (Permyakov et al. 2004).

The major component of α-la is unglycosylated. However, there is a minor glycosylated form (approximately 10%) with a mass spectrum that contains at least 15 discrete peaks (Slangen and Visser 1999). These arise from the glycosylation of asparagine 45.

A study concerning the allergenic properties of α-la showed that in 60% of the patients, allergic sera were specific for the intact α-la with only 40% binding to the peptides obtained after tryptic hydrolysis. Residue 17–58 was the most frequently recognized, followed by AA: 59–93, 99–108, and 109–123 (Maynard et al. 1997). The linear epitopes were identified by using sera of patients suffering from persistent allergies and their IgE to cow's milk > 100 kU(A)/L. IgE from the sera bound most strongly to residues AA: 1–16, 13–26, 47–58, and 93–102 (Järvinen et al. 2001).

β-Lactoglobulin has a molecular weight of 18 kDa (Natale et al. 2004) and belongs to the lipocalin superfamily. β-lg is named Bos d 5 as an allergen. It is capable of binding lipids, including retinol, β-carotene, saturated and unsaturated fatty acids, and aliphatic hydrocarbons, and transporting hydrophobic molecules, which is an important function (Godovac-Zimmermann et al. 1985, Kontopidis et al. 2004).

It is the most abundant fraction, making up 50% of the total whey protein. Under physiological conditions, β-lg exists as an equilibrium mixture of monomeric and dimeric forms. The proportion of monomers increases after heating to 70°C. Oligomers form below pH 6, with the largest one, an octamer, formed around pH 4.6 and dissociating below pH 3. Above pH 8, the protein irreversibly denatures, which may lead to aggregation. β-lg possesses three disulfide bridges and is present in several variants A, B, and C found in Jersey breed. β-lg is sensitive to thermal processes. Ehn et al. (2004) report that heating β-lg to 74°C and 90°C reduced IgE binding significantly. Heating to 90°C reduced IgE binding more extensively. However, full inhibition was always possible with high concentrations of the heated allergen, indicating that the IgE binding was not completely destroyed.

Chen et al. (2005) reported that almost 90% loss and denaturation of β-lg are observed in processed milk and that it is the major source of protein aggregation. Circular dichroism (CD) showed no significant conformational changes at temperatures below 70°C for as long as 480 s. The rapid changes of β-lg occurred between 80°C and 95°C. Fifty percent of the maximal changes could be reached within 15 s. Guyomarc'h et al. (2003) reported that large micellar aggregates, $4 \times 10^6$ Da are formed on heating milk that contained 3:1 ratios of β-lg and α-la together with κ-Casein and α-s2 Casein.

Proteolysis and use of monoclonal antibodies proved that β-lg possesses many allergenic epitopes spread all over the β-lg structure (Clement et al. 2002). Major human IgE epitopes for β-lg amino acid fragments are composed of residues AA: 41–60, 102–124, and 149–162; intermediate 1–8, 25–40, and 92–100; and minor 9–14, 84–91, 125–135, and 78–83 (Selo et al. 1999). Similar IgE epitope regions (AA: 21–40, 40–60, 107–117, and 148–168) were reported for rat as an animal model of β-lg allergy (Fritsche et al. 2005, Miller et al. 1999).

Lactoferrin has a molecular weight of about 67 kDa. Lactoferrin shows two transitions by differential scanning calorimetry, with the first peak at 65°C and the second peak at 92°C. These correspond to the denaturation of apo- and iron-loaded lactoferrin (Kulmyrzaev et al. 2005; Paulsson et al. 1993). Lactoferrin is a glycol-protein. If the carbohydrate moiety is cleaved, then the iron-binding activity is reduced. Lactoferrin has several antimicrobial roles (Vorland 1999) and its expression is increased in response to infection (Zheng et al. 2005). The main activity is the sequestration of iron. It may also protect cells from free radical damage by removing catalytic free iron. The antimicrobial peptide lactoferricin comprises of residues 17–41 of mature lactoferrin or 36–60 of the precursor. The peptide 265–284 also has antimicrobial activity (van der Kraan et al. 2005). In a study by Natale et al. (2004), 50% of 20 sera from cow's milk allergic patients aged 4 months to 14 months contained IgE against lactoferrin.

Bovine serum albumin (BSA) is named Bos d 6, as an allergen. It constitutes 5% of the total whey proteins. BSA is physically and immunologically very similar to human blood serum albumin. Serum albumin regulates the colloidal osmotic pressure of blood; binds several cations; and is the principal transporter of fatty acids, hormones, and bilirubin, which would otherwise be insoluble in plasma. In addition to being the most abundant plasma protein, its low level finds its way to milk. This protein was observed as a monomer and a dimer with respective molecular weights of 66,474 and 133,029 as estimated by electrospray ionization mass spectrometry. Such high masses may be due to the ions binding to water molecules (Wang et al. 2000). Three homologous domains, consisting of nine loops, are protected in the core and stabilized by 17 disulfide bridges, making the tertiary BSA structure relatively stable even during denaturation (Xiu and Ding 2004). Heating at 75°C and above produces disulfide-linked oligomers (Havea et al. 2000). Levi and Gonzalez Flecha (2002) argued that the dimer is noncovalent and need not involve a disulfide link. By contrast, Hunter and Carta (2001) suggested that the dimer is disulfide linked and can be removed by purification with an anion exchanger.

Restani et al. (2004) review IgE binding data using sera from beef allergic patients. They noted that reduction of the disulfides reduces but does not abolish IgE binding. Beretta et al. (2001) reported that sequential epitopes were able to resist proteolysis for 60 min when BSA was digested *in vitro* with pepsin at the ratio (enzyme to substrate) of 1:120 (w/w) and the region 524–542 is the region with strongest binding of human IgE. Anaphylaxis due to bovine serum albumin has also been reported in a patient injected with cells cultured in fetal calf serum (Mackensen et al. 2000).

The three-dimensional structure of bovine serum albumin has not been determined. Bovine serum albumin residues 126–144 (17-Amino-Acid Bovine Serum Albumin Peptide, ABBOS) have been reported to be responsible for the autoimmune reaction directed against pancreatic islet cells causing diabetes (Karjalainen et al. 1992). This remains controversial (Knip 2003, Persaud and Barranco-Mendoza 2004) but removal of this epitope as well as IgE binding is often an objective in producing infant formulas.

Immunoglobulin Bos d 7, IgG exists as an approximately 160 kDa disulfide-linked tetramer of two heavy and two light chains. Immunoglobulins are an important part of the humoral immune system and function by binding specifically to environmental agents such as viruses, bacteria, foods, and toxins. Li-Chan et al. (1995) reported that 59%–76% of native bovine IgG can be detected after commercial pasteurization during a mild heat treatment of milk such as heating to 72°C for at least 16 s, followed by rapid cooling. Some bovine IgG contains N-acetylgalactosaminylated N-linked sugar chains (Aoki et al. 1995).

The data pertain to the allergens that have been shown to bind IgE in sera from at least three patients with clinical manifestations of allergy to the food from which the allergen originated (Jenkins et al. 2007).

## REFERENCES

Aoki, N., Furukawa, K., Iwatsuki, K., Noda, A., Sato, T., Nakamura, R., and Matsuda, T. 1995. A bovine IgG heavy chain contains N-acetylgalactosaminylated N-linked sugar chains. *Biochem Biophys Res Commun* 210(2):275–280.

Beretta, B., Conti, A., Fiocchi A., Gaiaschi, A., Galli, C.L., Giuffrida, M.G., Ballabio, C., and Restani, P. 2001. Antigenic determinants of bovine serum albumin. *Int Arch Allergy Immunol* 126(3):188–195.

Bernard, H., Creminon, C., Yvon, M., and Wal, J.M. 1998. Specificity of the human IgE response to the different purified caseins in allergy to cow's milk proteins. *Int Arch Allergy Immunol* 115(3):235–244.

Bernard, H., Meisel, H., Creminon, C., and Wal, J.M. 2000. Post-translational phosphorylation affects the IgE binding capacity of caseins. *FEBS Lett* 467(2–3):239–244.

Busse, P.J., Järvinen, K.M., Vila, L., Beyer, K., and Sampson, H.A. 2002. Identification of sequential IgE-binding epitopes on bovine alpha(s2)-casein in cow's milk allergic patients. *Int Arch Allergy Immunol* 129(1):93–96.

Chatchatee, P., Jarvinen, K.M., Bardina, L., Beyer, K., and Sampson, H.A. 2001a. Identification of IgE- and IgG-binding epitopes on alpha(s1)-casein: Differences in patients with persistent and transient cow's milk allergy. *J Allergy Clin Immunol* 107(2):379–383.

Chatchatee, P., Jarvinen, K.M., Bardina, L., Vila, L., Beyer, K., and Sampson, H.A. 2001b. Identification of IgE and IgG binding epitopes on beta- and kappa-casein in cow's milk allergic patients. *Clin Exp Allergy* 31(8):1256–1262.

Chang, J.Y. 2004. Evidence for the underlying cause of diversity of the disulfide folding pathway. *Biochemistry* 43(15):4522–4529.

Chen, W.L., Hwang, M.T., Liau, C.Y., Ho, J.C., Hong, K.C., and Mao, S.J. 2005. Beta-lactoglobulin is a thermal marker in processed milk as studied by electrophoresis and circular dichroic spectra. *J Dairy Sci* 88(5):1618–1630.

Clement, G., Boquet, D., Frobert, Y., Bernard, H., Negroni, L., Chatel, J.-M., Adel-Patient, K., Creminon, C., Wal, J.-M., and Grassi, J. 2002. Epitopic characterization of native bovine b-lactoglobulin. *J Immunol Meth* 266:67–78.

Creamer, L.K. and Richardson, T. 1984. Anomalous behavior of bovine alpha s1- and beta-caseins on gel electrophoresis in sodium dodecyl sulfate buffers. *Arch Biochem Biophys* 234(2):476–486.

Creamer, L.K., Plowman, J.E., Liddell, M.J., Smith, M.H., and Hill, J.P. 1998. Micelle stability: Kappa-casein structure and function. *J Dairy Sci* 81(11):3004–3012.

Ehn, B.M., Ekstrand, B., Bengtsson, U., and Ahlstedt, S. 2004. Modification of IgE binding during heat processing of the cow's milk allergen beta-lactoglobulin. *J Agric Food Chem* 52(5):1398–1403.

Elsayed, S., Hill, D.J., and Do, T.V. 2004. Evaluation of the allergenicity and antigenicity of bovine-milk alphas1-casein using extensively purified synthetic peptides. *Scand J Immunol* 60(5):486–493.

Farrell, H.M. Jr., Jimenez-Flores, R., Bleck, G.T., Brown, E.M., Butler, J.E., Creamer, L.K., Hicks, C.L., Hollar, C.M., Ng-Kwai-Hang, K.F., and Swaisgood, H.E. 2004. Nomenclature of the proteins of cows' milk—sixth revision. *J Dairy Sci* 87(6):1641–1674.

Fritsche, R., Adel-Patient, K., Bernard, H., Martin-Paschoud, C., Schwarz, C., Ah-Leung, S., Wal, J.M. 2005. IgE-mediated rat mast cell triggering with tryptic and synthetic peptides of bovine beta-lactoglobulin. *Int Arch Allergy Immunol* 138:291–297.

Godovac-Zimmermann, J., Conti, A., Liberatori, J., and Braunitzer, G. 1985. Homology between the primary structures of beta-lactoglobulins and human retinol-binding protein: Evidence for a similar biological function? *Biol Chem Hoppe Seyler* 366(4): 431–434.

Guyomarc'h, F., Law, A.J., and Dalgleish, D.G. 2003. Formation of soluble and micelle-bound protein aggregates in heated milk. *J Agric Food Chem* 51(16):4652–4660.

Havea, P., Singh, H., Creamer, L.K. 2000. Formation of new protein structures in heated mixtures of BSA and alpha-lactalbumin. *J Agric Food Chem* 48(5):1548–1556.

Hakansson, A., Svensson, M., Mossberg, A.K., Sabharwal, H., Linse, S., Lazou, I., Lonnerdal, B., and Svanborg, C. 2000. A folding variant of alpha-lactalbumin with bactericidal activity against Streptococcus pneumoniae. *Mol Microbiol* 35(3):589–600.

Horne, D.S. 2002. Casein structure, self-assembly and gelation. *Curr Opin Colloid Interface Sci* 7(5–6):456–461. http://www. foodallergens.ifr.html

Hunter, A.K. and Carta, G. 2001. Effects of bovine serum albumin heterogeneity on frontal analysis with anion-exchange media. *J Chromatogr A* 937(1–2):13–19.

Järvinen, K.M., Chatchatee, P., Bardina, L., Beyer, K., and Sampson, H.A. 2001. IgE and IgG binding epitopes on alpha-lactalbumin and beta-lactoglobulin in cow's milk allergy. *Int Arch Allergy Immunol* 126(2):111–118.

Järvinen, K.M., Beyer, K., Vila, L., Chatchatee, P., Busse, P.J., and Samson, H.A. 2002. B-cell epitopes as a screening instrument for persistent cow's milk allergy. *J Allergy Clin Immunol* 110(2):293–297.

Jenkins, J.A., Breiteneder, H., and Mills, E.N.C. 2007. Evolutionary distance from human homologs reflects allergenicity of animal food proteins. *J Allergy Clin Immunol* 120:1399–1405.

Karjalainen, J., Martin, J.M., Knip, M., Ilonen, J., Robinson, B.H., Savilahti, E., Akerblom, H.K., and Dosch, H.M. 1992. A bovine albumin peptide as a possible trigger of insulin-dependent diabetes mellitus. *N Engl J Med* 327(5):302–307.

Knip, M. 2003. Cow's milk antibodies in patients with newly diagnosed type 1 diabetes: Primary or secondary? *Pediatr Diabetes* 4(4):155–156.

Kohno, Y., Honma, K., Saito, K., Shimojo, N., Tsunoo, H., Kaminogawa, S., and Niimi, H. 1994. Preferential recognition of primary protein structures of alpha-casein by IgG and IgE antibodies of patients with milk allergy. *Ann Allergy* 73(5):419–422.

Kontopidis, G., Holt, C., and Sawyer, L. 2004. Invited review: beta-lactoglobulin: Binding properties, structure, and function. *J Dairy Sci* 87(4):785–796.

Kulmyrzaev, A.A., Levieux, D., and Dufour, E. 2005. Front-face fluorescence spectroscopy allows the characterization of mild heat treatments applied to milk. Relations with the denaturation of milk proteins. *J Agric Food Chem* 53(3):502–507.

Levi, V. and Gonzalez Flecha, F.L. 2002. Reversible fast-dimerization of bovine serum albumin detected by fluorescence resonance energy transfer. *Biochim Biophys Acta* 1599(1–2):141–148.

Li-Chan, E., Kummer, A., Losso, J.N., Kitts, D.D., and Nakai, S. 1995. Stability of bovine immunoglobulins to thermal treatment and processing. *Food Res Int* 28:9–16.

Livney, Y.D., Verespej, E., and Dalgleish, D.G. 2003. Steric effects governing disulfide bond interchange during thermal aggregation in solutions of beta-lactoglobulin B and alpha-lactalbumin. *J Agric Food Chem*. 51(27):8098–8106.

Mackensen, A., Drager, R., Schlesier, M., Mertelsmann, R., and Lindemann, A. 2000. Presence of IgE antibodies to bovine serum albumin in a patient developing anaphylaxis after vaccination with human peptide-pulsed dendritic cells. *Cancer Immunol Immunother* 49(3):152–156.

Maynard, F., Jost, R., and Wal, J.M. 1997. Human IgE binding capacity of tryptic peptides from bovine alpha-lactalbumin. *Int Arch Allergy Immunol* 113(4):478–488.

McGuffey, M.K., Epting, K.L., Kelly, R.M., and Foegeding, E.A. 2005. Denaturation and aggregation of three alpha-lactalbumin preparations at neutral pH. *J Agric Food Chem* 53(8):3182–3190.

McKenzie, H.A. 1996. alpha-Lactalbumins and lysozymes. *EXS* 75:365–409.

Miller, K., Meredith, C., Selo, I., and Wal, J.M. 1999. Allergy to bovine β-lactoglobulin: Specificity of immunoglobulin E generated in the brown Norway rat to tryptic and synthetic peptides. *Clin Exp Allergy* 29:1696–1704.

Monaci, L., Tregoat, V., Van Hengel, A.J., and Anklam, E. 2006. Milk allergens, their characteristic and their detection in food. A review. *Eur Food Res Technol* 223:149–179.

Natale, M., Bisson, C., Monti, G., Peltran, A., Garoffo, L.P., Valentini, S., Fabris, C., Bertino, E., Coscia, A., and Conti, A. 2004. Cow's milk allergens identification by two-dimensional immunoblotting and mass spectrometry. *Mol Nutr Food Res* 48(5):363–369.

Paulsson, M.A., Svensson, U., Kishore, A.R., and Naidu, A.S. 1993. Thermal behavior of bovine lactoferrin in water and its relation to bacterial interaction and antibacterial activity. *J Dairy Sci* 76(12):3711–3720.

Pellegrini, A., Thomas, U., Bramaz, N., Hunziker, P., and von Fellenberg, R. 1999. Isolation and identification of three bactericidal domains in the bovine alpha-lactalbumin molecule. *Biochim Biophys Acta* 1426(3):439–448.

Permyakov, E.A. and Berliner, L.J. 2000. alpha-Lactalbumin: Structure and function. *FEBS Lett* 473(3):269–274.

Permyakov, S.E., Pershikova, I.V., Khokhlova, T.I., Uversky, V.N., and Permyakov, E.A. 2004. No need to be HAMLET or BAMLET to interact with histones: Binding of monomeric alpha-lactalbumin to histones and basic poly-amino acids. *Biochemistry* 43(19):5575–5582.

Persaud, D.R. and Barranco-Mendoza, A. 2004. Bovine serum albumin and insulin-dependent diabetes mellitus; is cow's milk still a possible toxicological causative agent of diabetes? *Food Chem Toxicol* 42(5):707–714.

Polverino de Laureto, P., Frare, E., Gottardo, R., Van Dael, H., and Fontana, A. 2002. Partly folded states of members of the lysozyme/lactalbumin superfamily: A comparative study by circular dichroism spectroscopy and limited proteolysis. *Protein Sci* 11(12):2932–2946.

Rasmussen, L.K., Hojrup, P., and Petersen, T.E. 1992. The multimeric structure and disulfide-bonding pattern of bovine kappa-casein. *Eur J Biochem* 207(1):215–222.

Rasmussen, L.K., Hojrup, P., and Petersen, T.E. 1994. Disulphide arrangement in bovine caseins: Localization of intrachain disulphide bridges in monomers of kappa- and alpha s2-casein from bovine milk. *J Dairy Res* 61(4):485–493.

Ramakrishnan, B. and Qasba, P.K. 2001. Crystal structure of lactose synthase reveals a large conformational change in its catalytic component, the beta-1,4-galactosyltransferase-I. *J Mol Biol* 310(1):205–218.

Redfield, C. 2004. NMR studies of partially folded molten-globule states. *Methods Mol Biol* 278:233–254.

Restani, P., Ballabio, C., Cattaneo, A., Isoardi, P., Terracciano, L., and Fiocchi, A. 2004. Characterization of bovine serum albumin epitopes and their role in allergic reactions. *Allergy* 59, 78:21–24.

Selo, I., Clement, G., Bernard, H., Chatel, J.-M., Creminon, C., Peltre, G., and Wal, J.-M. 1999. Allergy to bovine beta lactoglobulin: Specificity of human IgE to tryptic peptides. *Clin Exp Allergy* 29:1055–1063.

Slangen, C.J. and Visser, S. 1999. Use of mass spectrometry to rapidly characterize the heterogeneity of bovine alpha-lactalbumin. *J Agric Food Chem* 47(11):4549–4556.

Smyth, E., Clegg, R.A., and Holt, C. 2004. A biological perspective on the structure and function of caseins and casein micelles. *Int J Dairy Technol* 57(2–3):121–126.

Spuergin, P., Walter, M., Schiltz, E., Deichmann, K., Forster, J., and Mueller, H. 1997. Allergenicity of alpha-casein from cow, sheep, and goat. *Allergy* 52(3):293–298.

Wang, Y., Schubert, M., Ingendoh, A., and Franzen, J. 2000. Analysis of non-covalent protein complexes up to 290 kDa using electrospray ionization and ion trap mass spectrometry. *Rapid Commun Mass Spectrom* 14(1):12–17.

van der Kraan, M.I., van der Made, C., Nazmi, K., Van't Hof, W., Groenink, J., Veerman, E.C., Bolscher, J.G., and Nieuw Amerongen, A.V. 2005. Effect of amino acid substitutions on the candidacidal activity of L-Fampin. *Peptides* 7:265–284.

Veprintsev, D.B., Permyakov, S.E., Permyakov, E.A., Rogov, V.V., Cawthern, K.M., and Berliner, L.J. 1997. Cooperative thermal transitions of bovine and human apo-alpha-lactalbumins: Evidence for a new intermediate state. *FEBS Lett* 412(3):625–628.

Vila, L., Beyer, K., Jarvinen, K.M., Chatchatee, P., Bardina, L., and Sampson, H.A. 2001. Role of conformational and linear epitopes in the achievement of tolerance in cow's milk allergy. *Clin Exp Allergy* 31(10):1599–1606.

Vorland, L.H. 1999. Lactoferrin: A multifunctional glycoprotein. *APMIS*. 107(11):971–981.

Xu, Y. and Ding, Z. 2004. A novel method for simultaneous purification of albumin and immunoglobulin G. *Prep Biochem Biotechnol* 34(4):377–385.

Zheng, J., Ather, J.L., Sonstegard, T.S., and Kerr, D.E. 2005. Characterization of the infection-responsive bovine lactoferrin promoter. *Gene* 353(1):107–117.

## 6.2 ROLE OF MILK PROTEINS ORIGINATING FROM DIFFERENT ANIMALS IN THE INDUCTION OF AN ALLERGENIC REACTION

Barbara Wróblewska

Cow's milk (CM) allergy is quite frequent in the first years of human life. When breast-feeding is not possible, a CM substitute is usually provided for allergic subjects. Usually whey- and casein-based extensively hydrolyzed formulas or soy formulas are used. Cow milk hypoallergenic products are the most popular sub-stitute in west European countries. But in the United States, South Africa, and the Mediterranean, goat's milk is also a product for pediatric use (Maree 1978), donkey's milk in Asia, Africa, and eastern Europe (Vincenzetti et al. 2008).

There are studies revealing that milk from different mammalian species, except camel's milk, possesses identical kinds of proteins, which are characterized by simi-lar immunological properties (Restani et al. 1999, 2002). An official position of two European societies, ESPAGHN and ESPHACI (Høst et al. 1999), and the FDA (Food and Drug Administration) in the United States have not approved special formulas produced from milk other than cow's milk for people who suffer from cow's milk allergy. But there are some literature data concerning goat's, mare's, and donkey's milk as a basic resource for the production of hypoallergenic formulas.

Goat's milk (GM) allergy is usually associated with cow's milk allergy, with con-trary cases being a rather rare disorder (Bellioni-Businco et al. 1999). The major allergenic fraction of goat casein is β-Casein. The α-s-Casein, which is an important cow's milk allergen, is a minor one in goat's milk. The ratio of β-Casein to α-Casein is 70% and 30%, which is similar to human rather than cow's milk. This is probably the main reason why goat's milk and human milk are more readily digested by pep-sin than cow's milk. Goat and human β-Casein are more sensitive to proteolysis by pepsin than cow α-s-Casein. The peptide mapping of goat α-la and β-lg is different from that of cow's milk.

A study on the allergenicity of goat's milk performed on 26 children with proven IgE-mediated CMA showed that all the children had positive skin tests to both CM and GM, all had positive double-blind, placebo-controlled, food challenges (DBPCFCs); and 24 of the 26 had positive DBPCFCs to GM. These data indicated that GM is not an appropriate CM substitute for children with IgE-mediated CMA (Bellioni-Businco et al. 1999).

There are cases that indicate that goat protein allergens other than casein can be involved in food allergies to GM and even small quantities of protein can elicit clinical symptoms. A 27-year-old female patient experienced two episodes of urticaria after ingestion of goat's cheese. She tolerated cow's milk, dairy products, and sheep cheese but her skin tests were positive for goat's milk and goat's cheese (Tavares et al. 2007).

A study evaluated the possible use of goat's milk in patients with CM allergy by investigating the possible cross-reactivity between both milk proteins. Patients with cow's milk allergy were tested for tolerance to goat's milk protein. Only 25% of the patients showed adequate immediate and late oral tolerance and had negative results in immunological tests for adverse reactions. The conclusion was that the use of goat's milk cannot be recommended to patients with cow's milk allergy without pos-sible tolerance examinations conducted by a specialist. For the 25% of patients who tolerate goat's protein, GM could be an excellent substitute in children over 2 years of age (Infante Pina et al. 2003).

Sheep's milk (SM) and cheese made from sheep's milk may cause severe allergic reactions in children. In the literature data, there is an example of a 5-year-old atopic boy who experienced several anaphylactic reactions after eating food containing pecorino, a cheese made from sheep's milk. Skin-prick tests were strongly positive for sheep's buttermilk curd and pecorino sheep's cheese. Skin-prick tests for fresh sheep's milk and goat's milk were also positive but negative to all cow's milk proteins, whole pasteurized cow's milk, and cheese made from cow's milk. Specific IgE antibodies were negative for all cow's milk proteins (Calvani and Alessandri 1998).

Another example described a 2-year-old boy with allergy to sheep's and goat's milk proteins but not to cow's milk proteins. Sheep casein was probably the main allergen causing sensitization in this patient. The results suggest that sheep casein shows a high degree of cross-reactivity with goat casein but not with cow casein. The patient presented allergic symptoms caused by sheep's and goat's milk and cheese proteins. However, he was able to tolerate cow's milk and cow's milk dairy products without any side effects (Munoz Martin et al. 2004).

Donkey's milk (DM), used in some clinical trials as infant formula, is better adapted than cow's milk (Carroccio et al. 2000). Since it has been proved that donkey's milk is a good growth medium for probiotic lactobacilli strains because of its high content of lysozyme and lactose, Coppola et al. (2002) suggested that this milk be used for probiotic purposes. A high content of lactose is responsible for good palatability and intestinal absorption of calcium (Schaafsma 2003). DM lipid fraction is comparable to that of human milk since it has a high level of linoleic and linolenic acid. The latter is useful for the treatment of some atopic dermatitis (Horrobin 2000). The mineral composition of this milk is similar to mare's milk and human milk, except for very high levels of calcium and phosphorus. In contrast, the Ca/P ratio is very close to that of human milk (Salimei et al. 2004). The total protein content is rather low (13–28 mg/mL), similar to human and mare's milk. The whey proteins represent 35%–50% of the nitrogen fraction with $\alpha$-la (1.80 mg/mL), which has two isoforms, A and B, with different isoelectric points; $\beta$-lg with three genetic variants (3.75 mg/mL); and lysozyme (1.0 mg/mL) as the most important proteins (Vincenzetti et al. 2008). Among potentially allergenic milk components it was observed that the amount of $\beta$-lg was much lower than that in bovine milk, where $\beta$-lg can account for up to 50% of the total whey protein. In donkey's milk, the casein makes about 47.3% of the crude protein and the presence of $\alpha$-s1-like casein, $\beta$-like casein, $\kappa$-like casein, and gamma-like casein was reported (Salimei et al. 2004). Casein is considered as a predominant allergen in adults.

To date the problem of a cow milk allergy is resolved by the complete elimination of cow milk proteins from a diet, which is very difficult because of hidden allergens. Donkey's milk was proposed to a population of 46 selected children with cow's milk protein allergy, who could not resort to any cow's milk substitute. In a study by Monti et al. (2007), 38 children (82.6%) liked and tolerated donkey's milk, which helped them catch up on their growth, which was impaired during earlier cow's milk consumption. The degree of cross-reactivity of immunoglobulin E (IgE) with donkey's milk proteins was very weak and specific. Donkey's milk has been found to be a valid alternative to both IgE-mediated and non-IgE-mediated cow's milk protein allergies, including such aspects as its palatability and weight–height gain of consumers.

Mare's milk (MM) can be a cause of severe clinical manifestation, as has been described in the case of a 53-year-old woman. After her first mare's milk intake she developed pruritus on the palms and soles, generalized erythema, conjunctivitis, and intense dyspnea for 45 min. In fact, she had rhinoconjunctivitis and mild asthma sensitized to horse epithelium, but she had good tolerance to goat's milk and cow's milk both prior and after the incident. Immunoblotting with the patient's serum showed three bands of mare's milk recognized by IgE antibodies (caseins [23–36 kDa], β-lg [18 kDa], and α-la [15 kDa]) and only one band of horse epithelium (EquC1 [19 kDa] or EquC2 [18 kDa]). Although horse meat allergy has been related to hamster allergy, the anaphylaxis in this patient may be due to an association between a previous respiratory sensitization to animal epithelium and a later reaction with food allergens derived from the same animal. This may explain why the patient, previously sensitized to HE, had a reaction the first time she drank MM, although she may have had contact with the offending allergen by inadvertent contact in other foods. The allergenic proteins in MM are β-lg and α-la, which show no cross-reactions with the corresponding whey proteins in cow's milk (Robles et al. 2007).

Camel milk (CmM) is not popular in European or American diets. Traditionally, it is consumed in Africa and Middle Asia. Studies by Restani et al. (1999) showed that β-lg, one of the major milk allergens (Merin et al. 2001) and β-Casein were two proteins that were absent in camels' milk. CmM includes immunoglobulins that are similar to those in mothers' milk and protect infants from inflammation. This observation initiated an interest in camel's milk as a source of hypoallergenic milk proteins. CmM composition is different from that of ruminants, which could be associated with the phenotypic character of this animal, which belongs to *Tylopode* and not to ruminants. CmM contains about 2% of fat, consisting mainly of polyunsaturated fatty acids, which are completely homogenized and give the milk a smooth white appearance. The concentration of lactose is about 4.8%, which is easily metabolized even in the guts of patients with lactose intolerance. CmM is also rich in vitamin C, calcium, and iron (Shabo et al. 2005).

Cross-reactivity of milk proteins from different species is the main cause of similar immunoreactivity. Cross-reactivity indicates the homology in amino acid sequences and similar capacity of binding specific IgE antibodies. Weak cross-reactivity is usually observed between cow milk proteins and proteins from mares and donkeys.

The protein content in human milk is lower than in milk of ruminant dairy animals: cows, buffalos, yaks, camels, goats, sheep, and reindeers, but is closer to that of donkey's and mare's milk. Human milk caseins are homologous to donkey and mare milk proteins; weakly related to goat's and camel's milk; and show no relationship to cow, buffalo, and sheep milk proteins (El-Agamy 2007). The ratio of casein in the total protein is lower in human milk, and the amount of whey proteins is higher than in milk of cows, buffalo, and sheep but similar in donkey's and mare's milk. Specific properties, including a low level of soluble calcium, of milk produced by the above animals and of goat's result in the formation of soft curds during digestion in the infant's gut. Cow's and buffalo's milk yield hard curd, which is a desirable feature during cheese production.

A strong immunological relationship was found between human and donkey whey proteins, but with the other species only very weak homology was detected.

Human α-la is highly homologous to bovine α-la, with 66% identity (Aalberse and Stapel 2001). Human milk is free from β-lg, the main cow milk allergen, but in a mother's diet comprising cow milk or hidden milk allergens, β-lg is passed from the gut to the breast milk. Milk from nearly all the above species of animals (cow, buffalo, goat, mare, and donkey) contains various levels of β-lg. It is only camel's milk that like human milk, is free of β-lg.

Cross-reactivity at a 10% level was also found between polyclonal anti-bovine β-lg and α-la, in both the native and denatured forms, but no reaction was found with BSA (Baroglio et al. 1998).

The allergic potential of α-Caseins from bovine, sheep, and goat's milk shares more than 85% identical amino acids. Rat's, horse's, camel's, rabbit's, and human being's milk are identical and bear only 22%–41% homology to $\alpha_{s1}$-Casein bovine's milk (Jenkins et al. 2007). Analyses were performed on sera from children with an immediate-type allergy to cow's milk, children with atopy but without food allergy, and healthy children without atopy. The sera of cow's milk–allergic children showed significantly higher IgE and IgG bindings to α-Caseins from all the three species than the sera of the two other groups. All the groups showed an increased antibody binding to bovine α-Casein compared to the sheep and goat proteins, but the differences were significant only in the groups of atopic children and healthy controls. Furthermore, inhibition of the IgE binding to bovine α-Casein with α-Casein from cow, goat, and sheep revealed that the α-Casein from these species is highly cross-reactive as the differences in their primary structure are small. The research was concluded by a statement that milk of goat and sheep harbors an allergic potential and is not suitable as the nutrition for milk-allergic patients (Spuergin et al. 1997).

Cross-reactivity between β-lg and casein from cow and goat milk has also been detected (Sabbah et al. 1996).

## REFERENCES

Aalberse, R.C. and Stapel, S.O. 2001. Structure of food allergens in relation to allergenicity. *Pediatr Allergy Imunol* 12(Suppl. 14):10–14.

Baroglio, C., Giuffrida, M.G., Cantisani, A., Napolitano, L., Bernino, E., Fabris, C., and Conti, A. 1998. Evidence for a common epitope between bosine Ralpha-lactalbumin and beta-lactoglobulin. *Biol Chem* 379(12):1453–1456.

Bellioni-Businco, B., Paganelli, R., Lucenti, P., Giampietro, P.G., Perborn, H., and Businco, L. 1999. Allergenicity of goat's milk in children with cow's milk allergy. *J Allergy Clin Immunol* 103(6):1191–1194.

Calvani, M. Jr. and Alessandri, C. 1998. Anaphylaxis to sheep's milk cheese in a child unaffected by cow's milk protein allergy. *Eur J Pediatr* 157(1):17–19.

Carroccio, A., Cavataio, F., Montalto, G., and D'Amicio, A.L. 2000. Intolerance to hydro-lysated cow's milk proteins in infant: Characteristics and dietary treatment. *Clin Exp Allergy* 18:1597–1603.

Coppola, R., Salimei, E., Succi, M., Sorrentini, E., Nanni, M., and Ranieri, P. 2002. Behaviour of *Lactobacillus rhamnosus* strains in ass's milk. *Ann Microbiol* 52:55–60.

El-Agamy, E.I. 2007. The challenge of cow milk protein allergy. *Small Ruminant Res* 68(1–2):64–72.

Horrobin, D.F. 2000. Essential fatty acid metabolism and its modification in atopic eczema. *Am J Clin Nutr* 71:367–372.

Infante Pina, D., Tormo Carnice, R., and Conde Zandueta, M. 2003. Use of goat's milk in patients with cow's milk allergy. *An Pediatr (Barc)* 59(2):138–142.

Jenkins, J.A., Breiteneder, H., and Mills, C. 2007. Evolutionary distance from human homologs reflects allergenicity of animal food proteins. *J Allergy Clin Immunol* 120:1399–1405.

Maree, H.P. 1978. Goat milk and its use as a hypo-allergenic infant food. *Dairy Goat J* 56(5):62.

Merin, U., Bernstein, S.D., Bloch-Damti, N., Yagil, R., van Creveld, C., and Lindner, P. 2001. A comparative study of milk proteins in camel (*Camelus dromedarius*) and bovine colostrum. *Livestock Product Sci* 67:297–301.

Monti, G., Bertino, E., Muratore, M.C., Coscia, A., Cresi, F., Silvestro, L., Fabris, C., Fortunato, D., Giuffrida, M.G., and Conti, A. 2007. Efficacy of donkey's milk in treating highly problematic cow's milk allergic children: An in vivo and in vitro study. *Pediatr Allergy Immunol* 18(3):258–264.

Munoz Martin, T., De La Hoz Caballer, B., Maranon Lizana, F., Gonzalez Mendiola, R., Prieto Montano, P., and Sanchez Cano, M. 2004. Selective allergy to sheep's and goat's milk proteins. *Allergol Immunopathol (Madr)* 32(1):39–42.

Restani, G., Plebani, B., Cavagni, F., Poiesi, V., and Ugazio, G. 1999. Cross-reactivity between milk proteins from different animal species. *Clin Exp Allergy* 29(7):997.

Restani, P., Beretta, B., Fiocchi, A., Ballabio, C., and Galli, C.L. 2002. Cross-reactivity between mammalian proteins. *Ann Allergy Asthma Immunol* 89(6 Suppl. 1):11–15.

Robles, S., Torres, M.J., Mayorga, C., Rodriguez-Bada, J.L., Fernandez, T., Blanca, M., and Bartolome. 2007. Anaphylaxis to mare's milk. *Ann Allergy Asthma Immunol* 98(6):600–602.

Sabbah, A., Drouet, M., and Lauret, M.G. 1996. Western blotting or immunoblotting: application of the Alastst-Alablot to the study of cross reaction between cow's milk and goat's milk. *Allergy Immunol (Paris)* 28(10):335–339.

Salimei, E., Fantuz, F., Coppola, R., Chiofalo, B., Polidori, P., and Varisco, G. 2004. Composition and characteristic of ass's milk. *Animal Res* 53:67–78.

Schaafsma, G. 2003. Nutritional significance of lactose and lactose derivatives. In: Roginski H., Fuquay J.W., and Fox P.F. (Eds.), *Encyclopedia of Dairy Sciences* (Vol. 3. pp. 1529–1533). London: Academic Press.

Shabo, Y., Barzel, R., Margoulis, M., and Yagil, R. 2005. Camel milk for food allergies in children. *Israel Med Assoc J* 7:796–798.

Spuergin, P., Walter, M., Schiltz, E., Deichmann, K., Forster, J., and Mueller, H. 1997. Allergenicity of alpha-caseins from cow, sheep, and goat. *Allergy* 52(3):293–298.

Tavares, B., Pereira, C., Rodrigues, F., Loureiro, G., and Chieira, C. 2007. Goat's milk allergy. *Allergol Immunopathol (Madr)* 35(3):113–116.

Vincenzetti, S., Polidori, P., Mariani, P., Cammertoni, N., Fantuz, F., and Vita, A. 2008. Donkey's milk protein fractions characterization. *Food Chem* 106(2): 640–649.

## 6.3 CHANGES IN IMMUNOREACTIVITY AND ALLERGENICITY OF MILK ALLERGENS DURING TECHNOLOGICAL PROCESSES

Barbara Wróblewska and Lucjan Jędrychowski

Raw cow's milk is subject to many technological processes during milk production such as machine milking, cold storage, homogenization, heat treatment (pasteurization, ultrahigh-temperature processing [UHT]), and storage of packed products (pasteurized milk, UHT milk). During these processes, different interactions have been observed between milk components (lipid oxidation, lypolysis, proteolysis, activation and reactivation of some enzymes, destruction of microorganisms, whey protein denaturation, and Maillard reactions), leading to the formation of new chemical adducts, unknown to the immune system, which can affect reactions within a human organism (Korhonen and Korpela 1994, Morr and Richter 1988). Some allergenic properties have been thoroughly described on animal models, but controversial results have been obtained while observing the response to the human body, mainly regarding the inhibition of specific IgEs.

### 6.3.1 Thermal Processing

Boiling of milk is one of the most popular thermal processes, usually applied in a household. Thermal processes are common and popular because they are the oldest methods to improve the microbiological value of raw cow milk. On the one hand, this process can make proteins more edible by improving their intrinsic digestibility and modifying their functional properties (Jędrychowski et al. 2005, Korhonen 2002). But, on the other hand, this treatment causes Maillard's reaction (nonenzymatic browning) as a result of the binding between the lysine residues of proteins and the carbohydrates. Protein–sugar adducts may be recognized as foreign structures by the immune system and can become new allergens.

Heat denaturation via pasteurization or UHT processing can change the antigenic and allergenic properties of proteins. Among the milk proteins, α-la and β-lg are more sensitive to thermal treatments than casein, which is more stable. During an immunological reaction, antibodies recognize and interact with allergenic proteins through epitopes, originating from a few amino acids, on the molecule. Heating usually destroys most conformational epitopes by unfolding native proteins, leaving only the linear epitopes, which are mainly involved in allergenic incidents (Davis and Williams 1998). More intense processing conditions (like time, temperature) are associated with more extensive changes in immunoreactivity properties. Some studies have shown that during other thermal processes, e.g., ultrasounds and microwaves, the immunoreactivity of whey proteins α-la and β-lg is significantly reduced (Jędrychowski et al. 2005, Wróblewska and Jędrychowski 2001) (Table 6.3.1). In general heat treatment reduces the IgE reactivity as a result of unfolding mechanisms (Besler et al. 2001). Thermal processes are necessary to prepare raw milk as a base product to make hypoallergenic food and therefore should be combined with other processes like enzymatic hydrolysis.

### 6.3.2 Homogenization

The aim of homogenization is to reduce fat droplet size, which changes the structure of milk and may affect health-related properties (Michalski and Januel 2006). Research on an animal model has suggested that homogenization seems to favor hypersensitivity. Hypersensitive mice orally fed homogenized milk experienced an anaphylactic shock (Polusen and Hau 1987), increased milk-specific IgE production (Nielsen et al. 1989), increased intestinal segment mass, and demonstrated

**TABLE 6.3.1**

**Elimination of Immunoreactive Properties of Milk Proteins in Selected Technological Processes**

| Raw Material | Modification Method | Residual Immunoreactivity (%)[a] | |
|---|---|---|---|
| | | α-Lactalbumin | β-Lactoglobulin |
| Cow milk | Pasteurization (90°C/15 min) | 12.72 | 18.74 |
| Proteins | Ultrasonic treatment | 0.88 | 6.42 |
| | Microvalves (98°C/2 min) | 1.37 | 12.86 |

*Source:* Jędrychowski, L. et al., *Pol. J. Environ. Stud.*, 14(Suppl. II, Part I), 171, 2005. With permission.

[a] Calculated as % raw milk immunoreactivity.

mastocyte degranulation (Poulsen et al. 1990). Moreover, allergenicity increases with an increase in the fat content (Poulsen et al. 1987). Unhomogenized cow's milk induces few or no such symptoms and immune responses. However, when milk was given intravenously (Poulsen and Hau 1987) or subcutaneously (Poulsen et al. 1990), the reactions were identical regardless of the milk processing treatments.

### 6.3.3  ENZYMATIC MODIFICATION

The earliest commercial milk protein enzymatic modification dates back to the 1940s, when the first formulas for allergenic infants were made. The aims of this process were to reduce allergenicity as well as to change the functional properties of proteins while preserving their nutritional value for clinical use. Unfortunately the hydrolysates thus obtained were characterized by bitter taste, and for mainly this reason proteolysis, as a technological process, enjoyed very little popularity.

Enzymatic *in vitro* hydrolysis is carried out under moderate conditions involving pH 6–8 and temperature 40°C–60°C. An appropriate selection of enzymes makes it possible to obtain a product possessing the expected physicochemical and nutritional properties. During *in vitro* hydrolysis the following are used: proteolytic enzymes of animal (trypsin, chymotrypsin, pepsin, pancreatin), plant (papain, bromelain), bacterial (*Bacillus subtilis, Bacillus licheniformis*), and fungal (*Aspergillus oryzae*) origin. Ultrafiltration of enzymatically modified milk protein products removes the remaining trace amounts of intact proteins and suppresses allergenicity of milk (Thomas et al. 2007).

Investigations into an optimal baby formula for allergenic patients are continued until present. But nowadays enzymatic hydrolysis is an essential type of milk protein treatment to produce hypoallergenic formulas on an industrial scale. Depending on the degree of hydrolysis, there are production technologies for partially and extensively hydrolyzed products. However, no such product is completely free from allergenicity, and thereby cannot be guaranteed to be totally safe.

A synthetic amino acid mixture is the only completely hypoallergenic product, but it can be used only parenterally. Consumption of amino acids cannot stimulate oral tolerance in an organism.

The American Academy of Paediatrics recommends a new formula alongside conducting tests with DBPCFC samples, in which tolerance is confirmed in at least 90% of infants with formerly diagnosed milk allergy. Such an approach is shared by European organizations such as the European Society for Paediatric Allergology and Clinical Immunology (ESPACI); the Committee on Hypoallergenic Formulas and the European Society for Paediatric Gastroenterology, Hepatology and Nutrition (ESPGHAN); and the Committee on Nutrition (Høst et al. 1999).

After hydrolysis, peptides may re-associate to form aggregates, which may strengthen allergenic properties of milk or unmask potentially existing epitopes of the allergens (Thomas et al. 2007).

### 6.3.4 MODIFICATION OF MILK PROTEIN DURING LACTIC ACID FERMENTATION

Products obtained as a result of lactic acid fermentation are safe for people who require special diets. During fermentation, substrate proteins are modified under the effect of bacterial exogenous enzymes, which can considerably depress immunoreactivity (Table 6.3.2). During such a process, peptides with different amino acid sequences and single amino acids are formed. Fermentation involves natural and/or added microorganisms that hydrolyze sugars and proteins available in their surrounding medium during growth. The effect of microbial cultures on human

---

**TABLE 6.3.2**

**Changes in the Immunoreactive Properties of Milk Proteins upon Fermentation with Selected Cultures (the Best Results from 389 Strains and Cultures)**

| | Residual Immunoreactivity (%)[b] | |
|---|---|---|
| Species and Strain[a] | α-Lactalbumin | β-Lactoglobulin |
| Mesophilic culture 2957 SMADL | 0.06 | 8.95 |
| Mesophilic culture 14D | 0.99 | 0.67 |
| *Lactococcus lactis* ssp. *lactis biovar.* | 0.01 | 0.74 |
| *Lactococcus lactis* ssp. *lactis* w 83 | 0.18 | 1.37 |
| *Lactococcus lactis* ssp. *cremoris* 3z67 | 0.06 | 0.79 |
| *Lactococcus lactis* ssp. *cremoris* 32 | 0.01 | 0.70 |
| *Lactobacillus acidophilus* 67Ł | 0.09 | 1.46 |
| *Lactobacillus helveticus* 5V | 0.29 | 0.37 |

*Source:* Jędrychowski, L. et al., *Pol. J. Environ. Stud.*, 14(Suppl. II, Part I), 171, 2005. With permission.

[a] Strain and culture names as accepted by Rhodia-Biolacta in Olsztyn.

[b] Calculated as % raw milk immunoreactivity.

organisms is well documented (Parvez et al. 2006, Roessler et al. 2008, Vaarala 2003). Clinical studies have confirmed that consuming fermented milk products, e.g., yoghurt or kefir, reduces the level of immunoglobulin IgE in human sera. The therapeutic influence of bacteria relies on facilitating the quality change of precursor cells Th0 in Th1 and retaining the proportion between properties of Th1 and Th2 subpopulations.

Probiotics and their immunomodulative properties have been drawing an increasing interest (Table 6.3.2), but the results concerning their influence on food allergy patients are ambiguous. *In vivo* allergenicity tests allow us to observe only a slight attenuation of the immediate reaction to the provocation test. Nevertheless, fermented products have a slightly sour taste and pleasant aroma, which is very important for potential consumers (Jędrychowski and Wróblewska 1999).

The processes mentioned in the following section are not essential technological processes in the dairy industry. But research results suggest that they offer new possibilities, which may be applied to produce modified milk proteins in the future.

### 6.3.5 CHEMICAL MODIFICATION

The mechanisms of modification are different and depend on the chemical molecules used for the reactions. The anhydride of succinic acid reacts with lysine residues, α-amino groups of proteins and free thiol groups. During succinylation, proteins lose their globular structure and undergo aggregation by disulfide cross-binding with other whey proteins. Acetyl anhydride can modify tyrosine residues.

The results obtained with the ELISA method have shown that acetylation and succinylation were useful methods for modification of immunoreactive properties of whey allergens (Table 6.3.3). The addition of acetic or succinyl anhydride to milk proteins caused a significant reduction of α-la and β-lg immunoreactivity (Jędrychowski et al. 2005, Wróblewska and Jędrychowski 2002).

A promising method for reducing allergenicity relies on the polymerization of proteins with polyethylene glycol (PEG). Conjugation of whey proteins with nontoxic

---

**TABLE 6.3.3**

**Elimination of Immunoreactive Properties of Milk Proteins in Chemical Modifications (1 g of Modifying Agent/g Protein)**

| | Residual Immunoreactivity (%)[a] | | |
|---|---|---|---|
| Raw Material and Protein | After Acetylation | After Succinylation | After Addition of PEG |
| Cow Milk | | | |
| α-Lactalbumin | 0.01 | 0.02 | 0.12 |
| β-Lactoglobulin | 0.65 | 0.22 | 0.11 |

*Source:* Jędrychowski, L. et al., *Pol. J. Environ. Stud.*, 14(Suppl. II, Part I), 171, 2005. With permission.

[a] Calculated as % raw milk protein immunoreactivity.

and nonimmunogenic PEG has been applied to reduce immunoreactive properties of α-la and β-lg (Wróblewska and Jędrychowski 2002). The reduction of immunoreactivity depended on the number of polymer chains bound to the protein surface. The decrease in protein immunoreactivity could have been caused by covering the epitope area, i.e., the sites on the protein surfaces which have the ability to bind antibodies.

### 6.3.6 Gamma Irradiation

The application of gamma irradiation to reduce milk allergenicity is one of the unconventional methods proposed by Korean researchers (Byun et al. 2002). The results of their study show that allergenic epitopes were structurally altered by the gamma irradiation treatment and IgE did not recognize well the antigen-determinant sites on allergens. The researchers have suggested that this technology could be used to reduce allergenicity not only in milk but also in chicken egg albumin and shrimp tropomyosin.

### 6.3.7 Masking of Epitopes

Reduction of milk allergenicity is possible by a cross-linked reaction of milk proteins with microbial transglutaminase (m-TG) (Wróblewska et al. 2008). Diary products thus obtained possessed better functional properties with weaker syneresis and stronger curd. Also, the organoleptic properties of yoghurt prepared with m-TG make a favorable impression on potential allergic consumers.

## REFERENCES

Besler, M., Steinhard, H., and Paschke, A. 2001. Stability of food allergens and allergenicity of processed foods. *J Chromatogr B Biomed Sci Appl* 25: 207–228.

Byun, M.-W., Lee, J.-W., Yook, H.-S., Jo, C., and Kim, H.-Y. 2002. Application of gamma irradiation for inhibition of food allergy. *Radiat Phys Chem* 63: 369–370.

Davis, P.J. and Williams, S.C., 1998. Protein modification by thermal processing. *Allergy* 53(46): 102–105.

Høst, A., Koletzko, B., Dreborg, S., Muraro, A., Wahn, U., Aggett, P., Bresson, J.L., Hernell, O., Lafeber, H., Michaelsen, K.F., Micheli, J.L., Rigo, J., Weaver, L., Heymans, H., Strobel, S., and Vandenplas, Y. 1999. Dietary products used in infants for treatment and prevention of food allergy. Joint statement of the European Society for Paediatric Allergology and Clinical Immunology (ESPACI) Committee on Hypoallergenic Formulas and the European Society for Paediatric Gastroenterology, Hepatology and Nutrition (ESPGHAN) Committee on Nutrition. *Arch Dis Childhood* 81(1): 80–84.

Jędrychowski, L. and Wróblewska, B. 1999. Reduction of the antigenicity of whey proteins by lactic acid fermentation. *Food Agric Immunol* 11(1): 91–99.

Jędrychowski, L., Wróblewska, B., and Szymkiewicz, A. 2005. Technological aspects of food allergens occurrence in food products. *Pol J Environ Stud* 14(Suppl. II, Part I), 171–180.

Korhonen, H. 2002. Technology options for new nutritional concepts. *Int J Dairy Technol* 55(2): 79–88.

Korhonen, H. and Korpela, R. 1994. The effect of diary processes on the components and nutritional value of milk. *Scand J Nutr* 38: 166–172.

Michalski, M.-C. and Januel, C. 2006, Does homogenization affect the human health proper-ties of cow's milk? *Trend Food Sci Technol* 17: 423–437.

Morr, C.V. and Richter, R.L. 1988. Chemistry of processing. In N.P. Wong (Ed.), *Fundamentals of Dairy Chemistry*, pp. 739–766. New York: Van Nostrand Reinhold.

Nielsen, B.R., Poulsen, O.M., and Hau, J. 1989. Reagin production in mice: Effect of subcuta-neous and oral sensitization with untreated bovine milk and homogenized bovine milk. *In Vivo* 3(4): 271–274.

Parvez, S., Malik, K.A., Ah Kang, S., and Kim, H.-Y. 2006. Probiotics and their fermented food products are beneficial for health. *J Appl Microbiol* 100: 1171–1185.

Poulsen, O.M., Hau, J., and Kollerup, J. 1987. Effect of homogenization and pasteurization on the allergenicity of bovine milk analysed by murine anaphylactic shock model. *Clin Allergy* 17(5): 449–458.

Poulsen, O.M. and Hau, J. 1987. Homogenization and allergenicity of milk: Some possi-ble implication for the processing of infant formulae. *North Eur Food Diary J* 53(7): 239–242.

Poulsen, O.M., Nielsen, B.R., Basse, A., and Hau, J. 1990. Comparison of intestinal ana-phylactic reaction in sensitized mice challenged with untreated milk and homogenized bovine milk. *Allergy* 45(5): 321–326.

Roessler, (nee Klein) A., Friedrich, U., Vogelsang, H., Bauer, A., Kaatz, M., Hipler, U.C., Schmidt, I., and Jahreis, G. 2008. The immune system in healthy adults and patients with atopic dermatitis seems to be affected differently by a probiotic intervention. *Clin Exp Allergy* 38(1): 93–102.

Thomas, K., Herouet-Guicheney, C., Ladics, G., Bannon, G., Cockburn, A., Crevel, R., Fitzpatrick, J., Mills, C., Privalle, L., and Vieths, S. 2007. Evaluating the effect of food processing on the potential human allergenicity of novel proteins: International work-shop report. *Food Chem Toxicol* 45: 1116–1122.

Wróblewska, B. and Jędrychowski, L. 2001. Zmiany właęciwości immunoreaktywnych białek mleka krowiego w wybranych procesach termicznych i fermentacji mlekowej (in Polish). *Biotechnologia* 2(53): 54–56, 21–33.

Wróblewska, B. and Jędrychowski, L. 2002. Effect of conjugation of cow milk whey protein its polyethylene glycol on changes in their immunoreactive and allergic properties. *Food Agricult Immunol* 14: 155–162.

Wróblewska, B., Jędrychowski, L., Hajos, G., and Szabó, E. 2008. Influence of alcalase and transglutaminase hydrolysis on immunoreactivity of cow whey milk proteins. *Czech J Food Sci* 26(1): 15–23.

Vaarala, O. 2003. Immunological effects of probiotics with special reference to lactobacilli. *Clin Exp Allergy* 33(12): 1634–1640.

# 7 Egg Allergens

*Sabine Baumgartner and Patricia Schubert-Ullrich*

## CONTENTS

Hen's eggs of the species *Gallus domesticus* are known for their potential to induce allergic reactions in humans. Egg allergies represent one of the most frequent allergies in the population. Sensitization to egg with subsequent allergic symptoms in childhood often occurs without known oral exposure (NDA Opinions 2004). The frequency of hen's egg allergy is about three times higher in children than in adults (Besler and Mine 1999). While egg white is considered the major source of allergens, IgE-binding allergens have also been reported in the yolk. The amount of protein levels reported to induce adverse reactions in egg allergic individuals (threshold dose) ranges from 0.2 to 200 mg of protein (equivalent to 2–400 mg of food) (NDA Opinions 2004). The occurring allergic symptoms show great diversity and vary strongly between each individual.

## 7.1 CHARACTERISTICS OF MOST IMPORTANT ALLERGENS FROM EGG WHITE AND YOLK: THE BIOCHEMICAL, BIOLOGICAL, AND IMMUNOLOGICAL PROPERTIES OF MAIN EGG ALLERGENS

Main allergens of the egg white are already well characterized and have been classified by the International Union of Immunological Societies (IUIS), although major allergens especially present in egg yolk are still unassigned. Table 7.1 summarizes the characteristics of allergens found in egg white and egg yolk. Ovalbumin has found most scientific attention although it does not appear to be the most potent of the egg allergens. To date there is no evidence of significant differences in sensitization pattern of the various egg allergens in children or adults (Besler and Mine 1999). The results differ considerably with the applied diagnostic methods [dot-immunoblot, sodium

**TABLE 7.1**

**Egg Allergens of the Species *G. domesticus***

| | Nomenclature (by IUIS) | Content[a] (%) | Mr (kDa) | p*I* | Amino Acids | Carbohydrates | Biological Function |
|---|---|---|---|---|---|---|---|
| | | | | | **Egg White (Albumen)** | | |
| Ovomucoid | Gal d1 | 11 | 28 | 4.1 | 186 | ~25% | Serin-protease inhibitor |
| Ovalbumin | Gal d2 | 54 | 43–45 | 4.5 | 385 | ~3% | Serpin family |
| Ovotransferrin (=Conalbumin) | Gal d3 | 12–13 | 76–78 | 6.0 | 686 | 2.6% | Antimicrobial defense and iron-binding protein |
| Lysozyme | Gal d4 | 3.4–3.5 | 14 | 10.7 | 129 | 0% | 1,4-β-*N*-Acetyl-muramidase C |
| Serum albumin[b] | Gal d5 | | 69–70 | 4.6–4.8 | 592 | | Binding of water and Ca-, Na-, and K- cations, fatty acids, hormones, bilirubin, and drugs; regulation of the colloidal osmotic blood pressure |
| Ovomucin[c] | | 1.5–3.5 | 1800–8000 | 4.5–5.0 | | ~18%–33% | Glycosulfiprotein, antiviral, and antitumor properties |
| | | | | | **Egg Yolk** | | |
| Lipovitellins | | | 3–400 | | | | |
|   HDL | | 15 | | | | | |
|   LDL | | 65 | | | | | |
| Phosvitins | | 10 | ~175 | | 210 | | Glycophosphoprotein |
| Livetins | | 10 | 45–150 | | | | |
| α-Livetin[b] | Gal d5 | | 70 | 4.3–5.7 | | | |

*Source:* Besler, M. and Mine, Y., *Internet Symp. Food Allergens,* 1(4), 137, 1999. Available at: http://www.food-allergens.de

[a] In dried egg white or yolk, respectively.

[b] Serum albumin in egg white is identical to α-livetin in egg yolk.

[c] Data of ovomucin retrieved from Donovan et al. (1970), Walsh et al. (1988), and Carraro Alleoni (2006). HDL and LDL represent high- and low-density lipoprotein.

dodecyl sulfate polyacrylamide gel electrophoresis (SDS-PAGE) immunoblot, skin prick test (SPT), radio-allergosorbent test (RAST), crossed radio-immunoelectrophoresis (CRIE)]. For instance in case of ovomucoid, the sensitization frequencies vary between 34% and 97% of egg allergic patients depending on the diagnostic method used. These differences may be due to denaturing of the allergen during the blotting procedure, which could affect conformational epitopes. The lack of agreement in the literature on the allergenicity of hen egg proteins also may be partly due to the use of impure proteins (Walsh et al. 2005). Cross-contamination of proteins through the employed allergen preparations could give false results in nonseparating methods like SPT, RAST, and dot-blot. Therefore, highly purified allergen preparations should be used for correct diagnosis of sensitization. Isolation and purification of egg allergens is achieved by ion-exchange chromatography (IEC) and size-exclusion chromatography (SEC) (Ebbehoj et al. 1995; Besler et al. 1997), reversed-phase liquid chromatography (Awade 1996; Awade and Efstathiou 1999), gel permeation chromatography (GPC) (Awade and Efstathiou 1999), or capillary electrophoresis (Besler et al. 1998).

*Ovomucoid* (Gal d1) has been identified as one of the dominant allergens found in egg white and is the cause of most allergic reactions in children. Ovomucoid exhibits varying degrees of inhibitory activity toward a number of serine proteases. It is a highly glycosylated protein containing 20%–25% carbohydrate, with a molecular weight of 28 kDa and an isoelectric point (p$I$) of 4.1 (Besler and Mine 1999). Holen and Elsayed (1990) described two isoforms of ovomucoid in the p$I$ range of 4.4–4.6. Ovomucoid is composed of 186 amino acids that are arranged in three tandem domains (designated DI, DII, and DIII), each of 60 amino acids in length. A genetic variant with deletion of a dipeptide (at Val-134–Ser-135) occurs in approximately 20% of ovomucoid molecules (Kato et al. 1987). Each domain is cross-linked by three intradomain disulfide bonds; however, they lack any interdomain disulfide bonds. This unique structural characteristic might be responsible for its higher stability against proteolysis and heat, as well as its strong allergenicity (Mine et al. 2003). The third domain (DIII) shows significantly more human IgG- and IgE-binding activities than the first and second domains of ovomucoid in sera derived from egg allergic patients (Zhang and Mine 1998). Mine and Zhang (2002a) have determined the detailed sequential IgG and IgE epitope mapping in the whole ovomucoid molecules and have identified the amino acids within each of the IgG- and IgE-binding epitopes that are critical for immunoglobulin binding (G32 and F37) and, thus, have important roles on the antigenicity and allergenicity as well as on the structural integrity of ovomucoid DIII (Mine et al. 2003). Allergenicity studies on ovomucoid are rare. Some animal models with swine (Rupa et al. 2007) or mice (Hobson et al. 2007) were established but no double-blind placebo-controlled food challenge (DBPCFC) or determinations of minimum amounts inducing symptoms after ingestion of isolated ovomucoid have been performed to date because rigorous purification steps have to be applied to obtain very pure proteins for this purpose (Besler and Mine 1999; Poulsen et al. 2001). Only the specificities of patients' IgE antibodies against specific sequential epitopes of ovomucoid were evaluated as marker for the persistence of egg allergy (Järvinen et al. 2007).

*Ovalbumin* (Gal d2) is a major protein in egg white (Mine and Rupa 2004) and was one of the first proteins to be isolated in pure form (Hofmeister 1890). Its ready availability in large quantities has led to its widespread use as a standard preparation in studies of the structure and properties of proteins, and in experimental models of allergy. Although ovalbumin is probably one of the most studied antigens in immunology (Poulsen et al. 2001), its function as protein is still unknown. Huntington and Stein (2001) comprehensively summarized and discussed the structure and properties of ovalbumin. Ovalbumin is a glycoprotein with a relative molecular mass of 45 kDa. It belongs to the serpin family although it lacks any protease inhibitory activity. The amino acid sequence comprises 386 amino acids and the amino terminus of the protein is acetylated. Ovalbumin does not have a classical N-terminal leader sequence, although it is a secretory protein. Instead, the hydrophobic sequence between residues 21 and 47 may act as an internal signal sequence involved in transmembrane location. Heterogeneity in the electrophoretic behavior of ovalbumin is largely due to different degrees of phosphorylation at the amino acids S69 and S345. Three major fractions can be separated by IEC with, respectively two, one, and zero phosphate groups per ovalbumin molecule in an approximate ratio of 8:2:1 (Perlmann 1952).

The crystal structure of native hen ovalbumin shows an intact reactive center loop in the form of an exposed α-helix of three turns that protrudes from the main body of the molecule on two peptide stalks. The ovalbumin structure includes four crystallographically independent ovalbumin molecules and the position of the helical reactive center loop relative to the protein core differs by 2–3 Å between molecules. Although this shift is probably due to the different environments of the helices in the crystal lattice, it suggested that the reactive center loop is flexible in solution. Structural studies of serpins in various conformations have shown how the exceptional mobility of the serpin reactive center loop and their unique flexibility is essential for function. In contrary to inhibitory serpins, ovalbumin does not show evidence for a large conformational change following cleavage at its putative reactive center and appears to have lost the extreme mobility which is characteristic for its inhibitory ancestors.

Storage of eggs leads to a conformational change of ovalbumin to a thermally more stable form called "S-ovalbumin" shifting the midpoint of thermal denaturation ($T_m$) from 78°C to 86°C. The appearance of S-ovalbumin coincides with the loss of the "food value" of eggs during storage since eggs with high S-ovalbumin content have runny whites and do not congeal as effectively on cooking. S-Ovalbumin is easily formed *in vitro* by 20 h incubation at 55°C in 100 mM sodium phosphate, pH 10, the high pH and temperature increasing the rate of conversion. The increase in stability on conversion to the S-form results from a unimolecular conformational change and not a change in the chemical make-up of ovalbumin. The S-form differs from native ovalbumin only in its greater stability, compactness, and hydrophobicity. The chemically denatured states of native and S-ovalbumin also differ so that renaturation of S-ovalbumin does not lead to the native conformer. The preservation of the serpin fold and its metastability is presumably not accidental and the natural conversion of ovalbumin to the more stable S-form is likely to be functionally relevant. It is thus possible that ovalbumin plays a role in chick embryo development which is mediated by the natural metastability of ovalbumin (Huntington and Stein 2001).

*Ovotransferrin* (=*conalbumin*, Gal d3) comprises approximately 12%–13% of the egg white proteins and has a relative molecular mass of 77 kDa. It exhibits a low carbohydrate content of 2.6% and an isoelectric point of 6.0. Gal d3 is considered a minor allergen with a lower sensitization frequency compared to the two main egg allergens Gal d1 and Gal d2. Due to its iron-binding properties, ovotransferrin is involved in iron transport processes. It has antimicrobial and antiviral properties and plays an important role in the chicken's immunology. Ovotransferrin is also incorporated into the egg's shell. The biochemical characteristics, amino acid sequences, and chain forms are well known (Williams et al. 1982). Although ovotransferrin is highly cross-linked by disulfides, the apo form is not very stable to denaturants. Ovotransferrin is relatively stable to heating up to 60°C and 82°C depending on the isoforms (diferric and apo forms, respectively). IgE cross-reactivity might be expected with ovotransferrins from birds as the duck protein is 80% identical to that from chicken. No cross-reactivity is expected or reported for transferrins from liver (InformAll Database 2008).

*Lysozyme* (Gal d4) represents only around 3.5% of the total protein content of hen's egg white. It has a relative molecular mass of 14 kDa and an isoelectric point of 10.7. Lysozyme is regarded to be a minor allergen and its allergenicity is even rarer compared to Gal d3. Lysozyme plays an important part in the defense against bacterial infection of the egg. It is well known for its antibacterial properties but also exhibits antiviral, antitumor, and immunomodulatory activities. The biochemical characteristics like amino acid sequences, chain forms or the active center of lysozyme are well known (Canfield 1963). Lysozyme's stability has been studied by many methods and in many different conditions. The formation of adducts with sorbitol and other compounds has a stabilizing effect on lysozyme (Petersen et al. 2004). An increased stability of lyzozyme, e.g., against proteolysis, may decrease its allergenicity (So et al. 1997, 2001). In buffer without adducts, lysozyme was found to be most stable in the pH range of 3.5–5.0, where the denaturation temperature is reported to be 75°C–80°C (InformAll Database 2008). Lysozyme is used as food preservative as well as an active substance included in pharmaceutical preparations (Proctor 1988; Sava 1996). Since hen's egg white lysozyme is 95%–96% identical with sequences from the eggs of birds such as quail and turkey, and at least 78% identical to other known bird lysozymes, cross-reactivity to various bird eggs is highly probable (InformAll Database 2008)

Serum albumin present in egg white and α-livetin (Gal d5) present in egg yolk are identical (Williams 1962). The biological function of serum albumin comprises of binding to water; calcium-, sodium-, and potassium-cations; fatty acids; hormones; bilirubin; and drugs. It is also responsible for the regulation of the colloidal osmotic blood pressure. α-Livetin has a relative molecular mass of 70 kDa and an isoelectric point of 4.3–5.7 (Besler 1999). The protein consists of three homolog domains with domain I from amino acids 8 to 183, domain II from 202 to 375, and domain III from 394 to 573. α-Livetin is considered to be the most relevant allergen in the sensitization to egg proteins via the inhalation route (van Toorenenbergen et al. 1994; Quirce et al. 1998). IgE-binding to α-livetin occurs in 100% of patients with bird feather and egg yolk allergy. There are two further livetins with molecular weights of 42 kDa for β-livetin and about 150 kDa for γ-livetin. These two livetins find only little attention in scientific studies since they are considered to play an insignificant role in the allergenicity of egg.

*Ovomucin* comprises approximately 3.5% of egg white protein and is a heavily glycosylated protein with a carbohydrate content of up to 33%. It differs from other egg proteins because the molecule is extremely large. Relative molecular weights reported in literature vary from 1800 to 8300 kDa (Donovan et al. 1970; Walsh et al. 1988; Carraro Alleoni 2006; InformAll Database 2008). It contains a substantial amount of disulfide groups, sulfate ethers, large amounts of cystine (interconnected through intermolecular linkages), and 50% of the total sialic acid contents present in egg white. The egg white has two forms of ovomucin. The insoluble form characterizes the high viscosity of egg white's thin layer ovomucin, which has antiviral activity. The allergenicity of ovomucin is considered to be minor compared to the major allergens ovomucoid and ovalbumin. Ovomucin has not been identified as an allergen in most egg allergy studies. One reason might be that many extraction procedures for protein preparation include a dialysis step and a centrifugation in order to get a "mucin-free" solution to avoid mucin clogging chromatographic columns (InformAll Database 2008).

Low-density lipoproteins (LDLs) play only a minor role in the allergenicity of hen's eggs. Anet et al. (1985) have reported IgE-binding to some proteins in the LDL fraction of the egg yolk, but further characterization of these proteins is lacking. LDLs contain five major apoproteins with molecular weights of about 130, 80, 65, 60, and 15 kDa (Anton et al. 2003). LDLs are composed of about 12% of proteins and 87% of lipids, and present a spherical shape with a mean diameter of about 35 nm. LDLs are considered to be the main contributors to the exceptional emulsifying activity of hen egg yolk, which is an essential ingredient for the preparation of a large variety of food emulsions, such as mayonnaises, salad dressings, and creams. LDL solubility is high, whatever the medium conditions, because of their low density.

## 7.2   CHANGES IN IMMUNOREACTIVITY AND ALLERGENICITY OF EGG ALLERGENS DURING TECHNOLOGICAL PROCESSES

The stability of egg allergens and possible effects of food processing on the allergenicity of egg and egg-derived products have been comprehensively discussed (Besler et al. 2001; NDA Opinions 2004). Most egg allergic individuals react to cooked and raw eggs (Langeland 1982a,b). Rarely individuals may react only to raw eggs and can tolerate cooked eggs (Eigenmann 2000). These allergic individuals often exhibit lower egg-specific IgE levels (Boyano Martínez et al. 2001). Heating and freeze drying can reduce the clinical allergenicity in some patients (Urisu et al. 1997) but does not reliably prevent IgE-binding or clinical reactions. Heated or boiled eggs (90°C–100°C, 3–60 min) contain ovomucoid and ovalbumin with decreased, but clearly detectable antigenicity determined *in vitro* by radio-immunoelectrophoresis (RIEP) and RAST (Hoffman 1983; Anet et al. 1985) and *in vivo* in allergic patients by DBPCFC (Urisu et al. 1997). Heated ovomucoid-depleted egg white exhibited the lowest allergenicity, which indicates the importance of ovomucoid and heat-unstable antigens such as ovalbumin, ovotransferrin, and lysozyme in the pathogenesis of egg allergy (Urisu et al. 1997). Elevated temperatures above 100°C seem to be essential for the efficient reduction/removal of egg allergenicity. Leduc et al. (1999) investigated different pork meat pastes containing 2% dried egg white. In raw and in pasteurized pastes (70°C, 120 min) egg white allergens were detected by SDS-PAGE immunoblot and enzyme-allergosorbent test (EAST), while no allergens could be detected in sterilized paste (115°C, 90 min). Hydrolysis with digestive enzymes (pH 1.2) efficiently degrades ovotransferrin and ovomucoid (<10 min) whereas ovalbumin and phosvitin resists peptic digestion even after 1 h (Astwood et al. 1996). There are a number of reports investigating the effects of heat and chemical denaturation procedures on major egg allergens (Anet et al. 1985; Kahlert et al. 1992; Bernhisel-Broadbent et al. 1994; Elsayed and Stavseng 1994; Shimojo et al. 1994; Cooke and Sampson 1997; Sakai et al. 1998; Holen et al. 2001; Kato et al. 2001; Mine and Zhang 2002b; Gremel and Paschke 2007). It can be summarized that for egg only a few allergens are really labile to common industrial processing. Nevertheless, a combination of physical and enzymatic processing has reducing effects on the allergenicity of egg proteins due to an alteration within the conformational structure and destruction of linear amino acid sequences.

## 7.3   CROSS-REACTIVITY OF EGG ALLERGENS

Clinical cross-reactivity of egg allergens is generally restricted to other avian eggs (e.g., turkey, duck, goose, and seagull), but several cross-reacting proteins were also detected in chicken sera and meat. The probability of cross-reactions is likely to be affected by the interspecies relationships (NDA Opinions 2004). Allergic reaction and anaphylaxis have been reported after ingestion of edible birds' nests, a Chinese health-improving delicacy. Immunochemical characterization of a putative 66 kDa allergen was found to be homologous to ovoinhibitor, a serine protease inhibitor which is one of the allergens found in egg white. Birds' nest soups are increasingly being marketed worldwide and could be of clinical relevance to individuals with hens' egg allergies (NDA Opinions 2004). Microparticulated proteins present in Simplesse, a fat substitute, showed no difference in IgE-binding compared to native egg proteins when applied to sera from egg and/or cow milk allergic individuals (Sampson and Cooke 1992).

Patients with food allergies to egg yolk may also suffer from respiratory symptoms caused by bird exposure, called the "bird-egg syndrome" (NDA Opinions 2004). The bird-egg syndrome consists primarily of respiratory symptoms following exposure to bird, and secondarily of allergy symptoms after the ingestion of eggs. This syndrome displays a cross-sensitization to egg yolk and bird allergens (feathers, serum, droppings, and meat) mainly caused by the partially heat-labile α-livetin, which is a component of both egg yolk and birds' feathers. This phenomenon underlines the importance of the sensitization via the respiratory route in food allergy and is distinguished from the common egg allergy in children (Anibarro Bausela et al. 2000). Interestingly, in a study investigating the "bird-egg syndrome" patients with egg white allergy did not react with allergens in egg yolk or bird feather extract (Szepfalusi et al. 1994).

## REFERENCES

Anet, J., Back, J.F., Baker, R.S., Barnett, D., Burley, R.W., Howden, M.E. 1985. Allergens in the white and yolk of hen's egg. A study of IgE binding by egg proteins. *Int Arch Allergy Appl Immunol* 77:364–371.

Anibarro Bausela, B., Besler, M., Rancé, F., Szépfalusi, Z. 2000. Allergen data collection—Update: Bird-egg syndrome. *Internet Symp Food Allergens* 2(5):1–12. Available at: http://www.food-allergens.de.

Anton, M., Martinet, V., Dalgalarrondo, M., Beaumal, V., David-Briand, E., Rabesona, H. 2003. Chemical and structural characterisation of low-density lipoproteins purified from hen egg yolk. *Food Chem* 83:175–183.

Astwood, J.D., Leach, L.N., Fuchs, R.L. 1996. Stability of food allergens to digestion in vitro. *Nat Biotechnol* 14:1269–1273.

Awade, A.C. 1996. On hen egg fractionation: Applications of liquid chromatography to the isolation and the purification of hen egg white and egg yolk proteins. *Z Lebensm Unters Forsch* 202:1–14.

Awade, A.C., Efstathiou, T. 1999. Comparison of three liquid chromatographic methods for egg-white protein analysis. *J Chromatogr B* 723:69–74.

Bernhisel-Broadbent, J., Dintzis, H.M., Dintzis, R.Z., Sampson, H.A. 1994. Allergenicity and antigenicity of chicken egg ovomucoid (Gal d III) compared with ovalbumin (Gal d I) in children with egg allergy and in mice. *J Allergy Clin Immunol* 93:1047–1059.

Besler, M. 1999. Allergen data collection—Bird-egg syndrome (egg yolk, feathers). *Internet Symp Food Allergens* 1(2):81–92. Available at: http://www.food-allergens.de.

Besler, M., Mine, Y. 1999. Major hen's egg white allergen: Ovomucoid (Gal d 1). *Internet Symp Food Allergens* 1(4):137–146. Available at: http://www.food-allergens.de.

Besler, M., Steinhart, H., Paschke, A. 1997. Allergenicity of hen's egg-white proteins: IgE binding of native and deglycosylated ovomucoid. *Food Agric Immunol* 9:277–288.

Besler, M., Steinhart, H., Paschke, A. 1998. Immunological characterization of egg white allergens collected by capillary electrophoresis. *Food Agric Immunol* 10:157–160.

Besler, M., Steinhart, H., Paschke, A. 2001. Stability of food allergens and allergenicity of processed foods. *J Chromatogr B* 756:207–228.

Boyano Martínez, T., García-Ara, C., Díaz-Pena, J.M., Muñoz, F.M., García Sánchez, G., Esteban, M.M. 2001. Validity of specific IgE antibodies in children with egg allergy. *Clin Exp Allergy* 31:1464–1469.

Canfield, R. 1963. The amino acid sequence of egg white lysozyme. *J Biol Chem* 238:2698–2707.

Carraro Alleoni, A.C. 2006. Albumen protein and functional properties of gelation and foaming. *Sci Agric* (Piracicaba, Braz.) 63(3):291–298.

Cooke, S.K., Sampson, H.A. 1997. Allergenic properties of ovomucoid in man. *J Immunol* 159:2026–2032.

Donovan, J.W., Davis, J.G., White, L.M. 1970. Chemical and physical characterization of ovomucin, a sulfated glycoprotein complex from chicken eggs. *Biochim Biophys Acta* 207:190–201.

Ebbehoj, K., Dahl, A.M., Frokiaer, H., Norgaard, A., Poulsen, L.K., Barkholt, V. 1995. Purification of egg-white allergens. *Allergy* 50:133–141.

Eigenmann, P.A. 2000. Anaphylactic reactions to raw eggs after negative challenges with cooked eggs. *J Allergy Clin Immunol* 105:587–588.

Elsayed, S., Stavseng, L. 1994. Epitope mapping of region 11–70 of ovalbumin (Gal d I) using five synthetic peptides. *Int Arch Allergy Immunol* 104:65–71.

Gremel, S., Paschke, A. 2007. Reducing allergens in egg and egg products. In *Managing Allergens in Food*, eds. C. Mills, H. Wichers, K. Hoffmann-Sommergruber, Woodhead Publishing, Ablington, Cambridge, U.K., pp. 178–186.

Hobson, D.J., Rupa, P., Diaz, G.J., Zhang, H., Yang, M., Mine, Y., Turner, P.V., Kirby, G.M. 2007. Proteomic analysis of ovomucoid hypersensitivity in mice by two-dimensional difference gel electrophoresis (2D-DIGE). *Food Chem Toxicol* 45:2372–2380.

Hoffman, D.R. 1983. Immunochemical identification of the allergens in egg white. *J Allergy Clin Immunol* 71:481–486.

Hofmeister, F. 1890. Über die Darstellung von krystallisiertem Eieralbumin. *Zeitschr Physiol Chem* 14:165–174.

Holen, E., Elsayed, S. 1990. Characterization of four major allergens of hen-egg white by IEF/-SDS-PAGE combined with electrophoretic transfer and IgE-immunoautoradiography. *Int Arch Allergy Immunol* 91:136–141.

Holen, E., Bolann, B., Elsayed, S. 2001. Novel B and T cell epitopes of chicken ovomucoid (Gal d 1) induce T cell secretion of IL-6, IL-13, and IFN-gamma. *Clin Exp Allergy* 31:952–964.

Huntington, J.A., Stein, P.E. 2001. Structure and properties of ovalbumin. *J Chromatogr B* 756:189–198.

InformAll Database. 2008. Communicating about food allergies. Available at: http://www.foodallergens.ifr.ac.uk.

Järvinen, K.M., Beyer, K., Vila, L., Bardina, L., Mishoe, M., Sampson, H.A. 2007. Specificity of IgE antibodies to sequential epitopes of hen's egg ovomucoid as a marker for persistence of egg allergy. *Allergy* 62:758–765.

Kahlert, H., Petersen, A., Becker, W.M., Schlaak, M. 1992. Epitope analysis of the allergen ovalbumin (Gal d II) with monoclonal antibodies and patients' IgE. *Mol Immunol* 29:1191–1201.

Kato, I., Schrode, J., Kohr, W.J., Lakowski, M. Jr. 1987. Chicken ovomucoid: Determination of its amino acid sequence, determination of the trypsin reactive site, and preparation of all three of its domains. *Biochemistry* 26:193–201.

Kato, Y., Oozawa, E., Matsuda, T. 2001. Decrease in antigenic and allergenic potentials of ovomucoid by heating in the presence of wheat flour: Dependence on wheat variety and intermolecular disulfide bridges. *J Agric Food Chem* 49:3661–3665.

Langeland, T. 1982a. A clinical and immunological study of allergy to hen's egg white. II. Antigens in hen's egg white studied by crossed immunoelectrophoresis (CIE). *Allergy* 37:323–333.

Langeland, T. 1982b. A clinical and immunological study of allergy to hen's egg white. III. Allergens in hen's egg white studied by crossed radio-immunoelectrophoresis (CRIE). *Allergy* 37:521–530.

Leduc, V., Demeulemester, C., Polack, B., Guizard, C., Le-Guern, L., Peltre, G. 1999. Immunochemical detection of egg-white antigens and allergens in meat products. *Allergy* 54:464–472.

Mine, Y., Rupa, P. 2004. Immunological and biochemical properties of egg allergens. *Worlds Poult Sci J* 60:321–330.

Mine, Y., Zhang, J.W. 2002a. Identification and fine mapping of IgG and IgE epitopes in ovomucoid. *Biochem Biophys Res Commun* 292:1070–1074.

Mine, Y., Zhang, J.W. 2002b. Comparative studies on antigenicity and allergenicity of native and denatured egg white proteins. *J Agric Food Chem* 50:2679–2683.

Mine, Y., Sasaki, E., Zhang, J.W. 2003. Reduction of antigenicity and allergenicity of genetically modified egg white allergen, ovomucoid third domain. *Biochem Biophys Res Commun* 302:133–137.

NDA Opinions. 2004. Opinion of the scientific panel on dietetic products, nutrition and allergies on a request from the commission relating to the evaluation of allergenic foods for labelling purposes (Request No. EFSA-Q-2003-016). *EFSA J* 32:1–197.

Perlmann, G.E. 1952. Enzymatic dephosphorylation of ovalbumin and plakalbumin. *J Gen Physiol* 35:711–726.

Petersen, S.B., Jonson, V., Fojan, P., Wimmer, R., Pedersen, S. 2004. Sorbitol prevents the self-aggregation of unfolded lysozyme leading to and up to 13 degrees C stabilisation of the folded form. *J Biotechnol* 114:269–278.

Poulsen, L.K., Hansen, T.K., Noregaard, A., Verstergaard, H., Stahl Skov, P., Bindslev-Jensen, C. 2001. Allergens from fish and egg. *Allergy* 56(s67):39–42.

Proctor, V.A., Cunningham, F.E. 1988. The chemistry of lysozyme and its use as a food preservative and a pharmaceutical. *CRC Crit Rev Food Sci Nutr* 26:359–395.

Quirce, S., Diez-Gomez, M.L., Eiras, P., Cuevas, M., Baz, G., Losada, E. 1998. Inhalant allergy to egg yolk and egg white proteins. *Clin Exp Allergy* 28:478–485.

Rupa, P., Hamilton, K., Cirinna, M., Wilkie, B.N. 2007. A neonatal swine model of allergy induced by the major food allergen chicken ovomucoid (Gal d 1). *Int Arch Allergy Immunol* 146:11–18.

Sakai, K., Matsuoka, A., Ushiyama, Y., Shimoda, T., Ueda, N. 1998. Appearance of ovomucoid in coagulated egg yolk passing through from soluble fraction of coagulated egg white in boiled egg. *Arerugi* 47:1176–1181.

Sampson, H.A., Cooke, S. 1992. The antigenicity and allergenicity of microparticulated proteins: Simplesse®. *Clin Exp Allergy* 22:963–969.

Sava, G. 1996. Pharmacological aspects and therapeutic applications of lysozymes. *EXS* 75:433–449.

Shimojo, N., Katsuki, T., Coligan, J.E., Nishimura, Y., Sasazuki, T., Tsunoo, H., Sakamaki, T., Kohno, Y., Niimi, H. 1994. Identification of the disease-related T cell epitope of ovalbumin and epitope-targeted T cell inactivation in egg allergy. *Int Arch Allergy Immunol* 105:155–161.

So, T., Ito, H.O., Koga, T., Watanabe, S., Ueda, T., Imoto, T. 1997. Depression of T-cell epitope generation by stabilizing hen lysozyme. *J Biol Chem* 272:32136–32140.

So, T., Ito, H., Hirata, M., Ueda, T., Imoto, T. 2001. Contribution of conformational stability of hen lysozyme to induction of type 2 T-helper immune responses. *Immunology* 104:259–268.

Szepfalusi, Z., Ebner, C., Pandjaitan, R., Orlicek, F., Scheiner, O., Boltz-Nitulescu, G., Kraft, D., Ebner, H. 1994. Egg yolk alpha-livetin (chicken serum albumin) is a cross-reactive allergen in the bird-egg syndrome. *J Allergy Clin Immunol* 93:932–942.

Urisu, A., Ando, H., Morita, Y., Wada, E., Yasaki, T., Yamada, K., Komada, K., Torii, S., Goto, M., Wakamatsu, T. 1997. Allergenic activity of heated and ovomucoid-depleted egg white. *J Allergy Clin Immunol* 100:171–176.

van Toorenenbergen, A.W., Huijskesheins, M.I.E., Van Wijk, R.G. 1994. Different pattern of IgE binding to chicken egg yolk between patients with inhalant allergy to birds and food-allergic children. *Int Arch Allergy Immunol* 104:199–203.

Walsh, B.J., Barnett, D., Burley, R.W., Elliott, C., Hill, D.J., Howden, M.E.H. 1988. New allergens from hen's egg white and egg yolk. In vitro study of ovomucin, apovitellenin I and VI, and phosvitin. *Int Arch Allergy Immunol* 87:81–86.

Walsh, B.J., Hill, D.J., Macoun, P., Cairns, D., Howden, M.E.H. 2005. Detection of four distinct groups of hen egg allergens binding IgE in the sera of children with egg allergy. *Allergol Immunopathol* 33(4):183–191.

Williams, J. 1962. Serum proteins and the livetins in hen's-egg yolk. *Biochem J* 83:346–355.

Williams, J., Elleman, T.C., Kingston, I.B., Wilkins, A.G., Kuhn, K.A. 1982. The primary structure of hen ovotransferrin. *Eur J Biochem* 122:275–278.

Zhang, J.W., Mine, Y. 1998. Characterization of IgE and IgG epitopes on ovomucoid using egg-white-allergic patients' sera. *Biochem Biophys Res Commun* 253:124–127.

# 8 Fish Allergens

*Patrick Weber and Angelika Paschke*

## CONTENTS

## 8.1 CHARACTERISTICS OF THE MOST IMPORTANT ALLERGENS FROM FISH: THE BIOCHEMICAL, BIOLOGICAL, AND IMMUNOLOGICAL PROPERTIES OF MAIN SEAFOOD ALLERGENS

Probably the most known and most studied major fish allergen is named Gad c 1 (allergen M) (Poulsen et al. 2001). This highly water-soluble protein from Baltic cod fish (*Gadus callarias*) belongs to a family of calcium-binding proteins commonly known as parvalbumins (Poulsen et al. 2001). Currently, more than 20 parvalbumins from various fish species are classified as major allergens and have been adopted to the International Union of Immunological Societies (IUIS) allergen nomenclature, e.g., Sal s 1 (Atlantic salmon, *Salmo salar*) (Lindstroem et al. 1996), Tra j 1 (horse mackerel, *Trachurus japonicus*), Gad m 1 (Atlantic cod, *Gadus morhua*) (Das Dores et al. 2002b), Sco j 1 (mackerel, *Scomber japonis*), Sco a 1 (mackerel, *Scomber australasicus*), Sco s 1 (mackerel, *Scomber scombrus*) (Hamada et al. 2002b), Thu o 1 (bigeye tuna, *Thunnus obesus*), Ang j 1 (Japanese eel, *Anguilla japonica*) (Shiomi et al. 1999), The c 1 (pollock, *Theragra chalcogramma*), and Cyp c 1 (carp, *Cyprinus carpio*) (Wopfner et al. 2007).

Parvalbumins are acidic proteins that could be divided into two evolutionary lineages: $\alpha$-parvalbumins with a p$I \geq 5$ and $\beta$-parvalbumins with a p$I$ of $\leq 4.5$ (Goodman et al. 1979). Allergenic parvalbumins have molecular weights of approximately 10–13 kDa and, principally, belong to the $\beta$-parvalbumin lineage (Lindstroem et al. 1996; Hamada et al. 2002b; Chen et al. 2006).

Parvalbumins control the flow of $Ca^{2+}$ within the muscular sarcoplasm and, thus, play an important role in the muscle physiology (Taylor et al. 2004; Wild and Lehrer

2005). They appear in different isoforms mainly in fast twitching, white muscle tissues of fish but also in lower amounts in fish's dark muscle, swim bladder, and muscle tissues of all other vertebrates (Gerday 1982; Gerday et al. 1989; Kobayashi et al. 2006). Thus, fish mainly composed of dark meat, such as tuna or mackerel, was found to contain lower amounts of parvalbumin compared to fish with white meat (Hansen et al. 1997; Van Do et al. 2005; Chen et al. 2006). Different kinds of mackerel contain about 0.15–2 mg/g parvalbumin in the white but only 0.02–0.5 mg/g in the dark muscle (Kobayashi et al. 2006).

The tertiary structure of parvalbumin from carp consists of three homologous domains named AB, CD, and EF whereof the latter two are capable to bind $Ca^{2+}$ (Figure 8.1). This structure is conserved in parvalbumins from other species, e.g., cod and hake. Tryptic digest of Gad c 1 leads to highly cross-reactive fragments, corresponding to repeated IgE-binding epitopes alongside the protein's primary structure. Five peptides derived from amino acid residues 13–32, 33–44, 49–64, 65–83, and 88–113 were found to show immunological reactivity and, thus, were considered to bear allergenic epitopes of Gad c 1. Peptides 13–32 (AB), 49–64 (CD), and 88–113 (EF) are each part of one of the three domains, whereof peptides 49–64 and 88–113 were derived from the two calcium-binding domains (Elsayed and Apold 1983). The calcium-bound holoprotein was demonstrated to show a significantly higher allergenicity than the calcium-free apoprotein (Bugajska-Schretter et al. 1998). Peptides 33–44 and 65–83 are within the linkage region of domains AB + CD and CD + EF. Peptides derived from the domains and domain linkages, respectively, share a high sequence homology. Thus, it is generally accepted that the three domains descend from the same gene that has been triplicated during evolution (Elsayed and Apold 1983). Epitopes of parvalbumin are considered to be sequence epitopes because of their high stability as subsequently described (Elsayed and Aas 1971).

While parvalbumins are the most investigated fish allergens, several other fish proteins show IgE-binding properties to human sera. Various cod proteins, e.g., with molecular weights of 28, 41, and 49 kDa, react with sera from cod-allergic individuals as demonstrated in Figure 8.2 (Hansen et al. 1997; Bugajska-Schretter et al. 1998; Galland et al. 1998; Das Dores et al. 2002a,b). IgE-binding of proteins with molecular weights larger than parvalbumin also occur in several other species, such as 32, 46, and 80 kDa proteins in two tuna species, as well as proteins from mackerel, herring, carp, and plaice (Hansen et al. 1997; Yamada et al. 1999; Lian et al. 2006). These findings indicate the occurrence of species-specific allergens, while some of these antigens present dimeric or oligomeric parvalbumins (Das Dores

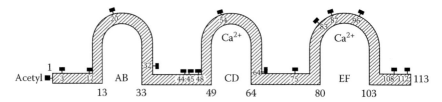

**FIGURE 8.1** Schematic illustration of Gad c 1. The sites of expected susceptibility to tryptic cleavage are indicated by quadrates. (Modified from Elsayed, S. and Apold, J., *Allergy*, 38, 451, 1983. With permission.)

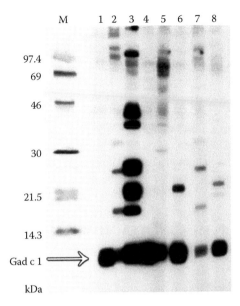

**FIGURE 8.2**  IgE-binding of human sera to aqueous cod fish extracts discovered by SDS-PAGE, followed by immunoblotting. M, molecular weight marker; 1–8, sera from patients allergic to fish. (Modified from Hansen, T.K. et al., *Ann. Allergy Asthma Immunol.*, 78, 191, 1997. With permission.)

et al. 2002b) or proteins with conserved parvalbumin epitopes (Helbling et al. 1999). Consequently, there is a large number of further possible fish allergens. Some of them seem able to elicit allergic reactions because of no or only weak sensitization of the respective individual to parvalbumin (Bernhisel-Broadbend et al. 1992a; James et al. 1997; Bugajska-Schretter et al. 1998). Unfortunately, the proper characterization of those possible allergens is still missing and, thus, clinical relevance is almost unclear. Only the immunogenic 41 kDa protein from cod was identified as aldehyde phosphate dehydrogenase (Das Dores et al. 2002a).

The IgE-binding property of fish collagen was also proven *in vitro* in fish-allergic patients (Sakaguchi et al. 1999, 2000; Hamada et al. 2001; André et al. 2003; Hamada et al. 2002a). Collagen is an intercellular component of connective tissue that provides strength and durability, supports soft tissues, and provides reinforcement during compression (Taylor et al. 2004). It is divided into more than 20 generic types, whereof type I is the main supporting collagen type in all vertebrates. High amounts of collagen type I are found in skin, bones, and swim bladder of fish. This collagen type consists of three alanine, glycine, and hydroxyproline-rich polypeptide chains ($\alpha$-chains) with a molecular weight between 80 and 125 kDa each. $\alpha$-Chains of type I collagen are divided with respect to their amino acid composition into $\alpha 1(I)$, $\alpha 2(I)$, and the fish-specific $\alpha 3(I)$ chain (Kimura et al. 1987). Three $\alpha$-chains build a stable triple helix with a molecular weight between 240 and 375 kDa, known as tropocollagen ($\gamma$-chain). Dimeric $\alpha$-chains, as they may occur after reduction of tropocollagen, have molecular weights of about 160–250 kDa ($\beta$-chain) (Hamada et al. 2002a). So far, there exist no evidence for the allergenicity of fish collagen and derived products, such as fish gelatine. Adverse reactions after contact with fish collagen or fish gelatine have not been reported (André et al. 2003; Hansen et al. 2004). Known cases of allergic reactions to gelatine were referred to mammalian gelatine (Wahl and Kleinhans 1989; Sakaguchi et al. 1996, 1999; Sakaguchi and Inouye 2001; Nakayama et al. 2004) or to gelatine with uncharacterized origin (Kelso et al. 1993; Sakaguchi et al. 1995, 1997; Nakayama et al. 1999; Wang and Sicherer 2005). No or only weak cross-reactivities occur between mammalian and fish gelatine and collagen (Kelso et al. 1993; Sakaguchi et al. 1999; Sakaguchi and Inouye 2000; Hamada et al. 2001; André et al. 2003). Thus, fish collagen and their products are currently considered to be of no risk for the triggering of allergic reactions and, thus, are not further discussed (Taylor et al. 2004).

## 8.2  CHANGES IN IMMUNOREACTIVITY AND ALLERGENICITY OF FISH ALLERGENS DURING TECHNOLOGICAL PROCESSES

Parvalbumins are stable against denaturation due to heat treatment, such as cooking, reducing agents, and against proteolysis at extreme pH (Elsayed and Aas 1971; Hansen et al. 1994; Taylor et al. 2004). However, extensive heat treatment as performed during the canning process of fish strongly reduces or eliminates the IgE-binding properties of parvalbumin. During the canning process, the cooked fish is treated with pressure and steam over a long period. The resulting product shows no detectable allergenicity at least in species such as tuna and salmon (Bernhisel-Broadbend et al. 1992b).

Cod parvalbumin Gad c 1 is described as a protein relatively resistant to enzymatic degradation. Nevertheless, treatment with proteolytic enzymes, particularly trypsin or pepsin, may cause a total reduction of detectable IgE-binding after treatment for 1 min (Untersmayr et al. 2004) and 2–3 h (Aas and Elsayed 1969). However, allergenicity after oral consumption of such degraded parvalbumin remains in a reduced extent (Untersmayr et al. 2007). Only partial reduction should be considered in the presence of other proteins. Furthermore, a strong impact of the pH is given, resulting in a rapid degradation of parvalbumin by pepsin under physiologic conditions (pH < 2.5) with no detectable IgE-binding capability but a complete resistance if pH excesses 2.75 (Untersmayr et al. 2004).

A method for the removal of parvalbumin due to its high water solubility is thorough washing of the fish meat. Such products (particularly surimi) present an allergen pattern different from the native fish species with reduced allergenicity due to no detectable parvalbumin but other allergens (Mata et al. 1994).

Other IgE-binding proteins than parvalbumin are more sensitive to heat treatment. Respective proteins from tuna or salmon significantly lose antigenicity already during cooking and, consequently, also during the canning process (Bernhisel-Broadbend et al. 1992a,b; Yamada et al. 1999). Tuna was found to demonstrate a total loss of IgE-binding after canning (Bernhisel-Broadbend et al. 1992a,b). However, a recent research on Indian fish demonstrated that fish species exist which express IgE-binding, nonparvalbumin proteins insensitive to cooking and/or frying (Chatterjee et al. 2006).

## 8.3 CROSS-REACTIVITY OF FISH ALLERGENS: INTERSPECIES CROSS-REACTIVITY

Cross-reactivities between different fish species are widely spread and thoroughly described. Their occurrence was demonstrated between various species, such as cod, carp, pollock, mackerel, herring, and salmon in diverse *in vitro* and *in vivo* experiments (De Martino et al. 1990; Bernhisel-Broadbend et al. 1992a; Hansen et al. 1997; Bugajska-Schretter et al. 1998; Helbling et al. 1999; Van Do et al. 2005). It is widely accepted that cross-reactivities between different fish species are mainly caused due to a well-conserved parvalbumin structure among various fish species and throughout the vertebrate kingdom (Table 8.1). The most conserved sequences lie in the regions that form the two calcium-binding sites, each containing binding epitopes for human IgE antibodies (Elsayed and Apold 1983; Chen et al. 2006). The homology decreases with decreasing zoological relationship. Consequently, cross-reactivities outside the fish species are rare and were reported between fish and frog parvalbumin only (Poulsen et al. 2001; Hilger et al. 2004).

The clinical relevance of these cross-reactivities is controversially discussed. Generally, fish-allergic individuals are suspected to be potentially allergic to all species of fish and are advised to avoid all kind of fish because of this structure conservation (Taylor et al. 2004). However, patients who are allergic to one or more species can orally tolerate some other species without symptoms (Bernhisel-Broadbend et al. 1992a; Hansen et al. 1997; Helbling et al. 1999). This fact is currently not really understood, at least because of the high occurrence of discrepancies between skin tests or *in vitro* assays and oral provocation tests. Patients allergic to fish show a far greater extent of cross-reactivity *in vitro* and in skin tests than after oral consumption (Bernhisel-Broadbend et al. 1992a). Thus, clinical relevant cross-reactivity after oral consumption had probably been overestimated in the past. The extent of tolerance to other fish species is hard to estimate. A Spanish workgroup reported that up to 40% of patients sensitized to one or more fish do not present symptoms on consuming other species (Torres et al. 2003). Currently, two explanations for the tolerance of some fish species in individuals allergic to fish are, first, the occurrence of species-specific allergens beside the common parvalbumins (Bernhisel-Broadbend et al. 1992a; Hansen et al. 1997) and, second, significantly different amounts of parvalbumins among the fish species.

## 8.4 GENETICALLY MODIFIED FISH AND FOOD ALLERGY PROBLEM

Genetical modification of fish is generally applied to achieve accelerated growth, increased feed efficiency, thermal tolerance, disease resistance, or high protein, low-fat fish by insertion of respective recombinant genes into newly fertilized fish eggs. Several species, such as salmon, carp (Muir 2004), tilapia (Rahman et al. 1998), catfish, charr, and loach (Nam et al. 2001) were successfully genetically modified. In doing so, researchers have currently chosen to focus on transfer of intrageneric or homologous DNA ("all-fish" DNA) construct into fish to increase the likelihood of social acceptance of transgenic fish (Pandian 2001). An example is the transfer

**TABLE 8.1**

**Parvalbumin Amino Acid Sequences of Various Vertebrates Compared with the Major Allergen Gad c 1 from Cod Fish (*G. callarias*)**

| Animal | | Amino Acid Sequence | Id. (%) | Pos. (%) |
|---|---|---|---|---|
| Cod | *G. callarias* | AFKGILSNADIKAAEAACFKEGSFDEDGFYAKVGL DAFSADELKKLFKIAD**EDKEGFIEEDE**LKLFLIAF AADLRALTDAETKAFLKAG**DSDGDGKIGVDEF**GA LVDKWGAKG | | |
| Carp | *C. carpio* | AF#GIL++ADI#AA###C####SFD###F+AKVGL #A#+#D++KK#F#+#D+**DK#GFIEEDE**LKLFL##F +A##RALTDAETKAFLKAG**DSDGDGKIGVDEF**#ALV | 68 | 77 |
| Catfish | *Ictalurus punctatus* | AF#G+L++ADI#AA##AC##+GSF+###F+#KVGL ###SAD++KK#F#I#D+**DK#GFIEEDE**LKLFL##F #+##RALTDAETK FLKAG**D+DGDGKIGVDEF**#+LV | 66 | 77 |
| Salmon | *S. salar* | ####################SF+###F+AKVGL #+#S+D++KK#F#+#D+**DK#GFIEEDE**LKLFL##F +A##RALTDAETKAFL##G**D#DGDG#IGVDEF**#A++ | 65 | 78 |
| Mackerel | *T. japonicus* | AFKG+L++AD+#AA###C##+#+FD###F+###GL #A#SAD++KK#F#I#D+**DK#GFIEEDE**LKLFL##F #A##RAL+DAETKAFLKAG**DSDGDGKIGVDEF**#A+V | 65 | 76 |
| Eel | *A. japonica* | AF#G+L#+ADI#AA##AC####SF+###F+AKVGL ###S#D++KK#F#I#D+**DK#GFIEEDE**LKLFL##F +###RALTD#ETKAFL+AG**D+DGDGKIG+DEF**#A+V | 63 | 74 |
| Pollock | *T. chalcogramma* | AF#GIL#+A++#AA##AC###GSFD###F+###GL ###S+D++KK#F#I#D+**D+##FIEE+E**LKLFL##F +A##RAL+DAETKAFLKAG**DSDGDGKIGVDEF**#A+V | 62 | 74 |
| Mackerel | *Scomber japonicus* | AF##+L#+A++#AA###C###GSFD###F+###GL ###S#DE+KK#F#I#D+**DK#GFIEE+E**LKLFL##F #A##RAL+DAETKAFLKAG**DSDGDGKIG+DEF**#A++ | 60 | 71 |
| Frog | *Xenopus laevis* | AF#G+LS#ADI#+A###C####SF+###F+A+#GL #+#SA#++K#+F#I#D+**D+#GFIEEDE**LKLFL##F +A##RALTDAETKAFL#AG**DSDGDGKIGV+EF**#ALV | 62 | 74 |
| Chicken | *Gallus gallus* | A###ILS##DI++A#++C####SF+###F++#VGL #+#+#D++KK+F#I#D+**DK#GFIEE+EL**+LFL##F ++#R#LT#AETKAFL#AG**D+DGDGKIGV+EF**#+LV | 54 | 73 |
| Mouse | *Mus musculus* | ####+LS##DIK#A##A#####SFD###F+##VGL ###+#DE+KK+F#I#D+**DK#GFIEEDEL**###L##F ++D#R#L+##ETK##L#AG**D#DGDGKIGV+EF**##LV | 53 | 63 |
| Human | *Homo sapiens* | ####+L+##DIK#A##A#####SFD###F+##VGL ###SAD++KK+F#+#D+**DK#GFIEEDEL**###L##F +#D#R#L+##ETK##+#AG**D#DGDGKIGVDEF**##LV | 52 | 63 |

*Source:* National Center of Biotechnology Information, Blast Sequence Analysis, www.ncbi.nlm.nih. gov/blast/, 2008)

#, no identity; +, amino acid that preserves the physiochemical properties of the respective Gad c 1 residue (conservative substitution); Id., amino acid identity compared to Gad c 1; Pos., = amino acid identity including conservative substitution; bold letters indicate $Ca^{2+}$-binding sites (Chen et al. 2006).

of a growth hormone gene from Chinook salmon to Atlantic salmon with a four- to sixfold increased growth (Muir 2004). Field-testing status of transgenic fish has been achieved in countries such as China, Israel, Hungary, New Zealand, United Kingdom, and United States (Pandian 2001). However, transgenic fish is currently not commercially available.

So far, fish allergy with respect to transgenic fish has not been focused on. Generally, the introduction of unforeseeable allergenicity is not given since transgenic fish is derived by introduction of intrageneric or homologous genes. Allergic reactions must be expected by individuals allergic to fish irrespective of the consumption of genetically modified or unmodified fish. Allergic individuals with no sensitization to fish but to other foodstuffs should be of no risk to react to genetically modified fish. On the other hand, the possibility that a fish-allergic individual tolerating a specific fish species will react to the same but genetically modified species is likely but currently unpredictable. Such reaction could be triggered by the transfer of a gene coding a species-specific allergen to another species. The likelihood of such a case is hard to overlook because there is practically no knowledge about those allergens as previously described. In this context, the transfer of fish genes into organisms other than fish, e.g., in order to produce food supplements, should be mentioned. This may introduce fish allergens into foods where fish is generally not expected. Concerning this matter, a pioneer work was done on the usage of a so-called ice structuring protein (ISP) gene isolated from ocean pout. This gene is commercially transferred into yeast in order to achieve high yields of ISP, e.g., for the ice cream industry. No allergenic potential was observed of this ISP in a thorough investigation (Bindslev-Jensen et al. 2003).

## REFERENCES

Aas, K. and Elsayed, S. M. 1969. Characterization of a major allergen (cod): Effect of enzymic hydrolysis on the allergenic activity. *J Allergy* 44(6):333–343.

André, F., Cavagna, S., and André, C. 2003. Gelatin prepared from tuna skin: A risk factor for fish allergy or sensitization? *Int Arch Allergy Immunol* 103:17–24.

Bernhisel-Broadbend, J., Holdford, S., and Sampson, H. A. 1992a. Fish hypersensitivity. I. In vitro and oral challenge results in fish-allergic patients. *J Allergy Clin Immunol* 89(3):730–737.

Bernhisel-Broadbend, J., Strause, D., and Sampson, H. A. 1992b. Fish hypersensitivity. II. Clinical relevance of altered fish allergenicity caused by various preparation methods. *J Allergy Clin Immunol* 90(4):622–629.

Bindslev-Jensen, C., Sten, E., Earl, L., Crevel, R. W. R., Bindslev-Jensen, U., Hansen, T. K., Stahl Skov, P., and Poulsen, L. K. 2003. Assessment of the potential allergenicity of ice structuring protein type III HPLC 12 using the FAO/WHO 2001 decision tree for novel foods. *Food Chem Toxicol* 41(1):81–87.

Bugajska-Schretter, A., Elfman, L., Fuchs, T., Kapiotis, S., Rumpold, H., Valenta, R., and Spitzauer, S. 1998. Parvalbumin, a cross-reactive fish allergen, contains IgE-binding epitopes sensitive to periodate treatment and $Ca^{2+}$ depletion. *J Allergy Clin Immunol* 101(1):67–74.

Chatterjee, U., Mondal, G., Chakraborti, P., Patra, H. K., and Chatterjee, B. P. 2006. Changes in the allergenicity during different preparations of pomfret, hilsa, bhetki and mackerel fish as illustrated by enzyme-linked immunosorbent assay and immunoblotting. *Int Arch Allergy Immunol* 141:1–10.

Chen, L., Hefle, S. L., Taylor, S. L., Swoboda, I. and Goodman, R. E. 2006. Detecting fish parvalbumin with commercial mouse monoclonal anti-frog parvalbumin IgG. *J Agric Food Chem* 54:5577–5582.

Das Dores, S., Chopin, C., Romano, A., Galland-Irmouli, A. V., Quaratino, D., Pascual, C., Fleurence, J., and Gueant, J. L. 2002a. IgE-binding and cross-reactivity of a new 41 kDa allergen of codfish. *Allergy* 57(Suppl. 72):84–87.

Das Dores, S., Chopin, C., Villaume, C., Fleurence, J., and Guéant, J. L. 2002b. A new oligomeric parvalbumin allergen of Atlantic cod (Gad m 1) encoded by a gene distinct from that of Gad c 1. *Allergy* 57(Suppl. 72):79–83.

De Martino, M., Novembre, E., Galli, L., de Marco, A., Botarelli, P., Marano, E., and Vierucci, A. 1990. Allergy to different fish species in cod-allergic children: In vivo and in vitro studies. *J Allergy Clin Immunol* 86:909–914.

Elsayed, S. and Aas, K. 1971. Characterization of a major allergen (cod)-observations on effect of denaturation on the allergenic activity. *J Allergy* 47(5):283–291.

Elsayed, S. and Apold, J. 1983. Immunochemical analysis of cod fish allergen M: Location of the immunoglobulin binding sites as demonstrated by the native and synthetic peptides. *Allergy* 38:449–459.

Galland, A. V., Dory, D., Pons, L., Chopin, C., Rabesona, H., Guéant, J. L., and Fleurence, J. 1998. Purification of a 41 kDa cod-allergenic protein. *J Chromatogr B* 706:63–71.

Gerday, C. 1982. Soluble calcium-binding proteins from fish and invertebrate muscle. *Mol Physiol* 2(1):63–88.

Gerday, C., Collin, S., and Gerardin-Otthiers, N. 1989. The amino acid sequence of the parvalbumin from the very fast swimbladder muscle of the toadfish (*Opsanus tau*). *Comp Biochem Physiol Part B: Biochem Mol Biol* 93B(1):49–55.

Goodman, M., Pechère, J. F., Haiech, J., and Demaille, J. G. 1979. Evolutionary diversification of structure and function in the family of intracellular calcium-binding proteins. *J Mol Evol* 13:331–352.

Hamada, Y., Nagashima, Y., and Shiomi, K. 2001. Identification of collagen as a new fish allergen. *Biosci Biotechnol Biochem* 65(2):285–291.

Hamada, Y., Nagashima, Y., Shiomi, K., Shimojo, N., Kohno, Y., Shibata, R., Nishima, S., Ohsuna, H., and Ikezawa, Z. 2003a. Reactivity of IgE in fish-allergic patients to fish muscle collagen. *Allergol Int* 52:139–147.

Hamada, Y., Tanaka, H., Ishizaki, S., Ishida, M., Nagashima, Y., and Shiomi, K. 2003b. Purification, reactivity with IgE and cDNA cloning of parvalbumin as the major allergen of mackerels. *Food Chem Toxicol* 41(8):1149–1156.

Hansen, T. K., Skov, S. P., Poulsen, L. K., and Bindslev-Jensen, C. 1994. Allergenic activity of processed fish. *Allergy Clin Immunol News Suppl* 2:445.

Hansen, T. K., Bindslev-Jensen, C., Skov, P. S., and Poulsen, L. K. 1997. Codfish allergy in adults: IgE cross-reactivity among fish species. *Ann Allergy Asthma Immunol* 78:187–194.

Hansen, T. K., Poulsen, L. K., Stahl Skov, P., Hefle, S. L., Hlywka, J. J., Taylor, S. L., Bindslev-Jensen, U., and Bindslev-Jensen, C. 2004. A randomized, double-blinded placebo-controlled oral challenge study to evaluate the allergenicity of commercial, food-grade fish gelatin. *Food Chem Toxicol* 42:2037–2044.

Helbling, A., Haydel, R., McCants, M. L., Musmand, J. J., El-Dahr, J., and Lehrer, S. B. 1999. Fish allergy: Is cross-reactivity among fish species relevant? Double-blind placebo-controlled food challenge studies of fish allergic adults. *Ann Allergy Asthma Immunol* 83:517–523.

Hilger, C., Thill, L., Grigioni, F., Lehners, C., Falagiani, P., Ferrara, A., Romano, C., Stevens, W., and Hentges, F. 2004. IgE antibodies of fish allergic patients cross-react with frog parvalbumin. *Allergy* 59:653–660.

James, J. M., Helm, R. M., Burks, A. W., and Lehrer, S. B. 1997. Comparison of pediatric and adult IgE antibody binding to fish proteins. *Ann Allergy Asthma Immunol* 79:131–137.

Kelso, J. M., Jones, R. T., and Yunginger, J. W. 1993. Anaphylaxis to measles, mumps, and rubella vaccine mediated by IgE to gelatin. *J Allergy Clin Immunol* 91(4):867–872.

Kimura, S., Ohno, Y., Miyauchi, Y., and Uchida, N. 1987. Fish skin type I collagen: Wide distribution of an α3 subunit in teleosts. *Comp Biochem Physiol* 88(B):27–34.

Kobayashi, A., Tanaka, H., Hamada, Y., Ishizaki, S., Nagashima, Y., and Shiomi, K. 2006. Comparison of allergenicity and allergens between fish white and dark muscles. *Allergy* 61:357–363.

Lian, Y., Zhigang, L., and Wen, A. 2006. Separation, purification and identification of major allergens in common carp. *Zhonggou Gonggong Weisheng* 22(8):947–949.

Lindstroem, C. D. V., Van Do, T., Hordvik, I., Endresen, C., and Elsayed, S. 1996. Cloning of two distinct cDNAs encoding parvalbumin, the major allergen of Atlantic salmon (*Salmo salar*). *Scan J Immunol* 44(4):335–344.

Mata, E., Favier, C., Moneret-Vautrin, D. A., Nicolas, J. P., Han-Ching, L., and Gueant, J. K. 1994. Surimi and native codfish contain a common allergen identified as a 63-kDa protein. *Allergy* 49:442–447.

Muir, W. 2004. The threats and benefits of GM fish. *EMBO Rep* 5(7):654–659.

Nakayama, T., Aizawa, C., and Kuno-Sakai, H. 1999. A clinical analysis of gelatine allergy and determination of its causal relationship to the previous administration of gelatin-containing acellular pertussis vaccine combined with diphtheria and tetanus toxoids. *J Allergy Clin Immunol* 103(2):321–325.

Nakayama, T., Kumagai, T., Pool, V., Mootrey, G., Chen, R. T., Gargiullo, P. M., Braun, M. M., Kelso, J. M., Yunginger, J. W., and Jacobson, R. M. 2004. Gelatin allergy. *Pediatrics* 113:170–171.

Nam, Y. K., Noh, J. K., Cho, Y. S., Cho, H. J., Cho, K. N., Kim, C. G., and Kim, D. S. 2001. Dramatically accelerated growth and extraordinary gigantism of transgenic mud loach *Misgurnus mizolepis*. *Transgenic Res* 10:353–362.

Pandian, T. J. 2001. Guidelines for research and utilization of genetically modified fish. *Curr Sci* 81(9):1172–1178.

Poulsen, L. K., Hansen, T. K., Nordgaard, A., Vestergaard, H., Stahl Skov, P., and Bindslev-Jensen, C. 2001. Allergens from fish and egg. *Allergy* 56(Suppl. 67):39–42.

Rahman, M. A., Mak, R., Ayad, H., Smith, A., and Maclean, N. 1998. Expression of a novel piscine growth hormone gene results in growth enhancement in transgenic tilapia (*Oreochromis niloticus*). *Transgenic Res* 7:357–369.

Sakaguchi, M. and Inouye, S. 2000. Systemic allergic reactions to gelatin included in vaccines as a stabilizer. *Jpn J Infect Dis* 53:189–195.

Sakaguchi, M. and Inouye, S. 2001. Anaphylaxis to gelatine-containing rectal suppositories. *J Allergy Clin Immunol* 108:1033–1034.

Sakaguchi, M., Ogura, H., and Inouye, S. 1995. IgE antibody to gelatine in children with immediate-type reactions to measles and mumps vaccines. *J Allergy Clin Immunol* 96:563–565.

Sakaguchi, M., Nakayama, T., and Inouye, S. 1996. Food allergy to gelatine in children with systemic immediate-type reactions, including anaphylaxis, to vaccines. *J Allergy Clin Immunol* 98:1058–1061.

Sakaguchi, M., Yoshida, T., Asahi, T., Aoki, T., Miyatani, Y., and Inouye, S. 1997. Development of IgE antibody to gelatine in children with systemic immediate-type reactions to vaccines. *J Allergy Clin Immunol* 99:720–721.

Sakaguchi, M., Hori, H., Ebihara, T., Irie, S., Yanagida, M., and Inouye, S. 1999. Reactivity of the immunoglobulin E in bovine gelatine-sensitive children to gelatins from various animals. *Immunology* 96:286–290.

Sakaguchi, M., Toda, M., Ebihara, T., Irie, S., Hori, H., Imai, A., Yanagida, M., Miyazawa, H., Ohsuna, H., Ikezawa, Z., and Inouye, S. 2000. IgE antibody to fish gelatine (type I collagen) in patients with fish allergy. *J Allergy Clin Immunol* 106:579–584.

Shiomi, K., Hamada, Y., Sekiguchi, K., Shimakura, K., and Nagashima, Y. 1999. Two classes of allergens, parvalbumins and higher molecular weight substances, in Japanese eel and bigeye tuna. *Fish Sci* 65(6):943–948.

Taylor, S. L., Kabourek, J. L., and Hefle, S. L. 2004. Fish allergy: Fish and products thereof. *J Food Sci* 69(8):R175–R180.

Torres, B., Martinez, C. J. F., and Tejero, G. J. 2003. Cross reactivity between fish and shellfish. *Allergol Immunopathol* 31(3):146–151.

Untersmayr, E., Poulsen, L. K., Platzer, M. H., Pedersen, M. H., Boltz-Nitulescu, G., Stahl Skov, P., and Jensen-Jarolim, E. 2004. The effect of gastric digestion on codfish allergenicity. *J Allergy Clin Immunol* 115(2):377–382.

Untersmayr, E., Vestergaard, H., Malling, H. J., Bjerremann Jensen, L., Platzer, M. H., Boltz-Nitulescu, G., Scheiner, O., Stahl Skov, P., Jensen-Jarolim, E., and Poulsen, L. K. 2007. Incomplete digestion of codfish represents a risk factor for anaphylaxis in patients with allergy. *J Allergy Clin Immunol* 119:711–717.

Van Do, T., Elsayed, S., Florvaag, E., Hordvik, I., and Endresen, C. 2005. Allergy to fish parvalbumins: Studies on the cross-reactivity of allergens from 9 commonly consumed fish. *J Allergy Clin Immunol* 116:1314–1320.

Wahl, R. and Kleinhans, D. 1989. IgE-mediated allergic reactions to fruit gums and investigation of cross-reactivity between gelatine and modified gelatine-containing products. *Clin Exp Allergy* 19:77–80.

Wang, J. and Sicherer, S. H. 2005. Anaphylaxis following ingestion of candy fruit chews. *Annals Allergy Asthma Immunol* 94:530–533.

Wild, G. L. and Lehrer, S. B. 2005. Fish and Shellfish Allergy. *Curr Allergy Asthma Rep* 5:74–79.

Wopfner, N., Dissertori, O., Ferreira, F., and Lackner, P. 2007. Calcium-binding proteins and their role in allergic diseases. *Immunol Allergy Clin N Am* 27(1):29–44.

Yamada, S., Nolte, H., and Zychlinsky, E. 1999. Identification and characterization of allergens in two species of tuna fish. *Ann Allergy Asthma Immunol* 82:395–400.

# 9 Seafood Allergen Overview: Focus on Crustacea

*Andreas Lopata and Samuel Lehrer*

## CONTENTS

## 9.1 SEAFOOD ALLERGY: INTRODUCTION TO THE NATURE AND IMMUNOBIOLOGICAL PROPERTIES OF THE MAIN SEAFOOD ALLERGENS

Seafood plays an important role in human nutrition and health. The growing international trade in seafood species and products has added to the popularity and frequency of consumption of a variety of seafood products across many countries.

233

The highest consumption of seafood in Europe appears to be found in Iceland, where the gross per capita consumption of crustacean and fish was about 91 kg live weight, followed by Portugal (59 kg), Norway (47 kg), Spain (43 kg), France (27 kg), United Kingdom (19 kg), Germany (13 kg) as compared to the United States (8 kg) (Administration NOaA 2007), and Australia (11 kg) (Canberra 2006). Importantly the imports of seafood from other countries often surpass their own productions. In the United States for example over 80% of its seafood is imported. The United States remains the third largest global consumer of fish and shellfish, behind Japan and China (Administration NOaA 2007).

Unfortunately this increased production and consumption of seafood has resulted in more frequent reporting of allergic health problems among consumers as well as processors of seafood. Allergic reactions to "shellfish," which comprises the groups of crustaceans and mollusks, are very common and the corresponding symptoms range from mild urticaria and oral allergy syndrome (OAS) to life-threatening ana-phylactic reactions (Lopata and Potter 2000; Sicherer et al. 2004; Wild and Lehrer 2005). The implicated allergens and their possible cross-reactivities are discussed below.

### 9.1.1 CLASSIFICATION OF SEAFOOD GROUPS

Patients with allergy to seafood may fail to identify the offending seafood species, often as a result of confusion regarding the diversity of seafood consumed and the different common names used to describe seafood. The three most important seafood groupings include the arthropods, mollusks, and pisces. The two invertebrate phyla of arthropods and mollusks are generally referred to as shellfish in the context of seafood consumption (Table 9.1). Most seafood species are edible and even more

**TABLE 9.1**

**Classification of Seafood Groups Causing Allergies, Representative Species, Common Symptoms Experienced, and Main Allergens Implicated**

| Phylum | Class | Common Name | Symptoms | Allergens |
|--------|-------|-------------|----------|-----------|
| Arthropods | Crustacean | Crab, rock lobster, prawn, shrimp, krill, barnacle | Urticaria | • Tropomyosin<br>• Arginine kinase<br>• ? |
| Mollusks | Gastropods | Abalone, snail, whelk | GI symptoms, larygoedema | • Tropomyosin<br>• ? |
| | Bivalves | Clam, oyster, mussel, cockles | Urticaria, OAS | • Tropomyosin<br>• ? |
| | Cephalopods | Squid (cuttlefish), octopus | Rhinitis, asthma | • Tropomyosin<br>• ? |
| Chordates | Osteichtyes (bony fish) | Salmon, hake, tuna, herring, carp | Anaphylaxis | • Parvalbumin<br>• ? |

?, indicates additional allergens not well characterized.

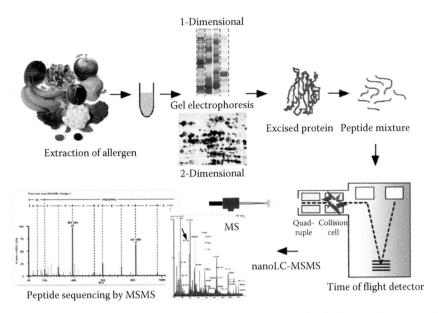

**FIGURE 3.4.1** Proteomic-based approach for identification of food allergens from natural source.

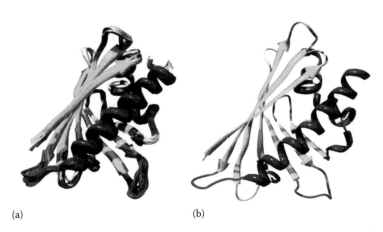

(a)                                                    (b)

**FIGURE 3.4.3** Cartoon representation of the three-dimensional structures of (a) Pru av 1 determined by NMR and (b) Api g 1 determined by x-ray crystallography. Pru av 1 represents an overlay of 22 chains retrieved from RCSB Protein Data Bank (accession number: 1e09), Api g 1 (2bk0). Highly flexible loops between β3-β4 and β7-α3 structures are depicted in blue, β-sheets in green, and α-helices in red.

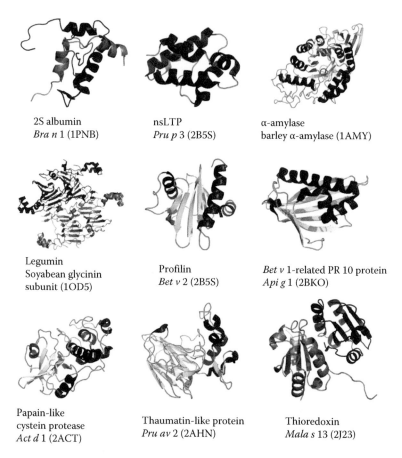

**2S albumin**
*Bra n* 1 (1PNB)

**nsLTP**
*Pru p* 3 (2B5S)

**α-amylase**
barley α-amylase (1AMY)

**Legumin**
Soyabean glycinin
subunit (1OD5)

**Profilin**
*Bet v* 2 (2B5S)

*Bet v* 1-related PR 10 protein
*Api g* 1 (2BKO)

**Papain-like**
cystein protease
*Act d* 1 (2ACT)

**Thaumatin-like protein**
*Pru av* 2 (2AHN)

**Thioredoxin**
*Mala s* 13 (2J23)

**FIGURE 14.2.1** Cartoon representation of the three-dimensional structure of allergens representative for distinct families. For single chain allergens alpha helical structures are presented in red, beta sheets in yellow, and turns in green. Chains of oligomeric proteins are shown in blue and orange. The PDB (www.pdb.org) codes are given in parenthesis.

exotic ones are consumed in small amounts around the world such as sea cucumber, jellyfish, and sea urchins (see Chapter 14.3).

Crustaceans, perhaps surprisingly, are classified as arthropods together with spiders and insects. Over 30,000 living crustacean species are found worldwide and a large number of varieties are consumed raw or cooked. Mollusks is a large and diverse group, subdivided into the classes Bivalve, Gastropods, and Cephalopods (Table 9.1) and comprises over 100,000 different species, including several economically important seafood groups such as mussels, oysters, abalone, snails, and squid (calamari). The last of the seafood groups are the fishes, which are the subject of another chapter.

### 9.1.2 ADVERSE REACTIONS TO SEAFOOD

Adverse reactions to seafood can also be generated via nonimmunological reactions. These reactions can result from exposure to the seafood itself or to various nonseafood substances present in the product (Table 9.2). Nonimmunological reactions among consumer of seafood as well as workers handling seafood can be triggered by a range of substances contained in seafood that include contaminants, parasites (e.g., *Anisakis*) (Audicana and Kennedy 2008; Nieuwenhuizen et al. 2006), protochordates (*Hoya*), bacteria (e.g., *Vibrio*; *Klebsiella*; *Pseudomonas*), viruses (e.g., hepatitis A), marine toxins (e.g., saxitoxins, ciguatera), and biogenic amines (e.g., histamine) (Auerswald et al. 2006). However, also ingredients such as preservatives, flavors, and colorings added during processing can cause adverse reactions such as chemical additives (sodium benzoate) (McCann et al. 2007), spices (e.g., mustard, paprika, flour additives, garlic) (Scholl and Jensen-Jarolim 2004), and some such as casein which are not ALWAYS obvious (hidden ingredients) (Lopata and Potter 2000).

---

**TABLE 9.2**
**Adverse Reactions to Seafood Produced by Various Substances**

| Etiology | Seafood Implicated | Clinical Symptoms | Time of Onset |
|---|---|---|---|
| Bacterial Salmonella, Vibrio, Aeromonas, Listeria | Fish, crustacean, mollusk | Dermatological Gastrointestinal Neurological Respiratory | Minutes to several hours |
| Viral Hepatitis A, Rota-, Astrovirus, small round viruses, etc. | Crustacean, mollusk | | |
| Parasites Anisakis Diphyllobothrium | All fish and cephalopods (e.g., squid) | | |
| Toxins Scombrotoxin | Fish, particularly with dark meat | | |
| Ciguatera toxin | Reef fish | | |
| Algae toxins | All mollusk species | | |
| Allergens | Fish, crustacean, mollusk | | |

---

### 9.1.3 Prevalence of Seafood Allergy

The prevalence of seafood allergy is usually higher when the consumption plays a greater part in the diet of the observed community. It is generally considered that crustacean and fish are among the four foods most commonly provoking severe food anaphylaxis. It is estimated that about 30,000 food-induced anaphylactic events are reported annually in the United States alone, of which about 200 are fatal. A recent study established surprisingly that seafood allergies are a significant health concern affecting approximately 6.5 million people in the United States—more than twice as common as peanut allergy. From the telephone survey among 14,948 individuals, 2% reported with shellfish allergy, and seafood allergy, was almost five times more common among adults compared to children (Sicherer et al. 2004) (Table 9.3). Of the subjects with allergies to crustaceans and mollusks only 38% and 49%, respectively reported reactions to multiple species and only 14% reacted to both shellfish groups, suggesting less cross-reactivity between the crustacean and mollusks. In France a study by Andre et al. (1994) among 580 patients with adverse reactions to food 34% demonstrated specific IgE to crab. A study by Crespo et al. (1995a) in Spain among 355 children established that 6.8% of patients reacted to crustaceans by skin prick test (SPT). A study from South Africa on 105 individuals with perceived adverse reactions to seafood confirmed sensitization to prawns and rock lobster in 47% and 44% of individuals, respectively (Zinn et al. 1997). Of the 131 positive reactions by ImmunoCAP, 50% reacted to four different crustacean species.

Seafood allergy is common in Western countries such as Europe, the United States, and Australia, but also in Asian countries allergic reactions to seafood and

---

**TABLE 9.3**

**Prevalence of Sensitization to Shellfish in Various Countries among Individuals (Adults and Children) with Food Allergy**

| Country | Number of Individuals Investigated | Prevalence (%) |
|---------|-----------------------------------|----------------|
| Philippines | 38 | 58 |
| South Africa | 105 | 55 |
| Singapore | 227 | 39 |
| France | 580 | 34 |
| Indonesia | 600 | 24 |
| Thailand | 202 | 22 |
| Taiwan | 392 | 21 |
| Singapore | 334 | 15 |
| Spain | 355 | 6.8 |
| United States[*] | 14,948 | 2.0 |

*Note:* A Survey among the General Population is Indicated by an Asterisk[*]. Sensitization Established by SPT and/or Quantification of Specific IgE Antibody.

particularly shellfish are significant among children and adults (Chiang et al. 2007; Goh et al. 1999; Hill et al. 1997, 1999). Furthermore, more seafood is readily available to a wider range of populations and countries due to improved transportation, shipping, and general globalization of food supply as well as increasing socioeconomic standards in regions such as Southern Europe. The likelihood of becoming sensitized to a particular food allergen seems to correlate with geographical eating habits, so seafood allergy to a particular seafood species is more prevalent in countries where this seafood is part of the stable diet.

### 9.1.4 CLINICAL FEATURES AND DIAGNOSTIC APPROACHES OF SEAFOOD ALLERGY

The pattern of allergic symptoms after ingestion of crustaceans appears similar to the symptoms experienced due to other foods. Reactions are immediate, reported mostly within 2 h; however, late phase reactions have been reported up to 8 h after ingestion, particularly to snow crab, cuttlefish, limpet, and abalone (Lopata et al. 1997; Villacis et al. 2006). Patients may have a single symptom but often there is a multiorgan involvement. Importantly respiratory reactions are often seen after ingestion of allergenic seafood and frequently anaphylactic reactions. Particular the OAS seems to be very often experienced by crustacean allergic subjects. Symptoms occur within minutes after ingestion of crustaceans and include itching and angioedema of the lips, mouth, and pharynx. Shrimp has also been implicated in food-dependent exercise-induced anaphylaxis (Zhang et al. 2006). It seems that atopic individuals are at greater risk of developing anaphylactic reactions.

The appearance of allergic symptoms results not only from ingestion of seafood, but can also be triggered from inhaling cooking vapors and handling seafood in the domestic as well as in the occupational environment (Goetz and Whisman 2000; Jeebhay et al. 2001; Taylor et al. 2000). Symptoms manifest mainly as upper and lower airway respiratory symptoms and dermatitis, while anaphylaxis is rarely seen with this type of exposure.

Importantly, there are a number of individuals who have reacted to seafood and wish to continue to eat seafood. Some even report taking an antihistamine before eating seafood as has been documented in studies on seafood allergic patients from South Africa. This is a very dangerous practice and the dangerous implications must be explained to the patients. It is therefore crucial to establish that any adverse reaction was indeed IgE-mediated and correctly identify the specific seafood species implicated in the adverse reaction. While a detailed history is essential, the identification of the implicated seafood species using specific diagnostic procedures is of importance, particularly if the seafood product is not properly identified. Sensitized individuals need to be advised about the potential dangerous consequences of continued exposure.

Diagnostic methods include SPT and quantification of specific IgE antibodies can be done using assays such as the ImmunoCAP or allergen-microarray. However, positive test results do not necessary confirm clinical sensitivity. Possible cross-reactivity between tropomyosin from crustacean and mollusks with tropomyosin from insects and mites may have clinical significance and is discussed below. Sampson and Ho (1997) attempted to establish IgE values to predict clinical reactivity to ingested fish, with 20 kU(A)/L. Wu and Williams (2004) reported that fatal anaphylaxis occurred after ingestion of three snails. A different study using double-blind placebo-controlled food challenge (DBPCFC) reported the accumulated amount of as little as 120 mg of dried snail caused a significant decrease in $FEV_1$ (Forced Expiratory Volume in the first second) (Pajno et al. 2002).

For crustacean Bernstein et al. (1982) reported that patients in a DBPCFC reacted to 14 g of shrimp. Similar results were confirmed by Daul et al. (1988) who reported that the equivalent dose of about four medium-sized shrimps (16 g) caused reactions in DBPCFC. The dose of protein was less than 32 mg of shrimp extract.

### 9.1.5   OCCUPATIONAL EXPOSURE TO SEAFOOD ALLERGENS

The fishing and fish processing industry has experienced tremendous growth in recent years. The Food and Agriculture Organization estimated that the number of people engaged in fishing, aquaculture, and related activities worldwide increased from about 13 million in 1977 to 38 million in 2002. Among these workers 52% worked aboard fishing trawlers, 32% were involved in aquaculture production (marine and freshwater), and 16% worked inland as capture fishers or in other land-based activities such as processing. Ninety-five percent of these workers were from developing countries, producing 58% of the seafood. Increased levels of production and processing of seafood have led and continue to lead to more frequent reporting of occupational health problems such as asthma and other allergic reactions. These occupational health problems result in increased incapacity and absenteeism among affected workers.

Occupational seafood allergy was documented for the first time in 1937, when a fisherman was reported to have developed asthma, angioedema, and conjunctivitis after handling codfish (De Besche 1937). Since then, coinciding with the significant growth in the seafood industry, seafood allergy symptoms ranging from rhinitis, conjunctivitis, asthma, urticaria, protein contact dermatitis, and occasional systemic anaphylactic reactions have been reported in seafood processing workers. The prevalence of occupational asthma in seafood processing workers is estimated to be between 2% and 36% and occupational protein contact dermatitis is 3%–11% (Howse et al. 2006; Jeebhay et al. 2001; Lehrer et al. 2003). From the limited scientific data available for all seafood groups, it seems that crustaceans produce a particular strong allergic response in the workplace with sensitization rates of up to 26% (SPT) for king-, rock-, and snow-crab (Desjardins et al. 1995; Hefle et al. 1995).

Allergic reactions to seafood are the result of exposure to seafood itself or to various nonseafood components present in the product. The composition of aerosols generated by snow crab and king crab processing was found to contain not only allergenic muscle proteins, but also crab exoskeleton, gills, kanimiso (internal organs) as well as background material such as sodium chloride crystals, cellulose, synthetic fibers, silicate, pigment constituent particles, and inorganic particles (silicon, aluminum, iron) (Desjardins et al. 1995). Most of the airborne particles are irregular and at least 30% are within the respirable range (<5 μm), which can reach the deeper areas of the lung. Environmental monitoring of seafood processing plants identified in addition to contaminated processing water (*Klebsiella pneumoniae* and

*Pseudomonas*) as well as elevated levels of endotoxin (>50 EU/m$^3$) are thought to be responsible for respiratory symptoms. Limited evidence from dose–response relation studies indicate that development of symptoms is related to duration and intensity of exposure (Jeebhay et al. 2001, 2005).

## 9.2  CHARACTERISTICS OF THE MOST IMPORTANT ALLERGENS FROM CRUSTACEANS: THE BIOCHEMICAL, BIOLOGICAL, AND IMMUNOLOGICAL PROPERTIES OF MAIN CRUSTACEANS AND SEAFOOD ALLERGENS

The major allergens responsible for ingestion-related allergic reactions due to crustaceans are tropomyosins, while mollusks seem to contain in addition to tropomyosin, other less well-characterized allergens (Table 9.4). It is to be noted that crustacean and mollusk allergens do not cross-react with fish allergens as these are mostly parvalbumins (further characterized in a different chapter).

Already in the early 1980s, Hoffman et al. identified a heat-stable IgE antibody-binding allergen in shrimps, which was later identified by Lehrer and coworkers in the brown shrimps as tropomyosin (Daul et al. 1994; Hoffman et al. 1981; Leung et al. 1994). Shrimp tropomyosin has a slightly acidic isoelectric point, seems to have minor glycan modifications and lacks cystein residues. Tropomyosin is a water-soluble and heat-stable protein with molecular weights ranging from 34 to 39 kDa. While tropomyosin migrates in sodium dodecyl sulfate polyacrylamide gel electrophoresis (SDS-PAGE) as a single band, the protein is in its native state as a coiled-coil homodimer with much higher molecular weight. Tropomyosin has a highly conserved amino acid sequence among different invertebrate organisms (see Section 9.5) and is present in muscle as well as in nonmuscle cells. It is present in all eukaryotic cells, where they are associated with the thin filament in muscle, and microfilaments in many nonmuscle cells. Tropomyosin together with actin and myosin plays a role in the contractile activities and morphology of these cells (Whitby and Phillips 2000). IgE-binding studies with various species and sensitized individuals demonstrated a variety of tropomyosin epitopes. This suggests the existence of species-specific epitopes in addition to common epitopes that may exist not only among crustaceans but also other invertebrates such as mollusks and insects (see Section 9.5).

Furthermore, it was shown that there are three different isoforms of tropomyosin relating to different functional needs (fast, slow-twitch, and slow-tonic), identified by amino acid sequence analysis (Motoyama et al. 2007). The fast isoform is mostly found in the abdominal muscle (tail), while the slow isoform is mainly associated with muscle obtained from the legs; however, both forms can be found in abdominal and leg muscle, with an amino acid homology of up to 100%.

In addition to tropomyosin other allergens were identified and characterized in crustaceans. Proteomic analysis of the black tiger shrimp *Penaeus monodon* has identified a novel allergen, Pen m 2 (Yu et al. 2003). Protein sequence analysis of Pen m 2 has interestingly shown the protein to be very similar to arginine kinase. It has been suggested that arginine kinase may be a new class of invertebrate pan allergens. Immunoblot analysis revealed the allergen to have a molecular weight of 40 kDa

**TABLE 9.4**

**Allergenic Tropomyosins Characterized from Crustacean and Mollusk Species**

| Source of Allergen | Allergen | Family | Molecular Weight (kDa) | Sequence Data | Recombinant Protein | Author |
|---|---|---|---|---|---|---|
| | | Crustaceans | | | | |
| Chinese spiny lobster (*Panulirus stimpsoni*) | Pan s 1 | Tropomyosin | 34 | cDNA | Yes | Leung et al. (1998b) |
| American lobster (*Homarus americanus*) | Hom a 1 | Tropomyosin | 34 | cDNA | Yes | Leung et al. (1998a) |
| Red crab (*Charybdis feriatus*) | Cha f 1 | Tropomyosin | 34 | cDNA | Yes | Leung et al. (1998a) |
| Sand shrimp (*Metapenaeus ensis*) | Met e 1 | Tropomyosin | 34 | cDNA | Yes | Leung et al. (1994) |
| Indian white shrimp (*Penaeus indicus*) | Pen i 1 | Tropomyosin | 34 | | No | Shanti et al. (1993) |
| Neptune rose shrimp (*Parapenaeus fissurus*) | Par f 1 | Tropomyosin | 39 | No | No | Lin et al. (1993) |
| Brown shrimp (*P. aztecus*) | Pen a 1 | Tropomyosin | 36 | cDNA | Yes | Daul et al. (1994), Reese et al. (1997) |
| Tiger shrimp (*P. monodon*) | Pen m 2 | Arginine kinase | 40 | cDNA | No | Yu et al. (2003) |
| White shrimp (*Litopenaeus vannamei*) | Lit v 2 | Arginine kinase | 40 | cDNA library | No | Garcia-Orozco et al. (2007) |
| Krill (*Euphausia superba*) | Eup s 1 | Tropomyosin | 38 | Yes | Yes | Nakano et al. (2008) |
| Krill (*E. pacifica*) | Eup p 1 | Tropomyosin | 38 | Yes | Yes | Nakano et al. (2008) |

**Mollusks**

| | | | | | | |
|---|---|---|---|---|---|---|
| Japanese common squid (*T. pacificus*) | Tod p 1 | Tropomyosin | 38 | 12 residue peptide | No | Miyazawa et al. (1996) |
| Pacific oyster (*Crassostrea gigas*) | Cra g 1 Cra g 2 | Tropomyosin | 35 | Peptide | No | Ishikawa et al. 1998b, 1999, 1997 |
| Marine snail (*Turbo cornutus*) | Tur c 1 | Tropomyosin | 35 | Peptide | No | Ishikawa et al. (1998a) |
| Abalone (*H. midae*) | Hal m 1 | Tropomyosin | 38 | No | No | Lopata et al. (1997) |
| Acorn barnacle (*Balanus rostratus*) | Bal r | Tropomyosin | 37 | cDNA | No | Suma et al. (2007) |
| Goose barnacle (*Capitulum mitella*) | Cap m | Tropomyosin | 37 | cDNA | No | Suma et al. (2007) |
| Brown garden snail (*Helix aspersa*) | Hel a 1 | Tropomyosin | 36 | cDNA | Yes | Asturias et al. (2002) |

(Garcia-Orozco et al. 2007; Yu et al. 2003). A number of proteins with molecular masses ranging from 8 to 89 kDa that bind serum IgE antibodies of allergic individuals have also been demonstrated, although not immunochemically identified. Similar observation was previously demonstrated in the brown shrimp (Lehrer et al. 1988).

Importantly, tropomyosin is not only a crustacean allergen but it has also been confirmed to be present in a number of mollusk species (Taylor 2008). Mollusk allergens have not been studied as well as those of fish or crustacean. However, it has become apparent that mollusks such as mussel, oyster, squid, limpet, and abalone are significant food allergens in exposed population. The first major allergen of mollusks was characterized in squid (*Todarodes pacificus*). The 38 kDa heat-stable protein, Tod p 1, revealed high homology with tropomyosin of snail and the allergenic tropomyosin (Met e 1) of shrimp. This suggested that Tod p 1 was a squid muscle tropomyosin. Subsequently, Lopata and coworkers have identified the major allergens in abalone (*Haliotis midae*), yielding MWs of 38 and 49 kDa (Hal m 1). Immunoblot and molecular analysis by other groups confirmed tropomyosin in other abalone species, as well as in snail, clam, oyster, mussel, scallop, octopus, whelk, and turban shell (Table 9.4). However, mollusks contain in addition other nontropomyosin allergens such as myosin heavy chain, hemocyanin, and amylase (Taylor 2008). Furthermore, arginine kinase as mentioned previously seems to be also allergenic in mollusks, accounting perhaps for an additional degree of cross-reactivity among these two seafood groups.

## 9.3 PROTEOMICS OF A NOVEL SHRIMP ALLERGEN

Tropomyosin is a major muscle protein present in all living animals and appears to be a highly conserved molecule. The structure is rather unique in that it is composed of two polypeptide chains, each in $\alpha$-helix formation coiled around on another in the so-called coiled-coil structure (Smillie et al. 1980). Tropomyosin had been identified as the major crustacean allergen in the muscle tissue of shrimp by three different research teams (Daul et al. 1993, 1994; Leung et al. 1994; Shanti et al. 1993). This allergen was characterized by deducing amino acid sequence from complementary DNA, and identified as muscle protein from the shrimp *Penaeus aztecus* (Pen a 1). While the amino acid sequence identity of tropomyosins to other nonshrimp invertebrate such as insects and mites is very high, and even to vertebrate tropomyosin, the latter one is nonallergenic (Ayuso et al. 1999a, 2000). Shanti et al. (1993) did identify two IgE-binding regions by analyzing IgE antibody reactivities of shrimp-allergic patients by using nine tryptic fragments of Pen e 1. Two peptides, nine-and six-amino acid residues long where identified as important, as they inhibited over 50% of specific IgE-binding to Pen e 1. Interestingly the smaller peptide region partially overlapped with one of the three IgE-binding sites which were subsequently identified by Reese et al. (1997) using a recombinant peptide library of Pen e 1. Using serum from shrimp-allergic subjects, four peptides of 13–21 amino acid length identified; however, all were located in the second half of the carboxy-terminal region of the protein. In order to identify areas on this molecule which contains IgE-binding regions, 36 overlapping peptides were synthesized that spanned the entire sequence of Pen a 1 (Ayuso et al. 1999b, 2002a). Testing sera from 18 shrimp-sensitized subjects for prevalence and intensity of IgE-binding, five major reactive regions were identified. The size of several IgE-binding regions and composition of two or more overlapping peptides suggested that they may contain more than one allergenic epitope. To identify the smallest sequence with maximal IgE-binding, shorter peptides were screened and finally eight IgE-binding epitopes were identified within the five IgE-binding regions of Pen a 1. Interestingly, the minimum IgE-binding peptide sites varied in length from 8 to 15 amino acid length, which was dependent on the specific region and the subject studied. Furthermore, the epitope for maximal IgE-binding capacity was followed by shorter or longer peptides, always with weaker IgE-reactivity for all subjects investigated.

Understanding the complex IgE-antibody reactivities on allergenic Pen a 1 was essential to generate peptides with reduced IgE-binding capacity. Importantly, many nonallergenic tropomyosins are naturally available that provided templates for amino acid substitutions. Based on the available nonallergenic homologues sequences, from the fish salmon as well as chicken and mammalian tropomyosin, mutated peptides were generated. All possible substitution combinations (up to five per peptide) were generated as overlapping peptides and tested with serum of individual subjects. The results were surprising and exciting. A single amino acid substitution could abolish, decrease, and even increase the IgE-reactivity of the modified peptides. Secondly, most of the critical amino acid substitutions that led to a decrease in IgE binding were in the center rather than the peripheral parts of the epitope. Furthermore, reduced binding was generally achieved with increasing the number of nonconservative amino acid (belonging to a different group) substitutions.

The identification of the major IgE-binding epitopes of Pen a 1 and the crucial amino acids within the epitopes for maximum IgE antibody-binding are fundamental for the development of hypoallergenic tropomyosin variants. This nonallergenic recombinant tropomyosin could now open the development of safer therapeutic tools for the treatment of shrimp-allergic patients. Subsequently Reese et al. (2006) produced a full-length recombinant tropomyosin (Pen a 1) from the Brown shrimp (*P. aztecus*) and compared the functional and immunological properties to the natural form. The secondary structure of natural and recombinant Pen a 1 by CD spectroscopy identified both proteins as α-helical confirmation. Most importantly the IgE antibody-binding reactivity was very similar to the natural form of this protein, as demonstrated by radio-allergosorbent test (RAST) and mast cell activation. These findings were the basis for future component-resolve diagnosis as well as allergen-specific immunotherapy, as these proteins demonstrated sensitizing potential in a murine model of shrimp allergy.

Subsequently the recombinant rPen a 1 is now available as ImmunoCAP (Phadia) and Microarray assay (VBC-diagnostics) and allows the specific diagnosis for IgE directed sensitivity to shrimp tropomyosin. Epitope identification of food allergens provides information on the structural basis of protein allergenicity and offers the possibility to reduce IgE binding. To date, immunotherapy of food allergies is not the course of treatment, because of the high risk of severe reactions. Because Pen a 1 is responsible for at least 75% of the shrimp-specific IgE antibodies and the detailed characterization of the antibody-binding epitopes, this proteins lends itself as model food allergen for future immunotherapy.

Based on the previous findings, Reese et al. (2005) produced a mutant of Pen a 1 (VR9-1 tropomyosin) using side-directed mutagenesis to substitute 12 important amino acids. The secondary structure of VR9-1 was not altered; however, the allergenic potency was reduced by 90%–98%, as demonstrated by using the functional rat-basophil assay (RBL). When comparing the activation of patient's serum IgE by VR9-1 in the RBL-assay with IgE antibodies from sensitized mice, it demonstrated that the reduction was much more pronounced in the murine model. These observations are probably explained by previous findings that in addition to the eight identified major epitopes additional IgE-binding sites exist (Ayuso et al. 2002a). Furthermore, the intraperitoneal route of sensitization of the mice renders a very specific antibody response to the identified major epitopes, while the oral route of sensitization of patients might generate antibodies to additional epitopes.

Exposure to crustacean and other invertebrate tropomyosins via the inhalation route might in addition generate these other IgE antibodies demonstrated in this study. Inhalational routes of sensitization have not been well documented but seems to be predominant in workers being sensitized in the food processing industry (Blotzer and Wuthrich 2004; Jeebhay et al. 2001, 2005; Roberts et al. 2002).

## 9.4   CHANGES IN ALLERGENICITY OF CRUSTACEAN ALLERGENS DURING FOOD PROCESSING

Food is subject to a large variety of processing conditions to prolong storage or improve sensory qualities. Many different processes are used, often in combination but can be generally categorized into thermal and nonthermal procedures. A recent workshop evaluated the effects of food processing on the allergenicity of food allergens (Thomas et al. 2007). Various food processes have been implemented to reduce allergenicity of certain foods, but very few studies focused on seafood.

Since tropomyosin of invertebrates is typically a lysine-rich protein (up to 12% in scallops) it reacts easily with reducing sugars through the Maillard reaction during food processing such as grilling, steaming, and roasting. Particularly, the brown color of dried seafood s is caused by the Maillard reaction. Studies on the effect of sugar residues on two different mollusk species showed opposite effects. Heating of scallops (a bivalve) in the presence of sugar residues increased the IgE-binding, as demonstrated by competitive enzyme-linked immunosorbent assay (ELISA) (Nakamura et al. 2005), while a decrease in allergenicity was observed for squid (calamari) in the presence of the reducing sugar ribose (Nakamura et al. 2006). The interpretations of these contradicting results are difficult as IgE-binding activity is not always correlated with clinical reactivity.

Nonthermal processes have been also investigated and an example is the gamma irradiation of crustacean and mollusks which resulted in reduced IgE-binding capacity of the allergens (Byun et al. 2000, 2002; Li et al. 2007) as well as high-intesity ultrasound treatment (Li et al. 2006) of shrimp. Meyer-Pittroff et al. (2007) suggest that pressure above 600 MPa causes reversible and irreversible changes to the secondary, quaternary, and tertiary structure, particularly in helical proteins, and demonstrated reduced allergenicity. Nevertheless, complete loss of allergenicity or allergen concentrations has not been demonstrated which is probably due to the fact that even small protein fragments of about 3.5 kDa can still cross-link mast cell IgE and elicit an allergic reaction (Thomas et al. 2007). Furthermore, the solubility and extractability of treated tropomyosin might be affected and results in under detection as has been demonstrated for radioactive-treated crustacean and mollusks (Sinanoglou et al. 2007). In addition it cannot be ruled out that processing has different effects on the less well-characterized shellfish allergens.

Most of the investigated processes to reduce allergenicity are purely on experimental basis but it is an important area of research for seafood allergy which has to be further explored. Furthermore, the challenge of maintaining the flavor and texture of seafood during these processes will be of importance.

### 9.4.1 DETECTION OF CRUSTACEAN ALLERGENS IN VARIOUS PRODUCTS

The labeling of foods containing material derived from crustaceans has already become mandatory in some countries such as in Europe, the United States, and Japan. Crustacean and fish have been previously recognized as important food allergens for labeling purpose (http://www.efsa.eu.int/science/nda/nda_opinions/catindex_en.html); however only recently the European Union adapted their guidelines to include mollusks as a separate food allergen, based on the limited cross-reactivity to crustacean allergens (http://www.efsa.europa.eu/EFSA/efsa_locale-11786207 53812_1178623594074.htm). A recent comparative study of two newly developed ELISA systems has demonstrated high sensitivity (1 μg/g food) as well as reasonable recovery and reproducibility rates (Sakai et al. 2008). Nevertheless, a certain degree of cross-reactivity to cockroach and mollusk tropomyosin has also been noted. This cross-reactivity might be of greater importance considering the large variety of tropomyosins identified in not only crustaceans but also mollusks (see below). Furthermore, the detection of processed crustacean rather than raw crustacean is dependent on the recognition of tropomyosin not only in the monomeric form but in addition possible oligomers and fragments of tropomyosin, which might still have allergenic activity.

Additional problems might not only arise with the different crustacean and mollusks species processed but with the increasing number of food, medical, and health products derived from crustacean. Chitin and chitosan are among the emerging materials which are being developed and applied widely in the food, biotechnology, pharmaceutical, and medial field (No et al. 2007). The main obstacle for the future use of this unique material is the residual amount of about 1% protein in industrial produced chitosan. Allergic reactions after using chitosan containing creams (Pereira et al. 1998) and food (Kato et al. 2005; Villacis et al. 2006) have been reported; however, the contribution of the thermo stabile tropomyosin or other yet unidentified crustacean allergens had not been demonstrated. Other pharmaceutical products derived from crustacean are glucosamine, a natural aminomonosaccharide, which is frequently used as therapeutic supplement for joint inflammations. It was previously indicated as a potential risk for shellfish sensitive individuals because it was derived from shellfish chitosan; however, Villacis et al. (2006) demonstrated no allergenic reactivity by using DBPCFC in 15 shrimp-allergic patients.

Food products can also be unexpectedly derived from crustacean. Surimi (seafood paste) is usually derived from fish, but can in some countries contain a variety of crustacean species (Hamada et al. 2000; Mata et al. 1994).

## 9.5   CROSS-REACTIVITY OF CRUSTACEAN ALLERGENS

### 9.5.1   Within Crustaceans

Tropomyosin is present in many organisms from phylogenetically unrelated vertebrates to invertebrates. While the sequence identity and functional similarity among different tropomyosins can be very high, vertebrate tropomyosins are nonallergenic. In fact, it is possible that vertebrate tropomyosins are generating immunological tolerance, which is demonstrated in no observed allergic reactions to meat tropomyosin (Ayuso et al. 1999a). It has been observed that cross-reactivity occurs frequently to foods within a certain group or family such as crab, lobster, shrimp, etc. among the crustaceans (Ayuso et al. 2002a; Lehrer 1987; Lehrer et al. 1988; Motoyama et al. 2006; Reese et al. 1999; Zhang et al. 2006), suggesting that cross-reactivity could occur between phylogenetically related organisms. In Figure 9.1, the amino acid identity of different allergenic crustacean and mollusk tropomyosin is compared with nonallergenic vertebrate tropomyosins. Crustacean species have very high homologies of up to 98% among the different shrimp, crab, and lobster species. Interestingly a recently identified barnacle tropomyosin demonstrates a much lower sequence identity with only 58% (Suma et al. 2007).

Molecular investigation of these allergens suggests that a high homology in the amino acid sequence of an allergen, i.e., the primary sequence, consequently results in a high homology of the 3D structure (protein folding) of the protein and thus potentially leading to cross-reactivity (Aalberse et al. 2001; Jenkins et al. 2007; Motoyama et al. 2007). Nevertheless, species-specific allergic reactions to particular crustacean species have been reported and are probably of clinical relevance. If these specific reactions are based on differential IgE responses to specific epitopes or perhaps a reflection of the first crustacean exposure is not known.

A recent review by Mills and coworkers (Jenkins et al. 2007) highlighted the position that almost all animal food allergens have homologs in the human proteome. Profile-based sequence homology methods were used to classify animal food allergens into Pfam families and their evolutionary and structural relationship were analyzed. In general the vertebrate tropomyosin sequences from other mammals, fish, and birds are very similar with over 90% homology and none of them has been reported to be allergenic. In contrast, allergenic tropomyosins are mainly found among the invertebrates such as crustaceans, insects, and some nematodes (Anisakis) and demonstrate maximal 54% sequence identity to human tropomyosin (Figure 9.1) (data retrieved from http://www.allergome.org/, GenBank and SwissProt). Furthermore, inhalant arthropod-derived tropomyosins share high sequence identities to crustacean tropomyosins with up to 84%. These allergenic tropomyosins are found in two cockroaches (Per a 7 and Bla g 7) as well as in the house dust mite (Der p 10 and Der f 10) (discussed below).

| | Species | Abbreviation | Crustaceans | | | | | | | | | | | | Cephalopods | | Bivalves | | | | Gastropods | Insects | | | Mites | | Nematode | Chicken | Human |
|---|---|---|---|---|---|---|---|---|---|---|---|---|---|---|---|---|---|---|---|---|---|---|---|---|---|---|---|---|---|
| | | | A | B | C | D | E | F | G | H | I | J | K | L | M | N | O | P | Q | R | S | T | U | V | W | X | Y | Z | AA |
| Crustaceans | Brown shrimp (*Penaeus aztecus*) | Pen a 1 | A | 100 | 100 | 99 | 89 | 89 | 97 | 91 | 92 | 92 | 92 | 98 | 58 | 63 | 63 | 57 | 55 | 57 | 63 | 61 | 81 | 82 | 67 | 80 | 80 | 72 | 54 | 53 |
| | Black tiger prawn (*Penaeus monodon*) | Pen m 1 | B | 100 | 100 | 99 | 89 | 97 | 97 | 91 | 92 | 92 | 98 | 93 | 58 | 63 | 63 | 57 | 55 | 57 | 63 | 61 | 81 | 82 | 67 | 80 | 80 | 72 | 54 | 53 |
| | Sand shrimp (*Metapenaeus ensis*) | Met e 1 | C | 99 | 99 | 100 | 89 | 90 | 87 | 87 | 92 | 92 | 98 | 85 | 57 | 62 | 62 | 55 | 54 | 56 | 63 | 60 | 80 | 81 | 67 | 80 | 80 | 71 | 53 | 51 |
| | Krill (*Euphausia superba*) | Eup s 1 | D | 89 | 89 | 89 | 100 | 90 | 84 | 85 | 85 | 88 | 98 | 94 | 58 | 63 | 63 | 57 | 55 | 57 | 64 | 61 | 81 | 82 | 66 | 75 | 75 | 70 | 51 | 51 |
| | Japanese mantis shrimp (*Oratosquilla oratoria*) | Squ o 1 | E | 89 | 97 | 90 | 90 | 100 | 92 | 93 | 93 | 93 | 94 | 90 | 57 | 64 | 64 | 57 | 57 | 58 | 64 | 61 | 81 | 82 | 67 | 81 | 80 | 73 | 54 | 53 |
| | Red crab (*Charybdis feriatus*) | Cha f 1 | F | 97 | 97 | 87 | 84 | 92 | 100 | 99 | 93 | 93 | 98 | 84 | 57 | 62 | 62 | 55 | 54 | 56 | 57 | 55 | 83 | 84 | 68 | 81 | 80 | 73 | 54 | 53 |
| | Sea crab (*Portunus sanguinolentus*) | Por s 1 | G | 91 | 91 | 87 | 85 | 93 | 99 | 100 | 99 | 99 | 97 | 85 | 59 | 64 | 64 | 57 | 56 | 57 | 63 | 60 | 82 | 83 | 67 | 81 | 81 | 74 | 54 | 55 |
| | Mud crab (*Scylla serrata*) | Scy s 1 | H | 92 | 92 | 92 | 85 | 93 | 93 | 99 | 100 | 100 | 92 | 94 | 59 | 64 | 64 | 57 | 56 | 58 | 63 | 60 | 82 | 83 | 67 | 82 | 79 | 74 | 54 | 54 |
| | Chinese mitten crab (*Eriocheir sinensis*) | Eri s 1 | I | 92 | 92 | 92 | 85 | 93 | 93 | 99 | 100 | 100 | 99 | 94 | 59 | 64 | 64 | 57 | 56 | 57 | 63 | 60 | 81 | 83 | 67 | 82 | 80 | 74 | 54 | 54 |
| | Chinese spiny lobster (*Panulirus stimpsoni*) | Pan s 1 | J | 98 | 98 | 98 | 98 | 94 | 98 | 97 | 92 | 99 | 100 | 93 | 57 | 62 | 62 | 56 | 55 | 56 | 64 | 60 | 80 | 81 | 67 | 80 | 80 | 71 | 54 | 52 |
| | American lobster (*Homarus americanus*) | Hom a 1 | K | 93 | 93 | 85 | 94 | 90 | 84 | 85 | 94 | 94 | 93 | 100 | 58 | 62 | 62 | 56 | 55 | 58 | 64 | 60 | 80 | 82 | 67 | 82 | 80 | 74 | 54 | 53 |
| | Acorn barnacle (*Balanus rostratus*) | Bal r 1 | L | 58 | 58 | 57 | 58 | 57 | 57 | 59 | 59 | 59 | 57 | 58 | 100 | 73 | 72 | 66 | 66 | 69 | 71 | 75 | 58 | 57 | 48 | 59 | 59 | 57 | 48 | 46 |
| Cephalopods | Octopus (*Octopus vulgaris*) | Oct v 1 | M | 63 | 63 | 62 | 63 | 64 | 62 | 64 | 64 | 64 | 62 | 62 | 73 | 100 | 91 | 70 | 69 | 71 | 80 | 79 | 62 | 62 | 58 | 63 | 63 | 63 | 51 | 81 |
| | Japanese flying squid (*Todarodes pacificus*) | Tod p 1 | N | 63 | 63 | 62 | 63 | 64 | 62 | 63 | 63 | 63 | 62 | 62 | 72 | 91 | 100 | 70 | 69 | 70 | 79 | 77 | 61 | 60 | 58 | 63 | 64 | 64 | 50 | 50 |
| Bivalves | Blue mussel (*Mytilus edulis*) | Myt e 1 | O | 57 | 57 | 55 | 55 | 57 | 55 | 57 | 57 | 57 | 56 | 56 | 66 | 70 | 70 | 100 | 94 | 69 | 74 | 71 | 57 | 57 | 48 | 55 | 55 | 55 | 49 | 45 |
| | Asian green mussel (*Perna viridis*) | Per v 1 | P | 55 | 55 | 54 | 55 | 57 | 54 | 56 | 56 | 56 | 55 | 55 | 66 | 69 | 69 | 94 | 100 | 69 | 75 | 71 | 56 | 56 | 48 | 54 | 54 | 55 | 45 | 45 |
| | Scallop (*Mimachlamys nobilis*) | Chl n 1 | Q | 57 | 57 | 56 | 57 | 58 | 56 | 57 | 58 | 57 | 56 | 58 | 69 | 71 | 70 | 69 | 69 | 100 | 72 | 69 | 55 | 55 | 50 | 58 | 58 | 58 | 47 | 47 |
| | Oyster (*Crassostrea gigas*) | Cra g 1 | R | 63 | 63 | 64 | 64 | 64 | 57 | 63 | 63 | 63 | 64 | 64 | 71 | 80 | 79 | 74 | 75 | 72 | 100 | 77 | 62 | 62 | 54 | 62 | 62 | 61 | 50 | 50 |
| Gastropods | California red abalone (*Haliotis rufescens*) | Hal ru 1 | S | 61 | 61 | 60 | 60 | 61 | 55 | 60 | 60 | 60 | 60 | 60 | 75 | 79 | 77 | 71 | 71 | 69 | 77 | 100 | 60 | 60 | 54 | 61 | 62 | 61 | 48 | 48 |
| Insects | Locusts (*Locusta migratoria*) | x | T | 81 | 81 | 80 | 81 | 81 | 83 | 82 | 82 | 81 | 80 | 80 | 58 | 62 | 61 | 57 | 56 | 55 | 62 | 60 | 100 | 89 | 64 | 79 | 79 | 70 | 53 | 51 |
| | American cockroach (*Periplaneta americana*) | Per a 7 | U | 82 | 82 | 81 | 82 | 82 | 84 | 83 | 83 | 83 | 81 | 82 | 57 | 62 | 60 | 57 | 56 | 55 | 62 | 60 | 89 | 100 | 65 | 79 | 79 | 69 | 52 | 50 |
| | Silverfish (*Lepisma saccharina*) | Lep s 1 | V | 67 | 67 | 67 | 66 | 67 | 68 | 67 | 67 | 67 | 67 | 67 | 48 | 58 | 58 | 48 | 48 | 50 | 54 | 54 | 64 | 65 | 100 | 64 | 63 | 60 | 45 | 45 |
| Mites | Dust mite (*Dermatophagoides pteronyssinus*) | Der p 10 | W | 80 | 80 | 80 | 75 | 81 | 79 | 80 | 80 | 82 | 80 | 82 | 59 | 63 | 63 | 55 | 54 | 58 | 62 | 61 | 79 | 79 | 64 | 100 | 96 | 73 | 53 | 53 |
| | Storage mite (*Lepidoglyphus destructor*) | Lep d 10 | X | 80 | 80 | 80 | 75 | 80 | 80 | 81 | 79 | 80 | 80 | 80 | 59 | 63 | 64 | 55 | 54 | 58 | 62 | 62 | 79 | 79 | 63 | 96 | 100 | 73 | 53 | 54 |
| Nematode | Herring worm (*Anisakis simplex*) | Ani s 3 | Y | 72 | 72 | 71 | 70 | 73 | 73 | 74 | 74 | 74 | 71 | 74 | 57 | 63 | 64 | 55 | 55 | 58 | 61 | 61 | 70 | 69 | 60 | 73 | 73 | 100 | 54 | 53 |
| Chicken | Chicken (*Gallus gallus*) | x | Z | 54 | 54 | 53 | 51 | 54 | 54 | 54 | 54 | 54 | 54 | 54 | 48 | 51 | 50 | 49 | 49 | 47 | 50 | 48 | 53 | 52 | 45 | 53 | 53 | 54 | 100 | 83 |
| Human | Human (*Homo sapiens*) | x | AA | 53 | 53 | 51 | 51 | 53 | 53 | 55 | 54 | 54 | 54 | 52 | 46 | 81 | 50 | 45 | 45 | 47 | 50 | 48 | 51 | 50 | 45 | 53 | 54 | 53 | 83 | 100 |

**FIGURE 9.1** Amino acid identities (in %) of Pen a 1 tropomyosin comparison with allergenic crustacean and other invertebrate tropomyosins and non-allergenic vertebrate tropomyosin. *Note:* x. not known. Compiled with the assistance of Dr. Natalie Nieuwenhuizen and Mr. Sandip Kamath (University of Cape Town and RMIT University).

## 9.5.2 BETWEEN CRUSTACEAN AND MOLLUSKS

A study conducted by Lehrer and Mccants (1987), demonstrated that crustacean sensitized sera had significant IgE antibody reactivity to oyster extract by RAST analysis, highlighting the cross-reactivity within shellfish. Crustacean allergic subjects often react to species of the mollusk group, such as squid (cuttlefish), abalone, limpet, squid, oyster, mussel, scallop, and clam. A study by Leung et al. (1996) confirmed the presence of a 38 kDa IgE-binding protein in all 10 mollusk species tested, using sera from nine crustacean allergic patients. This protein was subsequently identified as tropomyosin (Leung et al. 1996). Furthermore, varying reactivity of the sera with a number of other mollusk allergens was observed, such as oyster (Ishikawa et al. 1998b; Lehrer et al. 2003). Serological and clinical cross-reactivity is also often observed between crustaceans and the mollusk squid (*T. pacificus*) (Jeong et al. 2006; Miyazawa et al. 1996). This allergen was identified as Tod p 1 and is also a tropomyosin and seems to cross-react with other squid species (*Loligo vulgaris*) and also shrimp, lobster, and crab. Crespo's group showed in Spain that 9 of 10 children with sensitization to mollusks reacted by SPT and specific IgE to crustaceans (Crespo et al. 1995b).

Even though IgE cross-reactivity among crustaceans and mollusks are commonly reported until recently, limited work has been done on the molecular identity of these cross-reactive allergens. The amino acid sequence identity with shrimp tropomyosin is fairly low with 57% and 61% for mussels and abalone, respectively (Figure 9.1). The relationship of molecular cross-reactivity with clinical reactivity has however not been adequately defined.

## 9.5.3 BETWEEN SHELLFISH AND OTHER INVERTEBRATES

Allergic reactions in shellfish allergic patients to crustaceans and mollusks, as well as to mites and insects has been reported (Ayuso et al. 2002c; Banzet et al. 1992; Crespo et al. 1995b; Lehrer and Reese 1998; Martins et al. 1999; Oneil and Lehrer 1995; Petrus et al. 1997, 1999; Reese et al. 1999; vanRee et al. 1996b). This seemingly frequently encountered cross-reactivity is probably due to tropomyosin (as discussed) and may have significant clinical implications. This has been shown particularly for shellfish allergens and tropomyosins from insects and mites, which are all part of the phylum arthropod (Jeebhay et al. 2007; Lopata et al. 2005) (Figure 9.2). A recent study demonstrated sensitization to shrimp tropomyosin in orthodox Jews, who are prohibited by religious dietary laws from eating shellfish, which could be indicative of sensitization to tropomyosin from noncrustacean, such as house dust mites and cockroaches, via the inhalation route (Fernandes et al. 2003).

Clinical relevant cross-reactivity between crustacean and house dust mite allergens has been described (Witteman et al. 1994) and the term "mite–crustaceans–mollusk-syndrome" is sometimes used. The primary sensitization is believed mostly to be "respiratory" allergy to dust mites, which then sometimes causes food allergic reactions to crustaceans or mollusks in some individuals. However, there are also observations on allergy to mites or cockroaches possible occurring subsequent to

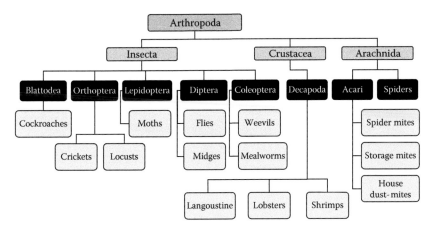

**FIGURE 9.2** Phylogenetic relationship between three different classes within the phylum arthropoda. The species shown in the different groups have all been implicated in allergic reactions (stinging insects excluded).

sensitization to crustaceans (Ayuso et al. 2002c). Comparing amino acid homologies, it becomes clear that Pen a 1 IgE-binding regions show high sequence homology with corresponding regions of Per a 7 and Der p 10 (60%–100%), suggesting similar IgE-binding epitopes in these different arthropods (Ayuso et al. 2002a,b). Using synthetic overlapping peptides spanning the length of the major shrimp allergen, Pen a 1, eight IgE-binding epitopes were identified. Four out of eight epitopes are identical to homologous regions in Der p 10 and Der f 10, and five out of eight are identical to homologous regions in Per a 7 (Reese et al. 2002). These findings were recently supported by two separate studies. During immunotherapy to house dust mites patients developed sensitization to shellfish tropomyosin, which did not exist before therapy (Pajno et al. 2002; Peroni et al. 2000; vanRee et al. 1996a,b). These immunological findings strongly indicate that the documented cross-reactivity between tropomyosins from different allergen sources can result in cellular activation and subsequently asthmatic reactions.

Other possible IgE-reactivity's to tropomyosin containing allergen sources have been documented, such as the cross-reactivity to the fish parasite Anisakis (Jeong et al. 2006; Lehrer and Reese 1998). The possible clinical cross-reactivity is supported by high sequence homology of crustacean and Anisakis nematode tropomyosin (Ani s 3) with 74% (Table 9.4) (Arlian et al. 2003; Asturias et al. 2000; Audicana and Kennedy 2008; Guarneri et al. 2007; Johansson et al. 2001).

In order to predict the evolutionary position of the different tropomyosins to each other a molecular phylogenetic tree was constructed (Figure 9.3). The phylogenetic tree of the alignment of a larger number of tropomyosin protein sequences clearly identifies clusters of related tropomyosin allergens (using the Clustal program; http:// www.ebi.ac.uk/clustalw/) (Chenna et al. 2003). This visualization of relationships supports the close immunological reactivities of crustacean tropomyosins to various insect and to a lower degree mite and mollusk tropomyosins. Most insect tropomyosins are closely related to their crustacean counterpart; however, a recent

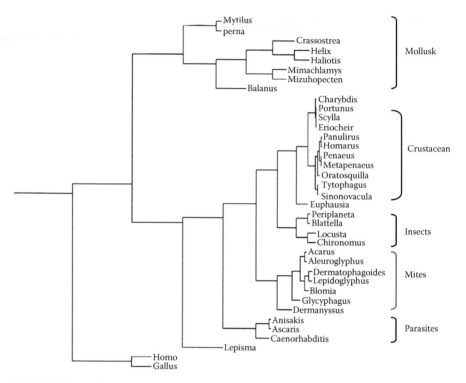

**FIGURE 9.3** Molecular phylogenetic tree for tropomyosin from various animals using the Clustal program (http://www.ebi.ac.uk/clustalw/). Compiled with the assistance of Dr. Natalie Nieuwenhuizen.

detailed analysis of tropomyosin from silverfish (Lepisma) (Barletta et al. 2005, 2007) revealed their distance with only up to 68% homology. While these studies did not demonstrate clinical reactivity to silverfish, patients with multiple sensitivity to crustacean and insects showed IgE-binding on immunoblots. A recent comparative study of two unusual allergenic tropomyosins highlighted the possible divergence of otherwise very closely related tropomyosins in the group of crustaceans. Although barnacles (Balanus) are members of the crustacean family, its tropomyosin has only 59%–61% sequence identity with decapod tropomyosin (Table 9.4). The low degree of homology is supported by the fact that an antilobster tropomyosin monoclonal antibody did not recognize barnacle tropomyosin (Suma et al. 2007) as well as several patients (with crustacean allergy). Furthermore, a previous study on clinically sensitized patients to barnacles, only one out of five patients was also diagnosed with shrimp allergy (Marinho et al. 2006).

A recent study by Marti et al. (2007) used an *in silico* motif-based allergenicity prediction protocol to generate a recombinant peptide which showed the same IgE-reactivity as shrimp full-length tropomyosin. This motif-generating algorithm may be used in the future to identify major IgE-binding structures of other coiled-coil proteins.

### 9.5.4 Conclusions

Crustaceans are a large and diverse group including over 30,000 different species of which a number of varieties are important food sources. The group of shellfish has gained recently more public health importance since the group of mollusks is designated as commonly allergenic foods in the European Union and Canada. The prevalence of crustacean allergy seems to vary largely between geographical locations, most probably as a result of seafood being part of the stable diet.

The major crustacean allergens are tropomyosin, although other allergens such as arginine kinase may play an important part in allergenicity. Tropomyosin seems to be the major allergen responsible for molecular and clinical cross-reactivity between crustaceans and mollusks, but also to other invertebrates such as house dust mites and insects. Shellfish allergens do not cross-react with fish allergens. However, allergic reactivity to fish might be triggered by the contaminating parasite Anisakis, resulting from cross-reactivity to invertebrate tropomyosin.

The allergenicity of crustacean allergens seems not reliably reduced by food processing. Future research on the molecular structure of tropomyosins with focus on the immunological and clinical reactivity will improve management of this life-threatening allergy, and is essential for future immunotherapy.

## REFERENCES

Aalberse, R.C., Akkerdaas, J.H., van Ree, R. 2001. Cross-reactivity of IgE antibodies to allergens. *Allergy* 56(6):478–490.

Administration NOaA. 2007. Seafood consumption increases in 2006. In: Administration NOaA, editor. Available at: http://www.publicaffairs.noaa.gov/releases2007/jul07/noaa07-r123.html.

Andre, F., Andre, C., Colin, L., Cacaraci, F., Cavagna, S. 1994. Role of new allergens and of allergens consumption in the increased incidence of food sensitizations in France. *Toxicology* 93(1):77–83.

Arlian, L.G., Morgan, M.S., Quirce, S., Maranon, F., Fernandez-Caldas, E. 2003. Characterization of allergens of *Anisakis simplex*. *Allergy* 58(12):1299–1303.

Asturias, J.A., Eraso, E., Martinez, A. 2000. Cloning and high level expression in *Escherichia coli* of an Anisakis simplex tropomyosin isoform. *Molecular and Biochemical Parasitology* 108(2):263–266.

Asturias, J.A., Eraso, E., Arlllam, M.C., Gomez-Bayon, N., Inacio, F., Martinez, A. 2002. Cloning, isolation, and IgE-binding properties of *Helix aspersa* (Brown garden snail) tropomyosin. *International Archives of Allergy and Immunology* 128(2):90–96.

Audicana, M.T., Kennedy, M.W. 2008. Anisakis simplex: From obscure infectious worm to inducer of immune hypersensitivity. *Clinical Microbiology Reviews* 21(2):360.

Auerswald, L., Morren, C., Lopata, A.L. 2006. Histamine levels in seventeen species of fresh and processed South African seafood. *Food Chemistry* 98(2):231–239.

Ayuso, R., Lehrer, S.B., Tanaka, L., Ibanez, M.D., Pascual, C., Burks, A.W., Sussman, G.L., Goldberg, B., Lopez, M., Reese, G. 1999a. IgE antibody response to vertebrate meat proteins including tropomyosin. *Annals of Allergy Asthma & Immunology* 83(5): 399–405.

Ayuso, R., Reese, G., Lehrer, S.B. 1999b. IgE-binding epitopes of Pen a 1 (shrimp tropomyosin): Localization of antigenic regions using overlapping peptides. *Journal of Investigative Medicine* 47(2):S66–S66.

Ayuso, R., Lehrer, S.B., Lopez, M., Reese, G., Ibanez, M.D., Esteban, M.M., Owilby, D.R., Schwartz, H. 2000. Identification of bovine IgG as a major cross-reactive vertebrate meat allergen. *Allergy* 55(4):348–354.

Ayuso, R., Lehrer, S.B., Reese, G. 2002a. Identification of continuous, allergenic regions of the major shrimp allergen Pen a 1 (tropomyosin). *International Archives of Allergy and Immunology* 127(1):27–37.

Ayuso, R., Reese, G., Arruda, L.K., Chapman, M.D., Lehrer, S.B. 2002b. Identification of IgE-binding epitopes in allergenic invertebrate tropomyosins Per a 7, Pen a 1 and Der p 10 with cockroach and shrimp-allergic sera. *Journal of Allergy and Clinical Immunology* 109(1):S94–S94.

Ayuso, R., Reese, G., Leong-Kee, S., Plante, M., Lehrer, S.B. 2002c. Molecular basis of arthropod cross-reactivity: IgE-binding cross-reactive epitopes of shrimp, house dust mite and cockroach tropomyosins. *International Archives of Allergy and Immunology* 129(1):38–48.

Banzet, M.L., Adessi, B., Vuitton, D.A. 1992. Allergic manifestations following eating snails in 12 patients with Acaris allergy—A new crossover allergy. *Revue Francaise D Allergologie Et D Immunologie Clinique* 32(4):198–202.

Barletta, B., Butteroni, C., Puggioni, E.M.R., Iacovacci, P., Afferni, C., Tinghino, R., Ariano, R., Panzani, R.C., Pini, C., Di Felice, G. 2005. Immunological characterization of a recombinant tropomyosin from a new indoor source, *Lepisma saccharina*. *Clinical and Experimental Allergy* 35(4):483–489.

Barletta, B., Di Felice, G., Pini, C. 2007. Biochemical and molecular biological aspects of silverfish allergens. *Protein and Peptide Letters* 14(10):970–974.

Bernstein, M., Day, J.H., Welsh, A. 1982. Double-blind food challenge in the diagnosis of food sensitivity in the adult. *Journal of Allergy and Clinical Immunology* 70:205–210.

Blotzer, I.C., Wuthrich, B. 2004. IgE-mediated food allergies: Classification based on the way of sensitization among 87 patients of the year 1998. *Allergologie* 27(5):191–202.

Byun, M.W., Kim, J.H., Lee, J.W., Park, J.W., Hong, C.S., Kang, I.J. 2000. Effects of gamma radiation on the conformational and antigenic properties of a heat-stable major allergen in brown shrimp. *Journal of Food Protection* 63(7):940–944.

Byun, M.W., Lee, J.W., Yook, H.S., Jo, C.R., Kim, H.Y. 2002. Application of gamma irradiation for inhibition of food allergy. *Radiation Physics and Chemistry* 63(3–6):369–370.

Canberra. 2006. *Australian Fisheries Statistics 2006*. In: Economics ABoAar, editor: Canberra, Australia.

Chenna, R., Sugawara, H., Koike, T., Lopez, R., Gibson, T.J., Higgins, D.G., Thompson, J.D. 2003. Multiple sequence alignment with the Clustal series of programs. *Nucleic Acids Research* 31(13):3497–3500.

Chiang, W.C., Kidon, M.I., Liew, W.K., Gohw, A., Tang, J.P.L., Chay, O.M. 2007. The changing face of food hypersensitivity in an Asian community. *Clinical and Experimental Allergy* 37(7):1055–1061.

Crespo, J.F., Pascual, C., Burks, A.W., Helm, R.M., Esteban, M.M. 1995a. Frequency of food allergy in a pediatric population from Spain. *Pediatric Allergy and Immunology* 6(1):39–43.

Crespo, J.F., Pascual, C., Helm, R., Sanchezpastor, S., Ojeda, I., Romualdo, L., Martinesteban, M., Ojeda, J.A. 1995b. Cross-reactivity of Ige-binding components between boiled Atlantic shrimp and German-cockroach. *Allergy* 50(11):918–924.

Daul, C.B., Morgan, J.E., Hughes, J., Lehrer, S.B. 1988. Provocation-challenge studies in shrimp-sensitive individuals. *Journal of Allergy and Clinical Immunology* 81(6):1180–1186.

Daul, C.B., Morgan, J.E., Lehrer, S.B. 1993. Hypersensitivity reactions to crustacea and mollusks. *Clinical Reviews in Allergy* 11(2):201–222.

Daul, C.B., Slattery, M., Reese, G., Lehrer, S.B. 1994. Identification of the major brown shrimp (Penaeus-Aztecus) allergen as the muscle protein tropomyosin. *International Archives of Allergy and Immunology* 105(1):49–55.

De Besche, A. 1937. On asthma bronchiale in man provoked by cat, dog, and different other animals. *Acta Medica Scandinavica* 42:237–255.

Desjardins, A., Malo, J.L., Larcheveque, J., Cartier, A., Mccants, M., Lehrer, S.B. 1995. Occupational Ige-mediated sensitization and asthma caused by clam and shrimp. *Journal of Allergy and Clinical Immunology* 96(5):608–617.

Fernandes, J., Reshef, A., Patton, L., Ayuso, R., Reese, G., Lehrer, S.B. 2003. Immunoglobulin E antibody reactivity to the major shrimp allergen, tropomyosin, in unexposed Orthodox Jews. *Clinical and Experimental Allergy* 33(7):956–961.

Garcia-Orozco, K.D., Aispuro-Hernandez, E., Yepiz-Plascencia, G., Calderon-de-la-Barca, A.M., Sotelo-Mundo, R.R. 2007. Molecular characterization of arginine kinase, an allergen from the shrimp *Litopenaeus vannamei*. *International Archives of Allergy and Immunology* 144(1):23–28.

Goetz, D.W., Whisman, B.A. 2000. Occupational asthma in a seafood restaurant worker: Cross-reactivity of shrimp and scallops. *Annals of Allergy Asthma & Immunology* 85(6):461–466.

Goh, D.L.M., Lau, Y.N., Chew, F.T., Shek, L.P.C., Lee, B.W. 1999. Pattern of food-induced anaphylaxis in children of an Asian community. *Allergy* 54(1):84–86.

Guarneri, F., Guarneri, C., Benvenga, S. 2007. Cross-reactivity of *Anisakis simplex*: Possible role of Ani s 2 and Ani s 3. *International Journal of Dermatology* 46(2):146–150.

Hamada, Y., Genka, E., Ohira, M., Nagashima, Y., Shiomi, K. 2000. Allergenicity of fish meat paste products and surimi from walleye pollack. *Journal of the Food Hygienic Society of Japan* 41(1):38–43.

Hefle, S.L., Bush, R.K., Lehrer, S.B., Malo, J.L., Cartier, A. 1995. Snow crab allergy—Identification of Ige-binding proteins. *Journal of Allergy and Clinical Immunology* 95(1): 332–332.

Hill, D.J., Hosking, C.S., Zhie, C.Y, Leung, R., Baratwidjaja, K., Iikura, Y., Iyngkaran, N., Gonzalez-Andaya, A., Wah, L.B., Hsieh, K.H. 1997. The frequency of food allergy in Australia and Asia. *Environmental Toxicology and Pharmacology* 4(1–2):101–110.

Hill, D.J., Hosking, C.S., Heine, R.G. 1999. Clinical spectrum of food allergy in children in Australia and South-East Asia: Identification and targets for treatment. *Annals of Medicine* 31(4):272–281.

Hoffman, D.R., Day, E.D., Miller, J.S. 1981. The major heat-stable allergen of shrimp. *Annals of Allergy* 47(1):17–22.

Howse, D., Gautrin, D., Neis, B., Cartier, A., Horth-Susin, L., Jong, M., Swanson, M.C. 2006. Gender and snow crab occupational asthma in Newfoundland and Labrador, Canada. *Environmental Research* 101(2):163–174.

Ishikawa, M., Shimakura, K., Nagashima, Y., Shiomi, K. 1997. Isolation and properties of allergenic proteins in the oyster *Crassostrea gigas*. *Fisheries Science* 63(4):610–614.

Ishikawa, M., Ishida, M., Shimakura, K., Nagashima, Y., Shiomi, K. 1998a. Purification and IgE-binding epitopes of a major allergen in the gastropod *Turbo cornutus*. *Bioscience Biotechnology and Biochemistry* 62(7):1337–1343.

Ishikawa, M., Nagashima, Y., Shiomi. K. 1998b. Identification of the oyster allergen Cra g 2 as tropomyosin. *Fisheries Science* 64(5):854–855.

Ishikawa, M., Nagashima, Y., Shiomi, K. 1999. Immunological comparison of shellfish allergens by competitive enzyme-linked immunosorbent assay. *Fisheries Science* 65(4):592–595.

Jeebhay, M.F., Robins, T.G., Lehrer, S.B., Lopata, A.L. 2001. Occupational seafood allergy: A review. *Occupational and Environmental Medicine* 58(9):553–562.

Jeebhay, M.F., Robins, T.G., Seixas, N., Baatjies, R., George, D.A., Rusford, E., Lehrer, S.B., Lopata, A.L, 2005. Environmental exposure characterization of fish processing workers. *Annals of Occupational Hygiene* 49(5):423–437.

Jeebhay, M.F., Baatjies, R., Chang, Y.S., Kim, Y.K., Kim, Y.Y., Major, V., Lopata, A.L. 2007. Risk factors for allergy due to the two-spotted spider mite (*Tetranychus urticae*) among table grape farm workers. *International Archives of Allergy and Immunology* 144(2):143–149.

Jenkins, J.A., Breiteneder, H., Mills, E.N.C. 2007. Evolutionary distance from human homologs reflects allergenicity of animal food proteins. *Journal of Allergy and Clinical Immunology* 120(6):1399–1405.

Jeong, K.Y., Hong, C.S., Yong, T.S. 2006. Allergenic tropomyosins and their cross-reactivities. *Protein and Peptide Letters* 13(8):835–845.

Johansson, E., Aponno, M., Lundberg, M., van Hage-Hamsten, M. 2001. Allergenic cross-reactivity between the nematode *Anisakis simplex* and the dust mites *Acarus siro*, *Lepidoglyphus destructor*, *Tyrophagus putrescentiae*, and *Dermatophagoides pteronyssinus*. *Allergy* 56(7):660–666.

Kato, Y., Yagami, A., Matsunaga, K. 2005. A case of anaphylaxis caused by the health food chitosan. *Arerugi*:1427–1429.

Lehrer, S.B. 1987. Seafood allergy—Immunological studies of shrimp hypersensitivity. *Southern Medical Journal* 80(9):2–2.

Lehrer, S.B., Mccants, M.L. 1987. Reactivity of Ige antibodies with crustacea and oyster allergens—Evidence for common antigenic structures. *Journal of Allergy and Clinical Immunology* 80(2):133–139.

Lehrer, S.B., Reese, G. 1998. Cross-reactivity between cockroach allergens and arthropod, nematode and mammalian allergens. *Revue Francaise D Allergologie Et D Immunologie Clinique* 38(10):846–850.

Lehrer, S.B., Ibanez, M.D., Mccants, M.L., Daul, C.B. 1988. Shrimp allergy—Identification and fractionation of allergens. *Journal of Allergy and Clinical Immunology* 81(1):189–189.

Lehrer, S.B., Ayuso, R., Reese, G. 2003. Seafood allergy and allergens: A review. *Marine Biotechnology* 5(4):339–348.

Leung, P.S.C., Chu, K.H., Chow, W.K., Ansari, A., Bandea, C.I., Kwan, H.S., Nagy, S.M., Gershwin, M.E. 1994. Cloning, expression, and primary structure of Metapenaeus-Ensis Tropomyosin, the major heat-stable shrimp allergen. *Journal of Allergy and Clinical Immunology* 94(5):882–890.

Leung, P.S.C., Chow, W.K., Duffey, S., Kwan, H.S., Gershwin, M.E., Chu, K.H. 1996. IgE reactivity against a cross-reactive allergen in crustacea and mollusca: Evidence for tropomyosin as the common allergen. *Journal of Allergy and Clinical Immunology* 98(5):954–961.

Leung, P.S.C., Chen, Y.C., Gershwin, M.E., Wong, H., Kwan, H.S., Chu, K.H. 1998a. Identification and molecular characterization of *Charybdis feriatus* tropomyosin, the major crab allergen. *Journal of Allergy and Clinical Immunology* 102(5):847–852.

Leung, P.S.C., Chen, Y.C., Mykles, D.L., Chow, W.K., Li, C.P., Chu, K.H. 1998b. Molecular identification of the lobster muscle protein tropomyosin as a seafood allergen. *Molecular Marine Biology and Biotechnology* 7(1):12–20.

Lin, R.Y., Shen, H.D., Han, S.H. 1993. Identification and characterization of a 30-Kd major allergen from Parapenaeus-Fissurus. *Journal of Allergy and Clinical Immunology* 92(6):837–845.

Li, Z.X., Linhong, C.L., Jamil, K. 2006. Reduction of allergenic properties of shrimp (*Penaeus Vannamei*) allergens by high intensity ultrasound. *European Food Research and Technology* 223(5):639–644.

Li, Z.X., Lin, H., Cao, L.M., Jamil, K. 2007. The influence of gamma irradiation on the allergenicity of shrimp (*Penaeus vannamei*). *Journal of Food Engineering* 79(3):945–949.

Lopata, A.L., Potter, P.C. 2000. Allergy and other adverse reactions to seafood. *Allergy & Clinical Immunology International* 12(6):271–281.

Lopata, A.L., Zinn, C., Potter, P.C. 1997. Characteristics of hypersensitivity reactions and identification of a unique 49 kd IgE-binding protein (Hal-m-1) in abalone (*Haliotis midae*). *Journal of Allergy and Clinical Immunology* 100(5):642–648.

Lopata, A.L., Fenemore, B., Jeebhay, M.F., Gade, G., Potter, P.C. 2005. Occupational allergy in laboratory workers caused by the African migratory grasshopper *Locusta migratoria*. *Allergy* 60(2):200–205.

Marinho, S., Morais-Almeida, M., Gaspar, A., Santa-Marta, C., Pires, G., Postigo, I., Guisantes, J., Martinez, J., Rosado-Pinto, J. 2006. Barnacle allergy: Allergen characterization and cross-reactivity with mites. *Journal of Investigational Allergology and Clinical Immunology* 16(2):117–122.

Marti, P., Truffer, R., Stadler, M.B., Keller-Gautschi, E., Crameri, R., Mari, A., Schmid-Grendelmeier, P., Miescher, S.M., Stadler, B.M., Vogel, M. 2007. Allergen motifs and the prediction of allergenicity. *Immunology Letters* 109(1):47–55.

Martins, L., Peltre, G., Pires, E., Faro, C., Inacio, F. 1999. Allergy to *Helix aspersa* (snail): Characterisation of the allergen repertoire. *Journal of Allergy and Clinical Immunology* 103(1):S104–S104.

Mata, E., Favier, C., Moneretvautrin, D.A., Nicolas, J.P., Ching, L.H., Gueant, J.L. 1994. Surimi and native codfish contain a common allergen identified as a 63-Kda protein. *Allergy* 49(6):442–447.

McCann, D., Barrett, A., Cooper, A., Crumpler, D., Dalen, L., Grimshaw, K., Kitchin, E., Lok, K., Porteous, L., Prince, E., Sonuga-Barke, E., O'Warner, J., Stevenson, 2007. Food additives and hyperactive behaviour in 3-year-old and 8/9-year-old children in the community: A randomised, double-blinded, placebo-controlled trial. *Lancet* 370(9598):1560–1567.

Meyer-Pittroff, R., Behrendt, H., Ring, J. 2007. Specific immuno-modulation and therapy by means of high pressure treated allergens. *High Pressure Research* 27(1):63–67.

Miyazawa, H., Fukamachi, H., Inagaki, Y., Reese, G., Daul, C.B., Lehrer, S.B., Inouye, S., Sakaguchi, M. 1996. Identification of the first major allergen of a squid (*Todarodes pacificus*). *Journal of Allergy and Clinical Immunology* 98(5):948–953.

Motoyama, K., Ishizaki, S., Nagashima, Y., Shiomi, K. 2006. Cephalopod tropomyosins: Identification as major allergens and molecular cloning. *Food and Chemical Toxicology* 44(12):1997–2002.

Motoyama, K., Suma, Y., Ishizaki, S., Nagashima, Y., Shiomi, K. 2007. Molecular cloning of tropomyosins identified as allergens in six species of crustaceans. *Journal of Agricultural and Food Chemistry* 55(3):985–991.

Nakamura, A., Watanabe, K., Ojima, T., Ahn, D.H., Saeki, H. 2005. Effect of Maillard reaction on allergenicity of scallop tropomyosin. *Journal of Agricultural and Food Chemistry* 53(19):7559–7564.

Nakamura, A., Sasaki, F., Watanabe, K., Ojima, T., Ahn, D.H., Saeki, H. 2006. Changes in allergenicity and digestibility of squid tropomyosin during the Maillard reaction with ribose. *Journal of Agricultural and Food Chemistry* 54(25):9529–9534.

Nakano, S., Yoshinuma, T., Yamada, T. 2008. Reactivity of shrimp allergy-related IgE antibodies to krill tropomyosin. *International Archives of Allergy and Immunology* 145(3):175–181.

Nieuwenhuizen, N., Lopata, A.L., Jeebhay, M.L.F., Herbert, D.R., Robins, T.G., Brombacher, F. 2006. Exposure to the fish parasite Anisakis causes allergic airway hyperreactivity and dermatitis. *Journal of Allergy and Clinical Immunology* 117(5):1098–1105.

No, H.K., Meyers, S.P., Prinyawiwatkul, W., Xu, Z. 2007. Applications of chitosan for improvement of quality and shelf life of foods: A review. *Journal of Food Science* 72(5):R87–R100.

Oneil, C.E., Lehrer, S.B. 1995. Seafood allergy and allergens—A review *Food Technology* 49(10):103–116.

Pajno, G.B., La Grutta, S., Barberio, G., Canonica, G.W., Passalacqua, G. 2002. Harmful effect of immunotherapy in children with combined snail and mite allergy. *Journal of Allergy and Clinical Immunology* 109(4):627–629.

Pereira, F., Pereira, C., Lacerda, M.H. 1998. Contact dermatitis due to a cream containing chitin and a carbitol. *Contact Dermatitis* 38(5):290–291.

Peroni, D.G., Piacentini, G.L., Bodini, A., Boner, A.L. 2000. Snail anaphylaxis during house dust mite immunotherapy. *Pediatric Allergy and Immunology* 11(4):260–261.

Petrus, M., Cougnaud, V., Rhabbour, M., Causse, E., Netter, J.C. 1997. Snail and house-dust mite allergy in children. *Archives De Pediatrie* 4(8):767–769.

Petrus, M., Nyunga, M., Causse, E., Chung, E., Cossarizza, G. 1999. Squid and house dust mite allergy in a child. *Archives De Pediatrie* 6(10):1075–1076.

Reese, G., Jeoung, B.J., Daul, C.B., Lehrer, S.B. 1997. Characterization of recombinant shrimp allergen Pen a 1 (Tropomyosin). *International Archives of Allergy and Immunology* 113(1–3):240–242.

Reese, G., Ayuso, R., Lehrer, S.B. 1999. Tropomyosin: An invertebrate pan-allergen. *International Archives of Allergy and Immunology* 119(4):247–258.

Reese, G., Ayuso, R., Leong-Kee, S.M., Plante, M., Lehrer, S.B. 2002. Epitope mapping and mutational substitution analysis of the major shrimp allergen Pen a 1 (tropomyosin). *Journal of Allergy and Clinical Immunology* 109(1):S307–S307.

Reese, G., Viebranz, J., Leong-Kee, S.M., Plante, M., Lauer, I., Randow, S., Moncin, M.S.M., Ayuso, R., Lehrer, S.B., Vieths, S. 2005. Reduced allergenic potency of VR9-1, a mutant of the major shrimp allergen Pen a 1 (tropomyosin). *Journal of Immunology* 175(12):8354–8364.

Reese, G., Schicktanz, S., Lauer, I., Randow, S., Luttkopf, D., Vogel, L., Lehrer, S.B., Vieths, S. 2006. Structural, immunological and functional properties of natural recombinant Pen a 1, the major allergen of Brown Shrimp, *Penaeus aztecus. Clinical and Experimental Allergy* 36(4):517–524.

Roberts G, Golder N, Lack G. 2002. Bronchial challenges with aerosolized food in asthmatic, food-allergic children. *Allergy* 57(8):713–717.

Sakai, S., Matsuda, R., Adachi, R., Akiyama, H., Maitani, T., Ohno, Y., Oka, M., Abe, A., Seiki, K., Oda, H. et al. 2008. Interlaboratory evaluation of two enzyme-linked immunosorbent assay kits for the determination of crustacean protein in processed foods. *Journal of AOAC International* 91(1):123–129.

Sampson, H.A., Ho, D.G. 1997. Relationship between food-specific IgE concentrations and the risk of positive food challenges in children and adolescents. *Journal of Allergy and Clinical Immunology* 100(4):444–451.

Scholl, I., Jensen-Jarolim, E. 2004. Allergenic potency of spices: Hot, medium hot, or very hot. *International Archives of Allergy and Immunology* 135(3):247–261.

Shanti, K.N., Martin, B.M., Nagpal, S., Metcalfe, D.D., Rao, P.V.S. 1993. Identification of Tropomyosin as the major shrimp allergen and characterization of its Ige-binding epitopes. *Journal of Immunology* 151(10):5354–5363.

Sicherer, S.H., Munoz-Furlong, A., Sampson, H.A. 2004. Prevalence of seafood allergy in the United States determined by a random telephone survey. *Journal of Allergy and Clinical Immunology* 114(1):159–165.

Sinanoglou, V.J., Batrinou, A., Konteles, S., Sflomos, K. 2007. Microbial population, physicochemical quality, and allergenicity of molluscs and shrimp treated with cobalt-60 gamma radiation. *Journal of Food Protection* 70(4):958–966.

Smillie, L.B., Pato, M.D., Pearlstone, J.R., Mak, A.S. 1980. Periodicity of alpha-helical potential in tropomyosin sequence correlates with alternating actin binding-sites. *Journal of Molecular Biology* 136(2):199–202.

Suma, Y., Ishizaki, S., Nagashima, Y., Lu, Y., Ushio, H., Shiomi, K. 2007. Comparative analysis of barnacle tropomyosin: Divergence from decapod tropomyosins and role as a potential allergen. *Comparative Biochemistry and Physiology Part B-Biochemistry and Molecular Biology* 147(2):230–236.

Taylor, S.L. 2008. Molluscan shellfish allergy. *Advances in Food and Nutrition Research* 54:139–177.

Taylor, A.V., Swanson, M.C., Jones, R.T., Vives, R., Rodriguez, J., Yunginger, J.W., Crespo, J.F. 2000. Detection and quantitation of raw fish aeroallergens from an open-air fish market. *Journal of Allergy and Clinical Immunology* 105(1):166–169.

Thomas, K., Herouet-Guicheney, C., Ladics, G., Bannon, G., Cockburn, A., Crevel, R., Fitzpatrick, J., Mills, C., Privalle, L., Vieths, S. 2007. Evaluating the effect of food processing on the potential human allergenicity of novel proteins: International workshop report. *Food and Chemical Toxicology* 45(7):1116–1122.

vanRee, R., Antonicelli, L., Akkerdaas, J.H., Garritani, M.S., Aalberse, R.C., Bonifazi, F. 1996a. Possible induction of food allergy during mite immunotherapy. *Allergy* 51(2):108–113.

vanRee, R., Antonicelli, L., Akkerdaas, J.H., Pajno, G.B., Barberio, G., Corbetta, L., Ferro, G., Zambito, M., Garritani, M.S., Aalberse, R.C., Bonifazi, F. 1996b. Asthma after consumption of snails in house-dust-mite-allergic patients: A case of IgE cross-reactivity. *Allergy* 51(6):387–393.

Villacis, J., Rice, T.R., Bucci, L.R., El-Dahr, J.M., Wild, L., DeMerell, D., Soteres, D., Lehrer, S.B. 2006. Do shrimp-allergic individuals tolerate shrimp-derived glucosamine? *Clinical and Experimental Allergy* 36(11):1457–1461.

Whitby, F.G., Phillips, G.N. 2000. Crystal structure of tropomyosin at 7 Angstroms resolution. *Proteins-Structure Function and Genetics* 38(1):49–59.

Wild, L.G., Lehrer, S.B. 2005. Fish and shellfish allergy. *Current Allergy and Asthma Reports* 5(1):74–79.

Witteman, A.M., Akkerdaas, J.H., Vanleeuwen, J., Vanderzee, J.S., Aalberse, R.C. 1994. Identification of a cross-reactive allergen (presumably tropomyosin) in shrimp, mite and insects. *International Archives of Allergy and Immunology* 105(1):56–61.

Wu, A.Y., Williams, G.A. 2004. Clinical characteristics and pattern of skin test reactivities in shellfish allergy patients in Hong Kong. *Allergy and Asthma Proceedings* 25(4):237–242.

Yu, C.J., Lin, Y.F., Chiang, B.L., Chow, L.P. 2003. Proteomics and immunological analysis of a novel shrimp allergen, Pen m 2. *Journal of Immunology* 170(1):445–453.

Zhang, Y., Matsuo, H., Morita, E. 2006. Cross-reactivity among shrimp, crab and scallops in a patient with a seafood allergy. *Journal of Dermatology* 33(3):174–177.

Zinn, C., Lopata, A., Visser, M., Potter, P.C 1997. The spectrum of allergy to South African bony fish (Teleosti)- Evaluation by double-blind, placebo controlled challenge. *South African Medical Journal* 87(2):146–152.

# 10 Nut Allergens

*Agata Szymkiewicz*

## CONTENTS

## 10.1 BACKGROUND

In the United States, an estimated 1%–2% of the population is allergic to peanuts, tree nuts (walnut, Brazil nut, cashew, and hazelnut), or both (Sicherer et al. 2001, 2003). Sicherer et al. (2003) found that self-reported peanut allergy had doubled among children between 1997 and 2002, and peanut allergies, tree nut allergies, or both continued to be reported by more than 3 million Americans. About 20% children outgrow peanut allergy (Skolnick et al. 2001), but tree nut allergy is generally thought to be lifelong and only approximately 9% of patients outgrow it (Fleischer et al., 2005). Allergies to nuts are severe, common, and lasting. Considering that the reactions are severe and the allergy is persistent, this represents an increasing health concern (Sicherer et al. 2003). Hypersensitivity to nuts is usually accompanied by allergy to other foodstuffs or aeroallergens (Arshad and Gant 2001). Typical of nut allergies are very severe anaphylaxis reactions, potentially even fatal, observed both in children and in adults. Nut allergy may be manifested in the form of oral allergy syndrome (OAS) or as rash, asthma fits, rhinitis, nausea, vomiting, upper respiratory tract swelling, or even cerebral symptoms (Pumphrey et al. 1999).

There are about 15 kinds of nuts known to potentially cause allergy. Nuts are defined as dry fruit from more than one pistil; they grow on trees which may be phylogenetically very distant. In the case of peanut, they belong to the *Leguminosae* (*Fabaceae*) family, of almond and pistachio to *Rosaceae*, of Brazil nut to *Lecithidaceae*, and of hazelnut to *Corylaceare* family.

## 10.2 BIOLOGICAL AND IMMUNOLOGICAL PROPERTIES OF MAIN NUT ALLERGENS

### 10.2.1 HAZELNUT ALLERGENS

Hazelnuts are used in a large variety of confectionery foods such as chocolates, nougat cookies, pralines, chopped nuts, nut spreads, and breakfast cereals. Ground hazelnuts can be added to cookies, cakes, and other desserts. Hazelnuts (*Corylus avellana*) make up a significant group of food allergens (Asero et al. 2004) and due to their extensive use in the food industry they may be a source of so-called hidden allergens (Fæste et al. 2006).

Among 383 patients with food allergy, 37% revealed positive reaction to hazelnut (Etesamifar and Wüthrich 1998), and among pollen-allergic patients as much as 53% (Eriksson et al. 1982). In the areas where birch trees are endemic, hazelnut allergy is most often manifested as mild OAS, both in children and in adults (Cudowska and Kaczmarski 2004). However, the route of clinically relevant sensitization to hazelnut in children can be nonpollen related (Flinterman et al. 2006). Children can be sensitized to hazelnut at an early age. In many cases, reactions are very serious and frequently correlated with sensitivity to peanut or other tree nuts (Pumphrey et al. 1999). So far it has not been univocally settled which major allergens, and of which kind of nut, are responsible for the primary sensitization in children with objective reactions to hazelnuts.

In birch pollen-exposed areas, hazelnut allergy has mainly been associated with cross-reactive IgE to birch allergens. The major hazelnut allergen (Cor a 1.04) is Bet-v-1-homologous protein (Breiteneder et al. 1989) as well as a minor 14 kDa hazelnut allergen (Cor a 2) related to birch profilin Bet v 2 (Ebner et al. 1995). Allergen Cor a 1.04 is a monomeric protein with a molecular mass of 18 kDa. The epitopes of hazelnut Cor a 1.04 are less related to hazel pollen allergen—Cor a 1 than to Bet v 1 from birch pollen (Lüttkopf et al. 2001). The isoform of Cor a 1 and Cor a 1.0401 is responsible for the majority of hazelnut allergies (Besler et al. 2001). This allergen is susceptible to protease activity and easily undergoes pepsin hydrolysis (Vieths et al. 1999). Cor a 1.04 is considered particularly as a thermolabile allergen that rapidly became denatured after heating (Schocker et al. 2000; Pastorello et al. 2002). Yet, Hansen et al. (2003) reported that roasting of the nuts at 140°C for 40 min did not completely remove IgE binding but reduced it by a factor of 100.

In areas without birches (the Mediterranean area), severe allergic reactions to hazelnut are more prevalent and linked to sensitization to the lipid transfer protein (LTP), allergen Cor a 8 (Schocker et al. 2004). Similarly, for walnut, LTP (allergen Jug r 3) was designated as the major allergen able to sensitize patients not allergic to pollen (Pastorello et al. 2004). The authors of the most recent studies claim, however, that in the case of children's sensitization to hazelnut, LTP can be a risk factor for objective symptoms in patients from a birch-endemic area (Flinterman et al. 2008). The IgE in patients serum with walnut allergy, which reacted with LTP, could be almost completely inhibited by peach ns-LTP (Asero et al. 2002; Pastorello et al. 2004). Cor a 8 and Jug r 3 have molecular mass of about 9–10 kDa and they are, like most nonspecific LTP, relatively stable against heating and proteolysis (Asero et al. 2000; Wigotzki et al. 2000; Pastorello et al. 2002).

Other important allergens occurring in hazelnut are proteins with molecular mass of 47, 32, and 35 kDa (Pastorello et al. 2002). The 35 kDa allergen, determined as Cor a 9, belongs to the *Cupin* family and is an acid subunit of 11S seed storage globulin with molecular mass of ca. 360 kDa. Conformational analysis revealed that consensual surface-exposed IgE-binding epitopes Cor a 9 exhibited some susceptible structural homology to account for IgE-binding cross-reactivity observed among other tree nut allergens (Jug r 4 of walnut, Ana o 2 of cashew nut) and peanut allergen Ara h 3 (Barre et al. 2007). Cross-reactivity between nut legumin allergens is described in greater detail in Chapter 11.7.2 concerning peanut allergy.

## 10.2.2  OTHER NUT ALLERGENS

Major walnut and Brazil nut allergens are 2S—albumins, Jug r 1, and Ber e 1 (9 kDa), respectively. They exhibit a 46.1% identity. Jug r 1 is an heterodimer composed of a large and a small subunit joined by disulfide bridges. Posttranslational processing of the 142 amino acids long precursor results in the two subunits, like in Brazil nut 2S albumin. Allergens from this group occur also in peanut (Ara h 2, 6, and 7) (Barre et al. 2005). 2S albumin proteins are a major allergen in cashew nut and this is a possible basis for cross-reactivity with walnut since Ana o 3 and Jug r 1 share an epitope with high sequence identity. One strongly reactive Ana o 3 epitope overlapped in amino acid position with the lone linear epitope of the large subunit of the English walnut allergen (Jug r 1) with which it shares considerable homology (81% similarity) (Robotham et al. 2005). All five amino acids, found to be critical or influential for IgE binding to the Jug r 1 epitope (Robotham et al. 2002), were conserved in Ana o 3 (100% similarity and 80% identity) (Robotham et al. 2005). MALDI–TOF mass spectroscopy of native Ana o 3 yielded molecular mass of 12 598 Da. Three native Ana o 3 large-subunit isoforms with molecular masses ranging from approximately 6 to 10 kDa were identified (Robotham et al. 2005). Linear epitope mapping revealed 16 immunreactive peptides, 4 of which produced strong signals. At least 8 linear epitopes were identified on the peptides. Some Ana o 3 epitopes shared positional overlapping with the IgE-binding regions of mustard and sesame 2S albumins (Robotham et al. 2005).

2S albumins are typically heterodimeric proteins with small and large subunits linked by disulfide bonds and they tend to be relatively resistant to denaturation and proteolysis. Moreno et al. (2005) reported that 2S albumin was very resistant to pepsin digestion under conditions simulating human gastric conditions. The intact protein as well as a fragment of over 6 kDa was observed after 2 h of digestion. The native and recombinant Ber e 1 were stable to digestion in simulated gastric fluid for over 15 min, with no fragments visible after 30 min (Alcocer et al. 2002; Murtagh et al. 2003). Ber e 1 retained its high resistance to digestion even following heating (100°C, 20 min) and cooling but reduction made Ber e 1 more susceptible to pepsin digestion (Koppelman et al. 2005; Moreno et al. 2005).

Albumins 2S occur in large quantities in nuts and they show high affinity of amino acid sequence; these proteins demonstrate a possible basis for cross-reactivity with tree nuts and peanuts or other seeds. IgE-binding epitopes of Ara h 2 are very similar to those present in the proteins of almond and Brazil nut, which may account for the high degree of sensitivity to nut of patients with peanut allergy (de Leon et al. 2007). This kind of cross-reactivity is described in greater detail in the chapter on peanut allergens.

Allergenic storage proteins of 2S type are also most likely to be responsible for cross-reactivity between nuts and sesame seeds. Sesame seeds contain ca. 20% protein of which 2S albumins make almost a quarter (Rajendran and Prakash 1988).

The 2S albumin precursor (β-globulin; accession no AF091841) was identified as the major sesame allergen, whereas the 11S globulin (α-globulin) was identified as a minor allergen (Beyer et al., 2002). These two storage sesame proteins serve as a source of amino acid during germination of seeds (Tai et al. 1999). It was shown that sesame allergen Ses i 2 has 38% homology to the walnut allergen Jug r 1, 40% homology to the Brazil nut Bre e 1, and 34% homology to the peanut allergen Ara h 2 (Beyer et al. 2002). It was identified as a peptide containing 71 amino acids (peptide B) that was the only fragment of sesame β-globulin that reacted positively in the dot-blot test with the serum samples which showed positive results in the Western blot with intact β-globulin. In this IgE-binding region of β-globulin identified at least nine different IgE-recognition sites and three of them appeared to be immunodominant IgE-binding epitopes (Wolff et al. 2004).

Sesame seeds commonly added to food become an increasingly frequent cause of allergic reactions in children and adults. Apart from the above described allergens recently there have been identified two important sesame seed allergens: two oleosins (Ses i 4 and Ses i 5) (Leduc et al. 2006) and Ses i 6 and Ses i 7, belonging to the 11S globulins (Beyer et al. 2007).

In contrast to tree nuts allergy (hazelnut, walnut, cashew, and Brazil nut), the chestnut allergy has been almost exclusively considered in the context of the latex-fruit syndrome. Class I chitinase with a hevein-like domain (Cas s 5) is considered to be the major chestnut allergen. Class I chitinase allergens are responsible for cross-reaction between chestnut (Cas s 5), avocado (Pers a1), banana (Mus a 1) and latex (Hev b 6.02). These allergens would be destroyed by boiling, but might survive digestion (Sánchez-Monge et al. 2000; Diaz-Perales et al. 2003). In chestnut allergy not linked to the latex-fruit syndrome an important role may be played by the allergen Cas s 8 (Sánchez-Monge et al. 2006) that belongs to nonspecific lipid transfer proteins (nsLTPs). It has also been reported to act as plant defense protein against bacterial and fungal infections and to form the PR14 family of pathogenesis related proteins.

## 10.3 CROSS-REACTIVITY OF NUT ALLERGENS

Despite the fact that tree nut allergy is often correlated with peanut allergy, it is still difficult to decide whether it follows from a specific response to the allergens which cross-bind to IgE or from hypersensitivity of a group of individuals who develop IgE-type response against nonrelated food allergens. A risk of cross-sensitization of peanut-sensitized individuals following intake of tree nuts and vice versa most likely results from the presence of allergenic glycoallergens like 2S albumins (Ara h 2 of peanut, Jug r 1 of walnut) or legumins (Ara h 3 of peanut, Cor a 9 of hazelnut) (Beardslee et al. 2000; de Leon et al. 2007) but it may also follow from the presence of vicilin allergens (Barre et al. 2008). The vicilin allergens of peanut–Ara h 1, hazelnut Cor a 11, walnut Jug r 2, and cashew nut (Ana o 1) share a very similar amino acid sequence, especially at their very C-termini, where most of the minor IgE-binding epitopes are concentrated (Burks et al. 1997; Shin et al. 1998). Most of the identified IgE-binding epitopes sharing similar amino acid sequences are rather well exposed on the surface of homotrimers, but they may actually be partly masked by, for instance, the extra-loop occurring in these allergens. As storage proteins allergenic seed vicilins occur in the form of glycoproteins (Kolarich and Altmann 2000; Lauer et al. 2004). The modeled N-glycans of Ara h 1 and other vicilins freely stand out of the molecular surface of homotrimers due to which they are more exposed than the respective peptide epitopes binding IgE. Most likely they play the role of conformational epitopes (glycol-epitopes), which may in part, account for the cross-reactivity between vicilin allergens of nuts. Glyco-epitopes may also mask epitopes binding IgE and lower their capability of reacting with antibodies (Barre et al. 2008). Vicilin allergens can be structurally changed not only by glycol-peptides but also by cross-reacting carbohydrate determinants (CCD) (Mari et al. 1999). Therefore, besides the serological aspect of the cross-reactivity between peanut and tree nuts, the clinical relevance of cross-reacting IgE in allergic individuals still remain to be resolved (van Ree 2004). The contradictions observed between cross-reactivity and cross-allergenicity which are responsible for the differences between patients sensitive but without clinical reactivity and allergic patients are so difficult to explain since they follow from many different factors such as the level of synthesized IgE, polymorphism of the FcɛRI receptors, balance of T regulatory cells, Th1/Th2 cells, etc. (Sicherer 2002; Bousquet et al. 2006).

## REFERENCES

Alcocer, M.J., Murtagh, G.J., Bailey, K. et al. 2002. The disulphide mapping, folding and characterisation of recombinant Ber e 1, an allergenic protein, and SFA8, two sulphur-rich 2S plant albumins. *J Mol Biol* 324:165–175.

Arshad, S.H. and Gant, C. 2001. Allergy to nuts: How much of a problem really is this? *Clin Exp Allergy* 31:5–7.

Asero, R., Mistrello, G., Roncarolo, D. et al. 2000. Lipid transfer protein: A pan-allergen in plant-derived foods that is highly resistant to pepsin digestion. *Int Arch Allergy Immunol* 122:20–32.

Asero, R., Mistrello, G., Roncarolo, D. et al. 2002. Immunological cross-reactivity between lipid transfer proteins from botanically unrelated plant-derived foods: A clinical study. *Allergy* 57:900–906.

Asero, R., Mistrello, G., Roncarolo, D., and Amato, S. 2004. Walnut-induced anaphylaxis with cross-reactivity to hazelnut and Brazil nut. *J Allergy Clin Immunol* 113:358–360.

Barre, A., Borges, J.P., Culerrier, R., and Rouge, P. 2005. Homology modelling of the major peanut allergen Ara h 2 and surface mapping of IgE-binding epitopes. *Immunol Lett* 100:153–158.

Barre, A., Jacquet, G., Sordet, C., Culerrier, R., and Rougé, P. 2007. Homology modelling and conformational analysis of IgE-binding epitopes of Ara h 3 and other legumin allergens with a cupin fold from tree nuts. *Mol Immunol* 44:3243–3255.

Barre, A., Sordet, C., Culerrier, R., Rance, F., Didier, A., and Rouge, P. 2008. Vicilin allergens of peanut and tree nuts (walnut, hazelnut, and cashew nut) share structurally related IgE-binding epitopes. *Mol Immunol* 45:1231–1240.

Beardslee, T.A., Zeece, M.G., Sarath, G., and Markwell, J.P. 2000. Soybean glycinin G1 acidic chain shares IgE epitopes with peanut allergen Ara h 3. *Int Arch Allergy Immunol* 123:299–307.

Besler, M., Steinhart, H., and Paschke, A. 2001. Stability of food allergenicity of processed foods-review. *J Chromatography B* 756:207–228.

Beyer, K., Bardina, L., Grishina, G., and Sapmson, H.A. 2002. Identification of sesame seed allergens by 2-dimensional proteomics and Edman sequencing: Seed storage proteins as common food allergens. *J Allergy Clin Immunol* 110:154–159.

Beyer, K., Grishina, G., Bardina, L., and Sampson, H.A. 2007. Identification of 2 new sesame seed allergens: Ses i 6 and Ses i 7. *J Allergy Clin Immunol* 119:1554–1556.

Bousquet, J., Anto, J.M., Bachert C. et al. 2006. Factors responsible for differences between asymptomatic subjects and patients presenting an IgE sensitization to allergens. A GA(2)LEN project. *Allergy* 61:671–680.

Breiteneder, H., Pettenburger, K., Bito, A. et al. 1989. The gene coding for the major birch pollen allergen Bet v 1 is highly homologous to a pea disease resistance response gene. *EMBO J* 8:1935–1938.

Burks, A.W., Shin, D., Cockrell, G., Stanley, J.S., Helm, R.M., and Bannon, G.A. 1997. Mapping and mutational analysis of the IgE-binding epitopes on Ara h 1, a legume vicilin protein and a major allergen in peanut hypersensitivity. *Eur J Biochem* 245:334–339.

Cudowska, B. and Kaczmarski, M. 2004. Diagnostic value of birch recombinant allergens (rBet v 1, profili r Bet v 2) in children with pollen-related food allergy. *Rocz Akad Med Bialymst* 49:111–115.

de Leon, M.P., Drew, A.C., Glaspole, I.N., Suphioglu, C., O'hehir, R.E., and Rolland, J.M. 2007. IgE cross-reactivity between the major peanut allergen Ara h 2 and tree nut allergens. *Mol Immunol* 44:463–471.

Diaz-Perales, A., Blanco, C., Sánchez-Monge, R., Varela, J., Carrillo, T., and Salcedo, G. 2003. Analysis of avocado allergen (Prs a 1) IgE-binding peptides generated by simulated gastric fluid digestion. *J Allergy Clin Immunol* 112:1002–1007.

Ebner, C., Hirschwehr, R., Bauer, L. et al. 1995. Identification of allergens in fruits and vegetables: IgE cross-reactivities with the important birch pollen allergens Bet v 1 and Bet v 2 (birch profilin). *J Allergy Clin Immunol* 95:962–969.

Eriksson, N.E., Formgren, H., and Svenonius, E. 1982. Food hypersensitivity in patients with pollen allergy. *Allergy* 37:437–443.

Etesamifar, M. and Wüthrich, B. 1998. IgE-vertmittele Nahrungs-mittelallergien bei 383 Patienten unter Berücksichtigung des oralen Allergie Syndroms. *Allergologie* 21:451–457.

Fæste, C.K., Holden, L., Plassen, C., and Almli, B. 2006. Sensitive time-resolved fluoroimmunoassay for the detection of hazelnut (*Corylus avellana*) protein traces in food matrices. *J Immunol Methods* 314:114–122.

Fleischer, D.M., Conover-Walker, M.K., Matsui, E.C., and Wood, R.A. 2005. The natural history of tree nut allergy. *J Allergy Clin Immunol* 116:1087–1093.

Flinterman, A.E., Hoekstra, M.O., Meijer, Y. et al. 2006. Clinical reactivity to hazelnut in children: Association with sensitization to birch pollen or nuts? *J Allergy Clin Immunol* 118:1186–1189.

Flinterman, A.E., Akkerdaas, J.H., Jager, C.F.D.H. et al. 2008. Lipid transfer protein-linked hazelnut allergy in children from a non-Mediterranean birch-endemic area. *J Allergy Clin Immunol* 121:423–428.

Hansen, K.S., Ballmer-Weber, B.K., Lüttkopf, D. et al. 2003. Roasted hazelnuts-allergenic activity evaluated by double-blind, placebo-controlled food challenge. *Allergy* 58: 132–138.

Kolarich, D. and Altmann, F. 2000. N-glycan analysis by matrix-assisted laser desorption/ionization mass spectrometry of electrophoretically separated nonmammalian proteins: Application to peanut allergen Ara h 1 and olive pollen allergen Ole e 1. *Anal Biochem* 285:64–75.

Koppelman, S.J., Nieuwenhuizen, W.F., Gaspari, M. et al. 2005. Reversible denaturation of Brazil nut 2S albumin (Ber e1) and implication of structural destabilization on digestion by pepsin. *J Agric Food Chem* 53:123–131.

Lauer, I., Foetisch, K., Kolarich, D. et al. 2004. Hazelnut (*Corylus avellana*) vicilin Cor a 11: Molecular characterization of a glycoprotein and its allergenic activity. *Biochem J* 383:327–334.

Leduc, V., Moneret-Vautrin, D.A., Tzen, J.T.C., Morisset, M., Guerin, L., and Kanny, G. 2006. Identification of oleosins as major allergens in sesame seed allergic patients. *Allergy* 61:349–356.

Lüttkopf, D., Müller, U., Skov, P.S. et al. 2001. Comparison of four variants of the major allergen in hazelnut (*Corylus avellana*) Cor a 1.04 with the major hazel pollen allergen Cor a 1.01. *Mol Immunol* 38:515–525.

Mari, A., Iacovacci, P., Afferni, C. et al. 1999. Specific IgE to cross-reactive carbohydrate determinants strongly affect the in vitro diagnosis of allergic diseases. *J Allergy Clin Immunol* 103:1005–1011.

Moreno, F.J., Mellon, F.A., Wickham, M.S., Bottrill, A.R., and Mills, E.N.C. 2005. Stability of the major allergen Brazil nut 2S albumin (Ber e 1) to physiologically relevant in vitro gastrointestinal digestion. *FEBS J* 272:341–352.

Murtagh, G.J., Archer, D.B., Dumoulin, M. et al. 2003. In vitro stability and immunoreactivity of the native and recombinant plant food 2S albumins Ber e 1 and SFA-8. *Clin Exp Allergy* 33:1147–1152.

Pastorello, E.A., Vieths, S., Pravettoni, V. et al. 2002. Identification of hazelnut major allergens in sensitive patients with positive double-blind, placebo-controlled food challenge results. *J Allergy Clin Immunol* 109:563–570.

Pastorello, A.E., Farioli, L., Pravettoni, V. et al. 2004. Lipid transfer protein and vicilin are important walnut allergens in patients not allergic to pollen. *J Allergy Clin Immunol* 114:908–914.

Pumphrey, R.S.H., Wilson, P.B., Faragher, E.B., and Edwards, S.R. 1999. Specific immunoglobulin E to peanut, hazelnut, and Brazil nut in 731 patients: Similar patterns found at all ages. *Clin Exp Allergy* 29:1256–1259.

Rajendran, S. and Prakash, V. 1988. Isolation and characterization of β-globulin low molecular weight protein fraction from sesame seeds (*Sesamum indicum*). *J Allergy Clin Immunol* 36:269–275.

Robotham, J.M., Teuber, S.S., Sathe, S.K., and Roux, K.H. 2002. Linear IgE epitope mapping of the English walnut (*Juglans regia*) major food allergen, Jug r 1. *J Allergy Clin Immunol* 109:143–149.

Robotham, J.M., Wang, F., Seamson, V. et al. 2005. Ana o 3, an important cashew nut (Anacardium occidental L) allergen of the 2S albumin family. *J Allergy Clin Immunol* 115:1284–1290.

Sánchez-Monge, R., Blanco, C., Perales, A.D. et al. 2000. Class I chitinases, the panallergens responsible for the latex-fruit syndrome, are induced by ethylene treatment and inactivated by heating. *J Allergy Clin Immunol* 106:190–195.

Sánchez-Monge, R., Blanco, C., López-Torrejón, G. et al. 2006. Differential allergen sensitization patterns in chestnut allergy with or without associated latex-fruit syndrome. *J Allergy Clin Immunol* 118:705–710.

Schocker, F., Lüttkopf, D., Müller, U., Thomas, P., Vieths, S., and Becker, W.M. 2000. IgE binding to unique hazelnut allergens: Identification of non pollen-related and heat-stable hazelnut allergens eliciting severe allergic reactions. *Eur J Nutr* 39:172–180.

Schocker, F., Lüttkopf, D., Scheurer, S. et al. 2004. Recombinant lipid transfer protein Cor a 8 form hazelnut: A new tool for in vitro diagnosis of potentially severe hazelnut allergy. *J Allergy Clin Immunol* 113:141–147.

Shin, D.S., Compadre, C.M., Maleki, S.J. et al. 1998. Biochemical and structural analysis of the IgE binding sites on Ara h 1, an abundant and highly allergenic peanut protein. *J Biol Chem* 273:13753–13759.

Sicherer, S.H. 2002. Food allergy. *Lancet* 360:701–710.

Sicherer, S.H., Furlong, T.J., Muñoz-Furlong, A., Burks, A.W., and Sampson, H.A. 2001. A voluntary registry for peanut and tree nut allergy: Characteristics of the first 5149 registrants. *J Allergy Clin Immunol* 108:128–132.

Sicherer, S.H., Muñoz-Furlong, A., Burks, A.W., and Sampson, H.A. 2003. Prevalence of pea-
    nut and tree nut allergy in the United States determined by means of random digit dial
    telephone survey. A 5-year follow-up study. *J Allergy Clin Immunol* 112:1203–1207.
Skolnick, H.S., Conover-Walker, M.K. Koerner, C.B., Sampson, H.A., Burks, A.W., and
    Wood, R.A. 2001. The natural history of peanut allergy. *J Allergy Clin Immunol*
    107:367–374.
Tai, S.S.K., Wu, L.S.H., Chen, E.C.F., and Tzen, J.T.C. 1999. Molecular cloning of 11S glonu-
    lin and 2S albumin, the two major seed storage proteins in sesame. *J Agric Food Chem*
    47:4932–4938.
van Ree, R. 2004. Clinical importance of cross-reactivity in food allergy. *Curr Opin Allergy
    Clin Immunol* 4:235–240.
Vieths, S., Reindl, J., Müeller, U., Hoffmann, A., and Haustein, D. 1999. Digestibility of pea-
    nut and hazelnut allergens investigated by a simple in vitro procedure. *Eur Food Res
    Technol* 209:379–388.
Wigotzki, M., Steinhart, H., and Paschke, A. 2000. Influence of varieties, storage and heat
    treatment on IgE-binding proteins in hazelnuts (Corylus avellana). *Food Agric Immunol*
    12:217–229.
Wolff, N., Yannai, S., Karin, N. et al. 2004. Identification and characterization of linear B-cell
    epitopes of β-globulin, a major allergen of sesame seeds. *J Allergy Clin Immunol*
    114:1151–1158.

# 11 Peanut (*Arachis hypogea*) Allergens

*Agata Szymkiewicz*

## CONTENTS

## 11.1 BACKGROUND

Peanut (*Arachis hypogea*) belongs to the Papilionacea family of the Fabales order, which also includes pea, bean, soybean, lupine, chickpea, and lentil (Duranti and Gius 1997, Makri et al. 2005).

In developed countries, peanut allergy affects about 0.4%–0.6% of children and 0.3%–0.7% of adults (Emmett et al. 1999, Sicherer et al. 1999) with increased prevalence (Sicherer et al.2003, Burks 2008). A cohort of children 4–5 years old (born between 1999 and 2000) from the United Kingdom have a rate of peanut allergy of 1.8% (Hourihane et al. 2007). There has been an increase in the observed incidence of peanut allergies in children over the recent years, which is thought to be the result of the growing popularity and use of peanut products by the population and the introduction of peanut products to children's diets at an early age (Burks 2003). Exposure to the peanut allergen is not easy to control in a pediatric population (Yu et al. 2006). Peanuts are generally eaten as snacks, after roasting, and are frequently components of snack bars, chocolates, and breakfast cereals; they are also often found in the Oriental (Chinese or Indian) cuisine (Furlong et al. 2001, Pomés et al. 2003, 2004). Studies indicate that ca. 1.5 million Americans suffer from allergy to peanut and every year about 30,000 patients are hospitalized due to symptoms of anaphylactic shock, of which 150–200 cases turn out to be fatal (Sampson 2003). Allergic reaction to peanut can be immediate (anaphylactic shock) or may occur after several hours. In majority of cases, allergic reactions are observed after taking peanuts, though in some cases the reaction may be triggered by saliva (kissing, utensils) (Maloney et al. 2006) or allergen inhaling (Kilanowski et al. 2006). It was proven that the main peanut allergen Ara h 1 is relatively easily cleaned from hands and tabletops with common cleaning agents and does not appear to be widely distributed in preschools or schools (Perry et al. 2004).

## 11.2  CHARACTERISTIC OF THE MOST IMPORTANT PEANUT ALLERGENS

Allergy to peanut is caused by proteins in the kernel. Like all seeds, peanuts are rich in protein, in particular the so-called storage proteins that serve as "source material" during the growth of a new plant. Some of these storage proteins have been shown to be the most important allergens: vicilins and albumins.

So far 9 (10) allergens have been identified in peanut. The major peanut allergen is Ara h 1, which is a vicilin; the other major allergen is Ara h 2 (2S albumin). These two allergens are the cause of 95% of peanut allergy reactions (Long 2002). Minor peanut allergens are arachin (legumin)—Ara h 3 and Ara h 4, profilin—Ara h 5, 2S albumins—Ara h 6 and Ara h 7, oleosin, agglutinin, and Ara h 8 (the Bet v 1 family). Sensitization to peanut generally occurs during infancy and very often persists throughout life. In this respect, peanut allergy differs from other current food allergies, e.g., to milk or egg proteins, which prevail in children but usually vanish in adults (Barre et al. 2005a).

The major peanut allergen Ara h 1, also known as conarachin, belongs to seed storage globulins. It is a 65 kDa glycoprotein with high mannose and complex N-glycans (van Ree et al. 2000) with acidic isoelectric point. Ara h 1, identified as a major peanut allergen in 1991 (Burks et al. 1991), and recombinant Ara h 1 were produced in 1995 (Burks et al. 1995). Ara h 1 is a homotrimeric protein belonging to the cupin superfamily, which contains structurally related proteins (vicilins) (Burks et al. 1994): phaseolin from kidney bean, canavalin from Jack bean, germin from barley or proglycinin from soybean (Lawrence et al. 1994, Ko et al. 2000, Woo et al. 2000, Adachi et al. 2001). The modeled vicilin monomers Ara h 1 consist of a cupin motif made of two tandemly arrayed modules related by a pseudodyad-axis. Each module consists of a $\tilde{\beta}$ barrel core domain built from two walls of antiparallel $\beta\alpha$-sheet associated to a loop domain which predominantly contains $\alpha$-helices. An $\alpha$-helix-containing linker region interconnects the two modules. The three cupin motifs of vicilin are putatively arranged in a homotrimeric structure around a threefold symmetry axis. (Barre et al. 2005b). Hydrophobic interactions were determined to be the main molecular force holding monomers together. Hydrophobic amino acids that contribute to trimer formation are at the distal ends of the three-dimensional structure where monomer–monomer contacts occur. The majority of the IgE-binding epitopes are also located in this region suggesting that they may be protected from digestion by the monomer–monomer contacts. On incubation of Ara h 1 with digestive enzymes, various protease-resistant fragments containing IgE-binding sites were identified. The highly stable nature of the Ara h 1 trimer, the presence of digestion-resistant fragments, and the strategic location of the IgE-binding epitopes indicate that the quaternary structure of protein may play a significant role in overall allergenicity (Shin et al. 1998, Maleki et al. 2000b).

Burks et al. (1997), using pooled serum IgE from a population of peanut-hypersensitive individuals, mapped 23 linear IgE-binding epitopes of Ara h 1. They found the following to be immunodominant epitopes: Ara h 1 25–34 (KSSPYQKK), Ara h 1 65–74 (EYDPRLVY), Ara h 1 89–98 (ERTRGRQP), and Ara h 1 498–507 (RRYTARLKEG). The other IgE epitopes identified were: Ara h 1 48–57 (QEPDDLKQKA), Ara h 1 89–98 (ERTRGRQP), Ara h 1 97–105 (GDYDDDRR), Ara h 1 107–116 (RREEGGRW), Ara h 1 123–132 (EREEDWRQ), Ara h 1 134–143 (EDWRRPSHQQ), Ara h 1 143–152 (PRKIRPEG), Ara h 1 294–303 (PGQFEDFF), Ara h 1 311–320 (YLQEFSRN), Ara h 1 325–334 (FNAEFNEIRR), Ara h 1 344–353 (QEERGQRR), Ara h 1 393–402 (DITNPINLRE), Ara h 1 409–418 (NNFGKLFEVK), Ara h 1 461–470 (GNLELV), Ara h 1 525–534 (ELHLLGFGIN), Ara h 1 539–548 (HRIFLAGDKDA), Ara h 1 551–560 (IDQIEKQAKDA), Ara h 1 559–568 (KDALAFPGSGE), Ara h 1 578–587 (KESHFVSARP), and Ara h 1 597–606 (EKESPEKED).

Shreffler et al. (2004) used an array of 213, 20 amino acid peptides with a 5-residue overlap from the sequences of Ara h 1, Ara h 2, and Ara h 3. They found that Ara h 1 contained 13 prominent IgE-binding regions including a new epitope comprising residues 361–385, which could not be found using pooled sera. However, they observed that no single epitope was recognized by more than 35% of their 77 individual peanut-allergic sera.

Another significant allergen identified in peanuts is Ara h 2. It is a glycoprotein with molecular mass of 17–19 kDa and isoelectric point pI of 5.2 (Burks et al. 1992). Currently, two isoforms of Ara h 2 have been identified (Chatel et al. 2003). Ara h 2 corresponds to delta conglutin, a member of the 2S albumin family. Homology-based molecular modeling of Ara h 2 and other 2S albumin allergens showed that they shared a common three-dimensional structural scaffold made of five α-helices arranged in a right-handed superhelix and connected by more or less extended loops. The three-dimensional fold is stabilized by disulphide bridges, which are conserved among all members of the 2S albumin superfamily (Clement et al. 2005). Ara h 2 readily differs from other 2S albumins by two additional loops at the N- and C-terminal ends of the polypeptide chain, respectively (Barre et al. 2005a).

Stanley et al. (1997) defined 10 linear epitopes of Ara h 2 as follows: 15-HASARQQWEL-24, 21-QWELQGDR-28, 27-DRRCQSQLER-36, 39-LRPCEQH LMQ-48, 49-KIQRDEDS-56, 59-RDPYSP-64, 65-SQDPYSPS-72, 118-LQGRQQ-122, 127-KRELRN-132, 143-QRCDLDVE-150.

The epitopes showed a fairly good exposure on the molecular surface of the three-dimensional model, but conformational analysis of the linear epitopes showed no structural homology of Ara h 2 with the corresponding regions of the other tree nut allergens (Barre et al. 2005a). It is suggested that the allergenic cross-reactivity observed between peanut and nut allergens depended on another ubiquitous seed storage protein, namely vicilin (Barre et al. 2005a). However, the latest studies using recombinant allergen Ara h 2 indicate that IgE specific for this peanut allergen cross-reacts with the proteins present in almond and Brazilian nut (de Leon et al. 2007). As an *in vitro* correlate of clinical reactivity, the basophil activation assay was used to demonstrate the biological activity of the recombinant form of Ara h 2 preparation, which demonstrates that Ara h 2 shares common IgE-binding epitopes with some tree nut allergens. Most likely, they are spatial epitopes which were not considered in the studies by Barre et al. (2005a). The presence of these common IgE-binding epitopes may contribute to the prevalence of cosensitization to peanut and tree nuts in peanut-allergic individuals (de Leon et al. 2007).

Ara h 1 and Ara h 2 are the most potent peanut allergens. Sera from over 90% peanut-allergic patients bound these proteins during immunoblotting (Burks et al. 1998). In general, *in vitro* studies with immunoblotting show that purified Ara h 1 binds IgE of subjects sensitive to peanut more strongly than Ara h 2. Nevertheless, it was demonstrated that Ara h 2 was functionally more potent and more relevant than Ara h 1 for most peanut-allergic patients on the basis of *in vitro* assay of specific IgE and ability to induce histamine release in basophils in allergic subjects (Koppelman et al. 2004, Palmer et al. 2005).

The remaining allergens occurring in peanuts are less significant. Two of them are Ara h 3 and Ara h 4, whose sequences are identical in 91% but which were named independently (normally, these would be named isoallergens). These allergens are seed storage proteins that belong to the 11S cupin superfamily.

The 11S storage globulin of peanut, named arachin is an oligomer with molecular mass of about 360 kDa. Like other legumins and glycinins, it is synthesized as approximately 60 kDa polypeptide chains, which form trimers. On the cleavage into 40 kDa N-terminal acid subunits and 20 kDa C-terminal basic subunits that remain disulphide linked, the trimers form a hexamer. An acidic and basic chain in the subunit are separated by a conserved Asn–Gly peptide bond. It is likely that arachin is, like other globulin storage proteins, thermostable.

Ara h 3 was originally identified as a glycinin. However, it turned out that this 14 kDa protein was a processed form of Ara h 3 following the translation of the expected whole protein (Eigenmann et al. 1996, Burks et al. 1998). Recently it is assumed that Ara h 3 contains a number of polypeptides which on SDS-PAGE of protein nut extract are visible within the molecular mass range of 14–45 kDa (Koppelman et al. 2003). The three-dimensional models built from the x-ray coordinates of the A3B4 glycinin soybean (PDB code 1OD5) performed for Ara h 3 and other legume allergens of nuts (Ana o 2, Bre e 1, Cor a 9, and Jug r 4) demonstrated that all these allergens contain a cupin motif made of two tandemly arrayed modules related by a pseudodyad-axis. In each module, two walls of antiparallel β-strands forming the core structure of the module associate to an extended loop containing three α-helices. Both modules are connected by a linker region made of two short stretches of α-helix to form the legumin protomer (Barre et al. 2007). The three-cupin motifs form a prism-shaped homotrimer similar to that in other legumes.

Rabjohn et al. (1999) reported four critical IgE-binding epitopes (IETWN PNNQEFECAG 33–47, GNIFSGFTPEFLEQA 240–254, VTVRGGLRILSPDRK 279–293, DEDEYEYDEEDRRRG 303–317) that were all in the N-terminal region of Ara h 3 and thus in the acid 40 kDa subunit. A recent study has shown that a basic subunit of Ara h 3 contains dominant immunoreactivity (Restani et al. 2005). Ara h 3 exhibits 62%–72% sequence identity with soybean and pea homologs (Rabjohn et al. 1999). Kang and Gallo (2007) found that Ara h 3 had higher amino acid sequence homology with soybean and other LegA proteins than with soybean G4 and other 11S globulin proteins. The epitope that binds cross-reactive peanut and soybean

IgE has been reported as SGFTPEFLEQAFQVD (Ara h 3 244–258) by Xiang et al. (2002).

Conformation analysis showed that the surface-exposed IgE-binding epitopes Ara h 3 exhibited some structural homology susceptible to account for the IgE-binding cross-reactivity observed among peanut and tree nut allergens (Jug r 4 of walnut, Cor a 9 of hazelnut, Ana o 2 of cashew nut). IgE-binding epitopes similar to these found in the 11S globulin allergens do not apparently occur in other vicilin allergens with the cupin-fold from peanut (Ara h 1) or nuts (Jug r 2 of walnut, Cor a 1 of hazelnut, Ana o 3 of cashew nut) (Barre et al. 2007).

Ara h 5 is a peanut allergen with molecular mass of 14 kDa and high thermostability. This minor allergen is an actin-binding protein of the cytoskeleton (Kleber-Janke et al. 1999) and it corresponds to the well-known plant allergen called profilin; it shows up to 80% of amino acid sequence identified in other profilins. Kleber-Janke et al. (2001) found that peanut profilin cross-reacted with profilin of cherry (Pru a 4) and less strongly with pear and celery profilins, whereas birch pollen profilin (Bet v 2) was not able to inhibit IgE-binding to peanut profilin. The Ara h 5 sequence shows an 83% identity with soybean Gly m 3. Recombinant peanut profilin was purified from *E. coli* using a poly-L-proline Sepharose column (Kleber-Janke et al. 2001).

Two other minor peanut allergens (Ara h 6 and Ara h 7) belong, like Ara h 2, to the 2S albumin family, which is thought to act as storage proteins. Whilst the homologous Ara h 2 is considered to be a major allergen, Ara h 6 is considered to be only a minor one, recognized by 38% of peanut-allergic sera while Ara h 7 was recognized by 43% of peanut-allergic sera (Kleber-Janke et al. 1999). Ara h 6 is approximately in 60% identical with Ara h 2 and is thus treated as a different allergen rather than as an isoallergen. However, there may occur some IgE cross-reactivity. Ara h 6 yields a protease-resistant core on digestion with trypsin and chymotrypsin which has a native-like structure (Lehmann et al. 2004). Ara h 7 may be less stable than Ara h 2 and Ara h 6 because only two disulphide bridges are conserved. Ara h 2 and Ara h 6 are 40%–50% identical with Ara h 7 throughout over 80% of the sequence. It is not clear if there is significant IgE cross-reactivity.

Ara h 8 is a monomer protein with molecular mass of 17 kDa, which belongs to the Bet v 1 family. Other peanut allergens, such as Ara h 2, Ara h 5, Ara h 6, and Ara h 7, have molecular mass of 14–18 kDa, which makes it difficult to identify allergenic proteins on immunoblots incubated with sera of allergic subjects. Ara h 8 may be a pathogenesis-related protein due to its sequence identical with several "bona fide" PR-10 proteins. Its precise function is not known but it may be a steroid-binding protein as is Bet v 1 (Markovic-Housley et al. 2003). Ara h 1 is a major peanut allergen for patients with concurrent birch pollen and peanut allergies. Mittag et al. (2004a) expressed Ara h 8 in *E. coli*. The recombinant Ara h 8 had a similar secondary structure to the recombinant Gly m 4 and Bet v 1. The sequence alignment revealed an amino acid sequence identity of 45.9% with Bet v 1 and 70.6% with Gly m 4. Mittag et al. (2004a) reported that Ara h 8 showed low stability to digestion by pepsin. Similarly low stability to gastric digestion was found for other Bet v 1-related allergens such as Mal d 1 or Cor a 1 (Jensen-Jarolim et al. 1999, Vieths et al. 1999). According to Mittag et al. (2004a) this might explain why allergic reactions in the majority of tested subjects were restricted to the oral cavity and might minimize the probability of sensitization to Ara h 8 through the gastrointestinal tract.

The last identified peanut allergen is oleosin with molecular mass of 16–17 kDa. Oleosins are the proteinaceous (Webster) components of plants' lipid storage bodies called "oil bodies." Oleosins are low molecular mass amphipathic proteins (15–26 kDa) with a long hydrophobic core, flanked by hydrophilic N- and C-terminal domains (Huang 1992, 1996) that act as emulsifiers for the storage of lipids in seeds (Pons et al. 2005). Pons et al. (2005) refined peanut oleosin and revealed predomiminance of α-helical structure, which may be assigned to the central region. Oleosin is regarded as a hidden allergen that might be the cause of hypersensitivity following consumption of oil refined from peanuts or products containing this oil. IgE reactivity of oleosin increased on roasting peanuts.

## 11.3   EFFECT OF TECHNOLOGICAL PROCESSES ON THE STABILITY OF PEANUT ALLERGENS

Technological treatment applied during food processing may result in changes in allergenic food properties. Thermal reactions such as roasting, curing, or various types of cooking can cause multiple nonenzymatic biochemical reactions to occur in food. One kind of most common reactions proceeding during thermal food treatment is the Maillard reactions (Maleki et al. 2003). The final products of these reactions play a significant role in shaping the smell and taste of ready food products. Peanuts are most often subject to roasting, which contributes to increasing the allergenicity of their main allergens. Both Ara h 1 and Ara h 2 from roasting peanuts bound higher levels of IgE. Maleki et al. (2001) observed a correlation between the level of increase in IgE binding and increase in carboxymethyl lysine modifications on the surface of the protein. The extract obtained from roasted peanuts reacted with sera of allergic subjects on the level ca. 90-fold higher than that observed for raw peanuts. Roasting resulted in forming highly stable Ara h 1 trimers. Ara h 1 purified from roasted peanuts was much less soluble than Ara h 1 from raw ones. Ara h 2 was thought to form intramolecular cross-links because of roasting, without forming higher order structures (Maleki et al. 2000a, 2001).

Maleki et al. (2003) showed that Ara h 2 was a weak trypsin inhibitor. The trypsin inhibitor activity of Ara h 2 increased 3.5-fold on roasting. The process also increased Ara h 2 resistance to trypsin digestion. Sen et al. (2002) showed that native, but not reduced Ara h 2, was resistant to proteases leaving a 10 kDa fragment. Ara h 2 was also observed to protect Ara h 1 against trypsin action and the protection intensity grew following roasting (Maleki et al. 2003). However, the protein's structure was altered, possibly with intramolecular cross-links. IgE-binding by Ara h 2 also survived roasting better than boiling or frying (Beyer et al. 2001). IgE-binding to profilin (Ara h 5) survived roasting, too.

Ara h 8 has a low resistance to roasting but is not fully inactivated by heat. Such partial thermal resistance was shown also for other food allergens that are homologues to Bet v 1, e.g., for Cor a 1 from hazelnut or Gly m 4 from soybean (Vieths et al. 2002, Mittag et al. 2004b).

### 11.3.1 PEANUT OIL

Peanut oil is widely used in pharmaceutical products, among others for the production of ointments and vitamins, or as bone cement for orthopedic surgeries. The ELISA results show that only crude oil contains significant amounts of protein, whereas in refined oils and pharmaceutical products no protein is detectable (below 0.3 ng/mL). On immunoblotting with sera of subjects allergic to peanut no reactivity was found (Peeters et al. 2004). Yet, there appears a new tendency in the production of edible oils. In general, crude plant oils contain numerous bioactive compounds that are removed on refining. New technologies are aimed at increasing the nutritional value of edible oils.

## 11.4 CROSS-REACTIVITY AMONG PEANUT AND OTHER MEMBERS OF THE LEGUME FAMILY

Peanut belongs to the legumes; due to phylogenetical and antigenical affinities among these plants a high level of cross-reactivity can be expected (Barnett et al. 1987, Bock et al. 1988, Eigenmann et al. 1996, Moneret-Vautrin et al.1999, Lifrani et al. 2005). Yet, available data do not confirm this assumption and they are often contradictory. There are described cases of subjects allergic to peanut in whom serologic cross-reactivity to other legumes was observed in *in vitro* studies. The research is focused mainly on seeking the relation between peanut and soybean allergens which are the cause of most allergic reactions induced by food in the United States, Great Britain, or Japan where their consumption is high (Bruijnzeel-Koomen et al. 1995). Indeed, the conducted studies do not seem to univocally confirm cross-reactivity among these legumes (Sicherer et al. 2000). In the Mediterranean and some Asian countries (India), where the consumption of lentil, chickpea, and pea is traditionally the highest, the problem of cross-reactivity between them is obvious (Pascual et al. 1999, Patil et al. 2001). The reports state that in Spain, 10% of patients suffering from food allergy display clinical symptoms following consumption of lentils (Crespo et al. 2001). Although it is assumed that clinical cross-reactivity between the proteins of legumes is relatively rare (Sicherer et al. 2000), over 70% of subjects allergic to pea, lentil, and chickpea show a positive reaction to proteins of all the studied seeds in open provocation tests (Ibañez et al. 2003). Hence, it can be supposed that the cross-reactivity among legumes should be considered in various aspects. It is commonly accepted that the seeds of some legumes, similarly to other food constituents, show cross-reactivity among them while others do not. Bonds et al. (2006) observed that the proteins of chickpea, split green pea, lentil, and soy reacted on membranes with antibodies highly specific against Ara h1, Ara h 2, and Ara h 3 with different intensity, but not all of the proteins in question reacted with serum IgE from allergic individuals.

Wensing et al. (2003) reported that three patients with histories of severe anaphylaxis after ingestion of pea had peanut-related symptoms that occurred due to cross-reactive IgE initially raised against pea allergens. The molecular basis for this cross-reactivity was vicilin homologues in pea and peanut (Ara h 1). Two patients also reported symptoms to other legumes (kidney bean, lentil, and others, but not to soybean). This might suggest that the affinity between proteins of the 7S type may be at least a partial cause of clinical reactivity between some legumes.

## 11.5   CROSS-REACTIVITY OF PEANUT AND LUPINE ALLERGENS

The United Kingdom-based Institute of Food Science & Technology recommends placing lupine flour on the list of 12 potentially allergic ingredients (peanut and soybean are already there). Lupine has been used in animal feeding for a long time but it was not until lupine flour started to be added to wheat flour (in the United Kingdom in 1996, in France at the end of 1997) that a rapid increase in the number of anaphylaxis episodes induced by consumption of products containing lupine proteins was observed. Sensitization can occur through oral route or through inhalation (Novembre et al. 1999, Crespo et al. 2001, Parisot et al. 2001, Moreno-Ancillo et al. 2005). The data presented by Peeters et al. (2007) showed that for 4 out of 6 (I think that it can b retained as such) subjects with lupine allergy the sensitizing dose was 1 mg or less to trigger subjective symptoms (oral allergy symptoms). For objective symptoms, the dose of 300 mg lupine flour resulted in modest-to-severe reactions to lupine in 5 out of 6 patients. This dose is similar to that determined for peanut (Wensing et al. 2002). Earlier studies informed about serological cross-reactivity between lupine and other members of the legume family (Barnett et al. 1987, Bernhisel-Broadbent and Sampson 1989, Lifrani et al. 2005) but clinical cross-reactivity is quite rare. Lupine allergy is most frequently related to allergy to peanut, soy, or pea (Moneret-Vautrin et al. 1999, Matheu et al. 1999, Radcliffe et al. 2005). Studies published in 2007 indicate that lupine flour allergy can occur as a separate entity, without evidence of clinical or laboratory cross-reactivity to other legumes (Peeters et al. 2007). Hence, it follows that lupine allergy might be the consequence of cross-reactivity after sensitization to peanut, other legumes, or *de novo* sensitization. In 1994 Hefle et al. reported a case of a 5 year old girl with peanut sensitivity who developed urticaria and angioedema following consumption of spaghetti-like pasta fortified with sweet lupine seed flour. They characterized proteins with molecular mass of ca. 21 kDa and in the range 35–55 kDa (SDS-PAGE) which reacted with IgE (Hefle et al. 1994). In some other study, it was shown that the strongest reaction with IgE was observed for lupine protein with molecular mass of ca. 43 kDa. However, this protein is not known to be a major peanut allergen. There were also identified bands at 13, 38, and 65 kDa that were not cross-reactive with peanut (Moneret-Vautrin et al. 1999). Peptide sequencing of the 50–66 kDa lupine proteins showed that multiple spots represent two highly similar proteins that are approximately in 47% identical with Ara h 1 and in 52% identical with β-conglycinins of soybean (Peeters et al. 2007). Since the spots reacted with peanut specific IgE very weakly or not at all, it can be supposed that 47% affinity is not sufficient to prove IgE bond affinity. Undoubtedly, lupine allergy and cross-reactivity with other legume allergens, particularly with peanut, is a problem much more complex than it was initially assumed and it requires further elucidation.

# REFERENCES

Adachi, M., Takenaka, Y., Gidamis, A.B., Mikami, B., and Utsumi S. 2001. Crystal structure of soybean proglycinin A1aB1b homotrimer. *J Mol Biol* 305:291–305.

Barnett, D., Bonham B., and Howden, M.E.H. 1987. Allergenic cross-reactions among legume foods — An in vitro study. *J Allergy Clin Immunol* 79:433–438.

Barre, A., Borges, J.-P., Culerrier, R., and Rougé, P. 2005a. Homology modelling of the major peanut allergen Ara h 2 and surface mapping of IgE-binding epitopes. *Immunol Lett* 100:153–158.

Barre, A., Borges, J.-P., and Rougé, P. 2005b. Molecular modelling of the major peanut allergen Ara h 1 and other homotrimeric allergens of the cupin superfamily: A structural basis for their IgE-binding cross-reactivity. *Biochimie* 87:499–506.

Barre, A., Jacquet, G., Sordet, C., Culerrier, R., and Rougé P. 2007. Homology modelling and conformational analysis of IgE-binding epitopes of Ara h 3 and other legumin allergens with a cupin fold from tree nuts. *Mol Immunol* 44:3243–3255.

Bernhisel-Broadbent, J. and Sampson, H.A. 1989. Cross-allergenicity in the legume botanical family in children with food hypersensitivity. *J Allergy Clin Immunol* 83:435–440.

Beyer, K., Morrow, E., Li, X.M. et al. 2001. Effects of cooking methods on peanut allergenicity. *J Allergy Clin Immunol* 107:1077–1081.

Bock, S.A., Atkins, F.M., and Sampson, H.A. 1988. Allergenic cross-reactivity among legume food. *J Allergy Clin Immunol* 82:310–312.

Bonds, R.S., Maleki, S.J., McBride, J., and Cheng, H. 2006. In vitro cross-reactivity of peanut allergens with other legumes. *J Allergy Clin Immunol* 11:154.

Bruijnzeel-Koomen, C., Ortolani, C., Aas, K. et al. 1995. Adverse reactions to food. Position paper. *Allergy* 50:623–635.

Burks, A.W. 2003. Peanut allergy: A growing phenomenon. *J Clin Invest* 111:950–952.

Burks, A.W. 2008. Peanut allergy. *Lancet* 371:1538–1546.

Burks, A.W., Williams, L.W., Helm, R.M., Connaughton, C., Cocrel, 1 G., and O'Brien, T.J. 1991. Identification of a major peanut allergen, Ara h 1, in patients with atopic dermatitis and positive peanut challenges. *J Allergy Clin Immunol* 88:72–179.

Burks, A.W., Williams, L.W., Connaughton, C., Cocrell, G., O'Brien, T.J., and Helm, R.M. 1992. Identification and characterization of a second major peanut allergen, Ara h II, with use of the sera of patients with atopic dermatitis and positive peanut challenges. *J Allergy Clin Immunol* 90:962–969.

Burks, A.W., Cockrell, G., Connaughton, C., and Helm, R.M. 1994. Epitope specificity and immunoaffinity purification of the major peanut allergen, Ara h 1. *J Allergy Clin Immunol* 93:743–750.

Burks, A.W., Cocrell, G., Stanley, J.S., Helm, R.M., and Bannon, G.A. 1995. Recombinant peanut allergen Ara h 1 expression and IgE-binding in patients with peanut hypersensitivity. *J Clin Invest* 96:1715–1721.

Burks, A.W., Shin, D., Cockrell, G., Stanley, J.S., Helm, R.M., and Bannon, G.A. 1997. Mapping and mutational analysis of the IgE-binding epitopes on Ara h 1, a legume vicilin protein and a major allergen in peanut hypersensitivity. *Eur J Biochem* 245:334–339.

Burks, A.W., Sampson, H.A., and Bannon, G.A. 1998. Review Article Series II. Peanut allergens. *Allergy* 53:725–730.

Chatel, J.M., Bernard, H., and Orson, F.M. 2003. Isolation and characterization of two complete Ara h 2 isoforms cDNA. *Int Arch Allergy Immunol* 131:14–18.

Clement, G., Boquet, D., Mondoulet, L., Lamourette, P., Bernard, H., and Wal, J.M. 2005. Expression in *Escherichia coli* and disulfide bridge mapping of PSC33, an allergenic 2S albumin from peanut. *Protein Expr Purif* 44:110–120.

Crespo, J.F., Rodriguez, J., Vives, R. et al. 2001. Occupational IgE-mediated allergy after exposure to lupine seed flour. *J Allergy Clin Immunol* 108:295–297

de Leon, M.P., Drew, A.C., Glaspole, I.N., Suphioglu, C., O'Hehir, R.E., and Rolland, J.M. 2007. IgE cross-reactivity between the major peanut allergen Ara h 2 and tree nut allergens. *Mol Immunol* 44:463–471.

Duranti, M. and Gius, C. 1997. Legume seeds: Protein content and nutritional value. *Field Crops Res* 53:31–45.

Eigenmann, P.A., Burks, A.W., Bannon, G.A., and Sampson, H.A. 1996. Identification of unique peanut and soy allergens in sera adsorbed with cross-reacting antibodies. *J Allergy Clin Immunol* 98:969–978.

Emmett, S.E., Angus, F.J., Fry, J.S., and Lee, P.N. 1999. Perceived prevalence of peanut allergy in Great Britain and its association with other atopic conditions and with peanut allergy in other household members. *Allergy* 54:380–385.

Furlong, T.J., DeSimone, J., and Sicherer, S.H. 2001. Peanut and tree nut allergic reactions in restaurants and other food establishments. *J Allergy Clin Immunol* 108:867–870.

Hefle, S.L., Lemanske, R.F.J., and Bush, R.K. 1994. Adverse reaction to lupine-fortified pasta. *J Allergy Clin Immunol* 94:167–172.

Hourihane, J.B., Aiken. R., Briggs, R. et al. 2007. The impact government advice to pregnant mothers regarding peanut avoidance on the prevalence of peanut allergy in United Kingdom children at school entry. *J Allergy Clin Immunol* 119:1197–1202.

Huang, A.H.C. 1992. Oil bodies and oleosins in seed. *Ann Rev Plant Physiol Plant Mol Biol* 43:177–200.

Huang, A.H.C. 1996. Oleosins and oil bodies in seed of other organs. *Plant Physiol* 110:1055–1061.

Ibañez, D., Martinez, M., Sanchez, J.J., and Fernández-Caldas, E. 2003. Legume: Cross-reactivity. *Allergol Immunopathol* 31:151–161.

Jensen-Jarolim, E., Wiedermann, U., Ganglberger, E. et al. 1999. Allergen mimotopes in food enhance type I allergic reactions in mice, *FASEB J* 13:1586–1592.

Kang, I.-K. and Gallo, M. 2007. Cloning and characterization of a novel peanut allergen Ara h 3 isoform displaying potentially decreased allergenicity. *Plant Sci* 172: 345–353.

Kilanowski, J., Stalter, A.M., and Gottesman, M.M. 2006. Preventing peanut panic. *J Pediatr Health Care* 20:61–66.

Kleber-Janke, T., Crameri, R., Appenzeller, U., Schlaak, M., and Becker, W.M. 1999. Selective cloning of peanut allergens, including profilin and 2S albumins, by phage display technology. *Int Arch Allergy Immunol* 119:265–274.

Kleber-Janke, T., Crameri, R., Scheurer, S., Vieths, S., and Becker, W. 2001. Patient-tailored cloning of allergens by phage display: Peanut (*Arachis hypogaea*) profiling, a food allergen derived from a rare mRNA. *J Chromatogr B* 756:295–305.

Ko, T.P., Day, J., and McPerson, A. 2000. The refined structure of canavalin from jack bean in two crystal forms at 2.1 and 2.0Å resolution. *Acta Crystallogr D* 56:411–420.

Koppelman, S.J., Knol, E.F., Vlooswijk, R.A.A. et al. 2003. Peanut allergen Ara h 3: Isolation from peanuts and biochemical characterization. *Allergy* 58:1144–1151.

Koppelman, S.J., Wensing, M., Ertmann, M., Knulst, A.C., and Knol, E.F. 2004. Relevance of Ara h1, Ara h 2, and Ara h 3 in peanut-allergic patients, as determined by immunoglobulin E Western blotting, basophil-histamine release and intracutaneous testing: Ara h 2 is the most important peanut allergen. *Clin Exp Allergy* 34:583–590.

Lawrence, M.C., Izard, T., Beuchat, M., Blagrove R.J., and Colman, P.M. 1994. Structure of phaseolin at 2.2Å resolution. Implications for a common vicilin/legumin and the genetic engineering of seed storage proteins. *J Mol Biol* 238:748–776.

Lehmann, K., Schweimer, K., Neudecker, P., and Rosch, P. 2004. Sequence-specific 1H, 13C and 15N resonance assignments of Ara h 6, an allergenic 2S albumin from peanut. *J Biomol NMR* 29:93–94.

Lifrani, A., Dubarry, M., Rautureau, M., Aattouri, N., Boyaka, P.N., and Tome, D. 2005. Peanut-lupine antibody cross-reactivity is not associated to cross-allergenicity in peanut-sensitized mouse strains. *Int Immunopharmacol* 5:1427–1435.

Long, A. 2002. The bolts of peanut allergy. *N Engl J Med* 346:1320–1322.

Makri, E., Papalamprou, E., and Doxastakis, G. 2005. Study of functional properties of seed storage proteins from indigenous European legume crops (lupin, pea, broad bean) in admixture with polysaccharides. *Food Hydrocoll* 19:583–594.

Maleki, S.J., Chung, S., Champagne, E.T., and Raufman, J.P. 2000a. The effects of processing and the allergenic properties of peanut proteins. *J Allergy Clin Immunol* 106:763–776.

Maleki, S.J., Kopper, R.A., Shin, D.S. et al. 2000b. Structure of the major peanut allergen Ara h 1 may protect IgE-binding epitopes from degradation. *J Immunol* 164:5844–5849.

Maleki, S.J., Chung, S., Champagne, E.T., and Raufman, J.P. 2001. Allergic and biophysical properties of peanut proteins before and after roasting. *Food Allergy Tolerance* 2:211–221.

Maleki, S.J., Viquez, O., Jacks, T. et al. 2003. The major peanut allergen, Ara h 2, functions as trypsin inhibitor, and roasting enhances this function. *J Allergy Clin Immunol* 112:190–195.

Maloney, J.M., Chapman, M.D., and Sicherer, S.H. 2006. Peanut allergen exposure through saliva: Assessment and interventions to reduce exposure. *J Allergy Clin Immunol* 118:719–724.

Markovic-Housley, Z., Degano, M., Lamba, D. et al. 2003. Crystal structure of a hypoallergenic isoform of the major birch pollen allergen Bet v 1 and its likely biological function as a plant steroid carrier. *J Mol Biol* 325:123–133.

Matheu, V., de Barrio, M., Sierra, Z., Gracia-Bara, M.T., Tornero, P., and Baeza, M.L. 1999. Lupine-induced anaphylaxis. *Ann Allergy Asthma Immunol* 83:406–408.

Mittag, D., Akkerdaas, J., Ballmer-Weber, B. et al. 2004a. Ara h 8 a Bet v 1-homologous allergen from peanut, is a major allergen in patients with combined birch pollen and peanut allergy. *J Allergy Clin Immunol* 114:1410–1417.

Mittag, D., Vieths, S., Vogel, L. et al. 2004b. Soybean allergy in patients allergic to birch pollen: clinical investigation and molecular characterization of allergens. *J Allergy Clin Immunol* 113:148–154.

Moneret-Vautrin, D.A., Guérin, L., Kanny, G., Flabbee, J., Frémont, S., and Morisset, M. 1999. Cross-allergrenicity of peanut and lupine: The risk of lupine allergy in patients allergic to peanuts. *J Allergy Clin Immunol* 104:883–888.

Moreno-Ancillo, A., Gil-Adrados, A.C., Dominguez-Noche, C., and Cosmes, P.M. 2005. Lupine inhalation induced asthma in a child. *Pediatr Allergy Immunol* 16:542–544.

Novembre, E., Moriondo, M., Bernardini, R., Rossi, M.E., and Vierucci A. 1999. Lupine allergy in a child. *J Allergy Clin Immunol* 103:1214–1216.

Palmer, G.W., Dibbern, D.A., Burks. et al. 2005. Comparative potency of Ara h 1 and Ara h 2 in immunochemical and functional assays of allergenicity. *Clin Immunol* 115:302–312.

Parisot, L., Aparicio, C., Moneret-Vautrin, D.A., and Guerin, L. 2001. Allergy to lupine flour. *Allergy* 56:918–919.

Pascual, C.Y., Fernandez-Crespo, J., Sanchez-Pastor, S. et al. 1999. Allergy to lentils in Mediterranean paediatric patients. *J Allergy Clin Immunol* 103:154–158.

Patil, S.P., Niphadkar, P.V., and Bapat, M.M. 2001. Chickpea: A major food allergen in the Indian subcontinent and its clinical and immunochemical correlation. *Ann Allergy Asthma Immunol* 87:140–145.

Peeters, K.A.B.M., Kunlst, A.C., Rynja, F.L., Bruijnzeel-Koomen, C.A.F.M., and Koppelman, S.J. 2004. Peanut allergy: Sensitization by peanut oil-containing local therapeutics seems unlikely. *J Allergy Clin Immunol* 113:1000–1001.

Peeters, K.A.B.M., Nordlee, J.A., Penninks, A.H. et al. 2007. Lupine allergy: Not simply cross-reactivity with peanut or soy. *J Allergy Clin Immunol* 120:647–653.

Perry, T.T., Conover-Walker, M.K., Pomes, A., Chapman, D.M., and Wood, R.A. 2004. Distribution of peanut allergen in the environment. *J Allergy Clin Immunol* 113:973–976.

Pomés, A., Helm, R.M., Bannon, G.A., Burks, A.W., Tsay, A., and Chapman, M.D. 2003. Monitoring peanut allergen in food products by measuring Ara h 1. *J Allergy Clin Immunol* 111:640–645.

Pomés, A., Vinton, R., and Chapman, M.D. 2004. Peanut allergen (Ara h 1) detection in foods containing chocolate. *J Food Prot* 67:793–798.

Pons, L., Chéry, C., Mrabet, N., Schohn, H., Lapicque, F., and Guéant, J.-L. 2005. Purification and cloning of two high molecular mass isoforms of peanut seed oleosin encoded by cDNAs of equal sizes. *Plant Physiol Biochem* 43:659–668.

Rabjohn, P., Helm, R.M., Stanley, J.S. et al. 1999. Molecular cloning and epitope analysis of the peanut allergen Ara h 3. *J Clin Invest* 103:535–542.

Radcliffe, M., Scadding, G., and Brown, H.M. 2005. Lupine flour anaphylaxis. *Lancet* 365:1360–1360.

Restani, P., Ballabio, C., Corsini, E. et al. 2005. Identification of the basic subunit of Ara h 3 as the major allergen in a group of children allergic to peanuts. *Ann Allergy Asthma Immunol* 94:262–266.

Sampson, H.A. 2003. Anaphylaxis and emergency treatment. *Pediatrics* 111:1601–1608.

Sen, M., Kopper, R., Pons, L., Abraham, E.C., Burks, A.W., and Bannon, G.A. 2002. Protein structure plays a critical role in peanut allergen stability and may determine immunodominant IgE-binding epitopes. *J Immunol* 169:882–887.

Shin, D.S., Compadre, C.M., Maleki, S.J. et al. 1998. Biochemical and structural analysis of the IgE-binding sites on Ara h 1, an abundant and highly allergenic peanut protein. *J Biol Chem* 273:13753–13759.

Shreffler, W.G., Beyer, K., Chu, T.H., Burks, A.W., and Sampson, H.A. 2004. Microarray immunoassay: Association of clinical history, in vitro IgE function, and heterogeneity of allergenic peanut epitopes. *J Allergy Clin Immunol* 113:776–782.

Sicherer, S.H., Munoz-Furlong, A., Burks, A.W., and Sampson, H.A. 1999. Prevalence of peanut and tree nut allergy in the US determined by a random digit dial telephone survey. *J Allergy Clin Immunol* 103:559–562.

Sicherer, S.H., Muñoz-Furlong, A., Burks, A.W., and Sampson, H.A. 2003. Prevalence of peanut and tree nut allergy in the United States determined by means of random digit dial telephone survey: A 5-year follow-up study. *J Allergy Clin Immunol* 112:1203–1207.

Sicherer, S.H., Sampson, H.A., and Burks, A.W. 2000. Peanut and soy allergy: A clinical and therapeutic dilemma – Review. *Allergy* 55:515–521.

Stanley, J.S., King, N., Burks, A.W. et al. 1997. Identification mutational analysis of the immunodominant IgE-binding epitopes of the major peanut allergen Ara h 2. *Arch Biochem Biophys* 342:244–253.

van Ree, R., Cabanes-Macheteau, M., Akkerdaas, J. et al. 2000. Beta(1,2)-xylose and alpha(1,3)-fucose residues have a strong contribution in IgE-binding to plant glycoallergens. *J Biol Chem* 275:11451–11458.

Vieths, S., Reindl, J., Muller, U., Hoffmann, A., and Haustein, D. 1999. Digestability of peanut and hazelnut allergens investigated by a simple in vitro procedure. *Eur Food Res Technol* 209:379–388.

Vieths, S., Scheurer, S., and Ballmer-Weber, B. 2002. Current understanding of cross-reactivity of food allergens and pollen. *Ann N Y Acad Sci* 964:47–68.

Woo, E.J., Dunwell, J.M., Goodenough, P.W., Marvier, A.C., and Pickersgill R.W. 2000. Germin is a manganese containing homohexamer with oxalate oxidase and superoxide dismutase activities. *Nat Strut Biol* 7:1036–1040.

Wensing, M., Knulst, A.C., Piersma, S., O'Kane, F., Knol, E.F., and Koppelman, S.J. 2003. Patients with anaphylaxis to pea can have peanut allergy caused by cross-reactive IgE to vicilin (Ara h1). *J Allergy Clin Immunol* 111:420–424.

Wensing, M., Penninks, A.H., Hefle, S.L., Koppelman, S.J., Bruijnzeel-Koomen, C.A.F.M., and Knulst, A.C. 2002. The distribution of individual threshold doses eliciting allergic reactions in a population with peanut allergy. *J Allergy Clin Immunol* 110:915–920.

Xiang, P., Beardslee, T.A., Zeece, M.G., Markwell, J., and Sarath, G. 2002. Identification and analysis of a conserved immunoglobulin E-binding epitope in soybean G1a and G2a and peanut Ara h 3 glycinins. *Arch Biochem Biophys* 408:51–57.

Yu, J.W., Kagan, R., Verreault, N. et al. 2006. Accidental ingestions in children with peanut allergy. *J Allergy Clin Immunol* 118:466–472.

# 12 Soy (*Glycine max*) Allergens

*Sabine Baumgartner and Patricia Schubert-Ullrich*

## CONTENTS

Interest in soybeans and their components has increased mainly because of the health benefits of soy-rich diets and potential protective influence of soy on the development of diseases (Friedman and Brandon 2001; Singh et al. 2008). Soy is a common dietary protein and soybean intake among adults in Europe is around 1–2 g/day according to a European multicenter dietary recall study (Keinan-Boker et al. 2002). Soy is also an excellent protein source and has been introduced in infant nutrition over 80 years ago as an alternative to cow's milk-based formulas and for the production of hypoallergenic formulas (Host and Halken 2004). However, adverse health effects such as allergies and other intolerance reactions have lead to a more critical view of the use of soybeans in nutrition and food production. For many years after the first adverse description in 1934, soy was considered a weak sensitizing protein on the basis of animal studies. Currently there is no doubt that soy protein is an important food allergen and at least as allergenic as cow's milk protein. Prevalence rates of 0.3%–0.4% in the general population have been quoted (NDA Opinion 2004).

Clinical reactions to soy are similar to those observed with cows' milk or egg allergy. Soy allergy may affect the skin, the gastrointestinal tract, the respiratory tract, and cause systemic anaphylaxis (Sampson 2000). Food allergy to soy proteins has been described mainly in young children with atopic dermatitis, who often outgrow their soy allergy after 1–2 years of dietary elimination, and many soy allergies have resolved by 3 years of age (Sampson and Scanlon 1989; Taylor and Kabourek 2003; NDA Opinion 2004). Individuals with severe peanut allergies often also react to soy proteins due to structural similarities of the allergens of soy and peanut.

In these coallergies, soy sensitivity is likely to be lost at an earlier stage (Foucard and Malmheden Yman 1999; Sicherer et al. 2000a; NDA Opinion 2004).

Food-based soy allergies are less frequent in adults, while respiratory allergy symptoms caused by inhalation of soybean dust are more common in adult patients. Such occupational allergies occur mostly in individuals working in soybean processing industries (e.g., bakeries) and originate from a sensitization to the soybean hull proteins Gly m 1 and Gly m 2. Asthma, rhinitis, and other allergic manifestations can occur in predisposed individuals with or without food allergy (Gonzalez et al. 2000; Quirce et al. 2000).

## 12.1 CHARACTERISTICS OF THE MOST IMPORTANT ALLERGENS FROM SOY: THE BIOCHEMICAL, BIOLOGICAL, AND IMMUNOLOGICAL PROPERTIES OF MAIN SOY ALLERGENS

Soybeans (soy seeds) contain approximately 37% of protein, of which at least 17 IgE-reactive proteins have been suggested as allergens (see Table 12.1) (Besler et al. 2001; NDA Opinion 2004; Wilson et al. 2005). Soy proteins are usually separated by fractionation using different solvents and ultracentrifugation. The 7S (euvicilins) and 11S (legumins) are the main fractions of the soy storage proteins. They contain the soy allergens β-conglycinin (7S) and glycinin (11S), both of them together counting for up to one-third of the total protein content in soybean. These two proteins are globular seed storage proteins (also called globulins) that belong to the cupin super family (Mills et al. 2002).

Furthermore, the soybean hull proteins Gly m 1 and Gly m 2, the soybean profilin Gly m 3, and Gly m 4 (also called Kunitz-trypsin inhibitor, formerly SAM 22) are officially accepted as soybean allergens according to the criteria of the International

## TABLE 12.1
### Soy Allergens

| | Nomenclature | MW (kDa) | Protein Fraction | Content[a] (%) | Biological Function and Characteristics |
|---|---|---|---|---|---|
| Hull protein | Gly m 1 | 7–7.5 | 60% ethanol soluble | <20 | Two isoallergens, lipid transfer protein, hydrophobic, inhalative allergen |
| | Gly m 1a (1.0101) | 7 | | | |
| | Gly m 1b (1.0102) | 7.5 | | | |
| Hull protein | Gly m 2 | 8 | | | Storage protein Inhalative allergen |
| Profilin | Gly m 3 | 14 | | | Profilin |
| n/a | n/a | 17 | 2S-Globulin fraction | | Water soluble |

**TABLE 12.1 (continued)**
**Soy Allergens**

| | Nomenclature | MW (kDa) | Protein Fraction | Content[a] (%) | Biological Function and Characteristics |
|---|---|---|---|---|---|
| Kunitz-trypsin inhibitor (SAM 22) | Gly m 4 | 20 | 2S-Globulin fraction | | Bet v 1-homologous (birch pollen) pathogenesis-related PR-10 family protein, water soluble |
| n/a | n/a | 18–21 | Whey fraction | | |
| n/a | Gly m Bd 28 K[c] | 28 | 7S-Globulin fraction | | Water soluble |
| Vacuolar protein (P34) | Gly m Bd 30 K (formerly Gly m 1) | 30 | 7S-Globulin fraction | 1–3 | Serine protease, immunodominant allergen, water soluble |
| n/a | n/a | 29–31 | Whey fraction | | |
| Soy lectin | n/a | 32 | | | Soybean agglutinin |
| n/a | n/a | 33–35 | 7S-Globulin fraction | | Water soluble |
| n/a | n/a | 35–38 | 7S-Globulin fraction | | Water soluble |
| n/a | n/a | 40–41 | 7S-Globulin fraction | | Water soluble |
| n/a | n/a | 47–50 | 7S-Globulin fraction | | Water soluble |
| n/a | n/a | 52–55 | 7S-Globulin fraction | | Water soluble |
| β-Conglycinin | n/a | 140–180 | 7S-Globulin fraction | <30[b] | Seed storage protein, water soluble, 3 subunits with 42–76 kDa |
| | Gly m Bd 60 K | 63–67 | | | α-Subunit of β-conglycinin |
| Glycinin | n/a | 320–360 | 11S-Globulin fraction | <30[b] | Seed storage protein, water soluble, 6 subunits with 58–62 kDa |

*Sources:* Based on Besler, M. et al., *J. Chromatogr. B*, 756, 207, 2001; NDA Opinion, *EFSA J.*, 32, 1, 2004; Wilson, S. et al., *Nutr. Rev.*, 63, 47, 2005.

[a] Amount of total protein in seeds.
[b] Sum of glycinin and β-conglycinin.
n/a, not assigned; MW, molecular weight.

Union of Immunological Societies Allergen Nomenclature Subcommittee (Ballmer-Weber et al. 2007). The latter two allergens together with the globulins β-conglycinin and glycinin are food allergens (Rihs et al. 1999; Mills et al. 2002; Mittag et al. 2004), whereas soy hull proteins have been described to be relevant in respiratory soy allergy acquired through inhalation of soy particles (Gonzalez et al. 1992, 2000).

*In vitro* IgE-binding studies performed with blood of patients suffering from soy allergy reported sensitivity to glycinin and Gly m 1 in over 90%, to Kunitz-trypsin inhibitor in 86%, and to profilin (Gly m 3) in 69% of all investigated cases. A number of reactivities to other not yet completely characterized moieties between 5 and 20 kDa have also been described (NDA Opinion 2004).

Although present only in relatively small amounts, the three soybean proteins Gly m Bd 60 K, Gly m Bd 30 K, and Gly m Bd 28 K represent major allergens in soy-sensitive patients (Ogawa et al. 2000). Many soy-sensitive patients will react to only one protein, although some, especially those with cross-reactivity to peanuts, will react to multiple proteins (Herian et al. 1990). The Gly m Bd 28 K protein is present in the 7S globulin fraction and is a vicilin-like glycoprotein that has a prevalence rate of around 25% in soybean-sensitive individuals. However, this allergen is not present in many soybean species. In fact, testing showed that only 20% of Japanese soybean varieties contained Gly m Bd 28 K (Bando et al. 1996). Antibodies against the α-subunit of β-conglycinin (Gly m Bd 60 K) is also found in approximately 25% of soybean-allergic patients' sera (Ogawa et al. 2000). Several IgE-binding studies showed that more than 65% of soy-sensitive patients react to Gly m Bd 30 K protein, only (Ogawa et al. 1993; Helm et al. 2000). Thus, even though it is a relatively minor seed constituent (less than 3% of the total seed proteins), Gly m Bd 30 K is regarded as the major (or immunodominant) soybean allergen.

The two main storage globulins, β-conglycinin (7S) and glycinin (11S), possess a common β-barrel structure which is characteristic for proteins of the cupin family. This characteristic protein structure has also been identified in other major plant food allergens, i.e., peanut, walnut, lentil, and coconut (Mills et al. 2002; Breiteneder and Mills 2005). Additionally, the 11S and 7S globulins of soy possess two structurally equivalent N-terminal and C-terminal domains. Each domain is composed of a β-barrel followed by a region of α-helices. Although the 11S and 7S globulins show high resemblance in their 3D structure, direct comparison of the protein sequences show only low similarity of around 35%–45% (Mills et al. 2002). The 11S globulins are hexameric heterooligomeric proteins of $M_r \sim 360$ kDa, with each subunit comprising an acidic 30–40 kDa polypeptide that is disulfide-linked to a 20 kDa basic polypeptide. The vicilin-like 7S globulins are typically trimeric proteins of $M_r \sim 150$–190 kDa, with subunit in the range of 40–80 kDa. Unlike the 11S globulins, the 7S globulins are frequently glycosylated, with one or two N-linked glycosylation sites being located in the C-terminal domain.

Globular storage proteins generally exhibit remarkable stability, especially thermal stability, which is common for proteins of the cupin superfamily. Globulins all share the tendency to form large thermally induced aggregates (heat-set gels), which form the basis of the widespread utilization of soy protein in foods (Mills et al. 2002).

Of the numerous allergens present in soybean, Gly m Bd 30 K, also known as P34 (formerly Gly m 1), has been classified as an immunodominant allergen. Sixty-five percent of soy-sensitive patients with atopic dermatitis exhibit an allergenic response to this protein (Wilson et al. 2005). The N-terminal amino acid sequence and the amino acid composition of Gly m Bd 30 K and P34 are identical and, therefore, they are considered similar proteins with interchangeable denomination. Gly m Bd

30 K is a monomeric, insoluble glycoprotein consisting of 257 amino acid residues attached by disulfide linkages in the 7S globulin protein fraction, and may play a role in protein folding (Bando et al. 1996). It has been previously characterized as an outlying member of the papain superfamily of cysteine proteases (Kalinski et al. 1990). Gly m Bd 30 K exhibits unique properties in that it possesses a glycine substitution at the position 38 cysteine amino acid in the active site, unlike all of the other proteases of this family. While other proteins of this family exhibit enzymatic activity, the absent catalytic action of cysteine suggests that its allergenicity may be structural in nature rather than induced by enzymatic activity (Kalinski et al. 1990; Herman et al. 2003).

The glycoprotein Gly m Bd 28 K was originally identified as a 28 kDa polypeptide in soybean seed flour. The full-length protein consists of 473 amino acids and contains a 23 kDa C-terminal polypeptide with an IgE-binding epitope. Xiang et al. (2004) found out that the C-terminal polypeptide of Gly m Bd 28 K is allergenic and apparently contains at least one immunodominant epitope near the edge of a cupin domain.

Knowledge of the severity of symptoms of soy allergy and the threshold dose of soy is most important and can have a major effect on food-labeling directives. However, most studies that address these questions have not been performed in a satisfactory way (Ballmer-Weber et al. 2007). And the opinions differ on whether soybean is a strong food allergen, or whether it shows lower allergenicity when compared to other food allergens. Comparisons of food allergen dose–response relationships for triggering allergic symptoms demonstrate a higher protein concentration threshold for soy (~100 times), indicating lower allergenic reactivity (Cordle 2004). Reported threshold levels for soy protein in food are in the low milligram range (0.0013–500 mg) (Sicherer et al. 2000b; Bindslev-Jensen et al. 2002; NDA Opinion 2004). The allergenicity of soy proteins are assessed *in vitro* with various immunological methods, and *in vivo* with skin prick tests, patch test, and challenge tests. *In vitro* tests however, do not precisely predict the allergenic effects in humans and at present there is no officially accepted threshold of immunogenic soy proteins in foodstuff. However, approaches to establish thresholds for major food allergens including soy have been discussed (FDA 2006). The threshold for allergens is usually very low, and a very small amount may be enough to trigger a reaction. A recommended level of 10 ppm for soy proteins in food (10 µg/g protein in foodstuff) should not be exceeded (EC 2000, 2002; Koppelman et al. 2004; Poms et al. 2004).

In order to decrease health risks in soy-sensitized individuals, reliable analytical methods for the determination of soy proteins in foodstuffs are necessary. To date enzyme-linked immunosorbent assays (ELISA) have been the preferred approach for allergen detection because of their high precision, simple handling, and good potential for standardization (Koppelman et al. 2004; Poms et al. 2004). Currently, three ELISA kits for soybean are commercially available (L'Hocine et al. 2007). The Tepnel Biosystems kit (ElisaTechnologies, Gainesville, FL) is a competitive ELISA that targets renatured soy proteins with a detection limit of <5000 mg/kg of food product. The Elisa Systems kit (Elisa Systems, Windsor, Australia) is based on a sandwich ELISA and determines the soy trypsin inhibitor in food samples with a claimed sensitivity of 1 mg/kg. The Veratox for Soy Flour Allergen (Neogen

Corporation, Lansing, MI) is a sandwich ELISA used for the quantitative analysis of minimally processed soy flour protein in food products such as cookies, crackers, chocolate bars, and cereals in the range of 2.5–25 mg/kg.

## 12.2   CHANGES IN IMMUNOREACTIVITY OF SOY ALLERGENS DURING TECHNOLOGICAL PROCESSES

The stability of soy allergens and their allergenicity in processed foods have been reviewed (Besler et al. 2001; Wilson et al. 2005). Structural studies of globulins gly-cinin and β-conglycinin showed that the double-stranded β-helix that comprises the cupin fold appears to be a remarkably stable structural motif, resisting both thermal denaturation and proteolysis (Mills et al. 2002). At elevated temperatures, soy globu-lins form large aggregates (heat-set gels) with only little change in their native-like β-sheet structures. Studies of the allergenic potential of several globulin fractions of soybean after heat treatment showed varying reduction of IgE-binding activities in radio-allergosorbent test (RAST) and enzyme-allergosorbent test (EAST) inhibition experiments, dependent on the temperature, duration, and the type of heating (e.g., microwave) (Burks et al. 1992; Müller et al. 1998; Besler et al. 2001). However, heat treatment is not efficient enough to reduce the allergenic potential to an acceptable level for secure soy consumption by soybean-sensitive individuals. In fact, the IgE-binding activity of the vacuolar protein (P34, Gly m Bd 30 K) has been reported to be enhanced by autoclave treatment that involves superheated steam (Yamanashi et al. 1995). Therefore, coupling heat treatment with a structure-modifying element, such as chemical modifications, may be more beneficial in the reduction of the allergenic properties of soybean.

Although glycinin and β-conglycinin are partially or fully insoluble between pH 3.5 and 6.5, both globulins are susceptible to proteolysis, but partly forming stable intermediates (Nielsen et al. 1988; Shutov et al. 1996; Lee et al. 2007). The 11S globulin of soy (glycinin) forms stable intermediates of $M_r \sim 280,000$, known as glycinin-T or glycinin-C, in which the quaternary structure of the native protein is largely retained (Shutov et al. 1996). Lee et al. (2007) observed, that the acidic polypeptide of the 11S globulin was effectively hydrolyzed, while basic polypeptide was more resistant leaving a highly immunoreactive peptide fragment of 20 kDa. The hydrolyzed fragments with molecular weight of less than 20 kDa showed no immunoreactivity (Lee et al. 2007). Stable intermediates also result from trypsinoly-sis of 7S globulins, such as β-conglycinin (Kamata et al. 1982). This stability plays an important role in permitting sufficient immunologically active fragments to pass down the gastrointestinal tract, and is responsible, in part at least, for the allergenic activity of these proteins.

Further approaches to reduce allergenicity of soybeans involves hydrolysis of the soy proteins by either enzymatic proteolysis or fermentation. Enzymatic hydrolysis is an effective way to reduce or even inactivate soy protein allergenicity, especially allergenicity related to Gly m Bd 30 K (Yamanashi et al. 1996; Tsumura et al. 1999; Penas et al. 2006). Van Boxtel et al. (2008) observed that the IgE-binding capacity of legumin allergens from peanuts (Ara h 3) and soybeans (glycinin) does not withstand peptic digestion. Consequently, these two allergens are likely unable to sensitize via the gastrointestinal tract and cause systemic food allergy symptoms. These proteins might thus be less important allergens than was previously assumed.

Fermentation hydrolyses proteins into smaller peptides that causes less allergenicity, because they are not recognized by IgE antibodies any more. Fermentation of soybean seed and flours by various mold strains and bacteria can even reduce IgE immunoreactivity up to 98%, which proves fermentation to be a promising technique for the production of hypoallergenic food ingredients (Yamanashi et al. 1995; Tsuji et al. 1997; Penas et al. 2006; Frias et al. 2008).

A relatively new approach to reduce or completely remove allergenicity of soy products involves genetic modification (Takahashi et al. 1994; Samoto et al. 1997). Herman et al. (2003) have successfully eliminated Gly m Bd 30 K, one of the immunodominant soy allergens by transgene-induced gene silencing, which prevents the accumulation of Gly m Bd 30 K protein in the genetically engineered soybean. Takahashi et al. (2003) have generated a soybean mutant line, whose seeds lack both glycinin and β-conglycinin. Interestingly, an increase of other proteins and free amino acids occurs in order to compensate for the nitrogen stored in the protein components that were removed. These overabundant proteins include Gly m Bd 30 K (P34), the immunodominant allergen in soybean.

The introduction of genetically modified (GM) plants, however, raises additional questions about the possibly changed allergenicity of foodstuffs produced thereof. Because the genetic modification ultimately results in the introduction of new proteins into the food plant, the safety, including the potential allergenicity, of the newly introduced proteins must be assessed. Various protocols have been developed to estimate the potential allergenicity of the introduced proteins. The evaluations focus on several scientific data including information concerning the amino acid sequence identity to known allergenic proteins, *in vitro* and/or *in vivo* immunological assays, and assessment of various physiochemical properties (Metcalfe et al. 1996; Taylor and Hefle 2001; Metcalfe 2003). However, none of these protocols can accurately assess the allergenic potential of foods or their components derived from GM plants. There is an eminent lack of data about the potential allergenicity of GM plant products and the need to accurately assess the allergenic potential of foods derived from GM plants in order to avoid potential health risks to allergic consumers (Nayak 2008).

## 12.3   USE OF SOY PROTEINS AS A SOURCE OF HYPOALLERGENIC FORMULAS

Consumption of soy is common in children and soy-based formulae were introduced in infant nutrition about 80 years ago. Since the 1970s, use of soy-based formulae became common, and in 1980s, U.S. consumption was around 25% of that of cows' milk-based formulae (NDA Opinion 2004). Soy is often introduced into the diet from an early age, often as a standard milk formula in healthy children and in children with suspected or proven cows' milk allergy as a hypoallergenic substitute. However, this practice is now discouraged since a significant number of children with cows' milk protein intolerance develop soy protein intolerance when soy milk is used in dietary management. Soy protein is reported to be at least as allergenic as cow's milk protein (AAP 1998; Barrett 2002; SCF 2003; Host and Halken 2004).

Most hypoallergenic formulas are processed by enzymatic hydrolysis of different protein sources such as soy or cow's milk or whey protein and followed by further processing such as heat treatment and/or ultrafiltration. Such hypoallergenic products, however, contain residual allergenicity. Only formulas based solely on amino acid mixtures are considered to be nonallergenic. Some extensively hydrolyzed soy protein products exhibit sufficiently reduced allergenicity which allows their usage as hypoallergenic alternative to pure amino acid mixtures for the treatment of high-risk or cow's milk-sensitized infants. It has been observed, that feeding high-risk infants with hypoallergenic formula combined with avoidance of solid foods during the first 4–6 months reduces the cumulative incidence of cow's milk protein allergy and atopic dermatitis as compared with standard cow's milk-based formula (Host and Halken 2004).

## 12.4 CROSS-REACTIVITY OF SOY PROTEINS

Cross-reactivity of soy allergens generally happens due to homology in the amino acid sequences found among various allergic proteins of different sources. This is the case with the vacuolar protein (P34), a major allergenic soy protein that shares approximately 70% sequence homology with peanut's main allergen (Ara h 1) and 50%–70% with the immunodominant cow's milk allergen (2-S1-casein). Due to this homology and close botanical relationship, peanuts and soybeans contain common allergenic components, and for this reason IgE antibodies to peanut proteins can also react with soybean proteins (Wilson et al. 2005). Patients with severe peanut allergy have been reported to react to soy proteins in 3%–6% of cases. However, there are contradictory reports on the true cause of severe life-threatening reactions related to soy allergy. A study in Sweden reported three anaphylactic deaths in patients aged 9–17 after consumption of meat products fortified with 2.2%–7% soy protein; these patients had a previously known allergy to peanuts but not to soybeans (Foucard and Malmheden Yman 1999). Exposure to hidden peanut as a trigger cannot be entirely ruled out (Sicherer et al. 2000a; NDA Opinion 2004). The following cross-reactivities against peanut and other legumes in soy allergic individuals have been described: peanut ~70%–90%, green pea ~80%, lima bean ~50%, string bean ~40%, and wheat flour ~86% in soybean-sensitized bakers (NDA Opinion 2004). The overall consensus from all these studies is, however, that in vitro cross-reactivities do not correlate with clinical reactivity.

Another example is Bet v 1, a major birch pollen allergen, which is a homologous protein to Gly m 4, the Kunitz-trypsin inhibitor (formerly SAM 22). Interestingly, sensitization against Bet v 1 occurs via the inhalation route while Gly m 4 is a food allergen with sensitization via the digestion route (Gonzalez et al. 2000; Kleine-Tebbe et al. 2002; Mittag et al. 2004). Two-thirds of highly Bet v 1-sensitized patients with birch pollen allergy also showed sensitization to Gly m 4, although only ~10% of those patients reported soy allergy (Mittag et al. 2004).

Several authors report coexisting clinical soy allergies in 5%–50% of patients with cows' milk allergies (NDA Opinion 2004). It is unclear whether soy allergy represents a *de novo* sensitization or a cross-reaction of a soy protein component with caseins from milk (Rozenfeld et al. 2002). However, due to homology in the amino acid sequences of soybean and cow's milk allergens of 50%–70%, cross-reactivity is likely (Wilson et al. 2005).

## REFERENCES

AAP. 1998. American Academy of Pediatrics. Committee on Nutrition. Soy protein-based formulas: Recommendations for use in infant feeding. *Pediatrics* 101:148–153.

Ballmer-Weber, B.K., Holzhauser T., Scibilia, J., Mittag, D., Zisa, G., Ortolani, C., Oesterballe, M., Poulsen, L.K., Vieths, S., Bindslev-Jensen, C. 2007. Clinical characteristics of soybean allergy in Europe: A double-blind, placebo-controlled food challenge study. *Allerg Clin Immunol* 119:1489–1496.

Bando, N., Tsuji, H., Yamanashi, R., Nio, N., Ogawa, T. 1996. Identification of the glycosylation site of a major soybean allergen, Gly m Bd 30 K. *Biosci Biotechnol Biochem* 60:347–348.

Barrett, J.R. 2002. Soy and children's health: A formula for trouble. *Environ Health Perspect* 110:A294–A296.

Besler, M., Steinhart, H., Paschke, A. 2001. Stability of allergens and allergenicity of processed foods. *J Chromatogr B* 756:207–228.

Bindslev-Jensen, C., Briggs, D., Osterballe, M. 2002. Can we determine a threshold level for allergenic foods by statistical analysis of published data in the literature? *Allergy* 57:741–746.

Breiteneder, H., Mills, E.N.C. 2005. Plant food allergens—Structural and functional aspects of allergenicity. *Biotechnol Adv* 23:395–399.

Burks, A.W., Williams, L.W., Connaughton, C., Cockrell, G., O'Brien, T.J., Helm, R.M. 1992. Allergenicity of peanut and soybean extracts altered by chemical or thermal denaturation in patients with atopic dermatitis and positive food challenges. *J Allergy Clin Immunol* 90:889–897.

Cordle, C.T. 2004. Soy protein allergy: Incidence and relative severity. *J Nutr* 134:1213S–1219S.

EC. 2000. European Commission. Food Labelling Directive. Off J L 109.

EC. 2002. European Commission. Food without fear: Amended food labelling directive allows consumers to discover details on allergens. Press release IP/02/1680, November 14, 2002.

FDA. 2006. Food and Drug Administration. Approaches to establish thresholds for major food allergens and for gluten in food. Available at http://www.cfsan.fda.gov/~dms/alrgn2.html.

Foucard, T., Malmheden Yman, I. 1999. A study on severe food reactions in Sweden—Is soy an underestimated cause of food anaphylaxis? *Allergy* 55:261–265.

Frias, J., Song, Y.S., Martinez-Villaluenga, C., Gonzalez de Mejia, E., Vidal-Valverde, C. 2008. Immunoreactivity and amino acid content of fermented soybean products. *J Agric Food Chem* 56:99–105.

Friedman, M., Brandon, D.L. 2001. Nutritional and health benefits of soy proteins. *J Agric Food Chem* 49:1069–1086.

Gonzalez, R., Polo, F., Zapatero, L., Caravaca, F., Carreira, J. 1992. Purification and characterization of major inhalant allergens from soybean hulls. *Clin Exp Allergy* 22:748–755.

Gonzalez, R., Duffort, O., Calabozo, B., Barber, D., Carriera, J., Polo, F. 2000. Monoclonal antibody-based method to quantify Gly m 1. Its application to assess environmental exposure to soybean dust. *Allergy* 55:59–64.

Helm, R.M., Cockrell, G., West, C.M., Herman, E.M., Sampson, H.A., Bannon, G.A., Burks, A.W. 2000. Mutational analysis of the IgE-binding epitopes of P34/Gly m1. *J Allergy Clin Immunol* 105:378–384.

Herian, A.M., Taylor, S.L., Bush, R.K. 1990. Identification of soybean allergens by immunoblotting with sera from soy-allergic adults. *Int Arch Allergy Appl Immunol* 92:193–198.

Herman, E.M., Helm, R.M., Jung, R., Kinney, A.J. 2003. Genetic modification removes an immunodominant allergen from soybean. *Plant Physiol* 132:36–43.

Host, A., Halken, S. 2004. Hypoallergenic formulas—When, to whom and how long: After more than 15 years we know the right indication! *Allergy* 59:45–52.

Kalinski, A., Weisemann, J.M., Matthews, B.F., Herman, E.M. 1990. Molecular cloning of a protein associated with soybean seed oil bodies that is similar to thiol proteases of the papain superfamily. *J Biol Chem* 265:13843–13848.

Kamata, Y., Otsuka, S., Sato, M., Shubaki, K. 1982. Limited proteolysis of soyabean beta-conglycinin. *Agric Biol Chem* 46:2829–2834.

Keinan-Boker, L., Peters, P.H., Mulligan, A.A., Nawarro, C., Slimani, N., Mattisson, I., Lundin, E., McTaggart, A., Allen, N.E., Overvad, K., Tjonneland, A., Clavel-Chapelon, F., Linseisen, J., Haftenberger, M., Lagiou, P., Kalapothaki, V., Ewangelista, A., Franca, G., Bueno-de-Mesquita, H.B., Van der Schouw, Y.T., Engeset, D., Skwie, G., Tormo, M.J., Ardanaz, E., Charrondiere, U.R., Riboli, E. 2002. Soy product consumption in 10 European countries: The European Prospective Investigation into Cancer and Nutrition (EPIC) study. *Public Health Nutr* 5:1217–1226.

Kleine-Tebbe, J., Vogel, L., Crowell, D.N., Haustein, U.F., Vieths, S. 2002. Severe oral allergy syndrome and anaphylactic reactions caused by a Bet v 1-related PR-10 protein in soybean, SAM 22. *J Allergy Clin Immunol* 110:797–804.

Koppelman, S.J., Lakemond, C.M.M., Vlooswijk, R., Hefle, S.L. 2004. Detection of soy proteins in processed foods: Literature overview and new experimental work. *J AOAC Int* 87:1398–1407.

Lee, H.W., Keum, E.H., Lee, S.J., Sung, D.E., Chung, D.H., Lee, S.I., Oh, S. 2007. Allergenicity of proteolytic hydrolysates of the soybean 11S globulin. *J Food Sci* 72(3):C168–C172.

L'Hocine, L., Boye, J.I., Munyana, C. 2007. Detection and quantification of soy allergens in food: Study of two commercial enzyme-linked immunosorbent assays. *J Food Sci* 72:C145–C153.

Metcalfe, D.D. 2003. Introduction: What are the issues in addressing the allergenic potential of genetically modified foods? *Environ Health Perspect* 111:1110–1113.

Metcalfe, D.D., Astwood, J.D., Townsend, R., Sampson, H.A., Taylor, S.L., Fuchs, R.L. 1996. Assessment of the allergenic potential of foods derived from genetically engineered crop plants. *Crit Rev Food Sci Nutr* 36:S165–S186.

Mills, E.N.C., Jenkins, J., Marigheto, N., Belton, P.S., Gunning, A.P., Morris, V.J. 2002. Allergens of the cupin superfamily. *Biochem Soc Trans* 30:925–929.

Mittag, D., Vieths, S., Vogel, L., Becker, W.M., Rihs, H.P., Helbling, A., Wüthrich, B., Ballmer-Weber, B.K. 2004. Soybean allergy in patients allergic to birch pollen: Clinical investigation and molecular characterization of allergens. *J Allergy Clin Immunol* 113:148–154.

Müller, U., Weber, W., Hoffmann, A., Franke, S., Lange, R., Vieths, S. 1998. Commercial soybean lecithins: A source of hidden allergens? *Z Lebensm Unters Forsch* 207:341–351.

Nayak, S.K. 2008. Food allergy with special reference to genetically modified foods: A review. *J Food Sci Technol* 45:14–19.

Nielsen, S.S., Deshpande, S.S., Hermodson, M.A., Scott, M.P. 1988. Comparative digestibility of legume storage proteins. *J Agric Food Chem* 36(5):896–902.

NDA Opinion 2004. Opinion of the scientific panel on dietetic products, nutrition and allergies on a request from the commission relating to the evaluation of allergenic foods for labelling purposes (Request No. EFSA-Q-2003-016). *EFSA J* 32:1–197.

Ogawa, T., Tsuji, H., Kitamura, K., Zhu, U.L., Hirano, H., Nishikawa, K. 1993. Identification of the soybean allergenic protein, Gly m Bd 30 K, with the soybean seed 34-kDa oil-body-associated protein. *Biosci Biotechnol Biochem* 57:1030–1033.

Ogawa, T., Samoto, M., Takahashi, K. 2000. Soybean allergens and hypoallergenic soybean products. *J Nutr Sci Vitaminol* 46:271–279.

Penas, E., Prestamo, G., Polo, F., Gomez, R. 2006. Enzymatic proteolysis, under high pressure of soybean whey: Analysis of peptides and the allergen Gly m 1 in the hydrolysates. *Food Chem* 99:569–573.

Poms, E.R., Klein, C.L., Anklam, E. 2004. Methods for allergen analysis in food: A review. *Food Add Contam* 21:1–31.

Quirce, S., Polo, F., Figueredo, E., Gonzalez, R., Sastre, J. 2000. Occupational asthma caused by soybean flour in bakers—Differences with soybean-induced epidemic asthma. *Clin Exp Allergy* 30:839–846.

Rihs, H.P., Chen, Z., Rueff, F., Petersen, A., Rozynek, P., Heimann, H., Baur, X. 1999. IgE binding of the recombinant allergen soybean profilin (rGly m 3) is mediated by conformational epitopes. *J Allergy Clin Immunol* 104:1293–1301.

Rozenfeld, P., Docena, G.H., Anon, M.C., Fossati, C.A. 2002. Detection and identification of a soy protein component that cross-reacts with caseins from cow's milk. *Clin Exp Immunol* 130:49–58.

Samoto, M., Fukuda, Y., Takahashi, K., Tabuchi, K., Hiemori, M., Tsuji, H., Ogawa, T., Kawamura, Y. 1997. Substantially complete removal of three major allergenic soybean proteins (Gly m Bd 30 K, Gly m Bd 28 K, and the alpha subunit of conglycinin) from soy protein by using a mutant soybean, Tohoku 124. *Biosci Biotechnol Biochem* 61:2148–2150.

Sampson, H.A. 2000. Food anaphylaxis. *Br Med Bull* 56:925–935.

Sampson, H.A., Scanlon, S.M. 1989. Natural history of food hypersensitivity in children with atopic dermatitis. *J Pediatr* 115:23–27.

SCF. 2003. Scientific Committee on Food. Report on the revision of essential requirements of infant formulae and follow-on formulae (opinion expressed on April 4, 2003).

Shutov, A.D., Kakhovskaya, I.A., Bastrygina, A.S., Bulmaga, V.P., Horstmann, C., Muntz, K. 1996. Limited proteolysis of P-conglycinin and glycinin, the 7s and 11s storage globulins from soybean (*Glycine max* (L.) Merr.) Structural and evolutionary implications. *Eur J Biochem* 241:221–228.

Sicherer, S.H., Sampson, H.A., Burks, A.W. 2000a. Peanut and soy allergy: A clinical and therapeutic dilemma. *Allergy* 55:515–521.

Sicherer, S.H., Morrow, E.H., Sampson, H.A. 2000b. Dose–response in double-blind, placebo-controlled oral food challenges in children with atopic dermatitis. *J Allergy Clin Immunol* 105:582–586.

Singh, P., Kumar, R., Sabapathy, S.N., Bawa, A.S. 2008. Functional and edible uses of soy protein products. *Comp Rev Food Sci Food Safety* 7:14–28.

Takahashi, K., Banba, H., Kikuchi, A., Ito, M., Nakamura, S. 1994. An induced mutant line lacking the α-subunit of β-conglycinin in soybean (*Glycine max* (L) Merril). *Breeding Sci* 44:65–66.

Takahashi, M., Uematsu, Y., Kashiwaba, K., Yagasaki, K., Hajika, M., Matsunaga, R., Komatsu, K., Ishimoto, M. 2003. Accumulation of high levels of free amino acids in soybean seeds through integration of mutations conferring seed protein deficiency. *Planta* 217:577–586.

Taylor, S.L., Hefle, S.L. 2001. Will genetically modified foods be allergenic? *J Allergy Clin Immunol* 107(5 suppl.):765–771.

Taylor, S.L., Kabourek, J.L. 2003. Soyfoods and allergies: Separating fact from fiction. *Soy Connect* 11:1–6.

Tsuji, H., Okada, N., Yamanashi, R., Bando, N., Ebine, H., Ogawa, T. 1997. Fate of a major soybean allergen, Gly m Bd 30K, in rice-, barley-, and soybean-koji miso (fermented soybean paste) during fermentation. *Food Sci Technol Int* (Tokyo) 3:145–149.

Tsumura, K., Kugimiya, W., Bando, N., Hiemori, M., Ogawa, T. 1999. Preparation of hypoallergenic soybean protein with processing functionality by selective enzymatic hydrolysis. *Food Sci Technol Res* 5:171–175.

Van Boxtel, E.L., van den Broek, L.A.M., Koppelman, S.J., Gruppen, H. 2008. Legumin allergens from peanuts and soybeans: Effects of denaturation and aggregation on allergenicity. *Mol Nutr Food Res* 52:674–682.

Wilson, S., Blaschek, K., de Mejia, E.G. 2005. Allergenic proteins in soybean: Processing and reduction of P34 allergenicity. *Nutr Rev* 63:47–58.

Xiang, P., Haas, E.J., Zeece, M.G., Markwell, J., Sarath, G. 2004. C-Terminal 23 kDa polypeptide of soybean Gly m Bd 28K is a potential allergen. *Planta* 220:56–63.

Yamanashi, R., Huang, T., Tsuji, H., Bando, N., Ogawa, T. 1995. Reduction of the soybean allergenicity by the fermentation with *Bacillus natto*. *Food Sci Technol Int* 1:14–17.

Yamanashi, R., Tsuji, H., Bando, N., Yamada, Y., Nadaoka, Y., Huang, T., Nishikawa, K., Emoto, S., Ogawa, T. 1996. Reduction of the allergenicity of soybean by treatment with proteases. *J Nutr Sci Vitaminol* (Tokyo) 42:581–587.

# 13 Wheat (*Triticum aestivum*) Allergens

*Joanna Leszczynska*

## CONTENTS

## 13.1 ALLERGENIC PROTEINS IN WHEAT AND CEREAL: THE BIOCHEMICAL, BIOLOGICAL, AND IMMUNOLOGICAL PROPERTIES OF MAIN CEREAL ALLERGENS

The most common wheat species used in food production is ordinary wheat, also called bread wheat (*Triticum aestivum*). It is an allohexaploid (AABBDD), in which the genomes were obtained by spontaneous hybridization of *T. turgidum* (AABB) and *Aegilops tauschii* (DD) about 10,000 years ago (Vasil, 2007). Other grown wheat species are tetraploidal durum wheat *T. durum*, used in pasta production and small amounts of hexaploidal spelt *T. spelta* and tetraploidal *T. polonicum* (Curtis et al. 2002).

Wheat grain endosperm contains 8%–12% of proteins. These proteins are divided into two groups: nongluten proteins (15%–20%) and gluten proteins, making up about 80%–85% of all proteins. Nongluten proteins (soluble proteins) are considered soluble in dilute salt solutions, and albumins (water soluble) and globulins (water insoluble) can be distinguished (Osborne, 1907); despite this some globulins are soluble in salt solutions only at increased temperatures (Singh and Shepherd, 1987), and some hydrophobic protein-binding lipids require more hydrophobic solvents (Singh et al., 1990). Gluten, described as a ductile substance left after washing out soluble compounds and starch granules from wheat dough, which according to mass consists of 75%–85% of proteins, 5%–10% of lipids, and carbohydrates. It is assumed that gluten means wheat proteins that are insoluble in salt solutions: gliadins and gluten-ins (Osborne, 1907).

Despite different sequences and repetitive motives, all gliadins have the same secondary structure of loose spirals which are a balanced compromise between the β-spiral and poly-L-proline structure (polyproline helix II) (Parrot et al., 2002), the balance is dependent on temperature, type of solvent, and hydration level (Miles et al., 1991). Similar sequences can be found in other proteins, mainly animal proteins such as elastin and collagen, and they are responsible for particular biomechanical properties connected to reverse β-spirals or β-sheet structures (Tatham and Shewry, 2000).

A high content of glutamine, proline, and phenylalanine residues is characteristic for ω-gliadins and they make up about 80% of these proteins. The types of ω1, 2- (so-called slow) and ω5-gliadins (fast) differ from each other by molecular weights (ca. 40kDa for ω1,2, ca. 50kDa for ω5-gliadins) and electrophoretic mobility. Most ω-gliadins do not contain cysteine residues, while Gln- and Pro-rich sequences dom-inate their structure, e.g., PQQPFPQQ. ω-Gliadins consist of large amounts of well-defined polyproline helixes with a lot of β turns, although the presence of α-helical structure has not been investigated (Blanch et al., 2003).

Apart from a few exceptions, α/β type gliadins contain six, while γ type has eight cysteine residues that are localized in C-terminal domains, creating three or four intracellular disulfide bonds, respectively (Grosch and Wieser, 1999). A little number of gliadins contains an odd number of cysteine residues, which is the result of some mutations. These proteins together with glutenins create polymers, and what follows by means of sequential fractionation is that they appear among gliadins as well as glutenins.

Decomposition of gliadins into types is strongly dependent on wheat specie (gen-otype) and crop conditions. The main ingredients are proteins of α/β (60%) and γ (30%) types, while ω-gliadins occur in low amounts (10%) (Wieser and Kieffer, 2001).

Glutenins are aggregated wheat gluten proteins bound by intermolecular disulfide bridges, which create polymers of molecular mass from 500 to above 10,000kDa, and these are the biggest known proteins in nature (Wieser et al., 2006). As a result of reduction of disulfide bonds glutenin subunits present similar solubility as glia-dins. The subunits of glutenins according to molecular weight were divided into two groups—low-molecular weight (LMW) and high-molecular weight (HMW) glute-nin subunits.

LMW glutenin subunits are the dominating group of the wheat protein fraction and make up about 20% of all gluten proteins (Wieser and Kieffer, 2001). In terms of molecular weight, amino acid content, and structure, glutenins are similar to α/β- and γ-gliadins. The N-terminal domain is rich in glutamine and prolamine repetitive units, such as QQQPPFS, whereas the C-terminal domain is homological to corre-sponding domains in α/β- and γ-gliadins. In LMW glutenins eight cysteine residues exist: six of them are located in homological places as in the case of both types of gliadins, and they create three intramolecular disulfide bonds; and two unique cysteine residues, unable to create intramolecular bonds due to steric reasons.

The properties of wheat dough are strongly dependent on the number of HMW subunits and their type, but the presence of type x subunits was said to be more significant (Wieser and Kieffer, 2001). Looking at dough quality and volume of obtained bread the most important is presence of Dx5 subunits (with additional Cys) and Bx7 (present in the highest number) (Wieser and Zimmermann, 2000). Wheat proteins can cause allergy. Their allergenicity is connected to the method of exposure, which can be inhalatory (through the respiratory chain), contact (through skin), and food (after consuming food product containing wheat) allergens.

Baker's asthma is a form of inhalatory allergy. It can be observed in asthma form or nose mucosa membrane inflammation (catarrh), with the creation of specific antibodies IgE against ingredients of wheat or rye flour. The presence of anti-wheat antibodies was discovered in almost 70% of bakers (Baur and Posh, 1998; Sander et al., 1999). For baker's asthma it is very characteristic that there exists plenty of different allergens, and patients show different, individual reactions to these allergens (Sutton et al., 1982; Sander et al., 2001). By using two-dimensional gel electrophoresis and immunoblotting, it was observed that among nongluten proteins, almost 70 proteins observed that bind IgE (Posh et al., 1995), but only a few of them were identified and molecularly characterized: the proteins of molecular weights 14 and 17 kDa, belonging to α-amylase/trypsin inhibitors, among them there are tetrameric subunits of α-amylase inhibitor (Sanchez-Monge et al., 1992; Armentia et al., 1993), two highly homologic dimeric α-amylase inhibitors (Armentia et al., 1993; Fränken et al., 1994; Amano et al., 1998), monomeric α-amylase inhibitor (Walsh and Howden, 1989; Armentia et al., 1993; Amano et al., 1998), homolog of barley trypsin inhibitor (Amano et al., 1998), 36 kDa peroxides (Sanchez-Monge et al., 1997; Yamashita et al., 2002), dehydrogenase homologs (glicerinaldehyde-3-phosphate) from *Hordeum vulgare* (Sander et al., 2001), isomerase homolog (triosephosphate) from *H. vulgare*, acyl-CoA oxidase (Posh et al., 1995; Weiss et al., 1997; Sander et al., 2001), fructose-biphosphate aldolase (Weiss et al., 1997), thioredoxin *h*B (Tri a 25) (Weichel et al., 2006a,b), and serpin/serine proteinase inhibitors (Sander et al., 2001). Despite the fact that 70%–80% of IgE-binding activity proteins from albumins and globulins are present (Walsh et al., 1985; Weiss et al., 1993), as inhalatory allergens also gluten proteins have been identified–mainly α- and ω5-gliadins (Sandiford et al., 1997).

Hydrolysates of wheat proteins that are added to the production of creams and hair-conditioners were identified as those evoking contact allergy symptoms, causing skin rash and reddening, in individuals having no previous symptoms connected to wheat products (Varjonen et al., 2000a; Pequet and Lauriere, 2003).

Consumption of wheat products or products enriched with wheat proteins may result in different symptoms. The most common are: urticaria, atopic dermatitis (AD), and wheat-dependent exercise-induced anaphylaxis (WDEIA), but AD is most common among children while urticaria and WDEIA refer to adults (Palosuo, 2003; Battais et al., 2005a,b).

The food allergen's ability to elicit an immunologic reaction on the intestinal mucosa is connected to its allergenic epitopes that evade degradation while going through the digestive system (Astwood et al., 1996). Allergenic reactions to food allergens are connected to symptoms' genesis in patients suffering from irritable bowel syndrome (Zwetchkenbaum and Burakoff, 1988). Gluten proteins are connected to allergy (related to IgE antibodies production) after wheat food consumption (Palosuo, 2003).

WDEIA is a serious affection where symptoms are not only connected to wheat protein consumption, but they also appear after the introduction of wheat proteins into the digestive track, and following physical effort. Research on IgE of patients suffering from WDEIA showed that wheat gliadins are responsible for the disease, as well as corresponding taxonomic prolamines of closely related cereals (Varjonen et al., 1997).

Analyzing sera of patients suffering from WDEIA the main allergen of this disease was found to be wheat $\omega$-gliadins. It was also shown that specific IgE antibodies against modified $\omega$5-gliadins undergo cross-reactions with $\gamma$- and $\omega$1,2-gliadins (Morita et al., 2000, 2001, 2003). Fast $\omega$-gliadins, also called $\omega$-gliadins type 1B (DuPont et al., 2000) or $\omega$-5 gliadins (Kasarda et al., 1983; Seilmeier et al., 2001), can be separated by means of RP HPLC into few dozens of proteins (Seilmeier et al., 2001). One of the fast $\omega$-gliadins, $\omega$5-gliadins, was identified as the main allergen in WDEIA disease (Palosuo et al., 1999).

Matsuo et al. have identified $\omega$5-gliadin linear epitopes recognized by IgE of patients suffering form WDEIA. QQXPQQQ (where X = I, F, or S) and QQSPEQQ are immunodominating fragments, while QQXPQQQ (X = L or Y) and PYPP are less reactive ones (Matsuo et al., 2004). Some of these characteristic motives occur also in sequences of other wheat proteins such as $\alpha$-, $\gamma$-, $\omega$1,2-gliadins, and glutenin LMW subunits (Anderson and Greene, 1997; Cassidy et al., 1998; Anderson et al., 2001), which can cross-react with IgE antibodies against $\omega$5-gliadin, but they are not present in proteins belonging to albumins and globulins, which are the main allergens in baker's asthma. Among wheat food allergens, proteins from $\alpha$- and $\gamma$-gliadin groups and LMW glutenin subunits (Watanabe et al., 1995; Maruyama et al., 1998) were identified, and a motif that is recognized by IgE antibodies, pentapeptide QQQPP, in LMW glutenin sequences was identified (Tanabe et al., 1996b).

$\omega$5-Gliadin protein was known to be an allergen in children suffering from an immediate type of allergy to wheat (Palosuo et al., 2001b). Cross-linking of $\omega$5-gliadin with transglutaminase after its previous digestion with pepsin and trypsin results in a significant increase in the amount of epitopes bound by IgE, both in *in vitro* as well as *in vivo* conditions (Palosuo et al., 2003).

LMW wheat albumins, belonging to the $\alpha$-amylase inhibitors family are related to baker's asthma (Gomez et al., 1990), however, they are not potential allergens causing the occurrence of symptoms after the consumption of wheat flour especially after thermal processing (Simonato et al., 2004). Although some authors defined these proteins as responsible for food allergy to wheat (James et al., 1997; Armentia et al., 2002), this form of allergy is connected to different allergens, mainly insoluble proteins (Sutton et al., 1982). Inhibitors of $\alpha$-amylase are present as main food allergens only in the case of atopic patients (Simonato et al., 2001). Among food allergens thioredoxin $h$B (Tri a 25) (Weichel et al., 2006b) and unspecific proteins responsible for lipids transport LPT (Battais et al., 2005a), LMW proteins (9 kDa), recognized in many of plant species as food allergens, have been identified (Asero et al., 2002).

More than 80% of patients suffering from AD to wheat and only 50% with wheat-dependent anaphylaxis and urticaria have serum IgE against proteins from albumin and globulin groups. Among people suffering from wheat-dependent urticaria, proteins from ω5-gliadins group-binding IgE occurred to be the main allergens in more than 50% of cases (Battais et al., 2005a).

James et al. have identified α-amylase inhibitor as an allergen in children with food allergy to wheat (James et al., 1997), also other research identified a lot of other nongluten proteins that are bound by IgE in this group of patients (Sutton et al., 1982; Jones et al., 1995; Varjonen et al., 1995). Moreover, it was found that in children with food allergy to wheat sera IgE antibodies against gliadins were present (Räsänen et al., 1994; Varjonen et al., 2000b; Battais et al., 2005a).

In the paper by Osman et al. (1998), the technique of phage imagining of short peptides obtained from gliadins was used in order to determine epitopes recognized by antibodies. Obtained peptides which were homologs to the primary structure of gliadin represented the antigens whose majority is concentrated on N-terminal fragments of gliadins.

The research on the binding reaction of gluten proteins with monoclonal antibodies against different fractions of wheat prolamines showed that antibodies of wide specificity were binding a lot of fragments of N-terminal α-gliadin, however first 24 amino acid residues showed antigenicity of N-terminal of α-gliadins domain (Sissons et al., 1999).

In case of γ-gliadins two regions showed high antigenicity, but both were contained in the domain with repeated motif. Other fragments recognized by monoclonal antibodies were CCQQL in C-terminal domain, containing two cysteine residues taking part in intracellular bonds and amphipathic nanopeptide DCQVMRQQC, located at the end of N-terminus of C-terminal domain. A small amount of monoclonal antibodies of various selectivity recognized epitopes from N-terminus of investigated prolamines (Skerritt et al., 2000).

Battais identified sequences of gliadin epitopes that are bound by IgE from patients allergic to wheat with utricaria, anaphylaxis, or WDEIA, with AD, allergy to deamidated proteins (Battais et al., 2005b).

## 13.2 MECHANISM AND PHYSIOLOGICAL INFLUENCES OF CEREAL GLUTEN ON ANATOMICAL PARTS OF THE SMALL INTESTINE: THE ROLE OF WHEAT PROTEINS IN INDUCTION OF OTHER DISEASES (DIARRHEA AND CELIAC DISEASE)

For the first time celiac disease (CD) was described in the first century A.C. (Adams, 1856), however in medical term it is used since the end of the nineteenth century (Gee, 1888).

Celiac disease, enteropathy of small intestine, is more common than it is expected. This is one of the most common food intolerances, occurring with frequency of

1:130–1:300 among European and U.S. population; however in South America, North Africa, and Asia it is hardly diagnosed (Di Cagno et al., 2004). Last research suggested that in the United Kingdom and Ireland the occurrence frequency is higher (1:80–1:122), while among Sahrawi (west Sahara) population every 20th person suffers from this disease (Ciclitira and Moodie, 2003).

Celiac disease is a genetically dependent disease. In people who are genetically predisposed, the consumption of cereal products containing gluten leads to atrophy of villi structure with compensational crypts hyperplasia and massive lymphocytic infiltration around the lamina propria of the mucosa. The consecutive introduction of gluten into the diet results in the recurrence of histopathological changes (Kaukinen et al., 2002).

The background of the disease has not yet been specified, probably because of the many different factors interacting: genetic, immunologic, metabolic, and environmental (Gianfrani et al., 2005; Cornell and Stelmasiak, 2007). The toxic theory assumes the existence of enzymatic disorders responsible for incorrect gluten digestion, which in nondigested form is toxic to bowel cells (enterocytes). Immunological mechanisms involved in the disease show that the body produces antigliadin antibodies, and that lymphocytic infiltration with a majority of T cells in the small intestine mucosa is present (confirmed by small intestine biopsy).

The following factors testify to the autoaggressive background of the disease: investigated specific antibodies in serum, e.g., IgAEMA, IgAARA, coexistence with other diseases having autoaggressive background such as ulcerative colitis, systemic lupus, and sarcoidosis. In case of people suffering from celiac disease, antibodies against other food antigens, e.g., against cow milk proteins or egg albumin were also present. Presence of these antibodies seems to be a secondary occurrence that is a result of the increased absorbance of these antigens by the damaged mucosa.

Individuals who inherit some copies of the human leukocyte antigen (HLA) gene more often suffer from celiac disease than the rest of the population. The strongest correlation to celiac disease is found in HLA DQ2 genes that are present in about 90%–95% of patients, while in the rest HLA DQ8 genes are present. However, these genes are also present in about 20%–40% of healthy people (Kaukinen et al., 2002; Ciclitira et al., 2005; Hourigan, 2006).

Although the relation between increased risk of falling sick with celiac disease and the presence of class I alleles HLA: HLA B8 is still valid, a higher association with celiac disease occurrence have class II HLA genes. More than 90% patients have celiac disease alleles Dqa1*0510 and DQb*0210, which occur in *cis* (haplotype DR17) or *trans* position (heterozygote DR11/7 or DR12/7). Patients who do not have this haplotype inherit DR4–DQ8 (Dqa1*0301 + DQb1*0302) genes. It seems that DQ2 genes show dose effect, which means that people who inherit two copies of DQ2 genes suffer from peracute course of the disease and initial symptoms than people being heterozygotes for DQ2.

The significant meaning of DQ2 and DQ8, in both inheritances as well as in celiac disease pathology, comes from the fact that these genes are coding proteins taking part in immunocompetent cell presentation of antigens to T-lymphocytes. T-lymphocytes that are isolated from the intestinal mucosa of patients with celiac disease with expression of tissue antigens DQ2 or DQ8 showed high affinity to some gliadin peptide fragments (Ciclitira et al., 2005; Hamer, 2005). Similar reaction has not been observed in the case of clones of T-lymphocytes that were isolated from people not suffering from CD. A lot of obtained result data seem to prove hypotheses suggesting that environmental factors may have influence on the disease. It is suggested that in people who are genetically predisposed it is possible to break tolerance to gluten during stimulation of the immunological system (e.g., digestion track infection, after surgeries), when intensified epithelium permeability occurs (neonates, during diarrhea caused by infections, during pregnancy). Increased epithelial permeability in these conditions leads to intensive antigen penetration among other gluten penetrates, what induces the cascade of steps resulting in villi structure atrophy (Williamson and Marsh, 2002). It is known that gluten antigenicity increases when it undergoes reaction with tissue transglutaminase (Ciclitira et al., 2005). This is an enzyme that is released in large amounts when tissues are damaged, and is responsible for regeneration processes (Koning et al., 2005). It can also undergo glutamine deamination. Gluten is glutamine-rich protein and its deamination in some specific areas makes it suitable to the structure of DQ2 and DQ8 antigens. It has to be pointed that the interactions between tissue transglutaminase and gliadin occur only in case of high supply of both substrates, which could explain the environmental hypothesis, pointing out unspecific damage of the intestinal epithelium as a stimulus breaking tolerance to gluten.

On subsequent exposure to prolamine, the cells that are responsible for antigen presentation show them to already allergic lymphocytes Th (Dewar et al., 2004; Periolo and Chernavsky, 2006), which then produce whole variety of cytokinins that have proinflammatory properties. Then cytokinins stimulate cytotoxic mechanisms that lead to villi atrophy and crypts expansion. Simultaneously T-lymphocytes activate B-lymphocytes that after conversion into plasmocytes produce highly sensitive and specific for noncured celiac disease endomysial antibodies in IgA class (IgAEmA), antibodies against tissue transglutaminase (IgAtTG) as well as antigliadin antibodies (AGA).

Some of the rarely occurring symptoms of CD are epilepsy, polyeuropathy, myelopathy, myopathy, and generalized or limited focuses of reduction of brain's grey matter with progressive dementia (Hadjivassiliou et al., 2007). The treatment for celiac disease is based on strict gluten-free diet excluding all wheat, rye, and barley products. It has now been proved that oat, advised to be avoided in the past, is not harmful for people with celiac disease (Holm et al., 2006). The products that can be included into the diet of celiac disease patients are naturally gluten-free ingredients such as processed gluten-free products of rice, maize, millet, soy, buckwheat, tapioca, or products containing wheat starch where gluten fraction is below 1 mg/100 g of dry mass. Epitopes related to celiac disease pathogenesis and allergy to wheat related to IgE seem to be different (Constantin et al., 2005).

Some of the peptide fragments were recognized as inducing toxic symptoms in patients with CD. Among them the following fragments can be found: 31–43 fragment from α-gliadin (Picarelli et al., 1999), 31–49 fragment from A-gliadin, one of the α-gliadin proteins (Sturgess et al., 1994), 56–75 fragment from α-gliadin (Fraser et al., 2003), 62–75 fragment from α2-gliadin (Shan et al., 2002), 33-meric epitope, corresponding to 57–89 fragment from α2-gliadin (Arentz-Hansen et al., 2000; Shan et al., 2002), 134–153 fragment from γ-gliadin (Aleanzi et al., 2001), and glutenin sequences (Wieser, 1996; van der Wal et al., 1999; Molberg et al., 2003)

## 13.3  CHANGES IN IMMUNOREACTIVITY OF WHEAT ALLERGENS DURING TECHNOLOGICAL PROCESSES

The structure of native gluten that is stabilized by disulfide bridges is constantly changing, from synthesis and proteins folding to final product achievement (e.g., bread) (Wieser et al., 2006). During bread-making process the state of polymers depends on three competitive factors: oxidation of free sulfhydryl groups that support glutenin polymerization, presence of glutathione, and gliadins with odd number of cysteine residues that block the polymerization, and reactions between glutenins and thiol compounds that cause gluten depolymerization. During dough mixing the main polymerizing oxidant is oxygen present in the air, similar effect can be achieved by adding other oxidizing agents such as potassium bromate(V), potassium iodate(V), or dehydroascorbic acid to prevent oxidative cross-linking of gluten proteins LMW compounds containing thiol groups such as cysteine or tripeptide glutathione (GSH), as they disturb creation of disulfide bridges (Hahn and Grosch, 1998; Grosch and Wieser, 1999; Koehler, 2003; Li et al., 2004). The reactions where disulfide bonds between gluten proteins are created or reorganized also occur while mixing wheat flour with water in order to obtain dough, with net protein required in bread production (Lindsay and Skerritt, 1999).

During bread production, apart from disulfide bonds between gluten proteins additional covalent bonds are also created. Among them we can distinguish dityrosine cross-linking (Tilley et al., 2001) and cross-linking between gluten proteins (tyrosine residues) and dehydroferulic acid of arabinoxylans (Piber and Koehler, 2005), and also noncovalent bonds influencing gluten aggregation and stabilization of created structure (Wieser et al., 2006).

In alkaline conditions, usually combined with thermal processing, racemization of amino acid residues can be observed and covalent cross-links such as dehydroalanine, lysinoalanine, and lanthionine are created (Friedman, 1999a,b). The bonds obtained that way are durable, and long-term protein processing in alkaline conditions leads to the decrease in nutrition value of the product, which is caused by the decrease in susceptibility of such created bonds to digestion. Severe thermal conditions during food processing might cause isopeptide cross-linking through condensation of lysine ε-amine group with asparagine or glutamine amide residue (Singh, 1991).

The influence of temperature on gliadin allergenicity has been investigated (Rumbo et al., 1996). Heating at 100°C for 5 min resulted in the increase of immunoreactivity while longer exposure resulted in a decreased. Other researches have not shown any dependence of wheat proteins allergenicity on cooking in boiling water temperature (Simonato et al., 2004). The increase followed by the decrease in gliadin immunoreactivity has been observed after microwave heating (Leszczyńska et al., 2003a), however, such result was only obtained for determination of immunoreactivity with the usage of commercial antigliadin antibodies. The measurements performed after microwave heating with the usage of the antibodies from patients allergic to wheat proteins showed an initial increase followed by a decrease, but further decrease had not been observed, and there was no high-level change of immunoreativity (Leszczyńska et al., 2003a).

The research conducted since 1970s showed that ionic radiation used for food preservation is an effective method of microorganism inactivation. The usage of irradiation does not require additional substances and it is a safe physical process that goes under full technological control (Farag and El-Khawas, 1998). Apart from unquestionable advantages, the main disadvantage of this method is induction of changes in radiated chemicals in the composition of food products. The influence of gamma irradiation on molecules is mainly connected to water radiolysis and its reactions with proteins. Radicals that are created may react with protein molecules causing physicochemical changes, such as amino acid residues transformation, cleavage of peptide and disulfide bonds, and cross-linking of chains resulting in aggregation (Cieśla et al., 2000). The usage of maximal dose of gamma irradiation (10 kGy) comes from Word Heath Organization (WHO) regulations of food decontamination and sterilization (WHO, 1988). Within the accepted limits for gamma irradiation usage it was observed that gamma irradiation treatment causes linear increase in gliadin immunoreactivity (Leszczyńska et al., 2003b).

Plenty of wheat prolamine epitopes contain one or more glutamine residues. The decrease of their immunoreactivity may be obtained by their deamidation. There are several methods known in order to conduct protein deamidation: by means of strong acids (Wagner and Gueguen, 1995), enzymes (Kato et al., 1987; Kumagai et al., 1998; Yong et al., 2004), or ion exchangers in cationic form (Shih, 1987; Kumagai et al., 2002, 2004). Acidic treatment is the simplest method from those presented above, however it causes uncontrolled hydrolysis of peptide bonds with the creation of peptides with characteristic bitter taste and reduction of protein properties. Due to the same reason usage of proteases is not recommended (Kato et al., 1987).

Glutaminases can be applied, but these enzymes do not affect asparagine residues as substrate (Yong et al., 2004). In case of gluten proteins, there exists another restriction; prolamines are insoluble in water solvents, while ethanol solvents cause enzyme inactivation. The application of ion exchange carriers seems to be the most convenient method with the smallest side effects (Kumagai et al., 2002).

Acidic deamidation of gluten proteins caused decrease in immunoreactivity of IgE from sera of patients with food allergy to wheat, however deamidation above 50% significantly limited protein-binding ability of IgE (Maruyama et al., 1998; Akiyama et al., 2006).

Usage of ionic exchanger allowed gliadin deamidation by 28% (Kumagai et al., 2001) and glutenins by 30% (Norimatsu et al., 2002). Kumagai et al. were investigating digestion of *in vitro* and *in vivo* deamidated gliadins. Deamidation increased gliadin digestivity by pancreatic enzymes in mice both *in vitro* and *in vivo*. Rabbit antigliadin did not show difference between pepsin hydrolysates of gliadin before and after as well as no difference between pancreatic hydrolysates of gliadins deamidated *in vivo*, but *in vitro* studies showed reduced bounding of these hydrolysates. However, the same researchers showed that deamidated gliadins can be only used for hypoallergenic flour for patients with food allergies (Kumagai et al., 2007).

The gentle deamidation of gluten proteins by acetic acid resulted in minor electrophoretic changes in gluten proteins, caused by partial proteolysis, especially when higher temperature were applied. Immunoreactivity of gluten proteins in relation to human IgA antigliadin antibodies was lowered even below 30% for unmodified proteins, however the immunoreactivity change has not been dependent on temperature of acidic deamidation but on how long the process lasted (Berti et al., 2007).

Enzymatic hydrolysis of wheat gluten in most cases leads to obtain hydrolysates of functional properties different to initial ones, which in most cases depends on molecular size and level of conducted hydrolysis (Drago and Gonzalez, 2001). Enzymatic modification of wheat proteins in *in vivo* conditions or during processing stage may additionally result in epitope changes so that they may not be recognized by the immunological system. Enzymatic modifications of wheat flour may cause food tolerance and this way reduces allergic response (Watanabe et al., 1994a).

The greatest problem connected to gluten protein immunoreactivity as well as with peptides which are responsible for inflammatory states in celiac disease is the presence of peptides containing proline that are resistant to proteolysis. The group of specific enzymes is required for hydrolysis of peptide bonds in which proline residue is present (Hausch et al., 2003).

Prolyl oligopeptidase (PEP) (EC 3.4.21.26) hydrolyses peptide bond on the inner side of the carbonyl residue of proline. High proline content in epitopes makes them resistant to digestive action of enzymes. PEP hydrolyzed 33-meric polypeptide (LQLQPFPQPQLPYPQPQLPYPQPQLPYPQPQPF) obtained from $\alpha$-gliadins (Shan et al., 2002). PEP obtained from *Aspergillus niger*, due to its high resistance to pepsin (Stepniak et al., 2006) is still investigated as an enzyme that can hydrolyze gluten in *in vitro* conditions.

Subtilisin (alkalase) (EC 3.4.21.62) used for gluten hydrolysis brought the highest hydrolysis level among all used enzymes. Usage of enzymes in an amount equal to 1% of the total amount of gluten proteins resulted in the creation of hydrolyzed polypeptides of molecular weights below 10 kDa (Kong et al., 2007). Subtilisin used for gliadins modification (0.01%) caused decrease in immunoreactivity below 50% of the initial values in case of tests where rabbit antigliadin antibodies were applied, while for tests with antibodies from human sera, hydrolyzed gliadins were hardly detectable (Leszczyńska et al., 2002). The electrophoretic profile of gliadins did not change after treatment with so small an amount of the enzyme, however LMW glutenin subunit epitopes (QQQPP) were hydrolyzed in 70%, no changes in physicochemical properties were observed.

Bromelain (EC 3.4.22.32) was used as an enzyme to hydrolyze gluten proteins. It was initially chosen due to its high ability to degrade this group of proteins and its low cost. The flour obtained after hydrolysis with bromelain showed significant decrease in gluten (glutenins) immunoreactivity (Tanabe et al., 1996a). However, bromelain undergoes cross-reactions with sera of patients with wheat allergy (Watanabe et al., 2000). Moreover, in other research studies gluten proteins hydrolyzed with bromelain instead of a decrease showed high increase in immunoreactivity in comparison to unmodified proteins (Leszczyńska et al., 2002).

Colagenase (EC 3.4.24.3): Wanatabe et al. obtained flour of lowered immunoreactivity of glutenin fraction by using collagenase of 0.1% and a longer process time than in the case of bromelain. This hypoallergic flour has then been used in bread production stopping carbon dioxide in bread structure (Watanabe et al., 1994a).

Actinase has been chosen to hydrolyze wheat flour allergens due to the fact that it does not undergo cross-reactions with patients' IgE, its low cost, and its starch hydrolyzing ability. Gluten in flour hydrolyzed with actinase presented low allergenicity (Watanabe et al., 1994b). To improve hypoallergenic flour production Wanatabe et al. introduced two-stage hydrolysis applying cellulase and actinase. Such obtained flour consisted of 96.4% of water-soluble polypeptides (Watanabe et al., 1994b). Gelatinization of obtained hypoallergic flour allowed for the production of noodles, cookies, pizza, and wafers with texture parameters similar to related products made of unmodified wheat flour (Watanabe et al., 2000).

Papain (EC 3.4.22.2) has been used to gluten proteins modification by Wang et al. (2007). Addition of enzyme was equal to 0.025% of mass of gluten (1500 U/g gluten). Gliadin fraction occurred to be more sensitive to papain action than glutenins, especially insoluble glutenins occurred to be resistant to hydrolysis. The content of gliadin fraction after 4-h hydrolyzation decreased by more than 50% (Wang et al., 2007). Lower enzyme to gliadins ratio (0.01%) resulted in immunoreactivity decrease by only about 20% (Leszczyńska et al., 2002).

Thioredoxin when combined with NADPH can effectively and specifically reduce disulfide bonds in proteins changing their biological characteristics. Gliadins from flour sample exposed to thioredoxin action lowered allergenic response in atopic dogs allergic to wheat (Buchanan et al., 1997). Similar results have been obtained by Waga et al. (2003). The immunoreactivity of gliadins decreased by a few times, while baking properties of flour did not change.

Application of enzymes for protein cross-linking is an alternative to chemical cross-linking and also they are safe to be used in food production and their activity does not change while thermal processing (baking, pasteurization, etc.).

Transglutaminase (EC 2.3.2.23) (TG) is an acylotransferase that has the ability to catalyze intra- and intermolecular cross-linking resulting in the creation of a peptide bond between lysine and glutamine residues (by creation of $\Sigma$-($\gamma$-Glu)-Lys with no loss of nutritional properties of lysine residues) (Seguro et al., 1996a). This enzyme can also catalyze incorporation of amine compounds through amid group of glutamine residue, which without availability of amines undergoes deamidation (Nielson, 1995). Due to escalating costs of enzymes, the most commonly used enzyme is transglutaminase, of microbiological origin, mainly produced by *Streptoverticulum* spp. (Seguro et al., 1996b) The most important feature of this exocellular enzyme is that its catalytic activity is $Ca^{2+}$ independent. A lot of cases when transglutaminase was used in order to improve functional properties of milk, meat, or fish proteins have been already described (Zhu et al., 1995; Motoki and Seguro, 1998).

Transglutaminase used in bread-making allows the improvement of functionality of flour proteins through creation of big, insoluble polymers (Larre et al., 2000; Bonet et al., 2005; Caballero et al., 2005). Among wheat proteins the most susceptible to cross-linking activity of transglutaminase are HMW glutenins (Larre et al., 2000; Gerrard et al., 2001; Bauer et al., 2003; Rosell et al., 2003), however as substrates for this enzyme LMW glutenins (Autio et al., 2005), $\alpha$-gliadins (Bauer et al., 2003), and even albumins and globulins (Gerrard et al., 2001) are also susceptible.

Gluten proteins from dough with bacterial TG in the amount 8–16 ppm do not show changes in SDS-PAGE electrophoretic characteristics (Tseng and Lai, 2002).

By using higher doses of transglutaminase, different wheat proteins were treated inequally (Gerrard et al., 2001). Among water-soluble proteins, the most influence of cross-linking agent can be observed on albumins that create complexes of HMW (even MW > 200 kDa) with no change in solubility compared to the initial substrates. Among albumin fraction mainly LMW proteins of MW < 55 kDa were cross-linking. Contrary to albumins, gliadins did not undergo cross-linking, however purified gliadin fraction undergoes such reaction (Alexandre et al., 1993). Aggregates can be also observed among glutenins, mainly HMW glutenins of molecular weight between 60 and 120 kDa (Gerrard et al., 2001).

Berti et al. examined transglutaminase influence on gliadin fraction proteins, both of native form as previously digested with trypsin (pH 8.0; E/S = 1/30, 3 h, 37°C, trypsin concentration 0.5 mg/mL). Low content of lysine residues did not have any influence on intermolecular-binding, so the influence of cysteamine as an acyl acceptor of amino acid residues was investigated. After TG treatment, both gliadins and trypsin-modified gliadins showed significant increase in immunoreactivity in relation to human antigliadin IgA, while cysteamine addition resulted in almost four times lower immunoreactivity than for proteins before TG treatment (Berti et al., 2007). The decrease in gluten allergenicity after treatment with microbial transglutaminase was also analyzed and described by other research groups (Watanabe et al., 1994a; Leszczyńska et al., 2006).

Although, transglutaminase used for protein cross-linking is of microbiological origin and differs from human transglutaminase by recognized glutamine residues in gliadins, both enzymes deamidate polypeptides with creation of structures that are recognized by antigliadin IgA (Berti et al., 2007).

A completely different influence on proteins can be observed after treatment with oxidating enzymes, and is limited to thiol–disulfide configuration. Glucose oxidase, laccase, peroxidase, and tyrosinase are oxidating enzymes applied in wheat protein cross-linking (Færgemand et al., 1998; Figueroa-Espinoza et al., 1999; Labat et al., 2001; Tilley et al., 2001; Mattinen et al., 2005; Mattinen et al., 2006; Selinheimo et al., 2007). Despite noticeable changes in wheat protein properties, no research on immunoreactivity of aggregates obtained after oxidative enzyme treatment has been performed so far.

Sourdough fermentation is conducted with application of lactic acid bacteria. The aim of the process is possibility to control processes when characteristic aromatic compounds are produced as well as stopping fermentation of yeast and other bacterial species and bread shelf-life improvement. Among spontaneously fermented sourdoughs large variety of lactic acid bacteria, both homo- and heterofermentative, has been isolated. Most of these bacteria belong to *Lactobacillus* specie (Rollan et al., 2005). Presence of lactic acid bacteria is related to higher proteolysis than just when yeast is added to the dough (Gobbetti et al., 1994). During fermentation, bacteria hydrolyze proteins with creation of short peptides and single amino acids, required for immediate growth and acidification, and they are also present as aromatic compound precursors in bakery products (Gobbetti et al., 1994, 1996a; Gobbetti, 1998; Rollan and de Valdez, 2001).

Proteolysis occurring in sourdough and its rheological consequences related to gluten degradation are mainly caused by wheat proteinases that are activated in low-pH conditions (Thiele et al., 2003; Loponen et al., 2004). Proteolytic activity of lactic acid bacteria depends on bacterial strain (Di Cagno et al., 2002), and it does not play crucial role in protein hydrolysis during fermentation (Thiele et al., 2002, 2003; Loponen et al., 2004). Stronger proteolysis performed by mixed cultures than by individual strains results from the action of the complex of proteolytic enzymes with wide specificity, produced by different strains of lactic acid bacteria (De Angelis et al., 2006).

The lactic acid bacterial growth is limited by dough pH (Gänzle et al., 1998; Thiele et al., 2004). Glutenin depolymerization during fermentation depends on the amount of glutathione produced by lactic acid bacteria (Bolotin et al., 1999). Heterofermentative lactic acid bacteria have the enzymatic ability to create LMW thiol compounds such as glutathione reductase in *Lactobacillus sanfrancisciensis* (von Olnhausen et al., 2002) and cystathionine γ-lyase in some of the *Lactobacillus* species (De Angelis et al., 2002).

During wheat flour fermentation using *L. perolens* and *L. sakei*, significant decrease in free thiol groups promoting oxidative gluten cross-linking was observed. In case of *L. sanfranciscensis* usage in fermentation, expression of gene coding glutathione reductase, which has the ability to reduce exocellular GSSG (oxidized form of glutathione) to GSH (reduced form of glutathione) takes place (Vermeulen et al., 2006).

During fermentation the degradation of HMW glutenins influenced by endogenic aspartyl proteases occurs, however at the same time gliadins undergo hydrolysis only to an insignificant level (Loponen et al., 2004). It is connected with the inability of aspartyl proteases to hydrolyze effectively proteins belonging to this group (Belozersky et al., 1989; Bleukx et al., 1998). Cysteine proteases from sprouting wheat grains have the ability to hydrolyze gliadins (Dunaevsky et al., 1989; Bottari et al., 1996) that are active in pH between 3.5 and 5.5 (Bottari et al., 1996), which is proper for protein hydrolysis in sourdough. During sprouting of cereal grains also many other proteases are synthesized (Jones, 2005), and they have specific abilities to hydrolyze substrates containing proline (Mikola, 1986; Simpson, 2001).

Rollan et al. examined the possibility to hydrolyze 31–43 fragment from α-gliadin, that is responsible for inflammatory response in people with celiac disease (Marsh et al., 1995), by *Lactobacillus plantarum* CRL 759 and CRL 778 bacteria. These bacteria hydrolyze wheat proteins, and this was observed by an increase in single amino acid concentration, mainly of basic and aromatic character, after 6-h fermentation of wheat flour. Both bacterial strains were characterized by wide spectra of peptidases activity, and among them dipeptidase and tripeptidase occurred to be useful for lactic acid bacterial growth in sourdoughs (Gobbetti et al., 1996b). The amount of synthetic peptide LGQQQPFPPQQPY, which correlates to α-gliadin fragment, was decreased by 73% (*L. plantarum* CRL 759) and 36% (*L. plantarum* CRL 778) (Rollan et al., 2005). Also other lactic acid bacteria such as *Lactobacillus alimentarius* 15M and *L. brevis* 14G by about 54%–50%, *L. sanfrancisco* 7A (43%), and *L. hilgardii* 51B (35%) are able to hydrolyze this peptide (Di Cagno et al., 2002). Also, other toxic gliadin peptides undergo degradation in lactic acid fermentation conditions (Rizzello et al., 2006). Even stronger effect was obtained when a mixed culture of lactic acid bacteria and yeast *Saccharomyces cerevisiae* was used to ferment wheat flour, however, introduction of yeast may result in cross-reactions occurrence between them and gluten proteins (Watanabe et al., 1995).

Another attempt to decrease immunoreactivity of fermented dough was usage of 30% of wheat flour while rest was substituted by oat, millet, or buckwheat flour (Di Cagno et al., 2004). During 24-h fermentation conducted by selected lactic acid bacteria: *L. alimentarius* 15M, *L. brevis* 14G, *L. sanfranciscensis* 7A, and *L. hilgardii* 51B gliadins were almost completely hydrolyzed whereas other cereal prolamines did not change. The same bacteria strains were used for pasta production from fermented wheat–buckwheat flour (3:7) (Di Cagno et al., 2005). Gliadins were almost completely hydrolyzed, and the amount of gluten determined by R5-ELISA test decreased six times. In both cases, for fermented bread and fermented pasta, significant decrease but not complete elimination of polypeptide immunoreactivity was observed while examined with antigliadin antibodies from people suffering from CD (Di Cagno et al., 2004; Di Cagno et al., 2005).

## 13.4 ADVANCES IN MODIFICATIONS OF BIOCHEMICAL PROPERTIES OF CEREAL ALLERGENS: THE EFFECT OF ENVIRONMENTAL STRESSES ON ALLERGIC PROPERTIES OF CEREAL PROTEINS AND THE PROBLEM OF SAFETY OF GENETICALLY MODIFIED CEREALS

Growth of Thésée specie of wheat was conducted in different conditions changing temperature and water stress (Daniel and Triboï, 2002). The linear accumulation of soluble proteins in the grain was observed till 400–550°Cd (the unit represents the product of temperature by days), while beyond this temperature immediate decrease in albumin and globulin amount was present together with an increase in the content of gluten proteins (mainly glutenins), indicating the end of the ripening process.

During drought, modifications of spare proteins occur faster, about 400°Cd (Daniel and Triboi, 2002). Immediate change in spare protein solubility arises from their delayed polymerization when insoluble aggregates are formed (Benetrix et al., 1994; Stone and Nicholas, 1996). Addition of N in the form of fertilizers after anthesis period leads to an increase in the protein content in grains, whereas temperature rise or drought can result in decrease in crop amount due to starch formation (Cassman et al., 1992; Fowler, 2003). The gliadin content increases with increase in protein content in grain and decrease in glutenins amount (Wieser and Seilmeier, 1998; Triboi et al., 2000). The proportional increase in albumin and globulin amount in relation to N addition or temperature increase has not been observed (Wieser and Seilmeier, 1998; Triboi et al., 2003).

Fertilization with nitrogen compounds leads to an increase in the ratio of proteins belonging to ω-gliadins and HMW glutenins among wheat proteins, while the ratio of γ-gliadins and LMW glutenins decreases (Wieser and Seilmeier, 1998). Other scientists did not observe changes in HMW and LMW glutenin ratio with increase of N addition (Luo et al., 2000; Triboi et al., 2000). The content of ω-gliadins increased with an increase in temperature and N addition, whereas the ratio of α-gliadins increased with an increase in temperature but decreased after N-fertilization, inversely to γ-gliadins (Daniel and Triboi, 2000).

In moderate temperatures addition of fertilizer containing nitrogen, phosphorus, and potassium (NPK) after anthesis resulted in an increase in protein content in grains, mainly influencing the speed of protein accumulation. This increase was related to an increase both in sulfur-poor ω-gliadins and HMW glutenins, as well as in S-rich α-gliadins, with little influence on γ-gliadins, and a decrease of LMW glutenins. In higher temperatures (38/24°C) addition of NPK showed no big influence on protein accumulation in evolving grains. Under these conditions protein content was independent on fertilization (Dupont et al., 2006).

Wheat enrichment in sulfur by fertilization under optimal growth conditions (temperature, humidity, nitrogen) did not influence the total amount of gluten proteins when sulfur content in grains was above 0.12%, however for lower sulfur contents amount of proteins decreased significantly (Wieser et al., 2004). Sulfur deficiency caused an increase of prolamines of sulfur-poor ω-gliadins (especially ω5-gliadins) resulting in an increase of this protein group from 12% to about 30% of gluten, making up the main gliadin fraction. Contrary to ω-gliadins, γ-gliadins that contain the highest amount of sulfur amino acids among all gluten proteins (3.9 mol%) were synthesized up to a lower degree. Minor increase was observed in case of glutenin HMW subunits. Under sulfur deficiency conditions, the gliadin/glutenin ratio was increased while the glutenin HMW/LMW ratio decreased (Wieser et al., 2004), resulting in a significant change in dough rheological properties (Zhao et al., 1999). During other research studies, no changes in glutenin HMW/LMW ratio were observed after fertilization with sulfur (Luo et al., 2000).

The protein content is also dependent on grain size. The content of glutenins decreases with decrease in grain size, while the lowest gliadin contents were observed in grains of medium size (Konopka et al., 2007).

Genetic modifications seem to be promising in food quality improvement, also toward food allergies treatment. So far, genetic modifications have been applied in order to study the increment of wheat resistance to herbicides, insects, and other pathogens, and increment of crop yield and improvement of flour baking quality and nutrition value (Vasil, 2007). Introducing changes in protein allergenicity has not been often used due to doubts related to this method.

Application of genetic modifications in order to decrease allergenicity of food products may be very limited. In case of multigenic protein families, (e.g., wheat) complete elimination is impossible, only partial decrease in immunoreactivity can be achieved. Also, no studies have determined the long-term stability of introduced genes, whose mutation may cause serious clinical consequences in allergic people consuming modified food products that they think is harmless to them.

## 13.5 CROSS-REACTIVITY OF WHEAT ALLERGENS

IgE antibodies against wheat thioredoxin *h*B (Tri a 25) obtained from sera of patients suffering from baker's asthma or food allergy cross-reacted with its homologs from maize Zea m 25, as well as at lower level with thioredoxin ZmTRX*h*2 from maize and human thioredoxin, which have the same epitopes (Weichel et al., 2006a). The allergy to wheat thioredoxin can be detectable in patients with inhalatory allergy to grass pollen when allergy to wheat does not occur (Weichel et al., 2006a).

Gluten proteins are closely related to rye and barley prolamines, which can cause cross reactions with IgE from patients with baker's asthma (Sandiford et al., 1995). The antigen similarity toward IgE was shown among ω5-gliadin, main allergen of WDEIA and one of the allergens responsible for baker's asthma (Sandiford et al., 1997), and barley γ-3 hordein and rye γ-35 and γ-75 secalins (Palosuo et al., 2001a).

Sandiford et al. showed identity of epitopes of gliadins and proteins belonging to albumins and globulins allowing the appearance of cross-reactivity (Sandiford et al., 1997).

## REFERENCES

Adams F. (Ed. and Trans.) 1856. *Aretaeus, the Cappadocian. The Extant Works*. Sydenham Society, London.

Akiyama, H., Sakata, K., Yoshioka, Y., Murata, Y., Ishihara, Y., Teshima, R., Sawada, J., Maitani, T. 2006. Profile analysis and immunoglobulin E reactivity of wheat protein hydrolysates. *Int Arch Allergy Immunol* 40:36–42.

Aleanzi, M., Demonte, A.M., Esper, C., Garcilazo, S., Waggener, M. 2001. Celiac disease: Antibody recognition against native and selectively deaminated gliadin peptides. *Clin Chem* 47:2023–2028.

Alexandre, M.C., Popineau, Y., Viroben, G., Chiarello, M., Lelion, A.P., Geugen, J. 1993. Wheat gamma-gliadin as a substrate for bovine plasma factor XIII. *J Agric Food Chem* 41:2008–2214.

Amano, M., Ogawa, H., Kojima, K., Kamidaira, T., Suetsugu, S., Yoshihama, M., Satoh, T., Samejima, T., Matsumoto, I. 1998. Identification of the major allergens in wheat flour responsible for baker's asthma. *Biochem J* 330:1229–1234.

Anderson, O.D., Greene, F.C. 1997. The α-gliadin gene family. II. DNA and protein sequence variation, subfamily structure, and origins of pseudogenes. *Theor Appl Genet* 95:59–65.

Anderson, O.D., Hsia, C.C., Torres, V. 2001. Wheat γ-gliadin genes: Characterization of ten new sequences and further understanding of γ-gliadin gene family structure. *Theor Appl Genet* 103:323–330.

Arentz-Hansen, H., Korner, R., Molberg, O., Quarsten, H., Vader, W., Kooy, Y.M. 2000. The intestinal T cell response to alpha-gliadin in adult celiac disease is focused on a single deaminated glutamine targeted by tissue transglutaminase. *J Exp Med* 191:603–612.

Armentia, A., Sanchez-Monge, R., Gomez, L., Barber, D., Salcedo, G. 1993. In vivo allergenic activities of eleven purified members of a major allergen family from wheat and barley flour. *Clin Exp Allergy* 23:410–415.

Armentia, A., Rodriguez, R., Callejo, A., Martin-Esteban, M., Martin-Santos, J.M., Salcedo, G., Pascual, C., Sanchez-Monge, R., Pardo, M. 2002. Allergy after ingestion or inhalation of cereals involves similar allergens in different ages. *Clin Exp Allergy* 32:1216–1222.

Asero, R., Mistrello, G., Roncarolo, D., Amato, S., Caldironi, G., Barocci, F., van Ree, R. 2002. Immunological cross-reactivity between lipid transfer proteins from botanically unrelated plant-derived foods: A clinical study. *Allergy* 57:900–906.

Astwood, J.D., Leach, J.N., Fuchs, R.L. 1996. Stability of food allergens to digestion in vitro. *Nat Biotechnol* 14:1269–1273.

Autio, K., Kruus, K., Knaapila, A., Gerber, N., Flander, L., Buchert, J. 2005. Kinetics of transglutaminase-induced cross-linking of wheat proteins in dough. *J Agric Food Chem* 53:1039–1045.

Battais, F., Courcoux, P., Popineau, Y., Kanny, G., Moneret-Vautrin, D.A., Denery-Papini, S. 2005a. Food allergy to wheat: Differences in immunoglobulin E-binding proteins as a function of age or symptoms. *J Cereal Sci* 42:109–117.

Battais, F., Mothes, T., Moneret-Vautrin, D.A., Pineau, F., Kanny, G., Popineau, Y., Bodinier, M., Denery-Papini, S. 2005b. Identification of IgE-binding epitopes on gliadins for patients with food allergy to wheat. *Allergy* 60:815–821.

Baur, X., Posh, A. 1998. Characterized allergens causing bakers' asthma. *Allergy* 53: 562–566.

Bauer, N., Koehler, P., Wieser, H., Schieberle, P. 2003. Studies on effects of microbial transglutaminase on gluten proteins of wheat. I. Biochemical analysis. *Cereal Chem* 80:781–786.

Belozersky, M.A., Sarbakanova, S.T., Dunaevsky, Y.E. 1989. Aspartic proteinase from wheat seeds: Isolation, properties and action on gliadin. *Planta* 177:321–326.

Benetrix, F., Kaan, F., Autran, J.C. 1994. Changes in protein complexes of durum wheat in developing seed. *Crop Sci* 34:462–468.

Berti, C., Roncoroni, L., Falini, M.L., Caramanico, R., Dolfini, E., Bardella, M.T., Elli, L., Terrani, C., Forlani, F. 2007. Celiac-related properties of chemically and enzymatically modified gluten proteins. *J Agric Food Chem* 55:2482–2488.

Blanch, E.W., Kasarda, D.D., Hecht, L., Nielsen, K., Barron, L.D. 2003. New insight into the solution structures of wheat gluten proteins from Raman optical activity. *Biochemistry* 42:5665–5673.

Bleukx, W., Brijs, K., Torrekens, S., Van Leuven, F., Delcour, J.A. 1998. Specificity of a wheat gluten aspartic proteinase. *Biochim Biophys Acta* 1387:317–324.

Bolotin, A., Mauger, S., Malarme, K., Ehrlich, S.D., Sorokin, A. 1999. Low-redundancy sequencing of the entire *Lactococcus lactis* IL1403 genome. *Antonie van Leeuwenhoek* 76:27–76.

Bonet, A., Caballero, P.A., Gomez, M., Rosell, C.M. 2005. Microbial transglutaminase as a tool to restore the functionality of gluten from insect-damaged wheat. *Cereal Chem* 82:425–430.

Bottari, A., Capocchi, A., Fontanini, D., Galleschi, L. 1996. Major proteinase hydrolysing gliadin during wheat germination. *Phytochemistry* 43:39–44.

Buchanan, B.B., Adamidi, C., Lozano, R.M., Mee, B.C., Somma, M., Kobrehel, K., Ermel, R., Frick, O.L. 1997. Thioredoxin-linked mitigation of allergic responses to wheat. *Proc Natl Acad Sci USA* 94:5372–5377.

Caballero, P.A., Bonet, A., Rosell, C.M., Gomez, M. 2005. Effect of microbial transglutaminase on the rheological and thermal properties of insect damaged wheat flour. *J Cereal Sci* 42(1):93–100.

Cassidy, B.G., Dvorak, J., Anderson, O.D. 1998. The wheat low-molecular-weight glutenin genes: Characterization of six new genes and progress in understanding gene family structure. *Theor Appl Genet* 96:743–750.

Cassman, K.G., Bryant, D.C., Fulton, A.E., Jackson, L.F. 1992. Nitrogen supply effects on partitioning of dry matter and nitrogen to grain of irrigated wheat. *Crop Sci* 32.1251–1258.

Ciclitira, P.J., Moodie, S.J. 2003. Coeliac disease. *Best Pract Res* 17(2):181–195.

Ciclitira, P.J., Ellis, H.J., Lundin, K.E.A. 2005. Gluten-free diet—What is toxic? *Best Pract Res* 19(3):359–371.

Cieśla, K., Roos, Y., Głuszewski, W. 2000. Denaturation process in gamma irradiated proteins studied by differential scanning calorimetry. *Radiat Phys Chem* 58:233–243.

Constantin, C., Huber, W.D., Granditsch, G., Weghofer, M., Valenta, R. 2005. Different profiles of wheat antigens are recognised by patients suffering from celiac disease and IgE-mediated food allergy. *Int Arch Allergy Immunol* 138:200–204.

Cornell, H.J., Stelmasiak, T. 2007. A unified hypothesis of coeliac disease with implications for management of patients. *Amino Acids* 33:43–49.

Curtis, B.C., Rajam, S., Macpherson, H.G. (Eds.) 2002. *Bread Wheat: Improvement and Production, FAO Plant Production and Protection Series*. No. 30, Food and Agriculture Organisation of the United Nations, Rome.

Daniel, C., Triboi, E. 2000. Effects of temperature and nitrogen nutrition on the grain composition of winter wheat: Effects on gliadin content and composition. *J Cereal Sci* 32.45–56.

Daniel, C., Triboï, E. 2002. Changes in wheat protein aggregation during grain development: Effects of temperature and water stress. *Eur J Agron* 16:1–12.

De Angelis, M., Curin, A.C., McSweeney, P.L., Faccia, M., Gobbetti, M. 2002. Lactobacillus reuteri DSM 20016: Purification and characterization of a cystathionine gamma-lyase and use as adjunct starter in cheesemaking. *J Dairy Res* 69:255–267.

De Angelis, M., Rizello, C.G., Fasano, A., Clemente, M.G., De Simone, C., Silano, M., De Vincenzi, M., Losito, I., Gobbetti, M. 2006. VSL#3 probiotic preparation has the capacity to hydrolyze gliadin polypeptides responsible for celiac sprue. *Biochim Biophys Acta* 1765:80–93.

Dewar, D., Pereira, S., Ciclitira, P.J. 2004. The pathogenesis of celiac disease. *Int J Biochem Cell Biol* 36:17–24.

Di Cagno, R., De Angelis, M., Lavermicocca, P., De Vincenzi, M., Giovannini, C., Faccia, M., Gobbetti, M. 2002. Proteolysis by sourdough lactic acid bacteria: Effects on wheat flour protein fractions and gliadin peptides involved in human cereal intolerance. *Appl Environ Microbiol* 68:623–633.

Di Cagno, R., De Angelis, M., Auricchio, S., Greco, L., Clarke, C., De Vincenzi, M., Giovannini, C., D'Archivio, M., Landolfo, F., Parrilli, G., Minervini, F., Arendt, E., Gobbetti, M. 2004. Sourdough bread made from wheat and nontoxic flours and started with selected lactobacilli is tolerated in celiac sprue patients. *Appl Environ Microbiol* 70:1088–1096.

Di Cagno, R., De Angelis, M., Alfonsi, G., De Vincenzi, M., Silano, M., Vincentini, O., Gobbetti, M. 2005. Pasta made from durum wheat semolina fermented with selected lactobacilli as a tool for a potential decrease of the gluten intolerance. *J Agric Food Chem* 53:4393–4402.

Drago, S.R., Gonzalez, R.J. 2001. Foaming properties of enzymatically hydrolysed wheat gluten. *Innov Food Sci Emerg Technol* 1:269–273.

Dunaevsky, Y.E., Sarbakanova, S.T., Belozersky, M.A. 1989. Wheat seed carboxypeptidase and joint action on gliadin of proteases from dry and germinating-seeds. *J Exp Bot* 40:1323–1329.

DuPont, F.M., Vensel, W.H., Chan, R., Kasarda, D.D. 2000. Characterization of the 1B-type ω-gliadins from *Triticum aestivum* cultivar Butte. *Cereal Chem* 77:607–614.

Dupont, F.M., Hurkman, W.J., Vensel, W.H., Tanaka, C., Kothari, K.M., Chung, O.K., Altenbach, S.B. 2006. Protein accumulation and composition in wheat grains: Effects of mineral nutrients and high temperature. *Eur J Agron* 25:96–107.

Farag, R.S., El-Khawas, K.H.A.M. 1998. Influence of gamma-irradiations and microwaves on the antioxidant property of some essential oils. *Int J Food Sci Nutr* 19:109–115.

Færgemand, M., Otte, J., Qvist, K.B. 1998. Cross-linking of whey proteins by enzymatic oxidation. *J Agric Food Chem* 46:1326–1333.

Figueroa-Espinoza, M.C., Morel, M.H., Surget, A., Rouau, X. 1999. Oxidative cross-linking of wheat arabinoxylans by manganese peroxidase. Comparison with laccase and horseradish peroxidase. Effect of cysteine and tyrosine gelation. *J Sci Food Agric* 79:460–463.

Fowler, D.B. 2003. Crop nitrogen demand and grain protein concentration of spring and winter wheat. *Agron J* 95:260–265.

Fränken, J., Stephan, U., Meyer, H.E., König, W. 1994. Identification of alpha-amylase inhibitor as a major allergen of wheat flour. *Int Arch Allergy Immunol* 104:171–174.

Fraser, J.S., Engel, W., Ellis, H.J., Moodie, S.J., Pollock, E.L., Wieser, H., Ciclitira, P.J. 2003. Coeliac disease: In vivo toxicity of the putative immunodominant epitope. *Gut* 52:1698–1702.

Friedman, M. 1999a. Chemistry, biochemistry, nutrition, and microbiology of lysinoalanine, lanthionine, and histidinoalanine in food and other proteins. *J Agric Food Chem*
47:1295–1319.

Friedman, M. 1999b. Chemistry, nutrition, and microbiology of D-amino acids. *J Agric Food
Chem* 47:3457–3479.

Gänzle, M.G., Ehmann, M., Hammes, W.P. 1998. Modeling of growth of *Lactobacillus sanfranciscensis* and *Candida milleri* in response to process parameters of the sourdough
fermentation. *Appl Environ Microbiol* 64:2616–2623.

Gee, S. 1888. On the celiac disease. *Saint Bartholomew's Hospital Reports*. London.
24:17–20.

Gerrard, J.A., Fayle, S.E., Brown, P.A., Sutton, K.H., Simmons, L., Rasiah, I. 2001. Effects of
microbial transglutaminase on the wheat proteins of bread and croissant dough. *J Food
Sci* 66:782–786.

Gianfrani, C., Auricchio, S., Troncone, R. 2005. Adaptive and innate immune response in
celiac disease. *Immunol Lett* 99:141–145.

Gobbetti, M. 1998. The sourdough microflora: Interactions between lactic acid bacteria and
yeast. *Trends Food Sci Technol* 9:267–274.

Gobbetti, M., Simonetti, M.S., Rossi, J., Cossignani, A., Corsetti, A., Damiani, P. 1994. Free
D- and L-amino acid evolution during sourdough fermentation and baking. *J Food Sci*
59:881–884.

Gobbetti, M., Smacchi, E., Fox, P., Stepaniak, L., Corsetti, A. 1996a. The sourdough microflora. Cellular localization of proteolytic enzymes in lactic acid bacteria. *Lebensm Wiss
Technol* 29:561–569.

Gobbetti, M., Smacchi, E., Corsetti, A. 1996b. The proteolytic system of *Lactobacillus
sanfrancisco* CB1: Purification and characterization of a proteinase, a dipeptidase, and
an aminopeptidase. *Appl Environ Microbiol* 62:3220–3226.

Gomez, L., Martin, E., Hernandez, D., Sanchez-Monge, R., Barber, D., Del Pozo, V., de
Andreas, B., Armentia, A., Lahoz, C., Salcedo, D. 1990. Members of the alpha-amylase
inhibitors family from wheat endosperm are major allergens associated with baker's
asthma. *FEBS Lett* 261:85–88.

Grosch, W., Wieser, H. 1999. Redox reactions in wheat dough is affected by ascorbic acid.
*J Cereal Sci* 29:1–16.

Hadjivassiliou, M., Chattopadhyay, A.K., Grunewald, R.A., Jarrot, J.A., Kandler, R.H., Rao,
D.G., Sanders, D.S., Wharton, S.B., Davies-Jones, A.B. 2007. Myopathy associated
with gluten sensitivity. *Muscle Nerve* 35:443–450.

Hahn, B., Grosch, W. 1998. Distribution of glutathione in Osborne fractions as affected by
additions of ascorbic acid, reduces and oxidised glutathione. *J Cereal Sci* 27:117–125.

Hamer, R.J. 2005. Coeliac disease: Background and biochemical aspects. *Biotech Adv*
23:401–408.

Hausch, F., Shan, L., Santiago, N.A., Gray, G.M., Khosla, C. 2003. Intestinal digestive resistance of immunodominant gliadin peptides. *Am J Physiol* 283:996–1003.

Holm, K., Maki, M., Vuolteenaho, N., Mustalahti, K., Ashorn, M., Ruuska, T., Kaukinnen, K.
2006. Oats in the treatment of childhood coeliac disease: A 2-year controlled trial and a
long-term clinical follow-up study. *Aliment Pharmacol Ther* 23(10):1463–1472.

Hourigan, C.S. 2006. The molecular basis of celiac disease. *Clin Exp Med* 6:53–59.

James, J.M., Sixbey, J.P., Helm, R.M., Bannon, G.A., Burks, A.W. 1997. Wheat alpha-amylase
inhibitor: A second route of allergic sensitization. *J Allergy Clin Immunol* 99:239–244.

Jones, B.L. 2005. Endoproteases of barley and malt. *J Cereal Sci* 42:139–156.

Jones, S.M., Magnolfi, C.F., Cooke, S.K., Sampson, H.A. 1995. Immunologic crossreactivity
among cereal grains and grasses in children with food hypersensitivity. *J Allergy Clin
Immunol* 96:341–351.

Kaukinen, K., Partanen, J., Maki, M., Collin, P. 2002. HLA-DQ typing in the diagnosis of celiac disease. *Am J Gastroenterol* 97:362–368.

Kasarda, D.D., Autran, J.C., Lew, E.J.L., Nimmo, C.C., Shewry, P.R. 1983. N-terminal amino acid sequences of ω-gliadins and ω-secalins: Implications for the evolution of prolamin genes. *Biochim Biophys Acta* 747:138–150.

Kato, A., Tanaka, A., Matsudomi, N., Kobayashi, K. 1987. Deamidation of food proteins by protease in alkaline pH. *J Agric Food Chem* 35:224–227.

Koehler, P. 2003. Effect of acid in dough: Reduction of oxidised glutathione with reactive thiol groups of wheat glutelin. *J Agric Food Chem* 51:4954–4959.

Kong, X., Zhou, H., Qian, H. 2007. Enzymatic hydrolysis of wheat gluten by proteases and properties of the resulting hydrolysates. *Food Chem* 102:759–763.

Koning, F., Schuppan, D., Cerf-Bebsussan, N., Sollid, L.M. 2005. Pathomechanisms in celiac disease. *Best Pract Res* 19(3):373–387.

Konopka, I., Fornal, Ł., Dziuba, M., Czaplicki, S., Nałęcz, D. 2007. Composition of proteins in wheat grain streams obtained by sieve classification. *J Sci Food Agric* 87:2198–2206.

Kumagai, H., Shizawa, Y., Sakurai, H., Kumagai, H. 1998. Influence of phytate removal and structural modification on the calcium-binding properties of soybean globulins. *Biosci Biotechnol Biochem* 62:341–346.

Kumagai, H., Norimatsu, Y., Hashizume, N., Sakurai, H., Kumagai, H. 2001. Deamidation of wheat-flour gliadin with ion-exchange resin. *Nippon Shokuhin Kagaku Kogaku Kaishi* 48:884–890.

Kumagai, H., Ishida, S., Koizumi, A., Sakurai, H., Kumagai, H. 2002. Preparation of phytate-removed, deamidated soybean globulins by ion exchangers and characterization of their calcium-binding ability. *J Agric Food Chem* 50:172–176.

Kumagai, H., Koizumi, A., Suda, A., Sato, N., Sakurai, H., Kumagai, H. 2004. Enhanced calcium absorption in the small intestine by a phytate-removed deamidated soybean globulin preparation. *Biosci Biotechnol Biochem* 68:1598–1600.

Kumagai, H., Suda, A., Sakurai, H., Kumagai, H., Arai, S., Inomata, N., Ikezawa, Z. 2007. Improvement of digestibility, reduction in allergenicity, and induction of oral tolerance of wheat gliadin by deamidation. *Biosci Biotechnol Biochem* 71:977–985.

Labat, E., Morel, M.H., Rouau, X. 2001. Effect of laccase and manganese peroxidase on wheat gluten and pentosans during mixing. *Food Hydrocoll* 15(1):47–52.

Larre, C., Denery, P.S., Popineau, Y., Deshayes, G., Desserme, C., Lefevre, J. 2000. Biochemical analysis and rheological properties of gluten modified by transglutaminase. *Cereal Chem* 77(1):32–38.

Leszczyńska, J., Łącka, A., Szemraj, J., Lukamowicz, J., Zegota, H. 2003a. The effect of microwave treatment on the immunoreactivity of gliadin and wheat flour. *Eur Food Res Technol* 217:387–391.

Leszczyńska, J., Łącka, A., Szemraj, J., Lukamowicz, J., Zegota, H. 2003b. The influence of gamma irradiation on the immunoreactivity of gliadin and wheat flour. *Eur Food Res Technol* 217:143–147.

Leszczyńska, J., Łącka, A., Pytasz, U., Szemraj, J., Lukamowicz, J., Lewiński, A. 2002. The effect of proteolysis on the gliadin immunogenicity. *Pol J Nutr Sci* 11/52 (SI2): 145–148.

Leszczyńska, J., Łącka, A., Bryszewska, M. 2006. The use of transglutaminase in the reduction of immunoreactivity of wheat flour. *Food Agric Immunol* 17(2):105–113.

Li, W., Tsiami, A., Bollecker, S., Schofield, D. 2004. Glutathione and related thiol compounds. II. The importance of protein bound glutathione and related protein-bound compounds in gluten proteins. *J Cereal Sci* 39:213–224.

Lindsay, M.P., Skerritt, J.H. 1999. The glutenin macropolymer of wheat flour doughs: Structure–function perspectives. *Trends Food Sci Technol* 10:247–253.

Loponen, J., Mikola, M., Katina, K., Sontag-Strohm, T., Salovaara, H. 2004. Degradation of HMW glutenins during wheat sourdough fermentations. *Cereal Chem* 81:87–93.

Luo, C., Branlard, G., Griffin, W.B., McNeil, D.L. 2000. The effect of nitrogen and sulphur fertilization and their interaction with genotype on wheat glutenins and quality parameters. *J Cereal Sci* 31:185–194.

Marsh, M.N., Morgan, S., Ensari, A., Wardle, T., Lobley, R., Mills, C., Auricchio, S. 1995. In vivo activity of peptide 31–43, 44–55, 56–68 of alfa-gliadin in gluten sensitive entheropathy (GSE). *Gastroenterology* 108:A871.

Maruyama, N., Ichise, K., Katsube, T., Kishimoto, T., Kawase, S., Matsumura, Y., Takeuchi, Y., Sawada, T., Utsumi, S. 1998. Identification of major wheat allergens by means of *Escherichia coli* expression system. *Eur J Biochem* 255:739–745.

Matsuo, H., Morita, E., Tatham, A.S., Korimoto, K., Horikawa, T., Osuna, H., Ikezawa, Z., Kaneko, S., Kohno, K., Dekio, S. 2004. Identification of the IgE-binding epitope in ω-5 gliadin, a major allergen in wheat-dependent exercise-induced anaphylaxis. *J Biol Chem* 279:12135–12140.

Mattinen, M.L., Kruus, K., Buchert, J., Nielsen, J.H., Andersen, H.J., Steffensen, C.L. 2005. Laccase-catalysed polymerization of tyrosine-containing peptides. *FEBS J* 272:3640–3650.

Mattinen, M.L., Hellman, M., Permi, P., Autio, K., Kalkkinen, N., Buchert, J. 2006. Effect of protein structure on laccase-catalysed protein oligomerization. *J Agric Food Chem* 54:8883–8890.

Mikola, L. 1986. Acid carboxypeptidases in grains and leaves of wheat *Triticum aestivum* L. *Plant Physiol* 81:823–829.

Miles, M.J., Carr, H.J., McMaster, T.J., I'Anson, K.J., Belton, P.S., Morris, V., Field, J.M., Shewry, P.R., Tatham, A.S. 1991. Scanning tunneling microscopy of a wheat seed storage protein reveals details of an unusual supersecondary structure. *Proc Natl Acad Sci USA* 88:68–71.

Molberg, O., Solheim-Flaete, N., Jensen, T., Lundin, K.E., Arentz-Hansen, H., Anderson, O.D. 2003. Intestinal T-cell responses to high-molecular-weight glutenins in celiac disease. *Gastroenterology* 125:337–344.

Morita, E., Yamamura, Y., Mihara, S., Kameyoshi, Y., Yamamoto, S. 2000. Food-dependent exercise-induced anaphylaxis: A report of two cases and determination of wheat γ-gliadin as the presumptive allergen. *Br J Dermatol* 143:1059–1063.

Morita, E., Kameyoshi, Y., Mihara, S., Hiragun, T., Yamamoto, S. 2001. γ-Gliadin: A presumptive allergen causing wheat-dependent exercise-induced anaphylaxis. *Br J Dermatol* 145:182–184.

Morita, E., Matsuo, H., Mihara, S., Morimoto, K., Savage, A.W.J., Tatham, A.S. 2003. Fast ω-gliadin is a major allergen in wheat-dependent exercise-induced anaphylaxis. *J Dermatol Sci* 33:99–104.

Motoki, M., Seguro, K. 1998. Transglutaminase and its use for food processing. *Trends Food Sci Technol* 9:204–210.

Nielson, P.M. 1995. Reactions and potential industrial applications of transglutaminase—Review of the literature and patents. *Food Biotechnology* 9:119–156.

Norimatsu, Y., Kumagai, H., Magai, R., Sakurai, H., Kumagai, H. 2002. Seamidation of wheat-flour gluten with ion-exchange resin and its functional properties. *Nippon Shokuhin Kagaku Kogaku Kaishi* 49:649–645.

Osborne, T.B. 1907. *The Protein of the Wheat Kernel*, Publ no. 84, Carnegie Institution of Washington, Washington D.C.

Osman, A.A., Uhlig, H., Thamm, B., Schneider-Mergener, J., Mothes, T. 1998. Use of the phage display technique for detection of epitopes recognized by polyclonal rabbit gliadin antibodies. *FEBS Lett* 433:103–107.

Palosuo, K. 2003. Update on wheat hypersensitivity. *Curr Opin Allergy Clin Immunol* 3:205–209.

Palosuo, K., Alenius, H., Varjonen, E., Koivuluhta, M., Mikkola, J., Keskinen, H., Kalkkinen, N., Reunala, T. 1999. A novel wheat gliadin as a cause of exercise-induced anaphylaxis. *J Allergy Clin Immunol* 103:912–917.

Palosuo, K., Alenius, H., Varjonen, E., Kalkkinen, N., Reunala, T. 2001a. Rye gamma-70 and gamma-35 secalins and barley gamma-3 hordein cross-react with omega-5 gliadin, a major allergen in wheat-dependent, exercise-induced anaphylaxis. *Clin Exp Allergy* 31:466–473.

Palosuo, K., Varjonen, E., Kekki, O.M., Klemola, T., Kalkkinen, N., Alenius, H., Reunala, T. 2001b. Wheat omega-5 gliadin is a major allergen in children with immediate allergy to ingested wheat. *J Allergy Clin Immunol* 108:634–638.

Palosuo, K., Varjonen, E., Nurkkala, J., Kalkkinen, N., Harvima, R., Reunala, T., Alenius, H.J. 2003. Transglutaminase-mediated cross-linking of a peptic fraction of omega-5 gliadin enhances IgE reactivity in wheat-dependent, exercise-induced anaphylaxis. *J Allergy Clin Immunol* 111:1386–1392.

Parrot, I., Huang, P.C., Khosla, C. 2002. Circular dichroism and nuclear magnetic resonance spectroscopic analysis of immunogenic gluten peptides and their analogs. *J Biol Chem* 277:455–472.

Pequet, C., Lauriere, M. 2003. New allergens in hydrolysates of wheat proteins. *Rev Fr Alergol Immunol Clin* 43:21–23.

Periolo, N., Chernavsky, A.C. 2006. Coeliac disease. *Autoimmunity Rev* 5:202–208.

Piber, M., Koehler, P. 2005. Identification of dehydro-ferulic acid-tyrosine in rye and wheat: Evidence for a covalent cross-link between arabinoxylans and proteins. *J Agric Food Chem* 53:5276–5284.

Picarelli, A., Di Tola, L., Sabbatella, M., Greco, L., Silano, R., De Vincenzi, M. 1999. 31–43 Amino acid sequence of the α-gliadin induces endomysial antibody production during in vitro challenge. *Scand J Gastroenterol* 34:1099–1102.

Posh, A., Weiss, W., Wheeler, C., Dunn, M.J., Görg, A. 1995. Sequence analysis of wheat grain allergens separated by two-dimensional electrophoresis with immobilized pH gradients. *Electrophoresis* 16:1115–1119.

Räsänen, L., Lehto, M., Turjanmaa, K., Savolainen, J., Reunala, T. 1994. Allergy to ingested cereals in atopic children. *Allergy* 49:871–876.

Rizzello, C.G., De Angelis, M., Coda, R., Gobbetti, M. 2006. Use of selected sourdough lactic acid bacteria to hydrolyze wheat and rye proteins responsible for cereal allergy. *Eur Food Res Technol* 223:405–411.

Rollan, G., de Valdez, G.F. 2001. The peptide hydrolase system of *Lactobacillus reuteri*. *Int J Food Microbiol* 70:303–307.

Rollan, G., De Angelis, M., Gobbetti, M., de Valdez, G.F. 2005. Proteolytic activity and reduction of gliadin-like fractions by sourdough lactobacilli. *J Appl Microbiol* 99:1495–1502.

Rosell, C.M., Wang, J., Aja, S., Bean, S., Lookhart, G. 2003. Wheat flour proteins as affected by transglutaminase and glucose oxidase. *Cereal Chem* 80:52–55.

Rumbo, M., Chirdo, F.G., Fossati, C.A., Anon, M.C. 1996. Influence of thermal treatment of food on the immunochemical quantification of gliadin. *Food Agric Immunol* 8:195–200.

Sanchez-Monge, R., Gomez, L., Barber, D., Lopez-Otin, C., Armentia, A., Salcedo, G. 1992. Wheat and barley allergens associated with bakers' asthma. Glycosylated subunits of the alpha-amylase-inhibitor family have enhanced IgE-binding capacity. *Biochem J* 281:401–405.

Sanchez-Monge, R., Garcia-Casado, G., Lopez-Otin, C., Armentia, A., Salcedo, G. 1997. Wheat flour peroxidase is a prominent allergen associated with baker's asthma. *Clin Exp Allergy* 27:1130–1137.

Sander, I., Merget, R., Leonhardt, L., Chen, Z., Raulf-Heimsoth, M., Baur, X. 1999. Prevalence of allergen-specific IgE in baker's asthma. *Allergy* 54 (Suppl. 52):50–51.

Sander, I., Flagge, A., Merget, R., Halder, T.M., Meyer, H.E., Baur, X. 2001. Identification of wheat flour allergens by means of 2-dimensional immunoblotting. *J Allergy Clin Immunol* 107:907–913.

Sandiford, C.P., Tee, R.D., Newman Taylor, A.J. 1995. Identification of crossreacting wheat, rye, barley and soya flour allergens using sera from individuals with wheat-induced asthma. *Clin Exp Allergy* 25:340–349.

Sandiford, C.P., Tatham, A.S., Fido, R., Welch, J.A., Jones, M.G., Tee, R.D., Shewry, P.R., Newman Taylor, A.J. 1997. Identification of the major water/salt insoluble wheat proteins involved in cereal hypersensitivity. *Clin Exp Allergy* 27:1120–1129.

Seguro, K., Kumazawa, Y., Kuraishi, C., Sakamoto, H., Motoki, M. 1996a. The ε-(γ-glutamyl) lisine moiety in crosslinked casein is an available source for lysine for rats. *J Nutr* 126:2557–2562.

Seguro, K., Nio, N., Motoki, M. 1996b. Some characteristics of a microbial protein cross-linking enzyme: Transglutaminase. In: Parris, N., Kato, A., Creamer, L.K., Pearce, J. (Eds.), *Macromolecular Interactions in Food Technology.* American Chemical Society, Washington D.C., pp. 271–280.

Seilmeier, W., Valdez, I., Mendez, E., Wieser, H. 2001. Comparative investigations of gluten proteins from different wheat species. II. Characterizations of ω-gliadins. *Eur Food Res Technol* 212:355–363.

Selinheimo, E., Autio, K., Kruus, K., Buchert, J. 2007. Elucidating the mechanism of laccase and tyrosinase in wheat bread making. *J Agric Food Chem* 55:6357–6365.

Shan, L., Molberg, O., Parrot, I., Hausch, F., Filiz, F., Gray, G.M., Sollid, L.M., Khosla, C. 2002. Structural basis for gluten intolerance in celiac sprue. *Science* 297:2275–2279.

Shih, F.F. 1987. Deamidation of protein in a soy extract by ion-exchange resin catalysis. *J Food Sci* 52:1529–1531.

Simonato, B., De Lazzari, F., Pasini, G., Polato, F., Giannattasio, M., Gemignani, C., Peruffo, A.D.B., Santucci, B., Plebani, M., Curioni, A. 2001. IgE binding to soluble and insoluble wheat flour proteins in atopic and nonatopic patients suffering from gastrointestinal symptoms after wheat ingestion. *Clin Exp Allergy* 31:1771–1778.

Simonato, B., Pasini, G., De Zorzi, M., Vergo, M., Curioni, A. 2004. Potential allergens in durum wheat semolina and pasta: Fate during cooking and digestion. *It J Food Sci* 16:151–163.

Simpson, D.J. 2001. Proteolytic degradation of cereal prolamins—The problem with proline. *Plant Sci* 161:825–838.

Singh, H. 1991. Modifications of food proteins by covalent crosslinking. *Trend Food Sci Technol* 2:196–200.

Singh, N.K., Shepherd, K.W. 1987. Solubility behaviour, synthesis, degradation and subcellular location of a new class of disulfide-linked proteins in wheat endosperm. *Aust J Plant Physiol* 14:245–252.

Singh, N.K., Donovan, G.R., Batey, I.L., MacRitchie, F. 1990. Use of sonification and size-exclusion high-performance liquid chromatography in the study of wheat flour proteins. I. Dissolution of total proteins in the absence of reducing agents. *Cereal Chem* 67:150–161.

Sissons, M.J., Blundell, M.J., Hill, A.S., Skerritt, J.H. 1999. Antibodies to N-terminal peptides of low $M_r$ subunits of wheat glutenin. I. Characterisation of the antibody response. *J Cereal Sci* 30:283–301.

Skerritt, J.H., Hill, A.S., Andrews, J.L. 2000. Antigenicity of wheat prolamins: Detailed epitope analysis using a panel of monoclonal antibodies. *J Cereal Sci* 32:259–279.

Stepniak, D., Spaenij-Dekking, L., Mitea, C., Moester, M., de Ru, A., Baak-Pablo, R., van Veelen, P., Edens, L., Koning, F. 2006. Highly efficient gluten degradation with a newly identified prolyl endoprotease: Implications for coeliac disease. *Am J Physiol Gastroenterol Liver Physiol* 291:G621–G629.

Stone, P.J., Nicholas, M.E. 1996. Varietal differences in mature protein composition of wheat resulted from different rates of polymer accumulation during grain filling. *Aust J Plant Physiol* 23:727–737.

Sturgess, R., Day, P., Ellis, J.H., Lundin, K.E.A., Gjertsen, H.A., Kontakou, M., Ciclitira, P.J. 1994. Wheat peptide challenge in celiac disease. *Lancet* 343:758–761.

Sutton, R., Hill, D.H., Baldo, B.A., Wrigley, C.W. 1982. Immunoglobulin E antibodies to ingested cereal flour components: Studies with sera from subjects with asthma and atopic eczema. *Clin Exp Allergy* 12:63–74.

Tanabe, S., Arai, S., Watanabe, M. 1996a. Modification of wheat flour with bromelain and baking hypoallergenic bread with added ingredients. *Biosci Biotechnol Biochem* 60:1269–1272.

Tanabe, S., Arai, S., Yanagihara, Y., Mita, H., Takahashi, K., Watanabe, M. 1996b. A major wheat allergen has a Gln-Gln-Gln-Pro-Pro motif identified as an IgE-binding epitope. *Biochem Biophys Res Commun* 219:290–293.

Tatham, A.S., Shewry, P.R. 2000. Elastomeric proteins: Biological roles, structures and mechanisms. *Trends Biochem Sci* 25:567–571.

Thiele, C., Gänzle, M.G., Vogel, R.F. 2002. Contribution of sourdough lactobacilli, yeasts, and cereal enzymes to the generation of amino acids in dough relevant for bread flavor. *Cereal Chem* 79:45–51.

Thiele, C., Gänzle, M.G., Vogel, R.F. 2003. Fluorescence labeling of wheat proteins for determination of gluten hydrolysis and depolymerization during dough processing and sourdough fermentation. *J Agric Food Chem* 51:2745–2752.

Thiele, C., Grassl, S., Gänzle, M. 2004. Gluten hydrolysis and depolymerization during sourdough fermentation. *J Agric Food Chem* 52:1307–1314.

Tilley, K.A., Benjamin, R.E., Bagorogoza, K.E., Okot-Kotber, B.M., Prakash, O., Kwen, H. 2001. Tyrosine cross-links: Molecular basis of gluten structure and function. *J Agric Food Chem* 49:2628–2632.

Triboi, E., Abad, A., Michelena, A., Lloveras, J., Ollier, J.L., Daniel, C. 2000. Environmental effects on the quality of two wheat genotypes. I. Quantitative and qualitative variation of storage proteins. *Eur J Agron* 13:47–64.

Triboi, E., Martre, P., Triboi-Blondel, A.M. 2003. Environmentally-induced changes in protein composition in developing grains of wheat are related to changes in total protein content. *J Exp Bot* 54:1731–1742.

Tseng, C.S., Lai, H.M. 2002. Physicochemical properties of wheat flour dough modified by microbial transglutaminase. *J Food Sci* 67:750–755.

van der Wal, Y., Kooy, M.C., van Veelen, P., Vader, W., August, S.A., Drijfhout, J.W., Pena, S.A., Koning, F. 1999. Glutenin is involved in the gluten-driven mucosal T cell response. *Eur J Immunol* 29:3133–3139.

Varjonen, E., Vainio, E., Kalimo, K., Juntunen-Backman, K., Savolainen, J. 1995. Skin-prick test and RAST responses to cereals in children with atopic dermatitis. Characterization of IgE-binding components in wheat and oats by an immunoblotting method. *Clin Exp Allergy* 25:1100–1107.

Varjonen, E., Vainio, E., Kalimo, K. 1997. Lifethreatening, recurrent anaphylaxis caused by allergy to gliadin and exercise. *Clin Exp Allergy* 27:162–166.

Varjonen, E., Petman, L., Makinen-Kiljunen, S. 2000a. Immediate contact allergy from hydrolysed wheat in a cosmetic cream. *Allergy* 55:294–296.

Varjonen, E., Vainio, E., Kalimo, K. 2000b. Antigliadin IgE-indicator of wheat allergy in atopic dermatitis. *Allergy* 55:386–391.

Vasil, I.K. 2007. Molecular genetic improvement of cereals: Transgenic wheat (*Triticum aestivum* L.). *Plant Cell Rep* 26:1133–1154.

Vermeulen, N., Kretzer, J., Machalitza, H., Vogel, R.F., Ganzle, M.G. 2006. Influence of redox-reactions catalysed by homo- and hetero-fermentative lactobacilli on gluten in wheat sourdoughs. *J Cereal Sci* 43:137–143.

von Olnhausen, S., Munscher, I., Brandt, M., Hammes, W. March 2002. *Oxidationsprozesse durch Laktobacillen in Sauerteigen, Fachsymposium der DGHM-Fachgruppe Lebensmittelmikrobiologie.* Karlsruhe, Germany.

Waga, J., Kaczkowski, J., Zientarski, J. 2003. Influence of thioredoxin-A on flour baking properties and gliadin immunoreactivity in spelt and common wheat genotypes. *Pol J Food Nutr Sci* 12:13–16.

Wagner, J.R., Gueguen, J. 1995. Effects of dissociation, deamidation, and reducing treatment on structural and surface active properties of soy glycinine. *J Agric Food Chem* 42:1993–2000.

Walsh, B.J., Howden, M.E. 1989. A method for the detection of IgE binding sequences of allergens based on a modification of epitope mapping. *J Immunol Methods* 121:275–280.

Walsh, B.J., Wrigley, C.W., Musk, A.W., Baldo, B.A. 1985. A comparison of the binding of IgE in the sera of patients with bakers' asthma to soluble and insoluble wheat-grain proteins. *J Allergy Clin Immunol* 76:23–28.

Wang, J., Zhao, M., Zhao, Q., Bao, Y., Jiang, Y. 2007. Characterization of hydrolysates derived from enzymatic hydrolysis of wheat gluten. *J Food Sci* 72:103–107.

Watanabe, M., Ikezawa, Z., Arai, S. 1994a. Fabrication and quality evaluation of hypoallergenic wheat products. *Biosci Biotechnol Biochem* 58:388–390.

Watanabe, M., Suzuki, T., Ikezawa, Z., Arai, S. 1994b. Controlled enzymatic treatment of wheat proteins for production of hypoallergenic flour. *Biosci Biotech Biochem* 58:388–390.

Watanabe, M., Tanabe, S., Suzuki, T., Ikezawa, Z., Arai, S. 1995. Primary structure of an allergen peptide occurring in the chymotryptic hydrolysate of gluten. *Biosci Biotechnol Biochem* 59:1596–1597.

Watanabe, M., Watanabe, J., Sonoyama, K., Tanabe, S. 2000. Novel method for producing hypoallergenic wheat flour by enzymatic fragmentation of the constituent allergens and its application to food processing. *Biosci Biotechnol Biochem* 64:2663–2667.

Weichel, M., Glaser, A.G., Ballmer-Weber, B.K., Schmid-Gendelmeier, P., Crameri, R. 2006a. Wheat and maize thioredoxins: A novel cross-reactive cereal family related to baker's asthma. *J Allergy Clin Immunol* 117:676–681.

Weichel, M., Vergoossen, N.J., Bonomi, S., Scibilia, J., Ortolani, C., Ballmer-Weber, B.K. 2006b. Screening the allergenic repertoires of wheat and maize with sera from double-blind, placebo-controlled food challenge positive patients. *Allergy* 61:128–135.

Weiss, W., Vogelmeier, C., Görg, A. 1993. Electrophoretic characterization of wheat grain allergens from different cultivars involved in bakers' asthma. *Electrophoresis* 14:805–81.

Weiss, W., Huber, G., Engel, K.H., Pethran, A., Dunn, M.J., Gooley, A.A. 1997. Identification and characterization of wheat grain albumin/globulin allergens. *Electrophoresis* 18:826–833.

WHO. 1988. *Food Irradiation. A Technique for Improving the Safety of Food.* WHO, Geneva.

Wieser, H., Bushuk, W., MacRitchie, F. 2006. The polymeric glutenins. In: Wrigley, C., Bekes, F., Bushuk, W. (Eds.), *Gliadin and Glutenin: The Unique Balance of Wheat Quality*, St. Paul American Association of Cereal Chemistry, St. Paul, MN, pp. 213–240.

Wieser, H. 1996. Relation between gliadin structure and coeliac toxicity. *Acta Paediatr* 412(85 Suppl.):3–9.

Wieser, H., Kieffer, R. 2001. Correlations of the amount of gluten protein types to the technological properties of wheat flours determined on a micro-scale. *J Cereal Sci* 34:19–27.

Wieser, H., Seilmeier, W. 1998. The influence of nitrogen fertilization on quantities and proportions of different protein types in wheat flour. *J Sci Food Agric* 76:49–55.

Wieser, H., Zimmermann, G. 2000. Importance of amounts and properties of high molecular weight subunits of glutenin for wheat quality. *Eur Food Res Technol* 210:324–330

Wieser, H., Gutser, R., von Tucher, S. 2004. Influence of sulphur fertilisation on quantities and proportions of gluten protein types in wheat flour. *J Cereal Sci* 40:239–244.

Williamson, D., Marsh, M.N. 2002. Celiac disease. *Mol Biotechnol* 22:293–299.

Yamashita, H., Nanba, Y., Onishi, M., Kimoto, M., Hiemori, M., Tsuji, H. 2002. Identification of a wheat allergen, Tri a Bd 36K, as a peroxidase. *Biosci Biotechnol Biochem* 66:2487–2490.

Yong, Y.H., Yamaguchi, S., Gu, Y.S., Mori, T., Matsumura, Y. 2004. Effects of enzymatic deamidation by protein-glutaminase on structure and functional properties of α-zein. *J Agric Food Chem* 52:7094–7100.

Zhao, F.J., Hawkesford, M.J., McGrath, S.P. 1999. Sulphur assimilation and effects on yield and quality of wheat. *J Cereal Sci* 30:1–17.

Zhu, Y., Rinzema, A., Tramper, J., Bol, J. 1995. Microbial transglutaminase—A review of its production and application in food processing. *Appl Microbiol Biotechnol* 44:277–282.

Zwetchkenbaum, J.F., Burakoff, R. 1988. Food allergy and the irritable bowel syndrome. *Am J Gastroenterol* 83:901–904.

# 14 Brief Characteristics of Other Important Food Allergens

*Lucjan Jędrychowski, Matthias Egger,*
*Michael Hauser, Georg Schmidt,*
*Nicole Wopfner, Fátima Ferreira,*
*Michael Wallner, and Andreas Lopata*

## CONTENTS

## 14.1 GENERAL CHARACTERISTICS OF MICROBIOLOGICAL ALLERGENS: ROLE OF BIOTECHNOLOGY THE DEVELOPMENT IN FOOD ALLERGY

Lucjan Jędrychowski

### 14.1.1 INTRODUCTION: GENERAL CHARACTERISTICS OF ALLERGENS OF MICROBIOLOGICAL ORIGIN

Development of biotechnology is often suggested as a remedy for the problem of meeting food requirements of humanity caused by distorted balance between the Siegel populations of humans and animals on the one hand and plant, i.e., food and fodder, production on the other (Bannon et al. 2008). In food production, especially in the case of the so-called functional food designed for human nutrition in specific disease conditions, there are often applied biotechnological processes. These processes, such as fermentation or processes involving activating native enzymes, e.g., seed germination, make it possible to enrich food with, among others proteins, lipids or vitamins, to modify raw material components, to increase product shelf life with simultaneous change of its sensory properties—all this through the use of microorganisms natural properties and enzymes. An example here are biotechnological processes used in the production of beverages from fermented milk (yoghurt, kefir, buttermilk, and cream), some fruit juices, wine, vegetable juices (red beetroot), brewing beer from malt, making cheese from mammal milk or soymilk, or pickling cabbage, cucumbers, or mushrooms. In the Far East there are numerous popular dishes prepared from fermented soybeans, e.g., Indonesian dish *tempeh* made with the use of *Rhizopus oligosporus*, Chinese *douchi*, or Japanese *hamanatto* made with *Aspergillus oryzae* as well as fermented soy paste: Chinese *jiang* or *chiang*, Japanese *miso*, or Indonesian *taucho* (Huang and Huang 1999).

The agents most often used for modifying biological or dietary food properties are microorganisms and enzymatic preparations. Chapter 1 and Sections 2.2, 2.4, and 2.5 discuss the role of microorganisms, both beneficial and harmful ones, in shaping the organism resistance mechanisms and also in forming the immunological response in cases of allergy at length.

As numerous studies have shown, application of biotechnological processes, especially those with the use of enzymatic preparations or microorganisms, may contribute to producing advantageous changes in antigenic, immunoreactive, and allergenic properties of food products. This seems to be confirmed by a wide use of proteolytic enzymatic preparations for the production of hypoantigenic and hypoallergenic formulas. Some biotechnological processes may lead to uncovering epitopes in proteins thus increasing allergenic properties and immunoreactivity of modified products (Jędrychowski et al. 2005).

Microorganisms used in biotechnological processes have been usually thoroughly characterized for their technological properties and labeled GRAS (generally regarded as safe), for instance, probiotic bacteria of the *Lactobacillus* and *Bifidobacterium* family. Progress in biotechnology and possibilities of using achievements in this field require a deep insight into biological properties, in this immunogenic and

**TABLE 14.1.1**

**Classification of Bacterial Allergens according to AllFam Database**

| Acc. | Protein Family Name | Number of Allergens |
|------|---------------------|---------------------|
| AF086 | Staphylococcal/streptococcal toxins | 6 |
| AF105 | Clostridial neurotoxins | 1 |
| AF091 | Diphtheria toxins | 1 |
| AF021 | Subtilisin-like serine proteases | 1 |
| AF024 | Trypsin-like serine proteases | 1 |

*Source:* Adapted from Radauer, C. et al., *J. Allergy Clin. Immunol.*, 121, 2008, 847—AllFam URL: http://www.meduniwien.ac.at/ allergens/allfam/. With permission.

allergenic, of the applied microorganisms as well as their metabolites (enzymes, toxins, and neurotoxins). This concerns also genetically modified organisms used in biotechnology.

AllFam database contains only proteins with experimentally confirmed allergenicity. Currently, as of September 2008, it comprises 1010 allergens. All defined bacterial allergens included in AllFam database have been grouped in 5 allergen families and they comprise 10 allergens in total (Table 14.1.1). The most numerous (6 allergens) is the group of *Staphylococcal/streptococcal* toxins of the *Staphylococcus aureus* family; due to contact allergens which they contain such as *Sta a* SEA, *Sta a* SEB, *Sta a* SEC, *Sta a* SED, *Sta a* SEE, *Sta a* TSST they pose the greatest allergenic threat.

In the *Corynebacterium diphtheriae* species there occurs iatrogenic allergen *Cor d* Toroid belonging to the Diphtheria family toxins; the remaining ones, another iatrogenic allergen *Clo t* Toxoid of the *Clostridium tetani* family neurotoxins of the *Bacillus lentus* species and inhalation allergen *Bac l* Subtilisin of the Trypsin-like serine proteases family, in *Streptomyces griseus* inhalation allergen *Str g* Pronase.

Mold allergens occur more abundantly than bacterial ones (Table 14.1.2). AllFam database contains 105 of them, classified into 39 families. They make a big group of compounds with highly diversified physiological and biochemical functions (Table 14.1.3). The most numerous group, containing as many as 17 mold allergens, has been classified as subtilisin-like serine proteases (Tables 14.1.3 and 14.1.4). What attracts attention is the fact that a substantial group of mold allergens is made by the following enzymes: Subtilisin-like serine proteases—17, enolases—9, thioredoxins—7, redoxins—6, Fe/Mn superoxide dismutases—5, and others) (Table 14.1.3).

### 14.1.2  Characteristics of Allergenic Properties of Selected Bacteria and Their Metabolites (Bacterial Enzymes)

There are a number of microorganisms containing allergenic compounds (Tables 14.1.1 through 14.1.4). They are microorganisms, and their metabolites (enzymes, toxins, and enzyme inhibitors), spores, or specific compounds are of molecular

**TABLE 14.1.2**

**Allergens Characteristic for the So-Called Environmental Mold Fungi**

| Phylum | Order | Species of the Mold | Allergens |
|---|---|---|---|
| Ascomycota | Dothideales | *Alternaria alternata* | *Alt a* 1, *Alt a* 3, *Alt a* 4, *Alt a* 5, *Alt a* 6, *Alt a* 7, *Alt a* 8, *Alt a* 10, *Alt a* 12, *Alt a* 13 |
| | | *C. cladosporioides* | *Cla c* 9 |
| | | *C. herbarum* | *Cla h* 2, *Cla h* 5, *Cla h* 6, *Cla h* 7, *Cla h* 8, *Cla h* 9, *Cla h* 10, *Cla h* 12 |
| | | *Curvularia lunata* | *Cur l* 1, *Cur l* 2, *Cur l* 3 |
| | Eurotiales | *A. flavus* | *Asp fl* 13 |
| | | *A. fumigatus* | *Asp f* 1, *Asp f* 2, *Asp f* 3, *Asp f* 4, *Asp f* 5, *Asp f* 6, *Asp f* 7, *Asp f* 8, *Asp f* 9, *Asp f* 10, *Asp f* 11, *Asp f* 12, *Asp f* 13, *Asp f* 15, *Asp f* 16, *Asp f* 17, *Asp f* 18, *Asp f* 22, *Asp f* 23, *Asp f* 27, *Asp f* 28, *Asp f* 29, *Asp f* 34 |
| | | *A. niger* | *Asp n* 14, *Asp n* 18, *Asp n* 25 |
| | | *A. oryzae* | *Asp o* 13, *Asp o* 21 |
| | | *P. brevicompactum* | *Pen b* 13, *Pen b* 26 |
| | | *P. chrysogenum* | *Pen ch* 13, *Pen ch* 18, *Pen ch* 20, *Pen ch* 31, *Pen ch* 33 |
| | | *P. citrinum* | *Pen c* 3, *Pen c* 13, *Pen c* 19, *Pen c* 22, *Pen c* 24, *Pen c* 30, *Pen c* 32 |
| | | *P. oxalicum* | *Pen o* 18 |
| Basidiomycota | Hymenomycetes | *Coprinus comatus* | *Cop c* 1, *Cop c* 2, *Cop c* 3, *Cop c* 5, *Cop c* 7 |
| | | *Psilocybe cubensis* | *Psi c* 1, *Psi c* 2 |
| | Urediniomycetes | *R. mucilaginosa* | *Rho m* 1, *Rho m* 2 |
| | | *Malassezia furfur* | *Mal f* 2, *Mal f* 3, *Mal f* 4 |
| | Ustilaginomycetes | *Malassezia sympodialis* | *Mal s* 1, *Mal s* 5, *Mal s* 6, *Mal s* 7, *Mal s* 8, *Mal s* 9, *Mal s* 10, *Mal s* 11, *Mal s* 12, *Mal s* 13 |

*Source:* Adapted from Radauer, C. et al., *J. Allergy Clin. Immunol.*, 121, 2008, 847—AllFam URL: http://www.meduniwien.ac.at/allergens/allfam/. With permission.

weight below 1 kDa (haptens). The role of enzymes in inducing hypoallergic reactions may be very different:

- They may sensitize as specific proteins characterized by the occurrence of suitable (linear or conformational) epitopes enabling reactions with receptors of the immunological system cells or antibodies produced by them.
- They can modify protective barriers of the immunological system (mucosa).
- They can modify nutrients thus exposing hidden epitopes.

**TABLE 14.1.3**
**Classification of Mold Fungi Allergens into Families according to AllFam Database**

| No. | Acc. | Protein Family Name | Number of Allergens |
|-----|------|---------------------|---------------------|
| 1. | AF021 | Subtilisin-like serine proteases | 17 |
| 2. | AF031 | Enolases | 9 |
| 3. | AF070 | 60S acidic ribosomal proteins | 7 |
| 4. | AF023 | Thioredoxins | 7 |
| 5. | AF131 | Redoxins | 6 |
| 6. | AF020 | Fe/Mn superoxide dismutases | 5 |
| 7. | AF002 | Heat-shock proteins Hsp70 | 4 |
| 8. | AF040 | Aldehyde dehydrogenases | 3 |
| 9. | AF038 | Cyclophilins | 3 |
| 10. | AF004 | Eukaryotic aspartyl proteases | 3 |
| 11. | AF010 | Glutathione S-transferases, C-terminal | 3 |
| 12. | AF061 | Prolyl oligopeptidase family | 3 |
| 13. | AF129 | Cerato-platanins | 2 |
| 14. | AF053 | Flavodoxins | 2 |
| 15. | AF079 | Glycoside hydrolase family 16 | 2 |
| 16. | AF080 | Glycoside hydrolase family 20 | 2 |
| 17. | AF110 | Nuclear transport factor 2 | 2 |
| 18. | AF113 | Ribonucleases N1 and T1 | 2 |
| 19. | AF028 | Short-chain dehydrogenases | 2 |
| 20. | AF029 | Zn-containing dehydrogenases | 2 |
| 21. | AF033 | $\alpha$-Amylases | 1 |
| 22. | AF055 | Calreticulin family | 1 |
| 23. | AF047 | Catalases | 1 |
| 24. | AF106 | Class 3 lipases | 1 |
| 25. | AF006 | Cytochromes c | 1 |
| 26. | AF108 | DJ-1/PfpI family | 1 |
| 27. | AF011 | Eukaryotic elongation factors 1 | 1 |
| 28. | AF109 | Fungalysin metalloproteases | 1 |
| 29. | AF076 | Glycoside hydrolase family 15 | 1 |
| 30. | AF083 | Glycoside hydrolase family 3 | 1 |
| 31. | AF081 | Oxidoreductases | 1 |
| 32. | AF042 | Heat shock proteins Hsp90 | 1 |
| 33. | AF001 | Helix-loop-helix DNA-binding domain | 1 |
| 34. | AF062 | Histidine acid phosphatases | 1 |
| 35. | AF014 | Lactate/malate dehydrogenases | 1 |
| 36. | AF073 | Pectate lyases | 1 |
| 37. | AF058 | Ribosomal proteins L3 | 1 |
| 38. | AF136 | Translationally controlled tumor proteins | 1 |
| 39. | AF071 | Xylanases | 1 |

*Source:* Adapted from Radauer, C. et al., *J. Allergy Clin. Immunol.*, 121, 2008, 847—AllFam URL: http://www.meduniwien.ac.at/allergens/allfam/. With permission.

## TABLE 14.1.4
## Inhalatory and Contact Allergens of Mold Origin of the Subtilisin-Like Serine Proteases Family

| Lp. | Allergen Systematic name | Allergen Source/ Mold Species | Allergen Character/ Exposure Way |
|-----|--------------------------|-------------------------------|----------------------------------|
| 1.  | Asp f 13   | A. fumigatus      | Inhalatory/respiratory tract |
| 2.  | Asp f 18   | A. fumigatus      |  |
| 3.  | Asp fl 13  | A. flavus         |  |
| 4.  | Asp n 18   | A. niger          |  |
| 5.  | Asp o 13   | A. oryzae         |  |
| 6.  | Cla c 9    | C. cladosporioides |  |
| 7.  | Cur l 18   | Cu. lunata        |  |
| 8.  | Pen c 1    | P. citrinum       |  |
| 9.  | Pen c 18   | P. citrinum       |  |
| 10. | Pen c 2    | P. citrinum       |  |
| 11. | Pen ch 13  | P. chrysogenum    |  |
| 12. | Pen ch 18  | P. chrysogenum    |  |
| 13. | Pen o 18   | P. oxalicum       |  |
| 14. | Rho m 2    | R. mucilaginosa   |  |
| 15. | Tri me 2   | Tr. mentagrophytes | Contact |
| 16. | Tri r 2    | Tr. rubrum        |  |
| 17. | Tri sc 2   | Tr. schoenleinii  |  |

Source: Adapted from Radauer, C. et al., J. Allergy Clin. Immunol., 121, 2008, 847—AllFam URL: http://www.meduniwien.ac.at/allergens/allfam/. With permission.

Some of the naturally occurring bacteria may be the cause of disease symptoms related to allergic hypersensitivity reactions (Table 14.1.1). Among the bacteria occurring in the natural environment and related mainly to the agricultural environment (hay mold, compost mold) some, such as *Faenia rectivirgula*, *Micropolyspora faeni*, *Thermoactinomyces vulgaris*, *Thermoactinomyces viridis* or those related to producing raw food materials (moldy sugar cane—*Thermoactinomyces sacchari*, vineyards—*Thermoactinomyces viridis)*, may cause hypersensitivity pneumonitis (Sikora et al. 2008).

In addition, enzymes produced on the industrial scale based on biotechnological processes may pose a health problem, which became evident in the end of the 1960s when production of alkaline thermostable enzymes, such as protease (subtilysine), amylase, cellulase or other preparations indispensable for detergent production and widely applied in the pharmaceutical, food, and light industry, started to be produced on the industrial scale (Quirce et al. 1992, Quirce and Sastre 1998, Vanhanen et al. 1996, 2001). Out of approximately 200 enzymatic preparations used for commercial purposes in the EU, the greatest number, i.e., 158 are used by the food industry, 64 for technical purposes, and 57 in the fodder industry. According to directive 62/548 by the European Parliament α-glucosidase, cellulase, exo-cellulohydrolase, α-amylase, and other amylases, phytase, papain, pepsin A, rennin, trypsin, chymotrypsin, bromelain, subtilysine, and other proteases belong to the group of increased risk R42 (i.e., enzymes which may cause allergy through inhalation). The aforementioned preparations, particularly proteases, may induce mucosa inflammation through activation of receptors and change in the functioning of Ca⁺⁺ flow and thus facilitate the onset of symptoms typical of allergy (Baur 2005).

Apart from enzymes naturally occurring in food products and microorganisms used for food processing about 100 enzymes with genetically modified properties should be taken into consideration.

### 14.1.3 CHARACTERISTICS OF MOLD ALLERGENS AND SOME MOLD-DERIVED PREPARATIONS

Molds abundantly occur in the natural world and are the source of many allergenic compounds (Tables 14.1.2 through 14.1.4).

The dominating sources of allergens are fungi of the *Alternaria, Aspergillus, Penicillium, Cladosporium,* and *Fusarium* species (Kurup 2003) (Table 14.1.2), which is reflected by public announcements about the inhalatory allergenic threats giving spore concentration in the air of the *Alternaria* and *Cladosporium* species. Patients sensitized to airborne fungi such as *Alternaria alternata* and *Cladosporium herbarum* often also show positive skin prick test results and specific serum IgE antibodies to yeast, *Pityrosporum ovale* (Leino et al. 2006).

Among mold allergens making the natural microflora of the natural world special mention should be made to vacuolar serine proteases ($m_w$ 34 kDa) and metaloproteases (*Asp f* 5, *Asp f* 6, *Asp f* 10, *Asp f* 11) synthesized by *A. fumigatus* (Shen et al. 2001). *A. flavus* and *A. oryzae* synthesize alkaline serine proteases (*Asp fl* 13, *Asp o* 13) (Shen et al. 1998). Allergenic proteases are also synthesized by the fungi of the *Penicillium* phylum, e.g., *P. chrysogenum, P. citrinum, P. brevicompactum,* and *P. oxalicum*. They comprise mainly vacuolar (*Pen ch* $m_w$ 18–32 and 34 kDa, *Pen c* 18, *Pen o* $m_w$ 18–34 kDa), and alkaline (*Pen ch* $m_w$ 13–34 kDa, *Pen c* $m_w$ 13–33 kDa) serine proteases (Shen et al. 1997, 2003) (Tables 14.1.2 and 14.1.4).

Allergens synthesized by the fungi of the *Trichophyton* phylum are serine proteases (*Tri t* 4 – prolyl oligopeptidase) with $m_w$ 83 kDa, responsible for allergic skin reactions (Kurup and Banerjee 2000). Among mold fungi occurring in agriculture, food production, and food industries which may induce hypersensitivity pneumonitis (HP) there are *A. clavatus* (moldy barley, malt, beer production, and moldy cheese production), *A. flavus* (moldy corn), *A. fumigatus* (vegetables, vegetable compost), *A. oryzae* (soy sauce brewing), *Cladosporium* (environment), *Mucor stolonifer* (moldy paprika pods), *Penicillium* sp., *P. casei, P. roqueforti* (cheese making), and *Botrytis cinarea* (moldy grapes) (Sikora et al. 2008).

The aforementioned facts seem to indicate that allergenic threat caused by mold fungi and other microorganisms is serious. Some of the mentioned mold fungi phyli are used in biotechnological processes aimed at targeted food processing (fermented products) or for obtaining metabolites applied in the food industry as food additives, which may increase the allergenic threat. Also enzymes themselves or mold-derived enzymatic preparations can be the source of food, inhalatory, or contact allergy.

Apart from the environmental fungi listed earlier, the food industry makes use of many technologically useful molds, for instance in cheese making or salami type sausage ripening. Molds and enzymes produced by them may trigger various hypoallergenic reactions. A study conducted in Germany demonstrated that in a group of 89 bakery workers 20% reportedly had conjunctivitis, 39%—rhinitis, and 37%—asthma symptoms; moreover, 22% of them had specific antibodies IgE against α-amylase produced by *A. oryzae*.

Among hydrolases with allergenic properties used in the food industry there are α-amylases, amyloglucosidases, glucoamylases, cellulases, hemicellulases, pectinases, lipoxygenases, and xylanases (Bindslev-Jensen et al. 2006, Cullinan et al. 1997, Houba et al. 1997, Kanerva and Vanhanen 1999, 2001, Scheibe et al. 2001). Most of these enzymes are synthesized by *A. oryzae* fungi or *Bacillus subtilis* bacteria.

Besides other enzymes, e.g., phytase obtained from *A. Niger*, alkaline serine protease (allergen—Asp f 13) from *A. fumigatus,* or xylanase and cellulase present in baking additives may induce allergic reactions such us inflammation of the respiratory tract or may cause asthma in bakers (Baur 2005, Baur and Posch 1998, Merget et al. 2001). Fungal amylase and xylanase, as plant-derived enzymes (promelain, papain), are known to induce rhinitis or occupational rhinitis (Sikora et al. 2008).

It should be, however, emphasized that like in the case of other allergens, also mold allergens are capable of causing cross-reactions with allergens characteristic for *A. oryzae* mold fungi (α-amylase and hemicellulase) in individuals sensitive to the allergens of *A. fumigatus* (Daniel and Triboi 2002). There were reported cases of bakers with occupational inhalatory allergy to α-amylase of fungal origin who developed hypersensitivity of the digestive tract due to consumption of bread made with the addition of this enzymatic preparation (Baur and Czuppon 1995, Kanny and Moneret-Vautrin 1995). Interestingly, α- and β-amylases, which are wheat flour allergens, do not show immunological cross-reactions with α-amylase produced by *Aspergillus* mold fungi (308).

### 14.1.4 OTHER MICROORGANISMS AND METABOLITES AS SOURCES OF ALLERGENS IN FOOD

Besides bacteria and molds yeast also can be a source of allergens, for instance *Saccharomyces cerevisiae* used for dough fermentation. The main allergens synthesized by yeast are enolase ($m_w$ 51 kDa), acidic proteases and mannan (Nittner-Marszalska et al. 2001), and yeast allergen—Mal f 1 (Zargari et al. 1999). Enolase, which takes part in saccharide transformations, is an allergen synthesized also by other kinds of fungi, e.g., *Rhodotorula mucilaginosa*, *Candida albicans*, *P. citrinum*, *A. fumigatus*, *C. herbarum*, or *Alternaria alternata* (Chang et al. 2002).

Allergenic proteases are synthesized also by *Epicoccum purpurascens* yeast (*Epi p* 1—$m_w$ 30 kDa serine protease) and *R. mucilaginosa* (*Rho m* 2—vacuolar serine protease) (Bottari et al. 1996). The aforementioned family of allergenic proteins also includes inhalatory allergen *Bac l Subtilisin* produced by *Bacillus lentu* bacteria. Aspartyl proteases ($m_w$ 44 kDa), inducing allergies of the respiratory tract and asthma, are synthesized by *Candida albicans* yeast (Ainsworth et al. 1983).

Recently the cases of severe allergic reactions to yeast, buckwheat, and macrogol were identified in Finland—patent blue and carmine dye have been noted in Finland (Alfola et al. 2006, Makinen-Kiljunen and Haahtela 2008).

A group of potential allergens is made up by the enzymes produced by genetically modified organisms (Baur 2005, Bindslev-Jensen et al. 2006). On the market there are about 100 enzymatic preparations obtained through genetic modification of microorganisms. It can be expected that the transfer of genes held responsible for the synthesis of a certain enzymatic protein with documented allergenicity into another organism will not change its immunomodulatory properties. Glucoamylases synthesized by *A. niger* coded by the genes whose donor is *Aspergillus* sp. 1 causes allergic skin reactions. Analogous allergenic properties are shown by lipase synthesized by *Aspergillus* sp. 1, a gene acceptor of this enzyme from *Thermomyces* sp.1 or *Fusarium* species. (Bindslev-Jensen et al. 2006).

Viruses, bacteria, and bacterial toxins may, according to Chegini and Metcalfe, cause gastrointestinal, skin, and systemic symptoms that can be confused with food allergy (Chegini and Metcalfe 2008).

Apart from microorganisms themselves and enzymes, their main metabolites, also other metabilites (toxins, neurotoxins, and inhibitors) have allergenic properties (Table 14.1.3). A wide use of nonpathogenic mold fungi in biotechnological production is related to, among others, the fact that they produce many valuable metabolites.

Allergenic properties of pathogenic fungi metabolites are relatively little known (Placinta et al. 1999).

The main metabolites of this group of fungi (*Fusarium, Aspergillus, Penicillium,* and *Alternaria)* are not only mycotoxins but also hormonally active compounds as well as enzymes, for instance amylase, chitinase, cellulase, glucanase, xylanase, or protease (Pawelzik et al. 1998).

### 14.1.5 APPLICATION OF MICROORGANISMS AND ENZYMES FOR MODIFYING ALLERGENIC PROPERTIES

A wide application of microorganisms and their metabolites, in the enzymatic preparations, in the food industry is commonly known. An important and interesting direction of their future use is modifying antigenic (allergenic) properties of food. An example here is the use of proteolytical enzymes for targeted destruction of epitopes in order to eliminate allergenic properties of some proteins applied for producing hypoantigenic and hypoallergenic formulas for infants and adults (Jędrychowski and Wróblewska 1999, Wróblewska and Jędrychowski 2002).

Chapters 6.3.3 and 6.3.4 discusses this problem in greater detail.

Moreover, other enzymes are becoming increasingly popular in modifying both animal and plant proteins, for example, enzymes capable of cross-linking such as disulfide osomerase, tiol osimerase, or most commonly used transglutaminase obtained mainly from *Streptoverticillum mobaraense* (Gerrard 2002).

Application of proteolytical enzymes and transglutaminase for modifying antigenic properties may bring about both lowering product allergenity and increasing allergic threat (Gerrard and Sutton 2005, Jędrychowski et al. 2005). Among many methods aimed at limiting the occurrence of allergic reactions in humans, those based on modifying immunoreactive properties of chemical components, especially of plant raw materials and food proteins, are particularly important.

### 14.1.5.1 The Possibility of Substrate Antigenic Modification in Fermentation Processes

Studies are conducted on the possibilities of using native enzymes or enzymes added during technological processes. The action of these enzymes can be observed in many fermentation processes, in seed germination (sprout production), or in the processes of enzymatic hydrolysis in a different extent. During seed germination, proteins undergo degradation, which lowers their immunoreactive properties as a result of the action of activated native proteolytical enzymes (Jędrychowski et al. 2005). Additional separating sprouts from seed leaves allows to lower immunoreactivity of sprouts alone by approximately 99% compared to reactivity of sprouts mixed with seed leaves (Jędrychowski et al. 2005).

On applying milk fermentation bacteria *Pediococcus pentosaceus*, *Lactococcus raffinolactis*, *Lactobacillus plantarum*, and mold fungi *R. microsporus var. oligosporus* and *Geotrichum candidum* for pea flour fermentation, Barkholt et al. (1998) obtained considerable though not complete reduction of antigenic activity against antibodies to pea profilin and birch allergen *Bet v* 1. The microorganisms used did not lower the allergenicity resulting from the presence of pea protease inhibitor or the presence of lectins.

The possibility of substrate antigenic modification in fermentation processes is also ascribed to yeast *Saccharomyces cerevisiae* (Diowksz 2003) and milk fermentation bacteria (LAB—lactic acid bacteria): *Lb. sanfranciscensis*, *Lb. plantarum*, and *Lb. brevis* (Gobbetti 1998), as well as to their symbiotic action especially during bread dough fermentation (Zotta et al. 2006). Bacteria of Lactobacillus kind: *Lb. alimentarius* 15M, *Lb. brevis* 14G, *Lb. sanfranciscensis* 7A, and *Lb. hilgardii* 51B and enzymes produced by them (like pepsin, trypsin, and pancreatin) are capable of hydrolysis of polypeptides occurring in wheat grains, which have to be eliminated from the diet of children and adults with celiac disease (Bleukx et al. 1997, Rizzello et al. 2006). Similar possibility of change in the fragment 31–43 of α-gliadin was observed for intracellular proteolytical enzymes *Lb. plantarum* CRL 759 and CRL 778 (Rollán et al. 2005) as well as enzymes of other bacteria *Bacillus subtilis* and mold *A. oryzae* (Wehrle et al. 1999). Endogenous enzymes of wheat kernels activated during germination cause beneficial changes in flour proteins (Muntz et al. 2001, Simpson 2001).

Decomposition of prolamines, including gluten, during milk fermentation was also confirmed in a study by Zotta et al. (2006), who, however, claim that proteo/peptidolytical activity of bread leavening bacteria such as *Lb. plantarum*, *Lb. curvatus*, *Leuconostoc mesenteroides*, and *Lb. pentosus* in combination with or without yeast is low compared to prolamines. Native proteolytical enzymes of cereals activated during seed germination of wheat, barley, or rye have a specific capability to hydrolyze allergenic prolamines thus lowering the possibility of occurring reactions typical of glutene in the flour obtained from such grain and its products (Kiyosaki et al. 2007, Thiele et al. 2004).

Besides, commercially available bacteria (*Bacillus subtilis*) and fungi (*A. oryzae*) enzymes, which are used in the bakery industry for obtaining dough elasticity, are capable of hydrolyzing glutene proteins (Wehrle et al. 1999). It was demonstrated that bread dough fermentation results in lowering allergenic properties of wheat proteins during their digestion by pepsin and pancreatinin (Simonato et al. 2001).

Yet another group of enzymes applied for modifying allergenic properties of cereals (glutene) are transglutaminase (EC.2.3.2.13) and praline peptidases. The latter are produced by some bacteria strains of milk fermentation of bread leavening, i.e., *Lactobacillus: L. brevis, L. brevis* ssp. *linderi, L. plantarum, L. delbruecki* ssp. *delbruecki, L. sanfranciscensis, L. alimentarius,* or *L. hilgardii* (Di Cagno et al. 2002, 2004) *Flavobacterium meningosepticum* (Shan et al. 2002), *A. niger, Aeromonas hydrophila, Sphingomonas capsule,* and *Myxococcus xanthus* (Shan et al. 2004, Stepaniak et al. 2006).

One of the methods increasing the efficiency of glutene hydrolysis in the human digestive tract is applying a mixture of endopeptidase, carboxydase, and aminopeptidase enzymes (Siegel et al. 2006).

## 14.1.6 PERSPECTIVES ON THE USE OF MICROORGANISMS AND ENZYMATIC PREPARATIONS FOR SHAPING HEALTH BENEFICIAL PROPERTIES OF FOOD PRODUCTS

In practice, progress in genomics, proteomics, and genetic engineering and its application favors improving the composition and properties of food products. In the near future, an important task of studies and application of their results will be searching for new as well as improving genetically recognized plants and microorganisms capable of biosynthesizing components with a definite biological activity. It may also be expected that the knowledge of beneficial effects of probiotic bacteria and the effect of their metabolites on consumers' health will be extended. Studies on enzymes selectively degrading protein allergens will be intensified and their results will be applied in practice.

Due to the increasing use of advances in biotechnology including those in the field of obtaining recombined proteins there is a potential possibility both to partly or totally reduce allergenicity and to create a significant threat through expression of hidden allergens (Moseley 2001). An example of possibility to lower allergenicity of food products is reducing the level of allergenic proteins by introducing copies of the appropriate gene but in the antisense orientation, or introducing a gene which modifies immunodominant epitopes of allergenic proteins. The former was used for lowering allergenicity of rice proteins (Nakamura and Matsuda 1996) and the latter for modifying by single-site amino acid substitution of two out of five immunodominant epitopes of Gly m Bd 30 K (soybean allergen) (Helm et al. 2000, Herman et al. 2003). A potential allergenic threat of genetic engineering may result from the transfer of protein genome with well recognized allergenic properties to new food products, or from the transfer of unknown protein allergens to new food products, or from the fact of incomplete knowledge of the cations of peripheral genes, particularly expression of proteins and their posttranslation modifications (e.g., glycation).

A potent research tool used in immunodetection methods are specific antibodies. At present, the possibilities in this field are broad-ranging, from little specific antibodies (most often showing affinity to several epitopes due to polyvalency), through antibody fragments obtained as a result of antibody fragmentation, chimerical antibodies, highly specific monoclonal antibodies, to antibodies obtained via recombination. One of the greatest advantages of the last technique mentioned is avoiding the troublesome, also for ethical reasons, phase of immunizing experiment animals and possibility to produce human antibodies useful in therapy of various diseases.

## REFERENCES

Ainsworth, C.C., Gale, M.D., and Baird, S. 1983. The genetic of β-amylase isozymes in wheat. Allelic variation among hexaploid varieties and intrachromsomal gene locatios. *Theor Appl Genet* 66(1): 39–49.

Airola, K., Petman, L., and Mäkinen-Kiljunen, S. 2006. Clustered sensitivity to fungi: Anaphylactic reactions caused by ingestive allergy to yeasts. *Ann Allergy Asthma Immunol* 97(3): 294–297.

Bannon, G.A., Astwood, J.D., Dobert, R.C., and Fuchs, R.L. 2008. Biotechnology and genetic engineering. In: *Food Allergy. Adverse Reactions to Foods and Food Additives*, 4th ed., D.D. Metcalfe, H.A. Sampson, and R.A. Simon, Eds., pp. 62–81. Blackwell Publishing, Malden, MA/Oxford, U.K.

Barkholt, V., Jørgensen, P.B., Sørensen, D., Bahrenscheer, J., Haikara, A., Lemola, E., Laitila, A., and Frøkiær, H. 1998. Protein modification by fermentation: Effect of fermentation on the potential allergenicity of pea. *Allergy* 53(Suppl 46): 106–108.

Baur, X. 2005. Enzymes as occupational and environmental respiratory sensitisers. *Int Arch Occup Environ Health* 78(4): 279–286.

Baur, X. and Czuppon, A.B. 1995. Allergic reaction after eating α-amylase (Asp o 2)-containing bread. A case report. *Allergy* 50(1): 85–87.

Baur, X. and Posch, A. 1998. Characterized allergens causing bakers' asthma. *Allergy* 53(6): 562–566.

Bindslev-Jensen, C., Stahl Skov, P., Roggen, E.L., Hvass, P., and Sidelmann Brinch, D. 2006. Investigation on possible allergenicity of 19 different commercial enzymes used in the food industry. *Food Chem Toxicol* 44(11): 1909–1915.

Bleukx, W., Roels, S.P., and Delcour, J.A. 1997. On the presence and activities of proteolytic enzymes in vital wheat gluten. *J Cereal Sci* 26(2): 183–193.

Bottari, A., Capocchi, A., Fontanini, D., and Galleschi, L. 1996. Major proteinase hydrolysing gliadin during wheat germination. *Phytochemistry* 43(1): 39–44.

Chang, Ch.-Y., Choua, H., Tamb, M.F., Tangc, R.-B., Laia, H.-Y., and Shena, H.-D. 2002. Characterization of enolase allergen from *Rhodotorula mucilaginosa*. *J Biomed Sci* 9(6): 645–655.

Chegini, S. and Metcalfe, D.D. 2008. Seafood toxins. In: *Food Allergy. Adverse Reactions to Foods and Food Additives*, 4th ed., D.D. Metcalfe, H.A. Sampson, and R.A. Simon, Eds., pp. 508–530. Blackwell Publishing, Malden MA/Oxford, U.K.

Cullinan, P., Cook, A., Jones, M., Cannon, J., Fitzgerald, B., and Newman, T.A.J. 1997. Clinical responses to ingested fungal α-amylase and hemicellulase in persons sensitized to *Aspergillus fumigatus*? *Allergy* 52(3): 346–349.

Daniel, C. and Triboi, E. 2002. Changes in wheat protein aggregation during grain development: Effects of temperatures and weather stress. *Eur J Agron* 16(1): 1–12.

Di Cagno, R., De Angelis, M., Auricchio, S., Greco, L., Clarke, C., De Vincenzi, M., Giovannini, C., D'Archivio, M., Landolfo, F., Parrilli, G., Minervini, F., Arendt, E., and Gobbetti, M. 2004. Sourdough bread made from wheat and nontoxic flours and started with selected *Lactobacilli* is tolerated in celiac patients. *Appl Environ Microbiol* 70(2): 1088–1096.

Di Cagno, R., De Angelis, M., Lavermicocca, P., De Vincenzi, M., Giovannini, C., Faccia, M., and Gobbetti, M. 2002. Proteolysis by sourdough lactic acid bacteria: Effects on wheat flour protein fractions and gliadin peptides involved in human cereal intolerance. *Appl Environ Microbiol* 68(2): 623–633.

Diowksz, A. 2003. Zakwas piekarski jako złożony układ biologiczny. *Przegl Piek Cuk* 9: 16–17.

Gerrard, J.A. 2002. Protein–protein crosslinking in food: Methods, consequences, applications. *Trends Food Sci Technol* 13(12): 389–397.

Gerrard, J.A. and Sutton, K.H. 2005. Addition of transglutaminase to cereal products may generate the epitope responsible for celiac disease. *Trends Food Sci Technol* 16(11): 510–512.

Gobbetti, M. 1998. The sourdough microflora: Interactions of lactic acid bacteria and yeasts. *Trends Food Sci Technol* 9(7): 267–274.

Helm, R.M., Cockrell, G., West, C.M., Herman, E.M., Sampson, H.A., Bannon, G.A., and Burks, A.W. 2000. Mutational analysis of the IgE-binding epitopes of P34/Gly m1. *J Allergy Clin Immunol* 105: 378–384.

Herman, E.M., Helm, R.M., Jung, R., and Kinney, A.J. 2003. Genetic modification removes an immunodominant allergen from soybean. *Plant Physiol* 132: 36–43.

Houba, R., van Run, P., Doekes, G., Heederik, D., and Spithoven, J. 1997. Airborne levels of alpha-amylase allergens in bakeries. *J Allergy Clin Immunol* 99(3): 286–292.

Huang, Y.-W. and Huang, C.-Y. 1999. Traditional Chinese functional foods. In: *Asian Foods: Science and Technology*, C.Y.W. Ang, K. Liu, and Y.-W. Huang, Eds., pp. 409–452. Technomic Publishing Company, Inc., Lancaster, PA.

Jędrychowski, L. and Wróblewska, B. 1999. Reduction of the antigenicity of whey proteins by lactic acid fermentation. *Food Agricult Immunol* 77: 91–99.

Jędrychowski, L., Wróblewska, B., and Szymkiewicz, A. 2005. Technological aspects of food allergens occurrence in food products. *Pol J Environ Stud* 14(Suppl. 2): 171–180.

Kanerva, L. and Vanhanen, M. 1999. Occupational protein contact dermatitis from glukoamylase. *Contact Dermatitis* 41(3): 171–173.

Kanerva, L. and Vanhanen, M. 2001. Occupational allergic contact urticaria and rhinoconjunctivitis from a detergent protease. *Contact Dermatitis* 45(1): 49–51.

Kanny, G. and Moneret-Vautrin, D.A. 1995. α-Amylase contained in bread can induce food allergy. *J Allergy Clin Immunol* 95(1): 132–133.

Kiyosaki, T., Matsumoto, I., Asakura, T., Funaki, J., Kuroda, M., Misaka, T., Arai, S., and Abe, K. 2007. Gliadain, a gibberellin-inducible cysteine proteinase occurring in germinating seeds of wheat, *Triticum aestivum* L., specifically digests gliadin and is regulated by intrinsic cystatins. *FEBS J* 274(8): 1908–1917.

Kurup, V.P. 2003. Fungal allergens. *Curr Allergy Asthma Rep* 3(5): 416–423.

Kurup, V.P. and Banerjee, B. 2000. Fungal allergens and peptide epitopes. *Peptides* 21(4): 589–599.

Leino, M., Reijula, K., Mäkinen-Kiljunen, S., Haahtela, T., Mäkelä, M.J., and Alenius, H. 2006. *Cladosporium herbarum* and *Pityrosporum ovale* allergen extracts share cross-reacting glycoproteins. *Int Arch Allergy Immunol* 140(1): 30–35.

Makinen-Kiljunen, S. and Haahtela, T. 2008. Eight years of severe allergic reactions in Finland: A register-based report. *World Allergy Org J* 1(11): 184–189.

Merget, R., Sander, I., Raulf-Heimsoth, M., and Baur, X. 2001. Baker's asthma due to xylanase and cellulase without sensitization to alpha-amylase and only weak sensitization to flour. *Int Arch Allergy Immunol* 124: 502–505.

Moseley, B.E.B. 2001. How to make foods safer—genetically modified foods. *Allergy* 56(Suppl. 67): 61–63.

Müntz, K., Belozersky, M.A., Dunaevsky, Y.E., Schlereth, A., and Tiedemann, J. 2001. Stored proteinases and the initiation of storage protein mobilization in seeds during germination and seedling growth. *J Exp Bot* 52(362): 1741–1752.

Nakamura, R. and Matsuda, T. 1996. Rice allergenic protein and molecular-genetic approach for hypoallergenic rice. *Biosci Biotech Biochem* 60: 1215–1221.

Nittner-Marszalska, M., Wojcicka-Kustrzeba, I., Bogacka, E., Patkowski, J., and Dobek, R. 2001. Skin prick test response to enzyme enolase of the baker's yeast (*Saccharomyces cerevisiae*) in diagnosis of respiratory allergy. *Med Sci. Monit* 7(1): 121–124.

Pawelzik, E., Permady, H.H., Weinert, J., and Wolf, G.A. 1998. Effect of *Fusarium*-contamination on selected quality criteria of wheat. *Getreide Mehl Brot* 52(5): 264–266.

Placinta, C.M., D'Mello, J.P.F., and Macdonald, A.M.C. 1999. A review of worldwide contamination of cereal grains and animal feed with *Fusarium* mycotoxins. *Animal Feed Sci Technol* 78(1): 21–37.

Quirce, S., Cuevas, M., Diez-Gomez, M., FernandezRivas, M., Hinojosa, M., Gonzalez, R., and Losada, E. 1992. Respiratory allergy to *Aspergillus* derived enzymes in bakers' asthma. *J Allergy Clin Immunol* 90: 970–978.

Quirce, S. and Sastre, J. 1998. Occupational asthma. *Allergy* 53: 633–641.

Radauer, C., Bublin, M., Wagner, S., Mari, A., and Breiteneder, H. 2008. Allergens are distributed into few protein families and possess a restricted number of biochemical functions. *J Allergy Clin Immunol* 121: 847–852—AllFam URL: http://www.meduniwien.ac.at/allergens/allfam/.

Rizzello, C.G., De Angelis, M., Coda, R., and Gobbetti, M. 2006. Use of selected sourdough lactic acid bacteria to hydrolyze wheat and rye proteins responsible for cereal allergy. *Eur Food Res Technol* 223(3): 405–411.

Rollán, G., De Angelis, M., Gobbetti, M., and De Valdez, G.F. 2005. Proteolytic activity and reduction of gliadin-like fractions by sourdough lactobacilli. *J Appl Microbiol* 99(6): 1495–1502.

Scheibe, B., Weiss, W., Bauer, C.P., and Görg, A. 2001. Electrophoretic and immunochemical determination of bioindustrial enzymes in apple juice. *Eur Food Res Technol* 212(6): 691–695.

Shan, L., Marti, T., Sollid, L.M., Gray, G.M., and Khosla, C. 2004. Comparative biochemical analysis of three bacterial prolyl endopeptidases: Implications for coeliac sprue. *Biochem J* 383(2): 311–318.

Shan, L., Molberg, Ø., Parrot, I., Haush, F., Filiz, F., Gray, G.M., Sollid, L.M., and Khosla, C. 2002. Structural basis for gluten intolerance in celiac sprue. *Science* 297(5590): 2275–2279.

Shen, H.D., Chou, H., Tam, M.F., Chang, C.Y., Lai, H.Y., and Wang, S.R. 2003. Molecular and immunological characterization of Pen ch 18, the vacuolar serine protease major allergen of *Penicillium chrysogenum*. *Allergy* 58(10): 993–1002.

Shen, H.D., Lin, W.L., Liaw, S.F., Tam, M.F., and Han, S.H. 1997. Characterization of the 33-kilodalton major allergen of *Penicillium citrinum* by using MoAbs and N-terminal amino acid sequencing. *Clin Exp Allergy* 27(1): 79–86.

Shen, H.D., Lin, W.L., Tam, M.F., Chou, H., Wang, C.W., Tsai, J.J., Wang, S.R., and Han, S.H. 2001. Identification of vacuolar serine proteinase as a major allergen of *Aspergillus fumigatus* by immunoblotting and N-terminal amino acid sequence analysis. *Clin Exp Allergy* 31(2): 295–302.

Shen, H.D., Lin, W.L., Tam, M.F., Wang, S.R., Tsai, J.J., Chou, H., and Han, S.H. 1998. Alkaline serine proteinase: A major allergen of *Aspergillus oryzae* and its cross-reactivity with *Penicillium citrinum*. *Int. Arch. Allergy Immunol* 116(1): 29–35.

Siegel, M., Bethune, M.T., Gass, J., Ehren, J., Xia, J., Johannsen, A., Stuge, T.B., Gray, G.M., Lee, P.P., and Khosla, C. 2006. Rational design of combination enzyme therapy for celiac sprue. *Chem Biol* 13(6): 649–658.

Sikora, M., Cartier, A., Aresery, M. et al. 2008. Occupational reactions to food allergens. In: *Food Allergy. Adverse Reactions to Foods and Food Additives*, 4th ed., D.D. Metcalfe, H.A. Sampson, and R.A. Simon, Eds., pp. 223–250. Blackwell Publishing, Malden, MA/Oxford, U.K.

Simonato, B., Pasini, G., Giannattasio, M., Perutto, A.D., De Lazzari, F., and Curioni, A. 2001. Food allergy to wheat products: The effect of bread baking and *in vitro* digestion on wheat allergenic proteins. A study with bread dough, crumb, and crust. *J Agric Food Chem* 49(11): 5668–5673.

Simpson, D.J. 2001. Proteolytic degradation of cereal prolamins—the problem with proline. *Plant Sci* 161(5): 825–838.

Stepniak, D., Spaenij-Dekking, L., Mitea, C., Moester, M., de Ru, A., Baak-Pablo, R., van Veelen, P., Edens, L., and Koning, F. 2006. Highly efficient gluten degradation with a newly identified prolyl endoprotease: Implications for celiac disease. *Am J Physiol Gastrointest Liver Physiol* 291(4): G621–G629.

Thiele, C., Grassl, S., and Gänzle, M. 2004. Gluten hydrolysis and depolymerization during sourdough fermentation. *J Agr Food Chem* 52(5): 1307–1314.

Vanhanen, M., Tuomi, T., Hokkanen, H., Tupasela, O., Tuomainen, A., Holmberg, P.C., Leisola, M., and Nordman, H. 1996. Enzyme exposure and enzyme sensitisation in the baking industry. *Occup Environ Med* 53(10): 670–676.

Vanhanen, M., Tuomi, T., Tiikkainen, U., Tupasela, O., Tuomainen, A., and Luukkonen, R., Nordman, H. 2001. Sensitisation to enzymes in the animal feed industry. *Occup Environ Med* 58(2): 119–123.

Wehrle, K., Crowe, N., van Boeijen, I., and Arendt, E.K. 1999. Screening methods for the proteolytic breakdown of gluten by lactic acid bacteria and enzyme preparations. *Eur Food Res Technol.* 209(6): 428–433.

Wróblewska, B. and Jędrychowski, L. 2002. Influence of technological and biological processes on the immunoreactivity of cow milk proteins. *Pol J Food Nutr Sci* 11/52(SI 2): 156–159.

Zargari, A., Schmidt, M., Lundberg, M., Scheynius, A., and Whitley, P. 1999. Immunologic characterization of natural and recombinant Mal f 1 yeast allergen. *J Allergy Clin Immunol* 103(5 Pt 1): 877–884.

Zotta, T., Piraino, P., Ricciardi, A., McSweeney, P.L.H., and Parente, E. 2006. Proteolysis in model sourdough fermentations. *J Agr Food Chem* 54: 2567–2576.

## 14.2 PLANT FOOD ALLERGENS

Matthias Egger, Michael Hauser, Georg Schmidt, Nicole Wopfner, Fátima Ferreira, and Michael Wallner

### 14.2.1 INTRODUCTION

Plant tissues consumed by humans contain thousands of different proteins. The number of genes expressed at mid endosperm development in wheat, for example, has been estimated within the range of 4000–8000. However, the number of proteins capable of eliciting an allergic response in atopic individuals is several orders of magnitudes lower in any given allergen source (Breiteneder and Radauer 2004). So far, the official allergen list of the International Union of Immunological Societies (IUIS) Allergen Nomenclature Subcommittee (www.allergen.org) comprises 122 plant-derived food allergens (see Table 14.2.1). In recent years there were several attempts of classifying these allergens by their source, biologic function (Breiteneder and Ebner 2000), protein fold (Aalberse 2000), or by protein families (Breiteneder and Ebner 2001, Shewry et al. 2002). Indeed, most of the plant-derived food allergens can be integrated into only a few protein families and superfamilies on the basis of sequence homology, which is related to conserved three-dimensional structures and possibly function (Breiteneder and Mills 2005b, Breiteneder and Radauer 2004).

## TABLE 14.2.1
## Plant-Derived Food Allergens

| Protein Family | | Botanical Family | Allergen Source | | Allergen Name |
|---|---|---|---|---|---|
| Prolamin superfamily | 2S albumins | *Brassicales* | Turnip | *B. rapa* | *Bra r* 1 |
| | | | Yellow mustard | *Sinapis alba* | *Sin a* 1 |
| | | | Oriental mustard | *B. juncea* | *Bra j* 1 |
| | | | Rape seed | *B. napus* | *Bra n* 1 |
| | | *Lamiales* | Sesame | *Sesamum indicum* | *Ses i* 1 *Ses i* 2 |
| | | *Ericales* | Brazil nut | *Bertholletia excelsia* | *Ber e* 1 |
| | | *Fabales* | Peanut | *Arachis hypogaea* | *Ara h* 2 *Ara h* 6 *Ara h* 7 |
| | | *Fagales* | Black walnut | *Juglans nigra* | *Jug n* 1 |
| | | | English walnut | *J. regia* | *Jug r* 1 *Jug r* 4 |
| | | *Malpighiales* | Castor bean | *Ricinus communis* | *Ric c* 1 |
| | | *Sapindales* | Cashew nut | *Anacardium occidentale* | *Ana o* 3 |
| | | | Pistachio | *Pistacia vera* | *Pis v* 1 |
| | nsLTPs | *Asparagales* | Asparagus | *Asparagus officinalis* | *Aspa o* 1 |
| | | *Poales* | Wheat | *Triticum aestivum* | *Tri a* 14 |
| | | | Maize | *Z. mays* | *Zea m* 14 |
| | | *Asterales* | Cultivated lettuce | *Lactuca sativa* | *Lac s* 1 |
| | | *Brassicales* | Cabbage | *B. oleracea* | *Bra o* 3 |
| | | *Fagales* | Hazelnut | *Corylus avellana* | *Cor a* 8 |
| | | | English walnut | *J. regia* | *Jug r* 3 |
| | | *Rosales* | Strawberry | *Fragaria ananassa* | *Fra a* 3 |
| | | | Apple | *Malus domestica* | *Mal d* 3 |
| | | | Apricot | *P. armeniaca* | *Pru ar* 3 |
| | | | Sweet cherry | *P. avium* | *Pru av* 3 |
| | | | European plum | *P. domestica* | *Pru d* 3 |
| | | | Peach | *P. persica* | *Pru p* 3 |
| | | | Pear | *Pyrus communis* | *Pyr c* 3 |
| | | | Red raspberry | *Rubus idaeus* | *Rub i* 3 |
| | | *Rosids incertae sedis* | Grape | *Vitis vinifera* | *Vit v* 1 |

*(continued)*

**TABLE 14.2.1 (Continued)**
**Plant-Derived Food Allergens**

| Protein Family | | Botanical Family | Allergen Source | | Allergen Name |
|---|---|---|---|---|---|
| | | *Sapindales* | Lemon | *Citrus limon* | *Cit l* 3 |
| | | | Tangerine | *Ci. reticuata* | *Cit r* 3 |
| | | | Sweet orange | *Ci. sinensis* | *Cit s* 3 |
| | | *Solanales* | Tomato | *Ly. esculentum* | *Lyc e* 3 |
| | α-amylases | *Poales* | Barley | *Hordeum vulgare* | *Hor v* 15 |
| | | | | | *Hor v* 16 |
| | Cereal prolamins | *Poales* | Barley | *H. vulgare* | *Hor v* 21 |
| | | | Wheat | *Tr. aestivum* | *Tri a* 19 |
| | | | | | *Tri a* 26 |
| | | *Poales* | Rye | *Secale cereale* | *Sec c* 20 |
| Cupin superfamily | Germins | *Sapindales* | Sweet orange | *Ci. sinensis* | *Cit s* 1 |
| | Vicillins | *Fabales* | Peanut | *Ar. hypogaea* | *Ara h* 1 |
| | | | Lentil | *Lens culinaris* | *Len c* 1 |
| | | | Pea | *Pisum sativum* | *Pis s* 1 |
| | | | | | *Pis s* 2 |
| | | *Fagales* | Black walnut | *J. nigra* | *Jug n* 2 |
| | | | English walnut | *J. regia* | *Jug r* 2 |
| | | *Lamiales* | Sesame | *Se. indicum* | *Ses i* 3 |
| | | *Sapindales* | Cashew nut | *Ana. occidentale* | *Ana o* 1 |
| | Legumins | *Fabales* | Brazil nut | *Be. excelsia* | *Ber e* 2 |
| | | | Peanut | *Ar. hypogaea* | *Ara h* 3 |
| | | | | | *Ara h* 4 |
| | | *Lamiales* | Sesame | *Se. indicum* | *Ses i* 6 |
| | | | | | *Ses i* 7 |
| | | *Sapindales* | Cashew nut | *Ana. occidentale* | *Ana o* 2 |
| | | | Pistachio | *P. vera* | *Pis v* 2 |
| Profilins | | *Bromeliales* | Pineapple | *An. comosus* | *Ana c* 1 |
| | | *Poales* | Barley | *H. vulgare* | *Hor v* 12 |
| | | | Rice | *Oryza sativa* | *Ory s* 12 |
| | | *Zingiberales* | Banana | *Musa x paradisiaca* | *Mus xp* 1 |
| | | *Apiales* | Celery | *Ap. graveolens* | *Api g* 4 |
| | | | Carrot | *Daucus carota* | *Dau c* 4 |
| | | *Cucurbitales* | Muskmelon | *Cucumis melo* | *Cuc m* 2 |
| | | *Fabales* | Peanut | *Ar. hypogaea* | *Ara h* 5 |
| | | | Soybean | *Glycine max* | *Gly m* 3 |
| | | *Fagales* | Hazelnut | *Co. avellana* | *Cor a* 2 |
| | | *Rosales* | Strawberry | *F. ananassa* | *Fra a* 4 |
| | | | Apple | *M. domestica* | *Mal d* 4 |
| | | | Sweet cherry | *P. avium* | *Pru av* 4 |
| | | | Almond | *P. dulcis* | *Pru du* 4 |

## TABLE 14.2.1 (continued)
## Plant-Derived Food Allergens

| Protein Family | Botanical Family | Allergen Source | | Allergen Name |
|---|---|---|---|---|
| | | Peach | *P. persica* | *Pru p* 4 |
| | | Pear | *Py. communis* | *Pyr c* 4 |
| | *Sapindales* | Sweet orange | *Ci. sinensis* | *Cit s* 2 |
| | | Lychee | *Litchi chinensis* | *Lit c* 1 |
| | *Solanales* | Bell pepper | *Ca. annuum* | *Cap a* 2 |
| | | Tomato | *Ly. esculentum* | *Lyc e* 1 |
| PR-10 (Bet v 1 related) | *Apiales* | Celery | *Ap. graveolens* | *Api g* 1 |
| | | Carrot | *Da. carota* | *Dau c* 1 |
| | *Fabales* | Peanut | *Ar. hypogaea* | *Ara h* 8 |
| | | Soybean | *G. max* | *Gly m* 4 |
| | | Mung bean | *Vigna radiata* | *Vig r* 1 |
| | *Fagales* | Hazelnut | *Co. avellana* | *Cor a* 1 |
| | *Rosales* | Strawberry | *F. ananassa* | *Fra a* 1 |
| | | Apple | *M. domestica* | *Mal d* 1 |
| | | Apricot | *P. armeniaca* | *Pru ar* 1 |
| | | Sweet cherry | *P. avium* | *Pru av* 1 |
| | | Pear | *Py. communis* | *Pyr c* 1 |
| | | Red raspberry | *Rubus idaeus* | *Rub i* 1 |
| Class I chitinases (hevein-like domain) | *Poales* | Wheat | *Tr. aestivum* | *Tri a* 18 |
| | *Brassicales* | Turnip | *B. rapa* | *Bra r* 2 |
| | *Laurales* | Avocado | *Persea americana* | *Pers a* 1 |
| Papain-like cysteine proteases | *Bromeliales* | Pineapple | *An. comosus* | *Ana c* 2 |
| | *Ericales* | Kiwi | *Ac. deliciosa* | *Act d* 1 |
| | *Fabales* | Soybean | *G. max* | *Gly m* 1 |
| Thaumatin-like proteins | *Ericales* | Kiwi | *Ac. deliciosa* | *Act d* 2 |
| | *Rosales* | Apple | *M. domestica* | *Mal d* 2 |
| | | Sweet cherry | *P. avium* | *Pru av* 2 |
| | *Solanales* | Bell pepper | *Ca. annuum* | *Cap a* 1 |
| Oleosin | *Lamiales* | Sesame | *Se. indicum* | *Ses i* 4 |
| | | | | *Ses i* 5 |
| Kunitz-type protease inhibitors | *Solanales* | Potato | *Solanum tuberosum* | *Sola t* 2 |
| | | | | *Sola t* 3 |
| | | | | *Sola t* 4 |
| Thioredoxins | *Poales* | Wheat | *Tr. aestivum* | *Tri a* 25 |
| | | Maize | *Z. mays* | *Zea m* 25 |

(*continued*)

**TABLE 14.2.1 (continued)**
**Plant-Derived Food Allergens**

| Protein Family | Botanical Family | Allergen Source | | Allergen Name |
|---|---|---|---|---|
| β-amylases | *Poales* | Barley | *H. vulgare* | *Hor v 17* |
| Cystatins | *Ericales* | Kiwi | *Ac. deliciosa* | *Act d 4* |
| Expansins | *Ericales* | Kiwi | *Ac. deliciosa* | *Act d 5* |
| | *Fabales* | Soybean | *G. max* | *Gly m 2* |
| Glycoside hydrolase | *Rosales* | Chinese-date | *Ziziphus mauritiana* | *Ziz m 1* |
| | *Solanales* | Tomato | *Ly. esculentum* | *Lyc e 2* |
| Isoflavone reductase | *Rosales* | Pear | *Py. communis* | *Pyr c 5* |
| Subtilisin-like serine protease | *Cucurbitales* | Muskmelon | *C. melo* | *Cuc m 1* |
| Berberine bridge enzymes | *Apiales* | Celery | *Ap. graveolens* | *Api g 5* |
| Chlorophyll-binding proteins | *Apiales* | Celery | *Ap. graveolens* | *Api g 3* |
| PR-1 proteins | *Cucurbitales* | Muskmelon | *C. melo* | *Cuc m 3* |
| Patatin family | *Solanales* | Potato | *S. tuberosum* | *Sola t 1* |
| Seed-specific biotinylated protein | *Fabales* | Lentil | *Lens culinaris* | *Len c 2* |
| 60S acidic ribosomal binding protein | *Rosales* | Almond | *P. dulcis* | *Pru du 5* |
| Unidentified | *Ericales* | Kiwi | *Ac. deliciosa* | *Act d 3* |

A few allergen databases have been constructed allowing an overview of allergens in general and of food allergens in particular. Interested readers are referred to their Web pages: www.meduniwien.ac.at/allergens/allfam/, www.allergome.org, www.allergenonline.com. Interestingly, many of the known plant food allergens are homologous to pathogenesis related (PR) proteins. These proteins represent a collection of 14 unrelated protein families, which by definition are induced upon environmental stress, pathogen infection, and antibiotic stimuli (Breiteneder and Radauer 2004, Hoffmann-Sommergruber 2002).

According to their clinical appearance, plant-derived food allergens can be distinguished in class 1 (complete food allergens) and class 2 (incomplete food allergens) food allergens. Class 1 food allergy mainly affects children and the sensitization process occurs via the gastrointestinal tract. Allergens eliciting this manifestation share special features like resistance to heat and gastric digestion. In contrast, class 2 food allergy is mainly seen in adults and develops as a consequence of allergic sensitization to inhalant allergens. This class of food allergens seems to be more sensitive to heat and digestive enzymes and therefore cannot cause per-orally sensitizations, but instead provokes allergic reactions in already sensitized patients due to IgE cross-reactivity. Thus, Class 2 food allergens are often termed nonsensitizing elicitors. Depending on their stability during the digestive process, they cause symptoms ranging from mild oral symptoms to anaphylactic shock and are responsible for the so called pollinosis-associated food allergy, where the pollen acts as primary sensitizing agent (Breiteneder and Ebner 2000, Egger et al. 2006, Sicherer 2001, Yagami 2002). So far, several clinical pollen-food syndromes (PFS) have been described, such as the birch-fruit, the celery-mugwort-spice, and the latex-fruit syndrome, which by its molecular background is comparable with PFS.

This section briefly describes the protein families known to contain plant food allergens. Allergenic members are discussed not only in terms of their structural characteristics, but also with regard to biologic function, cross-reactivity, and clinical relevance. A list of plant-derived food allergens identified so far, as acknowledged by the IUIS Allergen Nomenclature Sub-Committee, is given in Table 14.2.1. A list of publications referring to the first description of each of the 122 included allergens can be found on the IUIS Allergen Nomenclature Sub-Committee homepage (www.allergen.org). Three-dimensional structures of allergens representative for each allergen family are depicted in Figure 14.2.1.

### 14.2.2 THE PROLAMIN SUPERFAMILY

Named after cereal prolamins, which represent major storage proteins of cereal grains, the prolamin superfamily is characterized by high contents of proline and glutamine (Shewry et al. 2002). Allergens belonging to the prolamin superfamily are of low molecular weight (MW) and feature eight conserved cysteine residues and a similar three-dimensional structure rich in α-helices (Breiteneder and Radauer 2004, Kreis et al. 1985). They comprise three major groups of plant food allergens: seed storage 2S albumins found in tree nuts and seeds, defense-related nonspecific lipid transfer proteins (nsLTPs) found in some fruits and vegetables, and cereal α-amylase/trypsin inhibitors. In addition, a soybean hydrophobic protein *Gly m* 1 has been identified as an allergen and integrated into the prolamin superfamily.

Due to their stability to heat and gastrointestinal digestion, many allergens from the prolamin superfamily are important class 1 food allergens that may account for severe anaphylactic reactions (Breiteneder and Mills 2005c).

### 14.2.3 2S ALBUMINS

With exception of cereals, albumins and globulins make up the major group of seed storage proteins present in many dicotyledonous plant species (Shewry et al. 1995). Whereas albumins are water soluble at low salt concentrations, globulins dissolve at high salt conditions. In addition to their solubility, seed storage proteins are characterized and identified on the basis of sedimentation coefficient as 2S albumins and 7S and 11S globulins (Breiteneder and Ebner 2000). 2S albumins are small globular

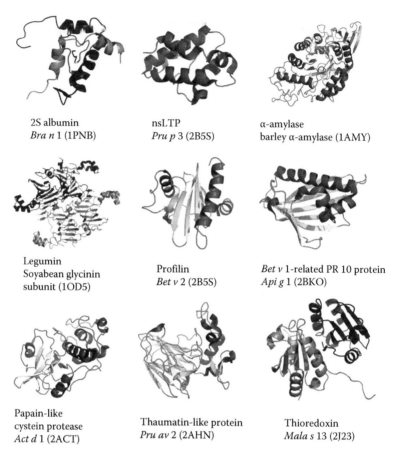

2S albumin
*Bra n* 1 (1PNB)

nsLTP
*Pru p* 3 (2B5S)

α-amylase
barley α-amylase (1AMY)

Legumin
Soyabean glycinin
subunit (1OD5)

Profilin
*Bet v* 2 (2B5S)

*Bet v* 1-related PR 10 protein
*Api g* 1 (2BKO)

Papain-like
cystein protease
*Act d* 1 (2ACT)

Thaumatin-like protein
*Pru av* 2 (2AHN)

Thioredoxin
*Mala s* 13 (2J23)

**FIGURE 14.2.1 (See color insert following page 234.)** Cartoon representation of the three-dimensional structure of allergens representative for distinct families. For single chain allergens alpha helical structures are presented in red, beta sheets in yellow, and turns in green. Chains of oligomeric proteins are shown in blue and orange. The PDB (www.pdb.org) codes are given in parenthesis.

proteins that are rich in arginine, glutamine, asparagine, and cysteine. They originate from several important food allergen sources like tree nuts and seeds such as Brazil nut, walnut, sesame, and mustard. The most characteristic feature of their amino acid sequence is the distribution of their eight cysteine residues in a conserved pattern (...C...C.../...CC...CXC...C...C) (Pantoja-Uceda et al. 2002). Due to their amino acid composition, their high content in the protein bodies of seeds and their mobilization during germination, a role as a nitrogen and sulfur donor has been proposed for these proteins. In addition, antifungal activity against a number of plant-pathogenic fungi has been shown for napins, the 2S albumins from radish (Terras et al. 1992). Furthermore, this family of proteins is subjected to modification after their synthesis. Typical 2S albumins, such as the napins from the Brassicaceae or the Brazil nut 2S albumin *Ber e* 1, are heterodimeric proteins consisting of two subunits of approximately 4 and 9 kDa, which are held together by conserved interchain disulfide bonds (Shewry et al. 1995). In addition to their biological interest, 2S albumins have been used by means of genetic engineering as carriers for the synthesis of biologically active peptides, as well as for improving the nutritional properties of grain crops by increasing their content of essential amino acids (Altenbach et al. 1992).

Many allergenic 2S albumins originate from the Brassicaceae family, i.e., oriental mustard seed *Bra j* 1, rapeseed *Bra n* 1, turnip *Bra r* 1, and yellow mustard seed *Sin a* 1. Furthermore, Brazil nut *Ber e* 1, black walnut *Jug n* 1, *Jug r* 1, and *Jug r* 4 from English walnut, *Ses i* 1 and *Ses i* 2 from sesame, *Ric c* 1 from castor bean, *Ana o* 3 from cashew nut, and *Pis v* 1 from pistachio have been included into the IUIS official allergen list.

Allergy to peanut is a significant health problem because of the high frequency of systemic allergic reactions. It is the most common cause of fatal and near-fatal food-induced anaphylaxis. Among the peanut allergens the glycoprotein *Ara h* 2, *Ara h* 6, and *Ara h* 7 belong to the conglutin protein family, which is related to the 2S albumin superfamily of seed storage proteins. Also soybean 2S albumins can cause serious health problems since soy products are used in an increasing number of aliments and can therefore augment the risk of atopic subjects to become sensitized. Additionally, IgE cross-reactivity between 2S albumins from rapeseed and mustard, as well as between members of the Brassicaceae family could be demonstrated (Monsalve et al. 1997, Pastorello et al. 1998, 2001). It was further reported that 2S albumins are stable proteins resistant to proteolysis by trypsin or simulated gastric fluid, which indicates that the intact allergens can enter the circulatory system constituting an important feature for their allergenic activity (Murtagh et al. 2002).

The 2S albumin family is an important class of common allergenic proteins in seeds. Their presence in almost all edible seeds must be taken into account because of the high incidence of possible clinical reactions occurring in sensitized people and because of the actual possibility of cross-reactivity among different proteins of the same class.

### 14.2.4    PLANT NONSPECIFIC LIPID TRANSFER PROTEINS

Lipid transfer proteins (LTP), originally named after their ability to transfer phospholipids between vesicles and membranes, can be divided into two types: those specific for certain classes of phospholipids and those that are able to accommodate several lipid classes, called nonspecific LTPs (nsLTPs) (Breiteneder and Mills 2005a). Plant nsLTPs are closely related basic proteins, unique to flowering plants. According to their molecular masses two subfamilies, the 9 kDa nsLTP1 and the 7 kDa nsLTP2 subfamily, can be classified. Various degrees of sequence identity (from 30% to 95%) are found between members of the LTP family from different species (Salcedo et al. 2004). nsLTPs are characterized by a common fold of four α-helices which are stabilized by four disulfide bonds forming a central hydrophobic tunnel where lipophilic molecules can bind. Nevertheless, it is now emerging that plant nsLTPs are not involved in intracellular lipid trafficking. Instead, plant evolution used the three-dimensional scaffold of nsLTPs in a promiscuous fashion for defense against fungi and bacteria by a mechanism that is still unknown. Indeed, in one instance, this hydrophobic tunnel has been lost completely. Thus, nsLTPs have been included as member of the heterogeneous collection of the PR protein families (Hoffmann-Sommergruber 2002, van Loon and van Strien 1999).

Plant nsLTPs are likely to act as potent food allergens (class 1 food allergens) because of their thermostability and extreme resistance to proteolysis as well as harsh pH conditions (Asero et al. 2000). They accumulate at high concentrations in the outer epidermal layers of plant organs explaining for instance the strong allergenicity of fruit peels compared to pulps as shown for Rosaceae fruits (van Ree 2002b). In fact, nsLTPs are considered major allergens especially in the Mediterranean area, where they are regarded as the most important allergens of Rosaceae fruits, such as apple *Mal d* 3, peach *Pru p* 3, and apricot *Pru ar* 3. For example, 60%–90% of Spanish peach allergic individuals show positive skin prick tests (SPT) to *Pru p* 3 (Fernandez-Rivas et al. 2003, Garcia-Selles et al. 2002). In contrast, the incidence of sensitization to nsLTPs in Central and Northern Europe is very limited. A recent study demonstrated that according to *in vitro* tests only 3% of German, but 100% of Italian patients were sensitized to the cherry nsLTP *Pru av* 3. However, the surprising geographical distribution pattern of sensitization to nsLTPs is still unexplained. Allergy to Rosaceae fruits in Central and Northern Europe seems rather associated with birch pollinosis and sensitization to *Bet v* 1 related allergens (Ebner et al. 1991, Scheurer et al. 1999). It is believed that sensitization to food nsLTPs is a consequence of food consumption and no epiphenomenon of pollen exposure. Nonetheless, there is evidence of IgE cross-reactivity between *Pru p* 3 and the mugwort pollen nsLTP *Art v* 3. Whether peach or pollen acts as primary sensitizing source is still a matter of debate (Lombardero et al. 2004, Pastorello et al. 2002). Other nsLTPs originating from the botanical family of Rosaceae comprise strawberry *Fra a* 3, plum *Pru d* 3, pear *Pyr c* 3, and raspberry *Rub i* 3. NsLTPs have a wide distribution and are considered as pan-allergens with sequences available from fruits, nuts, seeds, and vegetables. *Cor a* 8 has been demonstrated to be a clinically important hazelnut allergen causing severe allergic reactions in Spanish patients. Walnut *Jug r* 3, cabbage *Bra o* 3, and maize *Zea m* 14 nsLTPs were identified as major allergens cross-reacting with peach *Pru p* 3. Grape *Vit v* 1 was characterized and included as one elicitor of the proposed "LTP-associated-clinical-syndrome" that explains allergic cross-reactions to nsLTPs originating from multiple allergen sources (Vassilopoulou et al. 2007). Although allergic reactions to lettuce are not frequent, lettuce nsLTP *Lac s* 1 has been reported to cause anaphylaxis in susceptible individuals. In addition, the involvement of nsLTPs *Lyc e* 3 in tomato, *Aspa o* 1 in asparagus, and *Tri a* 14 in wheat allergy has been reported. Recently, nsLTPs originating from citrus fruits, i.e., *Cit l* 3 from lemon, *Cit r* 3 from tangerine, and *Cit s* 3 from sweet orange have been included into the official IUIS allergen list.

## 14.2.5 α-Amylases

A number of starch-converting enzymes belong to a single family termed the α-amylase family or family 13 hydrolases. This group of enzymes shares common characteristics such as an eight-stranded α/β barrel structure, the ability to hydrolyze 1,4-α-D-glucosidic linkages of attached polysaccharides in α-conformation, and conserved amino acid residues in the active sites of the enzymes (van der Maarel et al. 2002).

To date, several α-amylases have been identified in diverse organisms, e.g., *Aed a* 4 in yellow fever mosquito or *Der p* 4 in European house dust mite. Cereal α-amylases are important allergens for patients with baker's asthma involving the two crucial allergens from barley (*Hor v* 15 and *Hor v* 16). Some of these patients also show IgE reactivity to fungal α-amylases, e.g., *Asp o* 21 from Aspergillus, used as baking additives or present in mold contaminated flour.

### 14.2.6 CEREAL PROLAMINS

Cereal prolamins, named glutenins and gliadins in wheat, secalins in rye, and hordeins in barley, are major storage proteins of the cereal grain endosperm. These sulfur-rich proteins comprise an N-terminal domain of proline- and glutamin-rich repeats and a C-terminal domain responsible for intrachain disulfide bonds (Breiteneder and Radauer 2004). So far, γ-3 hordein (*Hor v* 21) from barley, *Sec c* 20 from rye, as well as *Tri a* 19 and *Tri a* 26 from wheat are included in the IUIS allergen list.

### 14.2.7 THE CUPIN SUPERFAMILY

Cupins, termed after their common conserved β-barrel fold ("cupa" is the Latin term for a small barrel), comprise a large superfamily of proteins sharing a common origin. Their evolution can be followed from bacteria to eukaryotes including animals and higher pants. Two functional classes can be divided: the monocupins and bicupins, containing one and two conserved cupin domains, respectively (Dunwell et al. 2004).

### 14.2.8 GERMINS

Monocupins include bacterial carbohydrate isomerases and epimerases as well as germins and germin-like proteins (GLPs). So far, *Cit s* 1 from orange is one of the few members of the germin family, which has been reported to act as an allergen.

### 14.2.9 VICILLINS

Mature 7/8S globulins (vicillins or 7S vicillin-like globulins) are homotrimeric proteins of about 150–190 kDa, which lack cysteines and therefore contain no disulfide bonds. Their detailed subunit compositions vary considerably due to differences in proteolytic processing and glycosylation of the monomers. The best characterized allergenic vicillin is the major peanut allergen *Ara h* 1, which is responsible for the majority of cases of fatal anaphylaxis induced by plant foods. Further allergenic vicillins include *Jug r* 2 from English walnut, *Jug n* 2 from black walnut, *Ana o* 1 from cashew nut, *Ses i* 3 from sesame, *Pis s* 1 and *Pis s* 2 from pea, and *Len c* 1 from lentil (Breiteneder and Radauer 2004, Dunwell et al. 2004).

### 14.2.10 LEGUMINS

Mature 11S globulins are hexameric proteins that are initially assembled and transported through the secretory system as intermediate trimers. In the protein storage vacuole, the subunits of these trimers are proteolytically processed to yield an acidic 30–40 kDa polypeptide linked by a disulfide bond to a basic polypeptide of about 20 kDa. Cleavage is accompanied by the transformation of two trimers into a mature hexameric 11S globulin. Allergenic legumins include the minor peanut allergens *Ara h* 3 and *Ara h* 4, previously described as distinct allergens with high sequence similarity to glycinins and now considered to be the same allergens. Other described legumins are *Cor a* 9 from hazelnut, *Ber e* 2 from Brazil nut, *Pis v* 2 from pistachio, *Ana o* 2 from cashew nut, soybean glycinin, and sesame *Ses i* 6 and *Ses i* 7 (Breiteneder and Radauer 2004, Dunwell et al. 2004).

### 14.2.11 PROFILINS

Profilins represent an allergen family of small 12–15 kDa cytosolic actin-binding proteins playing a key role in cell motility through the regulation of actin microfilament polymerization dynamics. In plant cells they are thus involved in processes like cytokinesis, cytoplasmatic steaming, cell elongation, and the growth of pollen tubes and root hairs (Ramachandran et al. 2000, Valster et al. 1997). Phosphoinositides and poly-L-proline stretches constitute additional profilin-binding domains. However, being involved in essential cellular processes, profilins can be found in all organisms examined so far, therefore being considered as pan-allergens, which are responsible for many cross-reactions between inhalant and nutritive allergen sources (Valenta et al. 1992, Witke 2004). In higher plants profilins constitute a family of highly conserved proteins displaying sequence identities of at least 75% even between members from distantly related organisms. However, as sequence conservation is reflected by highly similar three-dimensional structures, IgE cross-reactivity between profilins seems to be a result of the highly conserved three-dimensional profilin fold (Sankian et al. 2005). Profilins belong to the α-β class of proteins featuring mainly antiparallel beta sheets. In plants, profilin was first identified as allergen in birch pollen and designated as *Bet v* 2 (Valenta et al. 1991).

Various studies reported that about 20%–36% of all pollen-sensitized patients are allergic to profilin (Valenta et al. 1992, Wopfner et al. 2005). Since profilin-specific IgE cross-reacts with homologues from virtually every plant source, sensitization to these allergens is a risk factor for allergic reactions to multiple pollen sources and for the development of class 2 food allergy (Asero et al. 2003). As described for other class 2 food allergens, profilins are considered sensitive to heat denaturation and gastric digestion leading to allergic reactions which are usually confined as oral symptoms (e.g., pruritus, edema, pharyngitis) elicited by raw food (Breiteneder and Radauer 2004, Rodriguez-Perez et al. 2003). In contrast, celery profilin *Api g* 4 is known to be partially heat resistant, and might therefore also elicit allergic reactions after cooking (Ballmer-Weber et al. 2000, Jankiewicz et al. 1996).

To date, several plant food-derived profilins have been characterized, most of them being evidently involved in PFS. Hazelnut profilin *Cor a* 2 and the profilins from Rosaceae fruits strawberry *Fra a* 4, apple *Mal d* 4, cherry *Pru av* 4, almond *Pru du* 4, peach *Pru p* 4, and pear *Pyr c* 4, for example, are considered to cross-react with grass and/or birch pollen *Bet v* 2 profilin (van Ree et al. 1995). Reactions to celery *Api g* 4 and carrot *Dau c* 4 are observed in patients with concomitant birch- or mugwort pollen allergy (celery–mugwort–spice syndrome) (Egger et al. 2006). The ragweed–melon–banana association includes the melon and banana profilins *Cuc m* 2 and *Mus xp* 1, respectively. Furthermore, profilin is considered an important mediator in IgE cross-reactivity between pollen and exotic fruit, like lychee *Lit c* 1 (Fah et al. 1995, Willerroider et al. 2003) and pineapple *Ana c* 1. In addition, IgE binding profilins from peanut *Ara h* 5, soybean *Gly m* 3, orange *Cit s* 2, bell pepper *Cap a* 2, and tomato *Lyc e* 1 were produced as recombinant proteins. Finally, two profilins originating from the botanical family of Poaceae barley *Hor v* 12 and rice *Ory s* 12 have been identified and included into the official IUIS allergen list.

## 14.2.12   *Bet v* 1 Superfamily

The major birch pollen allergen *Bet v* 1 and its homologous allergens from other pollen as well as food sources belong to the PR-10 protein family. This group represents the largest of the three families within the *Bet v* 1 superfamily. The second group contains the ripening-related proteins and major latex proteins whereas the third group includes enzymes with S-noroclaurin synthase activity. However allergenic molecules were only found within the PR-10 proteins (Liscombe et al. 2005). Fifteen allergenic molecules of this family are officially listed in the IUIS database, 12 of them representing food allergens.

In general, the expression of PR-10 proteins in plants can be stress induced, though high levels of these proteins are also found in reproductive tissue such as pollen, fruits, or seeds. Despite a rather low amino acid sequence similarity of *Bet v* 1 and its allergenic homologues, a comparison of 3D structures of *Bet v* 1, *Api g* 1 from celery, and *Pru av* 1 from peach revealed a much conserved folding pattern of the allergens (Gajhede et al. 1996, Neudecker et al. 2001, Schirmer et al. 2005), which for sure affects the high level of patients' IgE cross-reactivity toward the *Bet v* 1 family members. Analysis of these structures showed that the allergen has an α-β fold with a solvent-accessible cavity traversing the protein. Resolving the crystal structure of a low IgE binding *Bet v* 1 isoform revealed two deoxycholate molecules bound to the cavity of the allergen. Structural similarities of deoxycholate with brassinosteroids (BRs), which are ubiquitous plant steroid hormones, indicated a role of *Bet v* 1 as plant steroid carrier (Markovic-Housley et al. 2003). Other studies demonstrated a much broader binding specificity of *Bet v* 1 toward a variety of biological ligands including fatty acids, flavonoids, and cytokinins (Mogensen et al. 2002). The role of *Bet v* 1 as carrier protein is supported by recent data from Mogensen et al. who demonstrated that the protein can bind to membranes, which might contribute to its role of transferring ligands between cells or tissues (Mogensen et al. 2007). Further, a ribonuclease activity has been reported for a PR-10 protein from hot pepper. Still the biological function of *Bet v* 1 is not fully understood (Park et al. 2004).

Food allergies caused by *Bet v* 1 related proteins are classified as class 2 allergies with *Bet v* 1 acts as sensitizing agent leading to the induction of highly cross-reactive IgE antibodies in atopic individuals. Among the foods most commonly implicated with *Bet v* 1-associated allergies are fruits of the Rosaceae (e.g., apple *Mal d* 1, pear *Pyr c* 1, peach *Pru p* 1, cherry *Pru av* 1, apricot *Pru ar* 1, and strawberry *Fra a* 1) or Fabaceae family (soybean *Gly m* 4, peanut *Ara h* 8, mung bean *Vig r* 1), but also nuts (hazelnut *Cor a* 1.04) and Apiaceae vegetables (celery *Api g* 1, carrot *Dau c* 1) display high levels of cross-reactivity toward the major birch pollen allergen. Most *Bet v* 1-like food allergens are relatively heat-labile and unstable toward digestion, therefore allergic symptoms are usually mild to moderate affecting mainly the oropharynx. However, severe forms of PFS including anaphylaxis have been attributed to the *Bet v* 1 homologue *Gly m* 4 from soybean (Breiteneder and Mills 2005c, Breiteneder and Radauer 2004). Clinically relevant cross-reactivity of *Bet v* 1 with homologous food allergens is not restricted to B-cells but also occurs at the T cell level. Allergens from apple, celery, and hazelnut have been demonstrated to potently activated pollen specific T-cells in primary blood mononuclear cells (PBMCs) from allergic individuals. *In vivo* this can lead to T-cell mediated late-phase cutaneous reactions such as atopic dermatitis following ingestion of food containing *Bet v* 1-related proteins. Moreover, T-cell cross-reactivity has not only been observed with the native food allergens but also with enzymatically degraded or heat-denatured proteins that could still induce T-cell proliferation and therefore provoke late-phase eczematous skin reactions in birch pollen allergic patients. Besides triggering late phase allergic reactions, T-cell activation following ingestion of food allergens could possibly boost pollen-specific T-cells in patients even outside the season and in the absence of IgE mediated reactions. This mechanism could be responsible for the maintenance of elevated *Bet v* 1-specific serum IgE titers throughout the year (Bohle 2007).

### 14.2.13   CLASS I CHITINASES AND THE HEVEIN-LIKE DOMAIN

Chitinases are enzymes that catalyze the hydrolysis of β-1,4-*N*-acetyl-D-glucosamine linkages in chitin polymers, thus playing a role in plant defense against fungal and insect pathogens (Kasprzewska 2003). Class IA/I and IB/II enzymes differ in the presence (IA/I) or absence (IB/II) of an N-terminal hevein-like chitin-binding domain. This domain is thought to be involved in recognition or binding of chitin subunits. Together with class IV chitinases, which also have a hevein domain, they share a homologous catalytic domain and make up the family 19 glycosyl hydrolases. Class III chitinases without, and class V chitinases with two hevein domains share a similar catalytic domain, building up the family 18 glycosyl hydrolases.

Due to the presence of the N-terminal hevein-like domain, class I chitinases, e.g., latex *Hev b* 11 (O'Riordain et al. 2002), and plant food allergens such as avocado *Pers a* 1 and chestnut *Cas s* 5 cross-react with the major latex allergen hevein (Karisola et al. 2005, Posch et al. 1997). Further, there are hints that class I chitinases from cherimoya, passion fruit, kiwi, papaya, mango, and tomato display IgE cross-reactivity with hevein (Diaz-Perales et al. 1999), although the catalytic domains of these allergens showed comparably low IgE binding activities (Diaz-Perales et al. 2003). As the hevein domain comprises most of the molecule's allergenicity, two more allergens should be mentioned although displaying no chitinase activity, i.e., *Bra r* 2 (turnip rape) with a prohevein-like domain composition (Hanninen et al. 1999) and the wheat germ agglutinin *Tri a* 18, a lectin, consisting of four hevein-like domains. In summary, most of the allergenicity of chitinases seems to be proceeded by the hevein-like domain. Due to their potentially high cross-reactivity these allergens are considered to play a role in the latex-fruit-syndrome.

## 14.2.14 Papain-Like Cysteine Proteases

Members of the papain family are widespread in nature and are cysteine proteases synthesized as inactive proenzymes with N-terminal pro-peptide regions. The pro-peptide plays an important role as inhibitor of enzymatic activity and for the correct folding of the newly synthesized protein. Mature enzymes are generally 25–28 kDa proteins (Coulombe et al. 1996). So far, a number of allergens belonging to the papain family have been identified including inhalant allergens such as the major dust mite allergen *Der p* 1 and also plant food allergens such as *Ana c* 2 bromelain from pineapple, *Act d* 1 actinidin, the major allergen from kiwi fruit, and *Car p* 1 papain from papaya (Mills et al. 2004). *Gly m* 1, a major allergen from soybean seed storage vacuoles shows sequence similarities to papain-like proteases but lacks enzymatic activity.

## 14.2.15 Thaumatin-Like Proteins

The family of thaumatin-like proteins (TLPs), also designated PR-5, can be classified into three groups: those produced in response to pathogen infection, in response to osmotic stress (osmotins), and antifungal proteins present in cereals (Breiteneder and Ebner 2000). The majority of TLPs has a molecular mass of about 20 kDa, consists mainly of antiparallel β-sheets, and is stabilized by eight disulfide bonds. TLPs are generally resistant to proteolytic degradation and pH- or heat-induced denaturation (Breiteneder 2004).

Among other allergen sources, allergenic TLPs can be found in several fruits such as apple *Mal d* 2, cherry *Pru av* 2, bell pepper *Cap a* 1, and kiwi *Act d* 2, as well as in orange and grape.

## 14.2.16 Oleosins

Oleosins are hydrophobic plant proteins found only in association with small storage oil drops. These oil bodies are discrete spherical organelles, mainly composed of triacylglycerols and are surrounded by a phospholipids/oleosin annulus. Several oleosins were lately described, confirming that all of them comprise three distinct domains: a conserved hydrophobic domain of about 70 amino acid residues being particularly rich in aliphatic amino acids flanked by an N- and a C-terminal domain, which are more hydrophilic with less conserved amino acid sequences. Allergenic oleosins were identified in sesame (*Ses i* 4 and *Ses i* 5), nuts (peanut and hazelnut oleosins), legumes, and seeds (Capuano et al. 2007, Leduc et al. 2006).

## 14.2.17 Kunitz-Type Protease Inhibitors

Protease inhibitors displaying a Kunitz-type domain protect plants against insect attacks, inhibiting enzymes of the digestive system, like trypsin. The Kunitz-type soybean trypsin inhibitor (STI) family consists mainly of protease inhibitors from legume seeds. They are expressed in different seeds (Deshimaru et al. 2002, Pando et al. 2001, Shee and Sharma 2007), and together with interleukin-1, heparin-binding growth factor, and histactophilin, they belong to the β-trefoil superfamily. All members of this family show very similar structures, but do not share sequence similarities with the STI family. Regarding allergenicity, the most prominent member of this group is the soybean trypsin inhibitor. Although only 20% of soybean allergic patients react with this soybean allergen, food-induced anaphylactic shocks have been reported (Burks et al. 1994, Moroz and Yang 1980). In addition to its presence in soy, the soybean trypsin inhibitor is also found as a contaminant in lecithin (Gu et al. 2001), which is widely used as emulgating agent and represents a potential risk for allergic patients. Furthermore, the soybean trypsin inhibitor is considered highly resistant to thermal and chemical denaturation (Roychaudhuri et al. 2004). Allergenic Kunitz-type protease-inhibitors have also been identified in potato, i.e., the cathepsin inhibitor *Sola t* 2, the cystein protease inhibitor *Sola t* 3, and the serine protease inhibitor *Sola t* 4. In enzyme-linked immunosorbent assays (ELISA), 51% of atopic children showed specific IgE to *Sola t* 2%, 43%, to 58% to different *Sola t* 3 isoforms, and 67% to *Sola t* 4, respectively.

### 14.2.18 THIOREDOXINS

Thioredoxins are small ubiquitous enzymes present in many species from Archaebacteria to man. They serve as general protein disulfide oxido-reductases interacting with a broad range of proteins. Allergenic thioredoxins have been identified in fungi as well as in plants. The thioredoxins from wheat (*Tri a* 25) and maize (*Zea m* 25) are related to baker's asthma, an occupational disease affecting 4%–10% of bakery workers in European countries (Holmgren 1995).

### 14.2.19 β-AMYLASES

β-Amylases are enzymes belonging to the group of exoamylases, which hydrolyze 1,4-α glucosidic linkages in starch-type polysaccharide substrates. These enzymes are found in a large variety of microorganisms as well as in plants where they can provoke allergic reactions as demonstrated for the barley allergen *Hor v* 17 (Horvathova et al. 2001, van der Maarel et al. 2002).

### 14.2.20 CYSTATINS

Cystatins belong to the cystatin superfamily of reversibly binding cysteine protease inhibitors, which can be subdivided into three animal and one plant cystatin family (Abrahamson 1994). Most phytocystatins are 12–14 kDa in size, contain no disulfide bonds, and show significant amino acid sequence similarity to the cystatin families of animal origin (Nagata et al. 2000). Plant seed cystatins are now understood as factors controlling germination by inhibition of endogenous cysteine proteinases. (Martinez et al. 2005). Oryzacystatin from rice seeds was identified as the first well-defined cystatin of plant origin (Abe et al. 1987). Although many cloning approaches led to the identification of various plant cytstatins including those of strawberry, sunflower, wheat, barley, corn, and soybean, phytocystatins eliciting allergic reactions were so far only found in kiwifruit (*Act d* 4), golden kiwi, and in the pollen of short ragweed (*Ambrosia artemisiifolia*) (Rogers et al. 1993).

## 14.2.21  EXPANSINS

Kiwellin (*Act d* 5) is a 28 kD allergen from kiwi fruits (*Actinidia chinensis*) related to ripening-related proteins from grape, potato, and rice. Comparative analysis of the hypothetical tertiary structure of kiwellin showed fold similarities with the major grass pollen allergen *Phl p* 1 (Ball et al. 2005), a cysteine-rich glycoprotein representing one of the most important aeroallergens known to date. Similarities were also found with Barwin-like proteins sharing a structural motif with various wound-induced and other pathogenesis-related proteins from potato, rubber trees, and tobacco (Tamburrini et al. 2005).

## 14.2.22  GLYCOSIDE HYDROLASES

Glycoside hydrolases are a widespread group of enzymes that hydrolyze glycosidic bonds. Based on sequence similarities the superfamily was classified into 85 subfamilies. The glycoprotein *Lyc e* 2, a fructofuranosidase from tomato, belongs to the glycoside hydrolase family 32 and represents a major allergen of tomato recognized by more than 50% of tomato allergic individuals. However, one-third of the sera from tomato allergic patients show glycan-specific antibodies leading to the speculation that the glycans of *Lyc e* 2 might contribute to its IgE binding properties (Kondo et al. 2001). The protein is highly concentrated in the red ripening stage of the fruit. If ripening is inhibited like in the ripening inhibitor mutant tomato, the accumulation of β-fructofuranosidase and consequently the serum IgE reactivity to the extract is reduced (Kitagawa et al. 2006). There are no reports of β-fructofuranosidases of other species that elicit allergy so far, though serum IgE cross-reactivity to molecules with similar carbohydrate moieties cannot be excluded.

Within the glycoside hydrolase subfamily 18, an additional plant food allergen has been identified, namely, *Ziz m* 1 from Chinese date, which belongs to the class III chitinases (Lee et al. 2006).

## 14.2.23  ISOFLAVONE REDUCTASES

Isovlavone reductases (IFR) belong to the nicotinamide adenine dinucleotide phosphate (NADP)-dependent oxidoreductases that are involved in plant secondary metabolism (Stammers et al. 2001). Allergens from this family include the minor birch pollen allergen *Bet v* 6, which has been demonstrated to cross-react with IFR from pear (*Pyr c* 5), lychee, and sharon fruit (Bolhaar et al. 2005, Karamloo et al. 1999, 2001). Additionally, *Bet v* 6-specific serum IgE recognized bands at the corresponding size in apple, mango, banana, and carrot extracts (Vieths et al. 1998). There are also reports on immunoreactive IFRs of orange and latex. Although these allergens are not considered as major allergens, IFRs can be classified as panallergens with members in pollen, fruits, and latex.

## 14.2.24  SUBTILISIN-LIKE SERINE PROTEASES

Subtilases comprise the second largest family of serine proteases characterized to date with members in Archaebacteria, eukaryotes, and even viruses. Surprisingly, the catalytic domains of subtilases display a high degree of sequence variability with exception of three catalytic residues (Asp-His-Ser). Apart from that, the structures show no further similarities (Siezen and Leunissen 1997).

Most allergens from this family are fungal allergens belonging to the subfamilies of alkaline or vacuolar serine proteases (Shen et al. 1999). So far, the only plant food allergen belonging to this family is *Cuc m* 1 (cucumisin) from muskmelon. Although homologues of cucumisin are reported in other plants like soybean, tomato, latex, rice, barley, etc. allergenicity and cross-reactivity require further proof.

### 14.2.25 BERBERINE BRIDGE ENZYMES

Berberine bridge enzyme (BBE) and berberine bridge-like enzymes are involved in the biosynthesis of numerous isoquinoline alkaloids. These flavoproteins catalyze the transformation of the N-methyl group of (S)-reticuline into the C-8 berberine bridge carbon of (S)-scoulerine (Facchini et al. 1996). The first allergen belonging to this family was found in Bermuda grass pollen. *Phl p* 4 from timothy grass also shows homology to BBEs (Dewitt et al. 2006), similar as *Api g* 5 from celery tuber, and a high MW allergen from *Brassica napus* pollen. All these allergens are glycoproteins and seem to bind human IgE if not exclusively, then prominently via their N-linked glycan moieties. For example, recombinant *Phl p* 4 produced in *Escherichia coli* displays a significantly lower IgE binding capacity compared to the natural, glycosylated allergen (Dewitt et al. 2006). *Api g* 5, the so far only known food allergen within this group, is considered to be involved in the celery–mugwort–spice syndrome. Carbohydrate analysis of the allergen revealed the presence of glycans carrying fucosyl and xylosyl residues, structures previously shown to bind IgE (Aalberse et al. 1981, Aalberse and van Ree 1997, van Ree 2002a).

### 14.2.26 CHLOROPHYLL BINDING PROTEINS

Celery *Api g* 3 isolated from a cDNA library with celery allergic patients' sera was identified as chlorophyll A/B binding protein. Chlorophylls A and B and chlorophyll A/B-binding proteins constitute the light-harvesting complex (LHC) of photosynthetic organisms. The LHC functions as light receptor capturing and delivering excitation energy to plant photosystems I and II. However, studies on the immunological characterization of *Api g* 3 still need to be performed (Bohle and Vieths 2004).

### 14.2.27 PATATIN FAMILY

The patatin family consists of various glycoproteins in plants making up more than 40% of the total soluble protein in potato tubers. Patatins serve as storage proteins and it has been demonstrated that they exhibit both lipid acyl hydrolase and acetyl transferase activities, which might be involved in tissue wounding responses. Further, recent studies report on antioxidant activities of the major potato allergen *Sola t* 1 (Seppala et al. 2000).

Moreover, potato patatin is homologous and cross-reacts with the major latex allergen *Hev b* 7. This could be one explanation for the association of potatoes with the latex-fruit syndrome.

## 14.2.28  CONCLUDING REMARKS

To date, around 9000 different protein families are defined within the protein database Pfam (http://www.sanger.ac.uk/Software/Pfam/which), which covers most of the known protein sequences. The 122 plant-derived food allergens included in the official IUIS allergen list can be assigned to only 22 of these protein families containing more or less members, though the growing knowledge about allergenic molecules will lead to the discovery of new allergens belonging to additional protein families. The muskmelon allergen *Cuc m* 3, for instance, is the only plant food allergen within the PR-1 family, which comprises many pollen allergens, thus delivering the first evidence of the involvement of this plant allergen family in food allergy (Asensio et al. 2004). In addition, the food allergen *Len c* 2 has been identified as seed-specific biotinylated protein in lentil and the almond allergen *Pru du* 5 as 60S acidic ribosomal protein. A novel kiwi allergen termed *Act d* 3 has been included in the official IUIS allergen list. So far, *Act d* 3 could not be assigned to a plant food allergen family.

The classification of plant food allergens into protein families based on biochemical and structural similarities will provide a new outlook on the molecules and might contribute to answer the question about allergenicity of different proteins. This will help to define clinically relevant allergenic molecules and explain cross-reactive phenomena between single food allergen sources as well as between food allergens and allergenic molecules of other origins (e.g., pollen).

## REFERENCES

Aalberse, R.C. 2000. Structural biology of allergens. *J Allergy Clin Immunol* 106: 228–238.

Aalberse, R.C., Koshte, V., and Clemens, J.G. 1981. Immunoglobulin E antibodies that cross-react with vegetable foods, pollen, and *Hymenoptera venom*. *J Allergy Clin Immunol* 68: 356–364.

Aalberse, R.C. and van Ree, R. 1997. Crossreactive carbohydrate determinants. *Clin Rev Allergy Immunol* 15: 375–387.

Abe, K., Emori, Y., Kondo, H., Suzuki, K., and Arai, S. 1987. Molecular cloning of a cysteine proteinase inhibitor of rice (oryzacystatin). Homology with animal cystatins and transient expression in the ripening process of rice seeds. *J Biol Chem* 262: 16793–16797.

Abrahamson, M. 1994. Cystatins. *Methods Enzymol* 244: 685–700.

Altenbach, S.B., Kuo, C.C., Staraci, L.C. et al. 1992. Accumulation of a Brazil nut albumin in seeds of transgenic canola results in enhanced levels of seed protein methionine. *Plant Mol Biol* 18: 235–245.

Asensio, T., Crespo, J.F., Sanchez-Monge, R. et al. 2004. Novel plant pathogenesis-related protein family involved in food allergy. *J Allergy Clin Immunol* 114: 896–899.

Asero, R., Mistrello, G., Roncarolo, D. et al. 2000. Lipid transfer protein: A pan-allergen in plant-derived foods that is highly resistant to pepsin digestion. *Int Arch Allergy Immunol* 122: 20–32.

Asero, R., Mistrello, G., Roncarolo, D. et al. 2003. Detection of clinical markers of sensitization to profilin in patients allergic to plant foods. *J Allergy Clin Immunol* 112: 427–432.

Ball, T., Edstrom, W., Mauch, L. et al. 2005. Gain of structure and IgE epitopes by eukaryotic expression of the major Timothy grass pollen allergen, Phl p 1. *FEBS J* 272: 217–227.

Ballmer-Weber, B.K., Vieths, S., Luttkopf, D. et al. 2000. Celery allergy confirmed by double-blind, placebo-controlled food challenge: A clinical study in 32 subjects with a history of adverse reactions to celery root. *J Allergy Clin Immunol* 106: 373–378.

Bohle, B. 2007. The impact of pollen-related food allergens on pollen allergy. *Allergy* 62: 3–10.

Bohle, B. and Vieths, S. 2004. Improving diagnostic tests for food allergy with recombinant allergens. *Methods* 32: 292–299.

Bolhaar, S.T., van Ree, R., Ma, Y. et al. 2005. Severe allergy to sharon fruit caused by birch pollen. *Int Arch Allergy Immunol* 136: 45–52.

Breiteneder, H. 2004. Thaumatin-like proteins—a new family of pollen and fruit allergens. *Allergy* 59: 479–481.

Breiteneder, H. and Ebner, C. 2000. Molecular and biochemical classification of plant-derived food allergens. *J Allergy Clin Immunol* 106: 27–36.

Breiteneder, H. and Ebner, C. 2001. Atopic allergens of plant foods. *Curr Opin Allergy Clin Immunol* 1: 261–267.

Breiteneder, H. and Mills, C. 2005a. Nonspecific lipid-transfer proteins in plant foods and pollens: An important allergen class. *Curr Opin Allergy Clin Immunol* 5: 275–279.

Breiteneder, H. and Mills, C. 2005b. Plant food allergens—structural and functional aspects of allergenicity. *Biotechnol Adv* 23: 395–399.

Breiteneder, H. and Mills, E.N. 2005c. Molecular properties of food allergens. *J Allergy Clin Immunol* 115: 14–23.

Breiteneder, H. and Radauer, C. 2004. A classification of plant food allergens. *J Allergy Clin Immunol* 113: 821–830.

Burks, A.W., Cockrell, G., Connaughton, C. et al. 1994. Identification of peanut agglutinin and soybean trypsin inhibitor as minor legume allergens. *Int Arch Allergy Immunol* 105: 143–149.

Capuano, F., Beaudoin, F., Napier, J.A. et al. 2007. Properties and exploitation of oleosins. *Biotechnol Adv* 25: 203–206.

Coulombe, R., Li, Y., Takebe, S. et al. 1996. Crystallization and preliminary X-ray diffraction studies of human procathepsin L. *Proteins* 25: 398–400.

Deshimaru, M., Hanamoto, R., Kusano, C. et al. 2002. Purification and characterization of proteinase inhibitors from wild soja (*Glycine soja*) seeds. *Biosci Biotechnol Biochem* 66: 1897–1903.

Dewitt, A.M., Andersson, K., Peltre, G., and Lidholm, J. 2006. Cloning, expression and immunological characterization of full-length timothy grass pollen allergen Phl p 4, a berberine bridge enzyme-like protein with homology to celery allergen Api g 5. *Clin Exp Allergy* 36: 77–86.

Diaz-Perales, A., Blanco, C., Sanchez-Monge, R. et al. 2003. Analysis of avocado allergen (Prs a 1) IgE-binding peptides generated by simulated gastric fluid digestion. *J Allergy Clin Immunol* 112: 1002–1007.

Diaz-Perales, A., Collada, C., Blanco, C. et al. 1999. Cross-reactions in the latex-fruit syndrome: A relevant role of chitinases but not of complex asparagine-linked glycans. *J Allergy Clin Immunol* 104: 681–687.

Dunwell, J.M., Purvis, A., and Khuri, S. 2004. Cupins: The most functionally diverse protein superfamily? *Phytochemistry* 65: 7–17.

Ebner, C., Birkner, T., Valenta, R. et al. 1991. Common epitopes of birch pollen and apples—studies by Western and Northern blot. *J Allergy Clin Immunol* 88: 588–594.

Egger, M., Mutschlechner, S., Wopfner, N. et al. 2006. Pollen-food syndromes associated with weed pollinosis: An update from the molecular point of view. *Allergy* 61: 461–476.

Facchini, P.J., Penzes, C., Johnson, A.G., and Bull, D. 1996. Molecular characterization of berberine bridge enzyme genes from opium poppy. *Plant Physiol* 112: 1669–1677.

Fah, J., Wuthrich, B., and Vieths, S. 1995. Anaphylactic reaction to lychee fruit: Evidence for sensitization to profilin. *Clin Exp Allergy* 25: 1018–1023.

Fernandez-Rivas, M., Gonzalez-Mancebo, E., Rodriguez-Perez, R. et al. 2003. Clinically relevant peach allergy is related to peach lipid transfer protein, Pru p 3, in the Spanish population. *J Allergy Clin Immunol* 112: 789–795.

Gajhede, M., Osmark, P., Poulsen, F.M. et al. 1996. X-ray and NMR structure of Bet v 1, the origin of birch pollen allergy. *Nat Struct Biol* 3: 1040–1045.

Garcia-Selles, F.J., Diaz-Perales, A., Sanchez-Monge, R. et al. 2002. Patterns of reactivity to lipid transfer proteins of plant foods and Artemisia pollen: An in vivo study. *Int Arch Allergy Immunol* 128: 115–122.

Gu, X., Beardslee, T., Zeece, M.J. et al. 2001. Identification of IgE-binding proteins in soy lecithin. *Int Arch Allergy Immunol* 126: 218–225.

Hanninen, A.R., Mikkola, J.H., Kalkkinen, N. et al. 1999. Increased allergen production in turnip (*Brassica rapa*) by treatments activating defense mechanisms. *J Allergy Clin Immunol* 104: 194–201.

Hoffmann-Sommergruber, K. 2002. Pathogenesis-related (PR)-proteins identified as allergens. *Biochem Soc Trans* 30: 930–935.

Holmgren, A. 1995. Thioredoxin structure and mechanism: Conformational changes on oxidation of the active-site sulfhydryls to a disulfide. *Structure* 3: 239–243.

Horvathova, V., Janecek, S., and Sturdik, E. 2001. Amylolytic enzymes: Molecular aspects of their properties. *Gen Physiol Biophys* 20: 7–32.

Jankiewicz, A., Aulepp, H., Baltes, W. et al. 1996. Allergic sensitization to native and heated celery root in pollen-sensitive patients investigated by skin test and IgE binding. *Int Arch Allergy Immunol* 111: 268–278.

Karamloo, F., Schmitz, N., Scheurer, S. et al. 1999. Molecular cloning and characterization of a birch pollen minor allergen, Bet v 5, belonging to a family of isoflavone reductase-related proteins. *J Allergy Clin Immunol* 104: 991–999.

Karamloo, F., Wangorsch, A., Kasahara, H. et al. 2001. Phenylcoumaran benzylic ether and isoflavonoid reductases are a new class of cross-reactive allergens in birch pollen, fruits and vegetables. *Eur J Biochem* 268: 5310–5320.

Karisola, P., Kotovuori, A., Poikonen, S. et al. 2005. Isolated hevein-like domains, but not 31-kd endochitinases, are responsible for IgE-mediated in vitro and in vivo reactions in latex-fruit syndrome. *J Allergy Clin Immunol* 115: 598–605.

Kasprzewska, A. 2003. Plant chitinases—regulation and function. *Cell Mol Biol Lett* 8: 809–824.

Kitagawa, M., Moriyama, T., Ito, H. et al. 2006. Reduction of allergenic proteins by the effect of the ripening inhibitor (rin) mutant gene in an F1 hybrid of the rin mutant tomato. *Biosci Biotechnol Biochem* 70: 1227–1233.

Kondo, Y., Urisu, A., and Tokuda, R. 2001. Identification and characterization of the allergens in the tomato fruit by immunoblotting. *Int Arch Allergy Immunol* 126: 294–299.

Kreis, M., Forde, B.G., Rahman, S. et al. 1985. Molecular evolution of the seed storage proteins of barley, rye and wheat. *J Mol Biol* 183: 499–502.

Leduc, V., Moneret-Vautrin, D.A., Tzen, J.T. et al. 2006. Identification of oleosins as major allergens in sesame seed allergic patients. *Allergy* 61: 349–356.

Lee, M.F., Hwang, G.Y., Chen, Y.H., Lin, H.C., and Wu, C.H. 2006. Molecular cloning of Indian jujube (*Zizyphus mauritiana*) allergen Ziz m 1 with sequence similarity to plant class III chitinases. *Mol Immunol* 43: 1144–1151.

Liscombe, D.K., MacLeod, B.P., Loukanina, N. et al. 2005. Evidence for the monophyletic evolution of benzylisoquinoline alkaloid biosynthesis in angiosperms. *Phytochemistry* 66: 2501–2520.

Lombardero, M., Garcia-Selles, F.J., Polo, F. et al. 2004. Prevalence of sensitization to Artemisia allergens Art v 1, Art v 3 and Art v 60kDa. Cross-reactivity among Art v 3 and other relevant lipid-transfer protein allergens. *Clin Exp Allergy* 34: 1415–1421.

Markovic-Housley, Z., Degano, M., Lamba, D. et al. 2003. Crystal structure of a hypoallergenic isoform of the major birch pollen allergen Bet v 1 and its likely biological function as a plant steroid carrier. *J Mol Biol* 325: 123–133.

Martinez, M., Abraham, Z., Gambardella, M. et al. 2005. The strawberry gene Cyf1 encodes a phytocyotatin with antifungal properties. *J Exp Bot* 56: 1821–189.

Mills, E.N., Jenkins, J.A., Alcocer, M.J. et al. 2004. Structural, biological, and evolutionary relationships of plant food allergens sensitizing via the gastrointestinal tract. *Crit Rev Food Sci Nutr* 44: 379–407.

Mogensen, J.E., Ferreras, M., Wimmer, R. et al. 2007. The major allergen from birch tree pollen, Bet v 1, binds and permeabilizes membranes. *Biochemistry* 46: 3356–3365.

Mogensen, J.E., Wimmer, R., Larsen, J.N. et al. 2002. The major birch allergen, Bet v 1, shows affinity for a broad spectrum of physiological ligands. *J Biol Chem* 277: 23684–23692.

Monsalve, R.I., Gonzalez de la Pena, M.A., Lopez-Otin, C. et al. 1997. Detection, isolation and complete amino acid sequence of an aeroallergenic protein from rapeseed flour. *Clin Exp Allergy* 27: 833–841.

Moroz, L.A. and Yang, W.H. 1980. Kunitz soybean trypsin inhibitor: A specific allergen in food anaphylaxis. *N Engl J Med* 302: 1126–1128.

Murtagh, G.J., Dumoulin, M., Archer, D.B. et al. 2002. Stability of recombinant 2 S albumin allergens in vitro. *Biochem Soc Trans* 30: 913–915.

Nagata, K., Kudo, N., Abe, K., Arai, S., and Tanokura, M. 2000. Three-dimensional solution structure of oryzacystatin-I, a cysteine proteinase inhibitor of the rice, *Oryza sativa* L. japonica. *Biochemistry* 39: 14753–14760.

Neudecker, P., Schweimer, K., Nerkamp, J. et al. 2001. Allergic cross-reactivity made visible: Solution structure of the major cherry allergen Pru av 1. *J Biol Chem* 276: 22756–22763.

O'Riordain, G., Radauer, C., Hoffmann-Sommergruber, K. et al. 2002. Cloning and molecular characterization of the *Hevea brasiliensis* allergen Hev b 11, a class I chitinase. *Clin Exp Allergy* 32: 455–462.

Pando, S.C., Oliva, M.L., Sampaio, C.A. et al. 2001. Primary sequence determination of a Kunitz inhibitor isolated from *Delonix regia* seeds. *Phytochemistry* 57: 625–631.

Pantoja-Uceda, D., Bruix, M., Santoro, J. et al. 2002. Solution structure of allergenic 2 S albumins. *Biochem Soc Trans* 30: 919–924.

Park, C.J., Kim, K.J., Shin, R. et al. 2004. Pathogenesis-related protein 10 isolated from hot pepper functions as a ribonuclease in an antiviral pathway. *Plant J* 37: 186–198.

Pastorello, E.A., Farioli, L., Pravettoni, V. et al. 1998. Sensitization to the major allergen of Brazil nut is correlated with the clinical expression of allergy. *J Allergy Clin Immunol* 102: 1021–1027.

Pastorello, E.A., Pompei, C., Pravettoni, V. et al. 2001. Lipid transfer proteins and 2S albumins as allergens. *Allergy* 56(Suppl. 67): 45–47.

Pastorello, E.A., Pravettoni, V., Farioli, L. et al. 2002. Hypersensitivity to mugwort (*Artemisia vulgaris*) in patients with peach allergy is due to a common lipid transfer protein allergen and is often without clinical expression. *J Allergy Clin Immunol* 110: 310–317.

Posch, A., Chen, Z., Wheeler, C. et al. 1997. Characterization and identification of latex allergens by two-dimensional electrophoresis and protein microsequencing. *J Allergy Clin Immunol* 99: 385–395.

Ramachandran, S., Christensen, H.E., Ishimaru, Y. et al. 2000. Profilin plays a role in cell elongation, cell shape maintenance, and flowering in Arabidopsis. *Plant Physiol* 124: 1637–1647.

Rodriguez-Perez, R., Crespo, J.F., Rodriguez, J. et al. 2003. Profilin is a relevant melon allergen susceptible to pepsin digestion in patients with oral allergy syndrome. *J Allergy Clin Immunol* 111: 634–639.

Rogers, B.L., Pollock, J., Klapper, D.G., and Griffith, I.J. 1993. Sequence of the proteinase-inhibitor cystatin homologue from the pollen of *Ambrosia artemisiifolia* (short ragweed). *Gene* 133: 219–221.

Roychaudhuri, R., Sarath, G., Zeece, M., and Markwell, J. 2004. Stability of the allergenic soybean Kunitz trypsin inhibitor. *Biochim Biophys Acta* 1699: 207–212.

Salcedo, G., Sanchez-Monge, R., Diaz-Perales, A. et al. 2004. Plant non-specific lipid transfer proteins as food and pollen allergens. *Clin Exp Allergy* 34: 1336–1341.

Sankian, M., Varasteh, A., Pazouki, N. et al. 2005. Sequence homology: A poor predictive value for profilins cross-reactivity. *Clin Mol Allergy* 3: 13.

Scheurer, S., Son, D.Y., Boehm, M. et al. 1999. Cross-reactivity and epitope analysis of Pru a 1, the major cherry allergen. *Mol Immunol* 36: 155–167.

Schirmer, T., Hoffimann-Sommergrube, K., Susani, M. et al. 2005. Crystal structure of the major celery allergen Api g 1: Molecular analysis of cross-reactivity. *J Mol Biol* 351: 1101–1109.

Seppala, U., Palosuo, T., Seppala, U. et al. 2000. IgE reactivity to patatin-like latex allergen, Hev b 7, and to patatin of potato tuber, Sol t 1, in adults and children allergic to natural rubber latex. *Allergy* 55: 266–273.

Shee, C. and Sharma, A.K. 2007. Purification and characterization of a trypsin inhibitor from seeds of *Murraya koenigii*. *J Enzyme Inhib Med Chem* 22: 115–120.

Shen, H.D., Tam, M.F., Chou, H., and Han, S.H. 1999. The importance of serine proteinases as aeroallergens associated with asthma. *Int Arch Allergy Immunol* 119: 259–264.

Shewry, P.R., Napier, J.A., and Tatham, A.S. 1995. Seed storage proteins: Structures and biosynthesis. *Plant Cell* 7: 945–956.

Shewry, P.R., Beaudoin, F., Jenkins, J. et al. 2002. Plant protein families and their relationships to food allergy. *Biochem Soc Trans* 30: 906–910.

Sicherer, S.H. 2001. Clinical implications of cross-reactive food allergens. *J Allergy Clin Immunol* 108: 881–890.

Siezen, R.J. and Leunissen, J.A. 1997. Subtilases: The superfamily of subtilisin-like serine proteases. *Protein Sci* 6: 501–523.

Stammers, D.K., Ren, J., Leslie, K. et al. 2001. The structure of the negative transcriptional regulator NmrA reveals a structural superfamily which includes the short-chain dehydrogenase/reductases. *Embo J* 20: 6619–6626.

Tamburrini, M., Cerasuolo, I., Carratore, V. et al. 2005. Kiwellin, a novel protein from kiwi fruit. Purification, biochemical characterization and identification as an allergen[*]. *Protein J* 24: 423–429.

Terras, F.R., Schoofs, H.M., De Bolle, M.F. et al. 1992. Analysis of two novel classes of plant antifungal proteins from radish (*Raphanus sativus* L.) seeds. *J Biol Chem* 267: 15301–15309.

Valenta, R., Duchene, M., Ebner, C. et al. 1992. Profilins constitute a novel family of functional plant pan-allergens. *J Exp Med* 175: 377–385.

Valenta, R., Duchene, M., Pettenburger, K. et al. 1991. Identification of profilin as a novel pollen allergen: IgE autoreactivity in sensitized individuals. *Science* 253: 557–560.

Valster, A.H., Pierson, E.S., Valenta, R. et al. 1997. Probing the plant actin cytoskeleton during cytokinesis and interphase by profilin microinjection. *Plant Cell* 9: 1815–1824.

van der Maarel, M.J., van der Veen, B., Uitdehaag, J.C. et al. 2002. Properties and applications of starch-converting enzymes of the alpha-amylase family. *J Biotechnol* 94: 137–155.

van Loon, L. and van Strien, E. 1999. The families of pathogenesis-related proteins, their activities, and comparative analysis of PR-1 type proteins. *Physiol Mol Plant Pathol* 55: 85–97.

van Ree, R. 2002a. Carbohydrate epitopes and their relevance for the diagnosis and treatment of allergic diseases. *Int Arch Allergy Immunol* 129: 189–197.

van Ree, R. 2002b. Clinical importance of non-specific lipid transfer proteins as food allergens. *Biochem Soc Trans* 30: 910–913.

van Ree, R., Fernandez-Rivas, M., Cuevas, M. et al. 1995. Pollen-related allergy to peach and apple: An important role for profilin. *J Allergy Clin Immunol* 95: 726–734.

Vassilopoulou, E., Zuidmeer, L., Akkerdaas, J. et al. 2007. Severe immediate allergic reactions to grapes: Part of a lipid transfer protein-associated clinical syndrome. *Int Arch Allergy Immunol* 143: 92–102.

Vieths, S., Frank, E., Scheurer, S. et al. 1998. D. Characterization of a new IgE binding 35-kDa protein from birch pollen with cross-reacting homologues in various plant foods. *Scand J Immunol* 47: 263–272.

Willerroider, M., Fuchs, H., Ballmer-Weber, B.K. et al. 2003. Cloning and molecular and immunological characterisation of two new food allergens, Cap a 2 and Lyc e 1, profilins from bell pepper (*Capsicum annuum*) and Tomato (*Lycopersicon esculentum*). *Int Arch Allergy Immunol* 131: 245–255.

Witke, W. 2004. The role of profilin complexes in cell motility and other cellular processes. *Trends Cell Biol* 14: 461–469.

Wopfner, N., Gadermaier, G., Egger, M. et al. 2005. The spectrum of allergens in ragweed and mugwort pollen. *Int Arch Allergy Immunol* 138: 337–346.

Yagami, T. 2002. Allergies to cross-reactive plant proteins. Latex-fruit syndrome is comparable with pollen-food allergy syndrome. *Int Arch Allergy Immunol* 128: 271–279.

## 14.3   OTHER INGESTED ANIMAL ALLERGENS: FROM FROGS TO INSECTS

Andreas Lopata

### 14.3.1   CHARACTERISTICS OF ADDITIONAL ALLERGENS CAUSING ALLERGIC REACTION AFTER INGESTION

It has been estimated that around 1%–2% of the population, and up to 8% of children suffer from some type of IgE-mediated food allergy. About eight types of foods are responsible for causing the majority of food allergies, including a number of foods of plant origin together with allergens of animal origin including cow's milk, egg, fish, and shellfish. Animal food allergens can be classified into three main families—the caseins (milk), the tropomyosins, and the EF-hand (Ca-binding) proteins (Jenkins et al. 2007). The latter two allergens are the major allergens found in crustacean and fish, respectively (Lehrer et al. 2003, Lopata and Potter 2000). The evolutionary relationships of each of these allergen superfamilies show that in general, proteins with a sequence identity to a human homolog above approximately 62% are rarely allergenic. These molecular observations are sustained by clinical cross-reactivity observations which are discussed in the following text.

### 14.3.2   MARINE ORGANISMS (EXCLUDING DECAPOD CRUSTACEAN, MOLLUSK, AND FISH)

Edible marine organisms are consumed around the world. More "exotic" creatures such as sea cucumber, jellyfish, sea urchins, and abalone are widely consumed in Asia and have more recently been introduced into the international cuisine.

*Sea urchins* are increasingly used as culinary products in Japanese and Korean cuisine. Two recent reports identified consumers with anaphylactic reactions after ingestion of sea urchin roe. Skin prick testing and ImmunoCAP analysis to fish, mollusks, and crustacean was negative, but positive by SPT to fresh sea urchin roe (Hickey 2007). Subsequently, Rodriguez et al. (2007) demonstrated that the major allergen is heat stable (by oral mucosa testing) and has a MW of approximately 118 kDa by immunoblotting.

Allergic reactions to seafood can also be caused by contaminants that induce sensitization. Anisakis (also called cod worm or herring worm) is a seafood-borne parasite that can cause not only infections (anisakiasis) but also allergic reactions in sensitized consumers. Whereas adult worms of Anisakis sp parasitize sea mammals, larval stages must pass through several intermediate hosts. Infectious stage larvae (L3) found within fish or cephalopods may be accidentally ingested (Audicana and Kennedy 2008). If ingested live, as a result of consumption of raw or undercooked fish, Anisakis L3 larvae can cause the zoonotic disease known as anisakiasis. This is usually an acute and transient infection, with the worm dying within a few weeks. Within hours of being ingested, Anisakis L3 penetrate the mucosal layers of the gastrointestinal tract, causing direct tissue damage that may lead to abdominal pain, nausea, and/or diarrhea. Importantly, some people develop an IgE-mediated "gastroallergic anisakiasis," which presents with clinical manifestations ranging from urticaria to life-threatening anaphylactic shock. This places gastroallergic anisakiasis on the borderline between parasitic infection and allergy (Audicana et al. 2002). Due to the heterogeneous clinical reactions and unawareness of this allergen source in seafood, allergic reactions to Anisakis are often misdiagnosed and mistaken for other diseases such as acute urticaria or fish allergy (Kasuya et al. 1990).

However, development of better diagnostic tools has resulted in an increase in the frequency of reports in many parts of the world including the United States, Canada, Europe, and Japan. In a randomized study among almost 5 million Japanese, a higher prevalence of sensitization was found to Anisakis than to seafood. Moreover, a Spanish study found that Anisakis as a hidden food allergen was the leading cause of food allergy in Spain. A recently developed murine model could demonstrate that occupational sensitization to Anisakis (Jeebhay et al. 2001) can be caused not only by previous infection with the live worm, but that exposure to allergenic proteins via ingestion or inhalation alone can cause sensitization (Nieuwenhuizen et al. 2006).

The current international regulations on food fish and products require the visual examination of the fish for visible parasites, and freezing at −35°C for >15 h prior marination. While this treatment will protect the consumer getting Anisakiasis, sensitization to Anisakis allergens is still possible. Recent studies showed that several Anisakis allergens are highly resistant to heat and pepsin treatment (Caballero and Moneo 2004). The high stability of these allergens was recently demonstrated by the detection of Anisakis allergens in the meat of chickens which were fed with fish meal, most probably containing Anisakis allergens (Armentia et al. 2006). Currently there are nine allergens from Anisakis characterized (Audicana and Kennedy 2008, Rodriguez-Perez et al. 2008), which are somatic or excretory–secretory products of the nematode. The molecular weight ranges from 15 to 154 kDa and several allergen classes were identified (see Table 14.3.1) (Audicana and Kennedy 2008).

The crustacea group is very large; however, most of the allergic reactions and characterized allergens are restricted to the decapods group, which are discussed in detail in Chapter 9. During the production of nori (dried seaweed used for e.g., sushi) often amphipods are found mixed in the sheets and the potential hazard to consumer has been investigated. When analyzed by ELISA and immunoblotting with sera from patients with shrimp allergy, a 37 kDa protein was identified as amphipod tropomyosin (Motoyama et al. 2007).

**TABLE 14.3.1**

**Allergen Sources and Putative Allergens Causing Allergic Reactions After Ingestion**

| Source of Allergen | Allergen Identified | Allergen Class | Molecular Mass (kDa) | Author |
|---|---|---|---|---|
| **Marine Organisms** | | | | |
| **Anisakis** (*Anisakis simplex*; *A. pegreffi*) | *Ani s* 1 | Kunitz-type serine protease inhibitor-like | 21–24 | Armentia et al. (2006); Audicana and Kennedy (2008); Jeebhay et al. (2001); Nieuwenhuizen et al. (2006) |
| | *Ani s* 2 | Paramyosin | 97 | |
| | *Ani s* 3 | Tropomyosin | 41 | |
| | *Ani s* 4 | Cysteine protease inhibitor | 9 | |
| | *Ani s* 5 | SXP/RAL protein | 15 | |
| | *Ani s* 6 | Serine protease inhibitor | | |
| | *Ani s* 7 | Glycoprotein | 139–154 | |
| | *Ani s* 8 | SXP/RAL protein | 15 | |
| | *Ani s* 9 | SXP/RAL-2 family | 14 | |
| **Sea urchin roe** | | | 118 | Hickey (2007); Rodriguez et al. (2007) |
| **Amphipods** (*Gammarus* sp.); (*Caprella equilibria*) | | Tropomyosin | 37 | Motoyama et al. (2007) |
| **Insects** | | | | |
| **Carmine Red (cochineal)** | | | | Acero et al. (1998) |
| (*Dactylopius coccus*) | | | 23, 38, 50, 88 | Chung et al. (2001) |
| **Caterpillar** (Hickory Tussock moth) | | | N.D. | Pitetti et al. (1999) |
| **Mealworm** (*Tenebrio molitor*); **Superworm** (*Zophobas morio*) | | | N.D. | Freye et al. (1996) |
| **Storage Mite** (Tyrophagus putrescentiae) | *Der f* 1 | | | Matsumoto et al. (1996) |
| **Mite** (*D. pteronyssinus*; *D. farinae*) | *Der p* 1 *Der f* 1 | Cysteine protease | 24 | SanchezBorges et al. (1997) |
| **Mite** (*D. farinae; T. entomophagus*) | *Der f* 1 | Cysteine protease | 24 | Blanco et al. (1997) |

**TABLE 14.3.1 (continued)**
**Allergen Sources and Putative Allergens Causing Allergic Reactions After Ingestion**

| Source of Allergen | Allergen Identified | Allergen Class | Molecular Mass (kDa) | Author |
|---|---|---|---|---|
| **Other Animals** | | | | |
| **European bee-eater (bird)** (*Merops apiaster*) | | Bee venom suspected | N.D. | Gulbahar et al. (2003) |
| **Frog** | | Parvalbumin (α-form) | 12 | Hilger et al. (2002) |
| **Frog (*Rana esculenta*)** | | Parvalbumin (β- form) | 12 | Hilger et al. (2004) |

*Note:* N.D. = Not determined.

### 14.3.3 INSECTS

There is steady growing evidence that environmental exposure to insects at home and in the workplace are the frequent causes of allergic sensitization (Arlian 2002). Subsequently clinical symptoms are mainly of respiratory nature, manifested in allergic rhinitis, asthma, and urticaria (Steen et al. 2004), and in some documented cases also via ingestion, causing systemic anaphylaxis.

Many species of insects are sources of potent allergens that induce IgE-mediated allergic reactions in sensitized humans. Current research data indicate the existence of numerous allergens which differ greatly among the diversity of insect species. More than 50% of all known animal species on earth are insects (currently over 800,000), highlighting the vast possibilities of unknown allergens (Auerswald and Lopata 2005). Consequently it is not surprising that detailed knowledge of the precise insect species (in particular geographical area), tissue source of allergen, and the molecular structure of the allergen can assist a great deal in the development of more sensitive tests to evaluate individuals with species specific allergy to insects.

Insects (and indeed all arthropods) are characterized by an exoskeleton and segmentations which produce large amounts of allergens found in respirable dust particulates or aerosol and can thereby contaminate food supplies. Sources of allergens are the dried, exuviate scales, hairs, fragmented dead remains, and metabolic products such as feces and silks (excluding allergic reactions to venom). An important source of allergens for many insect species appears to be the feces. It is perhaps not surprising that some investigators have documented some cross-reactivity of insects with the house dust-mite, where feces are also the main allergen source. Recently additional allergens were found in locusts (Lopata et al. 2005), raising the old question raised by Baldo of "pan-allergens" (Baldo and Panzani 1988, Panzani and Ariano 2001) between different insect species, which perhaps could also be found in the wings of many insects. Several major allergens of insects have been characterized using protein and cDNA analysis. All these allergens have high molecular weights (14–80 kDa), with some having enzymatic functions (proteases) and others are regulatory proteins (transferase; tropomyosins). Particularly tropomyosin is a candidate pan-allergen and is characterized in detail in Chapter 9. Interestingly the immunological findings of allergenic cross-reactivity between crustacean and insects support the suggestion by entomologists to group the crustacean and insects as "Pancrustacea" (Auerswald and Lopata 2005).

In general, sensitization to insects occurs in about 30% of individuals with high-risk exposure. Allergenic insects are not only found at home but frequently in various types of work places which favor the exposure to a number of insect species concurrently. Storage pests are also an important consideration in workers exposed at their workplace as demonstrated in recent studies from Spain and South Africa. Prevalence rates of up to 50% for insects such as cockroaches, mealworms, and mites were documented. While the sensitization to these insects most probably occurred via the inhalational route, cross-contamination of grain and subsequently the end-products can also be expected.

The realities of hidden-insect allergens in food products have recently been published with storage and house-dust mite contaminated flour triggering acute anaphylactic reactions in the consumer. In a case report by Matsumoto et al. (1996), a storage mite (*Tyrophagus putrescentiae*) was identified as the cause of systemic anaphylaxis in two patients. In a subsequent study on 30 subjects, systemic anaphylaxis precipitated by the ingestion of wheat-containing foods, caused symptoms such as breathlessness, angioedema, wheezing, and rhinorrhea (SanchezBorges et al. 1997). All subjects were SPT positive to house dust mites. The major house dust mite allergens *Der p* 1 and *Der f* 1 were detected in contaminated flour and subsequently identified in further 37% of 35 randomly selected flour samples. In a different study Blanco et al. (1997) conducted food challenges with contaminated flour and three of six subjects demonstrated systemic reactions and implicated two different mite species (*Dermatophagoides farinae and Thyreophagus entomophagus*).

To preserve food and enhance the visual life span of stored food, chemicals are often added. However, food additives can also be derived from unexpected animal products such a natural red dye. The red color carmine (E120) is extracted from the dried bodies of female cochineal insects and used as a coloring agent for food and cosmetics. Several cases of occupational asthma, allergic alveoli as well as food allergy have been reported and IgE mediated mechanisms demonstrated by skin-prick testing, leukocyte histamine release, RAST, and DBPCFC (Acero et al. 1998). A recent study by Chung et al. (2001) identified several IgE binding proteins by immunoblotting of cochineal extracts (23, 38, 50, 88 kDa), however, no universal protein was recognized by all three allergic patients.

A case report by Pitetti et al. (1999) described 10 pediatric patients with adverse reactions after eating caterpillars of a moth (Hickory Tussock moth), causing symptoms ranging from drooling to diffuse urticaria. The allergens responsible, however, were not identified.

In a study to investigate potential anaphylactic reactions of subjects with confirmed inhalant sensitization to insects, subjects were orally challenged with extracts of mealworm (*Tenebrio molitor*) and superworm (*Zophobas morio*). One of three subjects demonstrated allergic reactions by inhalation and ingestion of mealworm, the allergens were however not identified (Freye et al. 1996).

### 14.3.4 OTHER ANIMAL TISSUE

Contact with allergens may not always be obvious in allergic reactions. A case report from Turkey investigated the possible allergic sensitization to bee venom, via eating the European bee-eater (*Merops apiaster*). A man who frequently ate this type of bird developed oral allergy syndrome and breathing difficulties and was diagnosed by SPT and ImmunoCAP to be sensitized to bee venom. The bird's main diet includes bees, wasps, and hornets, and it consumes up to 250 bees per day. While this bird is apparently immune to the venom, it was suspected that venom allergens could be detectable in the bird's tissue and caused the allergic reaction.

The main cross-reactive allergen in fish is parvalbumin, as small calcium binding protein, which has recently been demonstrated to be cause also allergic reactions after ingestion of lower vertebrates. Over the past few years several reports indicated allergic reactions to frogs via inhalation and also via ingestion. A case of anaphylaxis after eating a frog from Indonesia (no species identified) was specifically directed to the α-form of parvalbumin (Hilger et al. 2002). No cross-reactivity to other frog or fish parvalbumin was demonstrated. However, a recent study by Hilger et al. (2004) investigated frog allergens in a case of a child with known allergy to fish, which presented with severe anaphylaxis after eating boiled frog legs (Romano et al. 2000). Inhibition studies with fish parvalbumin demonstrated that the child was sensitized to the β-form of parvalbumin from frog (*Rana esculenta*), which cross-reacted with fish parvalbumin. The cross-reactivity was confirmed by SPT and immunoblotting with fish allergic patients. Eleven of 12 tested sera demonstrated recognition mainly of the β-form of frog parvalbumin. This differential response is supported by protein sequence alignment studies which showed a sequence identify of 60% between cod parvalbumin and the β-form of *R. esculenta* parvalbumin, whereas the sequence identity to the α-form was only 45%. As the clinical relevance of this cross-reactivity has been demonstrated, parvalbumin could perhaps present a new family of pan-allergen, at least among lower vertebrates.

### REFERENCES

Acero, S., Tahar, A.I., Alvarez, M.J., Garcia, B.E., Olaguibel, J.M., and Moneo, I. 1998. Occupational asthma and food allergy due to carmine. *Allergy* 53(9): 897–901.

Arlian, L.G. 2002. Arthropod allergens and human health. *Annu Rev Entomol* 47: 395–433.

Armentia, A., Martin-Gil, F.J., Pascual, C., Martin-Esteban, M., Callejo, A., and Martinez, C. 2006. Anisakis simplex allergy after eating chicken meat. *J Invest Allergol Clin Immunol* 16(4): 258–263.

Audicana, M.T., Ansotegui, I.J., de Corres, L.F., and Kennedy, M.W. 2002. Anisakis simplex: Dangerous—dead and alive? *Trends Parasitol* 18(1): 20–25.

Audicana, M.T. and Kennedy, M.W. 2008. Anisakis simplex: From obscure infectious worm to inducer of immune hypersensitivity. *Clin Microbiol Rev* 21(2): 360–379.

Auerswald, L. and Lopata, A.L. 2005. Insects—diversity and allergy. *Curr Allergy Clin Immunol* 18(2): 58–60.

Baldo, B.A. and Panzani, R.C. 1988. Detection of IgE antibodies to a wide-range of insect species in subjects with suspected inhalant allergies to insects. *Int Arch Aller Appl Immunol* 85(3): 278–287.

Blanco, C., Quiralte, J., Castillo, R., Delgado, J., Arteaga, C., Barber, D., and Carrillo, T. 1997. Anaphylaxis after ingestion of wheat flour contaminated with mites. *J Aller Clin Immunol* 99(3): 308–313.

Caballero, M.L. and Moneo, I. 2004. Several allergens from Anisakis simplex are highly resistant to heat and pepsin treatments. *Parasitol Res* 93(3): 248–251.

Chung, K., Baker, J.R., Baldwin, J.L., and Chou, A. 2001. Identification of carmine allergens among three carmine allergy patients. *Allergy* 56(1): 73–77.

Freye, H.B., Esch, R.E., Litwin, C.M., and Sorkin, L. 1996. Anaphylaxis to the ingestion and inhalation of *Tenebrio molitor* (mealworm) and *Zophobas morio* (superworm). *Allergy Asthma Proc* 17(4): 215–219.

Gulbahar, O., Mete, N., Ardeniz, O., Onbasi, K., Kokuludag, A., Sin, A., and Sebik, F. 2003. Laryngeal edema due to European bee-eater (*Merops apiaster*) in a patient allergic to honeybee. *Allergy* 58(5): 453–453.

Hickey, R.W. 2007. Sea urchin roe (uni) anaphylaxis. *Ann Allergy Asthma Immunol* 98(5): 493–494.

Hilger, C., Grigioni, F., Thill, L., Mertens, L., and Hentges, F. 2002. Severe IgE-mediated anaphylaxis following consumption of fried frog legs: Definition of alpha-parvalbumin as the allergen in cause. *Allergy* 57(11): 1053–1058.

Hilger, C., Thill, L., Grigioni, F., Lehners, C., Falagiani, P., Ferrara, A., Romano, C., Stevens, W., and Hentges, F. 2004. IgE antibodies of fish allergic patients cross-react with frog parvalbumin. *Allergy* 59(6): 653–660.

Jeebhay, M.F., Robins, T.G., Lehrer, S.B., and Lopata, A.L. 2001. Occupational seafood allergy: A review. *Occup Environ Med* 58(9): 553–562.

Jenkins, J.A., Breiteneder, H., and Mills, E.N.C. 2007. Evolutionary distance from human homologs reflects allergenicity of animal food proteins. *J Allergy Clin Immunol* 120(6): 1399–1405.

Kasuya, S., Hamano, H., and Izumi, S. 1990. Mackerel-induced urticaria and Anisakis. *Lancet* 335(8690): 665–665.

Lehrer, S.B., Ayuso, R., and Reese, G. 2003. Seafood allergy and allergens: A review. *Mar Biotechnol* 5(4): 339–348.

Lopata, A.L., Fenemore, B., Jeebhay, M.F., Gade, G., and Potter, P.C. 2005. Occupational allergy in laboratory workers caused by the African migratory grasshopper *Locusta migratoria*. *Allergy* 60(2): 200–205.

Lopata, A.L. and Potter, P.C. 2000. Allergy and other adverse reactions to seafood. *Allergy Clin Immunol Int* 12(6): 271–281.

Matsumoto, T., Hisano, T., Hamaguchi, M., and Miike, T. 1996. Systemic anaphylaxis after eating storage-mite-contaminated food. *Int Arch Allergy Immunol* 109(2): 197–200.

Motoyama, K., Hamada, Y., Nagashima, Y., and Shiomi, K. 2007. Allergenicity and allergens of amphipods found in nori (dried laver). *Food Addit Contam* 24(9): 917–922.

Nieuwenhuizen, N., Lopata, A.L., Jeebhay, M.L.F., Herbert, D.R., Robins, T.G., and Brombacher, F. 2006. Exposure to the fish parasite Anisakis causes allergic airway hyperreactivity and dermatitis. *J Allergy Clin Immunol* 117(5): 1098–1105.

Panzani, R.C. and Ariano, R. 2001. Arthropods and invertebrates allergy (with the exclusion of mites): The concept of panallergy. *Allergy* 56: 1–22.

Pitetti, R.D., Kuspis, D., and Krenzelok, E.P. 1999. Caterpillars: An unusual source of ingestion. *Ped Emer Care* 15(1): 33–36.

Rodriguez-Perez, R., Moneo, I., Rodriguez-Mahillo, A., and Caballero, M.L. 2008. Cloning and expression of Ani s 9, a new Anisakis simplex allergen. *Mol Biochem Parasitol* 159(2): 92–97.

Rodriguez, V., Bartolome, B., Armisen, M., and Vidal, C. 2007. Food allergy to *Paracentrotus lividus* (sea urchin roe). *Ann Allergy Asthma Immunol* 98(4): 393–396.

Romano, C., Ferrara, A.M., Cislaghi, C., and Falagiani, P. 2000. Food allergy to frog. *Allergy* 55(6): 584–585.

SanchezBorges, M., CaprilesHulett, A., FernandezCaldas, E., SuarezChacon, R., Caballero, F., Castillo, S., and Sotillo, E. 1997. Mite-contaminated foods as a cause of anaphylaxis. *J Allergy Clin Immunol* 99(6): 738–743.

Steen, C.J., Carbonaro, P.A., and Schwartz, R.A. 2004. Arthropods in dermatology. *J Am Acad Dermatol* 50(6): 819–842.

## 14.4 FOOD ADDITIVES AS FOOD ALLERGENS

Lucjan Jędrychowski

### 14.4.1 GENERAL DESCRIPTION OF FOOD ADDITIVES

Worldwide food trade as well as customers' expectations regarding foodstuffs enforce implementation of measures which improve sensory, physicochemical, functional, and health-related characteristics of food products. Food producers themselves, aware of the importance of product quality, do not neglect the question of sensory, visual, and marketing features of food products. This, along with the required economic efficiency, encourages food manufacturers to use various additives in food processing technologies, which improve the characteristics of food products demanded by shoppers. In short, food additives play an important role in today's complex food supply.

"A food additive"—according to the Codex Alimentarius Commission (a joint FAO/WHO and the EEC organization)—"means any substance not normally consumed as a food by itself and not normally used as a typical ingredient of food, whether or not it has nutritive value, the intentional addition of which to food for a technological (including organoleptic) purpose in the manufacture, processing, preparation, treatment, packing, packaging, transport, or holding of such food results, or may reasonably be expected to result, directly or indirectly, in it or its by-products becoming a component of or otherwise affecting the characteristics of such foods. The term does not include contaminants or substances added to food for maintaining or improving nutritional qualities" (Codex Alimentarius Commission 1979, Council Directive 89/107/EEC).

Use of food additives is widespread and diverse, although some countries have undertaken to reduce it. Denmark was the first to introduce, in 1973, a legal ban on some food additives. In 1984, the ban was extended on food dyes. Norway and Sweden followed the Danish legislative solutions, introducing additional restrictions on food preservatives. However, none of the aforementioned countries has been consistent in imposing these laws and, as a result, consumption of food additives has increased (Madsen 1997).

The number of agents added to foodstuffs ranges between 2,000 and 20,000 (Bosso and Simon 2008). The database maintained by the U.S. Food and Drug Administration (FDA) Centre for Food Safety and Applied Nutrition (CFSAN), under the program The Priority-Based Assessment of Food Additives (PAFA), encompasses over 2000 substances directly added to food, whereas the Everything Added to Food in the United States (EAFUS) database quotes over 3500 components used in the United States as food additives (http://www.foodsafety.gov/~dms/eafus. html). It is estimated that a person consumes, in different amounts, about 12–60 various food additives in a single meal (Tuormaa 1994). Some food additives (benzoates, disulfides, IV sulfates, aspartame, dyes, and sodium glutamate) may cumulate in an organism and trigger symptoms of intolerance.

Continuous progress in food science, food chemistry, and technology has resulted in the discovery of many new substances which can fulfill numerous functions in foods.

Due to a large number of food additives used in the food manufacturing industry, depending on the type of a food product, expected functions, and characteristics of food additives, the latter are divided into several groups (types), for example:

- Acidity regulators (natural food acids, minerals, and organic acids)— E300–E399, E500–E599
- Antibiotics—E700–E799
- Anticaking agents—E500–E599
- Colors, (food colorings, food color modifying factors, e.g., color fixatives, color retention agents)—E100–E199
- Emulsifiers—E400–E499
- Firming agents
- Flavor enhancers—E600–E699
- Flour treatment agents (flour bleaches)
- Foaming and antifoaming agents
- Gelling agents
- Glazing agents
- Humectants
- Improving agents
- Mineral salts and additional chemicals—E1000–E1999
- Miscellaneous—E900–E999
- Others (such as flavors, other food products added in small quantities, e.g., plant proteins added to meat products, enzymatic products which modify physicochemical and sensory properties of foodstuffs)
- Preservatives (antioxidants)—E200–E299, E300–E399
- Propellants
- Seasonings
- Sequestrants
- Stabilizers—E400–E499
- Sweeteners (artificial sweeteners)
- Thickeners—E400–E499
- Vegetable gums

Similar categories, although not all of the aforementioned, are included in the Framework Directive 89/107/EEC (Council Directive 1989).

Colorings and dyes, preservatives (including insecticide sprays on fruits), emulsifying and stabilizing agents, antioxidants, synthetic and natural flavoring agents, additives improving specific sensory characteristics (sweet or sour taste), bleaching agents, e.g., to improve flour, are among the most popular food additives. The aforementioned division is made more complicated by the fact that some additives perform several functions. The available references contain many other food additive classification systems, for example, the one which divides such substances into three major groups, i.e., food additives affecting:

1. Physical or physicochemical properties ( buffers, anticaking agents, antifoaming and foaming agents, clouding/weighting agents, dispersing agents, enzymes, encapsulants, emulsifiers and stabilizers, glazing agents, dyes, raising agents, and thickeners)
2. Sensory properties (thickeners, emulsifiers and stabilizers, acidulants and buffers, clouding/weighting agents, dispersing agents, raising agents, antibrowning agents, sequestering agents, curing and pickling agents, humectants, flavor enhancers, colors, gelling agents, sweeteners, and flour improvers)
3. Shelf life (antioxidants, preservatives, antibrowning agents, sequestering agents, curing and pickling agents, and humectants)

Further in the aforementioned classification, many additives have overlapping functions.

Although many food ingredients do not correspond to the definition of food additives, mainly because they can occur as food products, for example, milk, eggs, wheat flour or starch, cornflour, etc., they can also perform the role of additives (David 1993). They can be thickeners, flavorings, condiments, acidity modifying agents, etc. The following foods can be given as examples:

Asparagus, seed and root, extract
Celery (*Apium graveolens* L.)—celery seed, celery seed extract solid, oil, oleoresin
Corn (*Zea mays* L.)—gluten, mint oil, silk, silk extract, cornstarch, corn steep liquor, corn syrup
Fatty acids
Garlic (*Allium sativum* L.)—garlic extract, dried garlic, oil
Cebula—susz
Milk—or chemically modified milk proteins, lactates, caseinians
Mustard (*Brassica* spp.), brown, mustard flour, extract, oil
Papain (*Carica papaya* L.)
Paprika (*Capsicum annuum* L.)—paprika oleoresin
Parmesan cheese, reggiano cheese
Parsley(*Petroselinum* spp.), oil, oleoresin
Passion (*Passiflora incarnata* L.)—passion flower, flower extract
Patchouli (*Pogostemon* spp.)—oil
Peach (*Prunus persica* sieb et zucc.)—peach kernel, peach kernel extract, peach leaves
Peanut (*Arachis hypogaea* L.) – oil, butter, stearine
Pectin

Starch—different kinds (potato, corn, and wheat starches) and many kinds of chemically modified starches (oxidized starches, phosphated distarch phosphate, etc.)

Whey—whey protein concentrate, delactosed, demineralized, partially demineralized and partially delactosed

They can be used in larger amounts in products such as sausages, cereals, flaked foods, concentrated foods, and the like.

A similar group of products which do not correspond strictly to the definition of food additives is composed of raw foods, which, owing to their sensory properties, are added in small quantities to proper food products (condiments, herbs, vegetables, and oils). They can, however, produce allergenic or nonallergenic hypersensitivity response.

Apart from the aforementioned food additives, used intentionally and inevitably in food products, foodstuffs can also contain unwanted components originating from (chemical) pollution or (microbiological) contamination (e.g., antigens of microbial cells and metabolites produced by microorganisms like enzymes, toxins), which likewise are not encompassed by the definition of food additives but can be harmful to human health when found in food products.

Substances obtained via biotechnological methods comprise a relatively new but rapidly developing group of food additives. An example of such additives could be milk protein coagulating enzymes used in cheese production and obtained with aid of GMOs (chymosin preparation obtained using genetically modified molds *Aspergillus niger* var. Awamori, bacteria Escherichia coli K-12, or yeast *Kluyveromyces marxianus* var. Lactis).

Food additives, and particularly added nutrients, are most often a source of the so-called hidden allergens in food products and, as such, constitute a serious health threat to consumers who suffer from allergenic hypersensitivity; they can even cause a life-threatening anaphylaxis (David 1993). For this reason, it is essential that use of food additives and food labeling be legally regulated.

Because of a large number and variety of food additives, an internationally accepted coding system known as the International Numbering System (determined by the Codex Alimentarius Committee) has been adapted. The so-called E-numbers signify that a given additive has been approved by the EU. However, the fact that different food additive classification systems exist in particular countries or in particular continents (Australia, Europe, and the United States) does not facilitate global discussion on this issue.

Locally, especially in the United Kingdom, Ireland, and central Europe, as well as among eco-food supporters, the term "E-number" is understood and used as a pejorative term for artificial food additives. Nonetheless, benefits derived from using food additives along with the "Westernalization of life" lead to an ever increasing average consumption of such substances (natural food additives and xenobiotics) (Tuormaa 1994).

In every country, the use of food additives in the food manufacturing and pharmaceuticals industries is preceded by obligatory toxicological assays, hedged with very stringent laws and strict hygienic and sanitary requirements, it is strictly monitored by authorized institutions, which should guarantee food safety.

On the other hand, allergenic and nonallergenic hypersensitivity caused by food additives is a relatively new issue and seems difficult to diagnose in clinical examinations, aspects related to such reactions should become a subject of in-depth research and be reflected in appropriate legal regulations.

To protect consumers from potential hypersensitivity, the European Union Commission Directive was announced regulating the content of food allergens on food labels (Directive 2006/142/EC). Sulfites are mentioned among 14 major food allergens, i.e., the ones that cause 90% of allergies. The EU Directive binds all food producers to declare the presence of sulfites in a food product if present in a concentration exceeding 10 mg/kg or 10mL/L, expressed as $SO_2$. Although sulfites (IV) of low molecular weight do not belong to haptens and cannot cause an allergenic reaction, they can be responsible for food hypersensitivity, whose underlying cause consists of pathogenic nonimmunological mechanisms (discussed in greater detail in Chapter 1).

Laws imposing food labeling are mainly addressed to people suffering from food allergies, thus labels must assure consumers that the labeled product is absolutely safe (van Hengel 2007).

- Laws regulating the issue of food additives are changing very dynamically in nearly all countries.

Amendments to legal regulations alongside continuous and dynamic developments in food producing technologies as well as discovery of new ingredients of useful properties—all these aspects make us perceive the question of food additives as a highly dynamic set of issues. One possible example pertains to recommendations concerning new additives approved for commercial use in Australia, which are deemed as causing uncertain reactions in humans (Table 14.4.2). The contents of particular EU Directives are available on the EU Web sites, at:

http://www.foodlaw.rdg.ac.uk/additive.htm
http://www.fsai.ie/legislation/food/legislation_foodadditives.asp#1

and the information about approved food additives (including new ones) can be found at

http://www.foodsafety.gov/~dms/eafus.html
http://www.fedupwithfoodadditives.info/information/additivesall.htm

## 14.4.2 ADVERSE REACTIONS TO FOOD ADDITIVES

Some of the food additives used, apart from performing their basic functions such as food quality improvement, can cause many health problems, for example, specific allergic or irritant reactions of various body systems (cutaneous, respiratory, gastrointestinal, and multisystem) (Fleischer and Leung 2008, McCann et al. 2007) as well as responses of the nervous system (migraine headaches, epilepsy, vertigo, and hemiplegia) (Weber 2008). Adverse, predominately hyperactive behavioral changes in children have been documented as associated with excess amounts of artificial food colorings and sodium benzoate preservatives in the diet (Bateman et al. 2004).

The mechanism of causing allergenic and nonallergenic hypersensitive response by food additives (mainly haptens) has not been completely clarified (Chapter 1 and Brostoff and Challacombe 2002, Metcalfe et al. 2008 discuss this in greater detail). McFadden has presented a hapten–atopic hypothesis that the increasing number of cases of atopic diseases observed during the last 40 years in Western countries is caused by consumption of processed products containing many artificially created haptens (McFadden et al. 2008). Chapter 1 discusses this theory in greater detail.

It is supposed that about 50 out of 350 permitted food additives in Australia are likely to cause adverse reactions (Table 14.4.1). Thus, food additives from Australia should be used with caution, if ever. The aforementioned group of new additives, untested as of yet, should be avoided or else used cautiously (Table 14.4.2). Other additives are unlikely to cause negative reactions (http://www.fedupwithfoodadditives.info/information/additivesall.htm).

Likewise, with great caution, food additives are treated in other countries, where attention is paid to possible adverse effects of such substances on human health (Tables 14.4.3 through 14.4.7).

The underlying problem caused by using food additives in foodstuffs is their effect on health safety of food consumers. Extremely divergent approaches appear in this context. Some neglect the effect of food additives in health because of their small concentration in food products and also because many of them have been widely used for centuries while others consider food additives as a great threat to human health.

In Europe, the EU Scientific Committee on Food (SCF) is responsible for food safety, including use of food additives. On an international level, the following organizations bear this responsibility: the Joint Expert Committee, from the Food and Agriculture Organization (FAO) and the World Health Organization (WHO), on Food Additives (JECFA) and the Codex Alimentarius Commission, which has produced new General Standards for Food Additives (GSFA). These organizations are responsible for establishing international standards for food industry and world trade as well as such indicators as "no-observed-adverse-effect level" (NOAEL) and the Acceptable Daily Intake (ADI) for each food additive, which are a measure of food safety.

The results of numerous research projects suggest that the question of food additives affecting man's health cannot be neglected, especially in the context of their influence on cancer incidence or possible occurrence of allergenic (Baldwin et al. 1997) and nonallergenic hypersensitivity reaction as well as their effect on the nervous system (hyperactivity), especially in children (Brostoff and Challacombe 2002, McCann et al. 2007, Metcalfe et al. 2008).

Cases of allergenic hypersensitivity caused by food additives are rather rare (0.03%–0.23% of population) (Wüthrich 1993) and difficult to diagnose (Spergel and Fiedler 2005). The prevalence rate of food-additive-induced asthma exacerbations obtained by using double-blind, placebo-controlled trails is about 5% (23%–67% of asthmatics believe that food additives exacerbate their asthma) (Bush and Montalbano 2008). One of the reasons why it is difficult to diagnose the exact effect of food additives is the fact that ingredients which appear in food products in very

**TABLE 14.4.1**

**List of Food Additives Deemed in Australia as the Ones to Avoid**

| Group | | EEC Number | Name | Remarks—Uses and Restrictions |
|---|---|---|---|---|
| Color additives | | 102 | Tartrazine, yellow | Dyes widely used in food |
| | | 104 | Quinoline yellow | industry. |
| | | 107 | Yellow 2G | Are often derived from raw |
| | | 110 | Sunset yellow | materials which are potential allergens. |
| | | 122 | Azorubine, carmoisine | Annatto (160b) is used as a |
| | | 123 | Amaranth | colorant in cheese, butter, |
| | | 124 | Ponceau 4R, brilliant scarlet | margarine, meats, and processed snacks. Annatto is |
| | | 127 | Erythrosine | believed to be harmful in |
| | | 128 | Red 2G | sensitive people; in rare cases it |
| | | 129 | Allura red | can cause allergic reactions |
| | | 132 | Indigotine, indigo carmine | (contact, urticaria, angioedema, asthma, and even anaphylaxis, |
| | | 133 | Brilliant blue | or delayed reaction type IV). |
| | | 142 | Food green S, acid brilliant green | |
| | | 151 | Brilliant black BN | |
| | | 155 | Brown HT, chocolate brown | |
| | | 160b | Annatto extracts, bixin, norbixin | |
| Preservatives | Sorbates | 200 | Sorbic acid | Sorbates and benzoates have |
| | | 201 | Sodium sorbate | been associated with a full |
| | | 202 | Potassium sorbate | range of food intolerance |
| | | 203 | Calcium sorbate | reactions. |
| | Benzoates | 210 | Benzoic acid | |
| | | 211 | Sodium benzoate | |
| | | 212 | Potassium benzoate | |
| | | 213 | Calcium benzoate | |
| | (Aka sulfites) | 220 | Sulfur dioxide | Sulfites are the biggest threat to |
| | | 221 | Sodium sulfite | asthmatics. Not to be confused |
| | | 222 | Sodium bisulfite | with sulfates (514–519), also |
| | | 223 | Sodium metabisulfite | known as sulfites. |
| | | 224 | Potassium metabisulfite | |
| | | 225 | Potassium sulfite | |
| | | 228 | Potassium bisulfite | |
| | Nitrates nitrites | 249 | Potassium nitrite | Nitrates and nitrites are used in |
| | | 250 | Sodium nitrite | processed meats to prevent |
| | | 251 | Sodium nitrate | bacterial growth and food |
| | | 252 | Potassium nitrate | poisoning. They are not completely safe. |

*(continued)*

**TABLE 14.4.1 (continued)**
**List of Food Additives Deemed in Australia as the Ones to Avoid**

| Group | EEC Number | Name | Remarks—Uses and Restrictions |
|---|---|---|---|
| Propionates | 280 | Propionic acid | Propionic acid and propionates may be used in bread (in Australia and the United States) and are permitted also in cheese, fruit, and vegetable products (in Australia). |
| | 281 | Sodium propionate | |
| | 282 | Calcium propionate | |
| | 283 | Potassium propionate | |
| Antioxidants | 310 | Propyl gallate | Gallates and TBHQ, BHA, and BHT are used to preserve vegetable oils and margarines. When vegetable oils are used in other products, these antioxidants are often unlisted because of the 5% labeling loophole. BHA and BHT can also leach into products from cereal wrappers and clingfilm. |
| | 311 | Octyl gallate | |
| | 312 | Dodecyl gallate | |
| | 319 | tert-Butylhydroquinone, TBHQ | |
| | 320 | Butylated hydroxyanisole, BHA | |
| | 321 | Butylated hydroxytoluene, BHT | |
| Vegetable gums and thickeners | 407 | Carrageenan | Vegetable gums are failsafe. Guar and xanthan are used extensively by coeliacs. Carrageenan (407) used in yoghurts, ice creams, and others has been linked to cancer, and is not recommended for consumption in large amounts. |
| Flavor enhancers | 620 | L-Glutamic acid | Made by fermentation or synthetically—enhances taste of meals, condiments, concentrated foods, soups, and sauces. MSG is classified by the FDA as generally recognized as safe (GRAS). Not recommended for consumption in large amounts due to ambiguous research results, especially regarding the possible neurotoxicity and neuroendocrine effects. Very few case reports of MSG-induced angioedema or urticaria have appeared in the literature. |
| | 621 | Monosodium L-glutamate (MSG) | |
| | 622 | Monopotassium L-glutamate | |

*Source:* Based on EAFUS, a Food Additive Database—http://www.foodsafety.gov/~dms/eafus.html; http://www.fedupwithfoodadditives.info/information/additivesall.htm

## TABLE 14.4.2
## List of Some New Food Additives Approved to Use in Australia, Which can Potentially Cause Health Problems in Humans

| Group | E Number Equivalent | Food Additive | Remarks |
|---|---|---|---|
| Carmel | 150 | Caramel | Caramel 150, according to possible chemical |
| | (150a) | (plain or spirit caramel) | modifications, may be divided into caramels 150 (sulfite ammonia caramel), 150a (plain |
| | (150b) | (caustic sulfite caramel) | or spirit caramel), 150b (caustic sulfite caramel), and 150c (ammonia caramel). Plain |
| | (150c) | (ammonia caramel) | caramel is considered failsafe. There is a report of sulfite ammonia caramel used widely in soft drinks like cola causing problems in extra sulfite sensitive people, particularly asthma patients. |
| Carotene | 160 | Carotene (others)— see listed below | 160e and 160f are too new to have been tested for behavioral toxicity. They might be safe |
| | 160e | β-apo-8′carotenal | like β-carotene (160a) or harmful like |
| | 160f | E-apo-8′carotenoic acid | annatto (160b). |
| | 161 | Xanthophylls, yellow | |
| | 161g | Canthaxanthin | β-apo 8′carotenal (160e), canthaxanthin (161g) and citranaxanthin (161i) are used in poultry feed to deepen the color of egg yolks. |
| | 161i | Citranaxanthin | There are a few reports of reactions. Canthaxanthin (161g) taken in large quantities in tanning tablets has been associated to retinal damage. It is used as a food color, in poultry feed and fed to farmed salmon and trout to color their flesh. |
| Flavoring substances | 627 631 635 | Disodium guanylate Disodium inosinate and Disodium 5′-ribonucleotides | Disodium guanylate (627), Disodium inosinate (631), and Disodium 5′-ribonucleotides (635), which is a combination of 627 and 631, are associated with skin rashes. |

*Source:* Based on http://www.fedupwithfoodadditives.info/information/additivesall.htm

small quantities (spices, condiments, additives, and other food products) may not be listed on food labels and can constitute the so-called hidden allergens. Another reason could be that same disease symptoms can be caused by different mechanisms. Food additives are typically haptens (usually characterized—beside natural food additives—by low molecular weight < 1 kDa). The mechanism of inducing allergenic and nonallergenic hypersensitivity reaction by haptens can be varied. This issue is discussed in more detail in Chapter 1 and by Kanerva (2002) and McFadden

**TABLE 14.4 3**

**Coloring Materials Used in Food Production which may Trigger Symptoms of Nonallergenic Hypersensitivity (Pseudoallergy-Adverse Reactions)**

| FD and C Dyes | E Number | Coloring Materials | Colors | Application |
|---|---|---|---|---|
| Yellow No. 5[b] | 102[a] | Tartrazine[b] | Lemon yellow | Not determined |
| | 104[a] | Quinoline yellow | Yellow | Not determined |
| Yellow No. 6[b] | 110[a] | Orange yellow S[b] | Orange yellow | Not determined |
| [b] | 120[a] | Carminic acid[b] | Red | Not determined |
| | 122[a] | Azorubine (azo dye) | Red | Not determined |
| Red No. 2[b] | 123[a] | Amaranth (azo dye)[b] | Red | Used as coloring in wines, alcohols, and roe (prohibited in the United States) |
| | 124[a] | Cochineal red A (azo dye) | Red | Not determined |
| Red No. 3[b] | 127[a] | Erythrosine BS (non-azo dye)[b] | Red | Used as coloring in cherry products and in fruit salad containing cherries |
| | 128[a] | Red 2G | Red | Used as coloring in sausages or meat products containing plant food components |
| | 129[a] | Allura red | Red | Not determined |
| | 151[a] | Brilliant black PN | Black | Not determined |
| | 154[a] | Brown FK | Brown | Used as coloring in cured herring products manufactured in the Great Britain and Norway |
| | 155[a] | Brown HT, chocolate brown | Brown | Not determined |
| [b] | 160 (b)[b] Natural | Annatto extracts, bixin, norbixin | Orange–yellow | Extracted from the seeds of the tree *Bixa orellana*, used as coloring in cheese, snack foods, and cereals |

**TABLE 14.4.3 (continued)**
**Coloring Materials Used in Food Production which may Trigger Symptoms of Nonallergenic Hypersensitivity (Pseudoallergy-Adverse Reactions)**

| FD and C Dyes | E Number | Coloring Materials | Colors | Application |
|---|---|---|---|---|
| | 180[a] | Lithol rubine | Red | Used as coloring in edible cheese outer layer |
| Red No. 4[b] | | Ponceau[b] | | |
| Blue No. 1[b] | | Brilliant blue[b] | | |
| Blue No. 2[b] | | Indigotin[b] | | |
| [b] | Natural | Carmine[b] | Red | Derived from bodies of female cochineal insects (*Nopalea coccinellifera*), used to color liqueur Campari |
| [b] | Natural | Saffron[b] | Dark yellow–orange | Derived from crocus plant, used to color cheese, liqueur, sauces, soups, rice dishes, some cakes. |

[a] Based on Consumers Federation, Food Additives, 2nd edn., Consumers Federation Poland, Warsaw, 1999 (in Polish).
[b] Mentioned as additives associated with adverse reaction by Bosso and Simon 2008.

et al. (2008). Besides, the mechanism of additive-induced urticaria, angioedema, and anaphylaxis has been more thoroughly described by Bosso and Simon (2008), while general aspects regarding physiological mechanisms of the appearance of allergenic and nonallergenic hypersensitivity as well as medical aspects of food allergies are discussed in Chapter 1 and, in much greater detail, in the work of Brostoff and Challacombe (2002).

The presence of other components in a food product, from the point of view of an allergologist, requires deep knowledge of both allergies and technologies of food production (biotechnology) and food chemistry. It is so because of allergenic components that should be taken into consideration, both those that originate from specific allergenic characteristics of a main food product (see, the main chapters of this book) and the ones that occur as a result of intentional addition of substances or accidental contamination of a given food product.

## 14.4.3 SPICES: ADDITIVES ASSOCIATED WITH ADVERSE REACTION

Spices are well-known and popular additives to food, which improve the taste and flavor of food products. They are most often aromatic parts of plants (roots, leaves,

**TABLE 14.4.4**

**Preservatives Used as Food Additives, which may Trigger Symptoms of Nonallergic Hypersensitivity**

| E Number | Preservatives | Application |
|---|---|---|
| 200 | Sorbic acid | Acidity regulators. The main applications of E201–E203 are |
| 201 | Sodium sorbate | not determined. |
| 202 | Potassium sorbate | Sorbates (E200–E203) have been associated with the full |
| 203 | Calcium sorbate | range of food intolerance reactions |
| 210 | Benzoic acid | Benzoic acid used as a preservative in fish products, salads, |
| 211 | Sodium benzoate[a] | fruit juices, fats. It can enhance the allergic reaction. The |
| 212 | Potassium benzoate | main applications of E211–E213 are not determined. |
| 213 | Calcium benzoate | Benzoates (E211–E213) have been associated with the full |
| | | range of food intolerance reactions. |
| 214–219 | Esters and salts of (PHB) *p*-Hydroxybenzoic acid[a] | Used as a preservative in fish products, salads, and fruit and vegetable products. |
| 220 | Sulfur dioxide[a], sulfite anhydride | Used as a preservative and antioxidant in wines, dried fruits, and potato products. |
| 221 | Sodium sulfite[a] | Sulfites are the biggest threat to asthmatics. |
| 222 | Sodium hydrogen sulfite | Not to be confused with sulfates (514–519), |
| 223 | Sodium metabisulfite[a] | Also known as sulfites. |
| 224 | Potassium metabisulfite[a] | |
| 226 | Calcium sulfite | |
| 227 | Calcium bisulfite | |
| 228 | Potassium bisulfite | |
| 230 | Diphenyl | Food additive for the preservation against molds in, e.g., lemon and orange peels or in direct packages. It can trigger contact allergy. |
| 231 | *ortho*-Phenyl phenol | Application as that of E 230 |
| 239 | Hexamethylenetetramine | Used in stabilization of Provolone cheeses. |
| 280 | Propionic acid (and propionates) | Food additive for the preservation against molds in, e.g., cheese products, in bread, fruit, and vegetable products, |
| 281 | (Sodium propionate) | production of fruit flavors (It has been permitted in the EU |
| 282 | (Calcium propionate) | countries again since 1996.) |
| 283 | (Potassium propionate) | |

*Source:* Based on Consumers Federation, *Food Additives*, 2nd edn., Consumers Federation Poland, Warsaw, 1999 (in Polish).

[a] Mentioned as additives associated with adverse reaction by Bosso and Simon 2008.

flowers, bark, seed fruits, and buds) or plant components (oils, ethereal oils, and extracts). Some spices can be added to food or eaten directly (onion, garlic, cayenne pepper, and green pepper). Others are added in small quantities to foodstuff, which is why determination of their threshold levels (the lowest dose of an allergen needed to induce an allergenic reaction under controlled conditions) is not easy. Spices, like

## TABLE 14.4.5
## Other Food Additives Used as Agents Modifying Functional Properties which may Trigger Symptoms of Nonallergenic Hypersensitivity

| E Number | Food Additive | Application and Allergenic Hazard |
|---|---|---|
| 405 | Propylene glycol alginate | Concentrating agent, emulsifier, and foam stabilizer |
| 410 | Locust bean gum | Derived from Carob or Locust bean tree *Ceratonia siliqua.* |
| | | Concentrating and gelling agent. It is supposed to trigger the allergenic hypersensitivity. Used in lollies, cordials, essences, some flour products, dressings, fruit juice drinks, and as a caffeine-free chocolate substitute. |
| 412 | Guar gum | Concentrating and stabilizing agent. It is seldom supposed to trigger the allergic reaction. |
| 413 | Tragacanth | Concentrating agent. |
| 414 | Acacia, (gum arabic). | Concentrating and stabilizing agent, emulsifier derived from the sap of Acacia Senegal. |
| 417 | Tara gum | Thickener, concentrating and stabilizing agent from tara legume seeds. |
| 466 | Sodium carboxymethyl cellulose, | Naturally occurring thickener, concentrating and stabilizing agent. |
| 1105 | Lysozyme | Preservative and enzymatic preparation used in cheese production. |

*Source:* Based on Consumers Federation, *Food Additives*, 2nd edn., Consumers Federation Poland, Warsaw, 1999 (in Polish).

other raw foods, depending on an allergen-inducing agent (hapten or protein), may cause different disease symptoms originating from nonallergenic hypersensitivity reaction (e.g., skin or lips or oral mucosa). Contact with spices may result in irritant contact dermatitis and allergenic hypersensitive reaction (contact, and/or immediate or delayed allergy, systemic allergen contact dermatitis, contact urticaria, protein contact dermatitis, chemical photosensitivity reactions of phototoxic character, or photoallergic reactions) (Ale and Maibach 2000, Kanerva 2002, Kanerva et al. 1996, Niinimäki 1984, 2000, Niinimäki and Hannuksela 1981, van Bever et al. 1989).

In the International Classification of Diseases (ICD) coding, there are 21 diagnostic descriptions (codes) to characterize and classify food allergic reactions across Europe (Opinion of the Scientific Panel 2004). There are known cases of immediate allergy to spices, especially to allergens found in mustard, celery seeds, dill, caraway, anis, and paprika (Kanerva et al. 1996, Niinimäki 1981). Among vegetables, also used as spices, which can cause contact dermatitis (type IV allergy) are carrots, celeries, chicory, garlic, horseradish, and onion (Kanerva 2002).

It has been found out that patients with food allergy demonstrated as asthma tend to indicate a more severe disease constellation and more serious, life-threatening food allergenic reactions. It seems interesting that susceptible patients may even

**TABLE 14.4.6**

**Antioxidants and Oxidizers Used as Food Additives, which may Trigger Symptoms of Nonallergenic Hypersensitivity (See Also Table 14.4.1)**

|  | E Number | Food Additive | Application and Allergic Hazard |
|---|---|---|---|
| Antioxidants | 223 | Sodium metabisulfite | Synthetic preservative and antioxidant sulfites are the biggest threat to asthmatics |
|  | 224 | Potassium metabisulfite | Application as that of E223 |
|  | 310 | Propyl gallate | Antioxidant for use in margarine and peanut butter. It is suspected to trigger symptoms of hypersensitivity reaction |
|  | 311 | Octyl gallate | Antioxidant for use in margarine and peanut butter |
|  | 312 | Dodecyl gallate | Antioxidant for use in margarine and other food products |
|  | 320 | Butylated hydroxyanisole, BHA[a] | Application as that of E 310 |
|  | 321 | Butylated hydroxytoluene, BHT[a] | Application as that of E310 |
| Oxidizer |  | Ammonium persulfate | Flour color improver |
|  |  | Benzoyl peroxide | Oxidizer for use in bleaching oils and flours |

*Source:* Based on Consumers Federation, *Food Additives*, 2nd edn., Consumers Federation Poland, Warsaw, 1999 (in Polish).

[a]　Mentioned as additives associated with adverse reaction by Bosso and Simon 2008.

react to a causative food or additive on inhalation, without ingestion (Spergel and Fiedler 2005).

Among well-known spice allergens are diallyl disulfide and Allicin (garlic allergens, *Allium sativum*), eugol (nutmeg, cloves, and Jamaica pepper), cinnamic aldehyde (cinnamon), dipentene (caraway, cardamom, and spearmint), and linalool (basilica, coriander) (Kanerva 2002).

Other spices, too, for example, mustard, paprika, flour additives, and garlic (Dannaker and White 1987, Scholl and Jensen-Jarolim 2004) as well as many food products, such as milk proteins (casein), whey proteins (α-lactalbumin, β-lactoglobulin), and wheat proteins, which are not always obvious food ingredients (hidden ingredients) (Lopata and Potter 2000, Chapters 6 and 13), may cause adverse reactions.

Among the most popular spices and herbs used in food and food-related industries which are known to induce adverse reactions (oral allergy, rhinitis, dermatitis, and occupational asthma) are some aromatic herbs (Forrer et al. 2005, Lemière et al. 1996), garlic (Lybarger et al. 1982, Sikora et al. 2008), coriander, mace, ginger paprika (Hafner et al. 1992, van Toorenbergen and Dieges 1985), cinnamon (Malten 1979, Uragoda 1984,), ginseng (Lee et al. 2006), and curry (Hafner et al. 1992).

## Table 14.4.7
## Flavor Enhancers and Synthetic Flavoring Substances Used as Food Additives

| Group | E number CAS RN or Other Code | Food Additive |
|---|---|---|
| Flavor enhancers | 620 | L-Glutamic acid |
| | 621 | Monosodium L-glutamate (MSG)[a] |
| | 622 | Monopotassium L-glutamate |
| | 623 | Calcium L-diglutamate |
| | 624 | Monoamonium L-glutamate |
| | 625 | Magnesium L-diglutamate |
| Synthetic flavoring substances | 000075-07-0 | Acetalaldehyde |
| | 000513 86-182.60 | Acetoin |
| | 00049912-7 | Aconitic acid |
| | 004180-23-8 | Anethole (*trans*-anethole) |
| | 000100-52-7 | Benzaldehyde |
| | 000107-92-6 | *N*-Butyric acid (butyric acid) |
| | 000099-49-0 | D- or L-Carvone (carvone) |
| | 000104-55-2 | Cinnamaldehyde |
| | 005392-40-5 | Citral |
| | 000112-31-2 | Decanal |
| | 000431-03-8 | Diacetyl |
| | 000141-78-6 | Ethyl acetate |
| | 000105-54-4 | Ethyl butyrate |
| | | Ethyl vanilin |
| | 000097-53 | Eugenol |
| | 000106-24-1 | Geraniol |
| | 000105-87-3 | Geranyl acetate |
| | 000060-01-5 | Glycerol tributyrate |
| | 005989-27-5 | Limonene (D-limonene) |
| | 000078-70-6 | Linalool |
| | 000115-95-7 | Linalyl acetate |
| | 000617-48-1 | Malic acid |
| | 000134-20-3 | Methyl anthranilate |
| | 000077-83-8 | 3-Methyl-3-phenyl glycidic acid ethyl ester |
| | 000120-57-0 | Piperonal |
| | 000121-33-5 | Vanillin (E107) |

*Sources:* Based on Consumers Federation, *Food Additives*, Second edition, Consumers Federation Poland, Warsaw, 1999 (in Polish); Modified from Kanerva, L., Skin contact reactions to food and spices, In *Food Allergy and Intolerance*, Brostoff, J. and Challacombe, S.J., Eds., Saunders, London, Edinburgh, New York, Philadelphia, St Louis, Sydney, Toronto, 2002; EAFUS: A Food Additive Database—http://www.foodsafety.gov/~dms/eafus.html

[a]  Mentioned also as additives associated with adverse reaction by Bosso and Simon (2008).

Many other food ingredients, such as antioxidants, preservatives, flavors and colorings, and chemical additives, added during food processing, can also cause adverse reactions (McCann et al. 2007). Their addition to a food product is usually very small, which creates a problem when trying to determine their threshold levels. The suggested maximum doses for additives used in challenge protocols are 150 mg for aspartame, 250 mg for BHA/BHT, 2.5 g for MSG, 50 mg for nitrates/nitrites, 100 mg for parabens/benzoates, 100 mg for sulfites, and 50 mg for yellow dyes nos. 5 and 6 (Bosso and Simon 2008).

### 14.4.4 ANTIOXIDANTS ASSOCIATED WITH ADVERSE REACTIONS

Antioxidants make up a large group of food additives, as they can prevent spoilage of easily oxidizable substances (containing much fat or oil). Typical examples of antioxidants used as food additives are the synthetic antioxidants butylated hydroxyanisole (BHA) and butylated hydroxytoluene (BHT), widely used in packaged foods (Directive 2006/52/EC). It has been discovered that these antioxidants can cause adverse reaction in the upper and lower respiratory tract (not well documented), utricarial reactions (very common), and delayed hypersensitivity reactions (well documented) (Weber 2008a).

Some antioxidants (sulfites) are also used as bleaching agents (cherries, hominy, and pectins) and for the development of translucency (in lemon, orange, grapefruit, and citron peel). Sulfites are also applied (in a 10–100 ppm concentration) in the food industry for inhibition of unwanted microflora (in wines, corn wet-milling, and corn syrup), inhibition of nonenzymatic browning (dried fruits, potatoes, and other vegetables), inhibition of enzymatic browning (pre-peeled raw potatoes, some fruits, and vegetables), dough conditioning (frozen pie and pizza crust). Although sulfites are removed in further processes (especially thermal ones), they create a large threat, particularly to people suffering from asthma in whom they can induce attacks. Due to frequent hypersensitivity reactions to sulfites, they have been classified in the EU regulations as a major allergy-inducing food component (Directive 2003/89/EC 2003). Different laws apply to addition of sulfites to food products in different countries, for example, in the United States they are no longer used in beer production, whereas earlier they were applied to prevent undesirable, oxidative flavor changes. However, they are still used in meat processing (Taylor et al. 2008). Moreover, in the United States it is acceptable to use sulfites as food additives in order to extend shelf life of maize grains, light color of dried fruits, to halt "wild" fermentation of wines, to prevent development of undesirable microflora during fermentation, and in order to prevent oxidation of wine dyes.

Sulfite sensitivity primarily affects a relatively small subgroup of asthmatic population (Bosso and Simon 2008), Salicylates can also cause allergenic hypersensitivity reactions (Sainte-Laudy 2001).

### 14.4.5 PRESERVATIVES ASSOCIATED WITH ADVERSE REACTIONS

Preservatives are among the most widespread food additives, as they inhibit growth and development of bacteria and molds, thus extending the shelf life of food products. The way they affect the durability of food products is varied, for example, benzoates act by inhibiting enzymatic pathways of microorganisms and their spores. Many preservatives (Table 14.4.4), and particularly parabens (methylparaben and propylparaben), benzoates (benzoic acid and sodium benzoate), and sorbic acid, can cause allergic contact dermatitis, urtocaria, asthma, and angioedema (Fahrenholz and Smith 2008, Jacobson 1991, Rietschel and Flower 1995, Worm et al. 2000, 2001).

Disulfides, applied mainly as food and drink preservatives, are found in numerous products: bread additives, tea, sweets, seafood, jams, jellies, dried fruit and vegetables, fruit juices, vegetable preserves, potato powder, frozen potatoes, and soup concentrates may be a direct reason of nonallergenic hypersensitivity (Taylor et al. 2008).

There are known cases (albeit not many) of anaphylactic/anaphylactoid reactions to benzoates and parabens, although no systematic anaphylaxis has been observed after orally ingested parabens. Moreover, asthmatic reactions caused by benzoates and parabens have been reported (Fahrenholz and Smith 2008).

### 14.4.6 FLAVORING ADDITIVES ASSOCIATED WITH ADVERSE REACTIONS

Among flavorings and fragrances, which can be present in foodstuffs or occur during technological food processing and cause contact urticaria are benzaldehyde, benzoil acid (preservatives), cinnamon-based components (cassia—cinnamon oil, cinnamic acid, cinnamic aldehyde, menthol, and vanillin). Condiments and spices which may cause such reactions include cinnamon, cayenne pepper, caraway, coriander, curry, pepper (*Capsicum annum*), and thyme (Ale and Maibach 2000, Kanerva 2002, Malten 1979), synthetic or natural flavoring substances (Table 14.4.5), such as cinnamic aldehyde present as a cinnamon component, an additive to cakes and sweets, other flavorings and fragrances, flavors in ice creams, soft drinks, flavored beers, chewing gums, and toothpaste. Cinnamic aldehyde is one of the allergens responsible for contact dermatitis, especially among cooks, bakers, and candy makers (Kanerva 2002).

### 14.4.7 COLORINGS AS ADDITIVES ASSOCIATED WITH ADVERSE REACTIONS

Many natural and artificial colorings (especially the natural ones because of the character of the antigen), used as color improvers in food products can be associated with adverse reaction, including allergenic hypersensitivity (Bosso and Simon 2008) (Table 14.4.3). Adverse hyperactive behavioral changes in children have been documented as caused by excess amounts of artificial food colorings and sodium benzoate preservatives in the diet (Bateman et al. 2004).

In some countries, use of certain colorings has been limited as they can potentially cause adverse reaction. The European Union, for example, banned in 1996 the following colorings (with few exceptions): erythrosine E127 (since 1992 it has been allowed to be used only in fruit preservatives containing black cherries, at a maximum concentration of 150–200 mg/kg), canthaxanthine E161 (allowed only in Strasburg sausages, max. 15 mg/kg), tartrazine E102 (not allowed in cakes, sweets, ice creams, and hard cheeses in Poland).

Since 1976 amaranth dye (E123) has been banned in the United States, whereas in Poland it can be added to food, e.g., wines, spirits, and caviar.

The color of some kinds of wines and drinks (e.g., Campari wine and liqueur) can be enhanced by adding natural food dyes (carmine E120, cochineal red E124) or synthetic colorings (indigo carmine E132). It has been found out that all these food dyes can induce allergenic hypersensitivity reactions. Natural food dyes (extracts obtained from female cochineal insects—*Dactylopius coccus*) have been determined to contain allergenic proteins of a molecular weight of 23–88 kDa (Chung et al. 2001).

There are many scientific reports (although typically not recent ones) on tartrazine, azo, and non-azo dyes, which suggest that these colorings can cause adverse reactions (albeit not so frequently < 1%) (Nettis et al. 2003). There have been rare cases of urticaria or asthma developed after ingesting tartrazine or other azo dyes, but the relationship between the cause and illness symptoms is generally overestimated, as it is based on earlier studies (Nettis et al. 2003, Stevenson 2008, van Bever et al. 1989). It has also been identified that patent blue and carmine dye induced severe allergic reactions (Makinen-Kiljunen and Haahtela 2008).

In general, it is possible to notice highly different approaches in different countries to the use of food dyes associated with adverse reactions.

### 14.4.8  GLUTAMIC ACID AND MONOSODIUM GLUTAMATE

Glutamic acid is a substance obtained by fermentation or via chemical synthesis. It is also a natural food component present in proteins as a nonessential dicarboxylic amino acid (in Camembert cheeses it occurs in a concentration of about 1%). Glutamic acid enhances the taste of meals, condiments, soups, and sauces. Monosodium glutamate (MSG) is classified by the FDA as "generally recognized as safe" (GRAS). However, it is not recommended to consume too much of glutamic acid, or to eat it too often, due to ambiguous results of the relevant research, especially the ones regarding possible neurotoxicity and neuroendocrine effects. There are reports on very few cases (not clearly documented) of MSG-induced angioedema or urticaria in the literature (Woessner 2008). On the other hand, it has been demonstrated that MSG causes other than allergenic symptoms, such as headache, chest tightness, nausea, sweating, or a burning sensation along the back of the neck (Bosso and Simon 2008).

Many taste-improving substances (Table 14.4.5) can be a cause of undesirable responses or allergenic reactions, although such cases are rare.

### 14.4.9  OTHER IMPORTANT FOOD ADDITIVES ASSOCIATED
###            WITH ADVERSE REACTIONS

Although the list of food additives associated with adverse reactions is long, many researchers have suggested that only some allergenic reactions (like urticaria, angioedema, and anaphylaxis related to ingestion of food additives) are relatively common (as expressed as less than a percent of the general population) (Bosso and Simon 2008, Wüthrich 1993). Many of the data on this issue are rather dated (Malten 1979, Uragoda 1984, van Bever et al. 1989) or not well documented (Stevenson 2008).

Further Bateman comments critically on previous reports that suggested that artificial food additives such as coloring and benzoate preservatives are potentially linked to hyperactivity in children (Bateman et al. 2004).

In contrast, it seems that the number of allergies caused by food additives is underestimated due to diagnostic difficulties. Thus, it is recommendable to approach the use of food additives, especially those that have been indicated as causing adverse reactions, with great caution.

Among the food additives mentioned as associated with adverse reaction (most frequently dermatitis) are sodium metabisulfite (White et al. 1982), persulfate (Hafner et al. 1992), acetylsalicylic acid (Sainte-Laudy 2001), aspartame, sorbit acid, propyl gallate, dodecyl gallate, karaya gum (Sikora et al. 2008) (Tables 14.4.1 and 14.4.4).

Aspartame (a low calories sweetener) can also trigger urticaria (nettle rash), itchy hives, and swelling of the body (Bosso and Simon 2008).

The new additives allowed to be used in Australia (627—disodium guanylate, 631—disodium inosinate, and 635—disodium 5′-ribonucleotides) are associated with occurrence of skin rashes in hypersensitive persons (Table 14.4.2).

Yeast extract, hydrolyzed vegetable protein (HVP), and hydrolyzed plant protein (HPP) as natural additives are a way in which manufacturers include MSG without having to declare it on the label and for this reason they are a health threat created by hidden allergens. Baker's yeast (*Saccharomyces cerevisiae*), yeast preparation, and yeast extract which are widely used by the food industry as flavoring in, for example, powdered and readymade sauces and soups can develop multiple anaphylactic reactions after ingestion in mold-allergic patients (Airola et al. 2006).

The wide spectrum of the enzymes employed as (food) additives are increasingly used in food, feed, and biotechnology industry. Some of them ($\alpha$-amylase, $\beta$-amylase, and cellulase) are allergens known for their ability to induce skin and respiratory allergic symptoms (Quirce et al. 1992, Quirce and Sastre 1998, Vanhanen et al. 1996, 2001).

Another group of additives which participate in causing allergenic and nonallergenic hypersensitivity response are lecithin and gums, which are classified as emulsifiers and stabilizers.

Lecithin is typically made from soybeans and eggs and therefore may contain allergenic proteins originating from the aforementioned raw materials. Reactions to soy lecithin are rare, even in soy-allergic people, since the level of this additive is usually very low in most foods. Likewise, oils (especially cold pressed ones) may contain trace amounts of proteins from the raw materials they are produced from.

Gums (guar, tragacanth, xanthan, carrageenan, acacia (Arabic), and locust bean) are generally known to cause allergenic reactions when present in foods (Table 14.4.5). Many of these gums are known to worsen asthma, particularly in the occupational setting, when airborne. It has been identified that macrogol induced severe allergic reactions (Makinen-Kiljunen and Haahtela 2008). Also two cases of anaphylaxis to Macrogol 6000 (polyethylene glycol) after ingestion drug tablets was observed by Hyry et al. (2006).

In addition, two cases of anaphylaxis to Macrogol 6000 (polyethylene glycol) after ingestion drug tablets was observed (Hyry et al. 2006).

A serious threat to health, also in persons who are not hypersensitive to allergens, is created by antibiotics present in food products. It has been confirmed that penicillin in particular as well as other antibiotics of the group of $\beta$-lactams (penicillins, cephalosporins, and four smaller ones: monobactams, carbapenems, oxacephems, and clavams) have very strong immunogenic properties. Within β-lactam antibiotics strong cross reaction has been demonstrated between

- Penicillin and cephalosporins
- Penicillin and carbapenems
- Cephalosporins and monobactams

In the food chain, antibiotics can originate from animal fodder or from animals previously treated with penicillin, which are finally used to obtain foodstuffs: cow milk or eating meat, eggs, and fish. Allergy caused by penicillin is relatively frequent as it is estimated to strike 1%–10% of the general population. The most frequent symptoms of allergy to antibiotics are urticaria, erythema, asthma, and Quincke's oedema. A systemic response such as anaphylactic shock is less common. Ninety-five percent of mild allergenic reactions are mainly caused by the main chemical chain (β-lactam and trazolidin rings). The side-chain which implicated far less often: about 5% anaphylactic shock cases.

The mechanism of allergenic effect produced by antibiotics, which are low molecular weight compounds, is similar to that of other haptens (see Chapter 1). Antibiotics are able to react between β-lactam ring and amino groups of protein, forming immunogenic conjugates which can induce production of antibodies and, consequently, evoking an immunological reaction of an organism.

### 14.4.10 CONCLUSIONS

Many studies, both older (often though to be poorly documented) and newer ones (e.g., Bosso and Simon 2008) suggest that many food additives may cause adverse reaction such as allergenic and nonallergenic hypersensitivity (hyperactivity, vaso-motor swelling of labia, eyelid, foot, and hand). Thus, we must not neglect the risk of potentially negative effect of food additives on human health. More detailed research, especially on molecular mechanisms causing allergic hypersensitivity reactions, is needed. The research should be supported by analytical and technological methods as well as clinical diagnostics.

### REFERENCES

Airola, K., Petman, L., and Mäkinen-Kiljunen, S. 2006. Clustered sensitivity to fungi: Anaphylactic reactions caused by ingestive allergy to yeasts. *Ann Allergy Asthma Immunol* 97(3): 294–297.

Ale, S.I. and Maibach, H.I. 2000. Occupational contact urticaria. In: *Handbook of Occupational Dermatology*, L., Kanerva, P., Elsner, J.E., Wahlberg, and H.I. Maibach, Eds., pp. 200–216. Springer-Verlag, Berlin, Heidelberg, New York.

Baldwin, J.L., Chou, A.H., and Solomon, W.B. 1997. Popsicle-induced anaphylaxis due to carmine dye allergy. *Ann Allergy Asthma Immunol* 79: 415–419.

Bateman, B., Warner, J.O., Hutchinson, E. et al. 2004. The effects of a double blind, placebo controlled, artificial food colourings and benzoate preservative challenge on hyperactivity in a general population sample of preschool children. *Arch Dis Childhood* 89: 506–511.

Bosso, J.V. and Simon, R.A. 2008. Urticaria, angiodema, and anaphylaxis provoked by food and drug additives. In: *Food Allergy. Adverse Reactions to Foods and Food Additives*, 4th ed., D.D. Metcalfe, H.A. Sampson, and R.A. Simon, Eds., pp. 340–352. Blackwell Publishing, New York.

Brostoff, J. and Challacombe, S.J. 2002. *Food Allergy and Intolerance*, 2nd ed. Saunders, London/Edinburgh/New York/Philadelphia/St Louis/Sydney/Toronto.

Bush, R.K. and Montalbano, M.M. 2008. Asthma and food additives. In: *Food Allergy. Adverse Reactions to Foods and Food Additives*, 4th ed., D.D. Metcalfe, H.A. Sampson, and R.A. Simon, Eds., pp. 335–339. Blackwell Publishing, New York.

Chung, K., Baker, J.R., Baldwin, J.L., and Chou, A. 2001. Identification of carmine allergens among three carmine allergy patients. *Allergy* 56(1): 73–77.

Codex Alimentarius Commission. 1979. Guide to the Safe Use of Food additives.

Commission Directive 2006/142/EC of 22 December 2006 amending Annex IIIa of Directive 2000/13/EC of the European Parliament and of the Council listing the ingredients which must under all circumstances appear on the labeling of foodstuffs. *Official Journal of the European Union*. L 368/110 EN. 23.12.2006.

Consumers Federation, 1999. *Food Additives*, 2nd ed. Consumers Federation Poland, Warsaw (in Polish).

Council Directive of December 21, 1988 on the approximation of the laws of the Member States concerning food additives authorized for use in foodstuffs intended for human consumption. (89/107/EEC) 1989L0107—EN—10.09.1994—001.001

Dannaker, C.J. and White, I.R. 1987. Cutaneous allergy to mustard in a salad maker. *Contact Dermatitis* 16: 212–214.

David, T.J. 1993. *Food and Food Additive Intolerance in Childhood*. Blackwell Scientific Publications, Oxford.

Directive 2003/89/EC of the European Parliament and of the Council of November 10, 2003 (amending Directive 2000/13/EC as regards indication of the ingredients present in foodstuffs. *Official Journal of the European Union* L 308/15, 25.11.2003.

Directive 2006/52/EC of the European Parliament and of the Council of July 5, 2006 amending Directive 95/2/EC on food additives other than colors and sweeteners and Directive 94/35/EC on sweeteners for use in foodstuffs. *Official Journal of the European Union*. L 204/10.

EAFUS: A Food Additive Database, http://www.foodsafety.gov/-dms/eafus.html

Fahrenholz, J.M. and Smith, K.M. 2008. Adverse reaction to benzoates and parabens. In: *Food Allergy. Adverse Reactions to Foods and Food Additives*, 4th ed., D.D. Metcalfe, H.A. Sampson, and R.A. Simon, Eds., pp. 394–402. Blackwell Publishing, New York.

Fleischer, D.M. and Leung, D.Y.M. 2008. Eczema and food hypersensitivity. In: *Food Allergy. Adverse Reactions to Foods and Food Additives*, 4th ed., D.D. Metcalfe, H.A. Sampson, R.A. Simon, Eds., pp. 110–123. Blackwell Publishing, New York.

Forrei, A., Marco, F.M., Andreu, C., and Sempere, J.M. 2005. Occupational asthma to carmine in a butcher. *Int Arch Allergy Immunol* 138: 243–250.

Hafner, J., Riess, C.E., and Wuthrich, B. 1992. Protein contact dermatitis from paprika and curry in Cook. *Contact Dermatitis* 26: 51–52.

Hyry, H., Vuorio, A., Varjonen, E., Skyttä, J., and Mäkinen-Kiljunen, S. 2006. Two cases of anaphylaxis to Macrogol 6000 after ingestion of drug tablets. *Allergy* 61(8): 1021.

Jacobson, D.W. 1991. Adverse reaction to benzoates and parabens. In: *Food Allergy. Adverse Reactions to Food and Food Additives*. D.D. Metcalfe and H.A. Sampson, Eds., pp. 276–287. Blackwell Scientific, Boston, MA.

Kanerva, L. 2002. Skin contact reactions to food and spices. In: *Food Allergy and Intolerance*, 2nd ed., J. Brostoff and S.J. Challacombe, Eds., pp. 631–645. Saunders, London.

Kanerva, L., Estlander, T., and Jolanki, R. 1996. Occupational allergic contact dermatitis from spices. *Contact Dermatitis* 35: 157–162.

Lee, J.V., Lee, Y.D. Bahn, J.W., and Park, H.S. 2006. A case of occupational asthma and rhinitis caused by Sanyak and Korean ginseng dust. *Allergy* 61: 392–393.

Lemière, C., Cartier, A., Lehrer, S.B., and Malo, H. 1996. Occupational asthma caused by aromatic herbs. *Allergy* 51: 647–649.

Lopata, A.L. and Potter, P.C. 2000. Allergy and other adverse reactions to seafood. *Allergy Clin Immunol Int* 12(6): 271–281.

Lybarger, J.A., Gallagher, J.S., Pulver, D.W. et al.1982. Occupational asthma by inhalation and ingestion of garlic. *J Allergy Ciln Immunol* 69: 448–454.

Madsen, C. 1997. Chemicals in food and allergy: Fact and fiction. *Environ Toxicol Pharmacol* 4(1–2): 115–120.

Makinen-Kiljunen, S. and Haahtela, T. 2008. Eight years of severe allergic reactions in Finland: A register-based report. *World Allergy Org J* 1(11): 184–189.

Malten, K.E. 1979. Four bakers showing positive patch-tests to a number of fragrance materials, which can also be used as flavors. *Acta Derm Venereol Suppl* 59: 117–121.

McCann, D., Barrett, A., Cooper et al. 2007. Food additives and hyperactive behaviour in 3-year-old and 8/9-year-old children in the community: A randomised, double-blinded, placebo-controlled trial. *Lancet* 370(9598): 1560–1567.

McFadden, J., White, J.M.L., Basketter, D., and Kimber, I. 2008. Reduced allergy rates in atopic eczema to contact allergens used in both skin products and foods: Atopy and the "hapten-atopy hypothesis." *Contact Dermatitis* 58(3): 156–158.

Metcalfe, D.D., Sampson, H.A., and Simon, R.A., Eds. 2008. *Food Allergy. Adverse Reactions to Foods and Food Additives*, 4th ed. Blackwell Publishing Ltd., New York.

Nettis, E., Colanardi, M.C., Ferrannini, A., and Tursi, A. 2003. Suspected tartrazine induced acute urticaria/angiodema is only rarely reproduced by oral rechallenge. *Clin Exp Allergy* 33: 1725–1729.

Niinimäki, A. 1984. Delayed-type allergy to spices. *Contact Dermatitis* 11: 34–40.

Niinimäki, A. 2000. Spices. In: *Handbook of Occupational Dermatology*, L. Kanerva, P. Elsner, J.E. Wahlberg, and H.I. Maibach, Eds., pp. 767–770. Springer-Verlag, Berlin/Heidelberg/New York.

Niinimäki, A. and Hannuksela, M. 1981. Immediate skin test reactions to spices. *Allergy* 36: 487–493.

Opinion of the Scientific Panel on Dietetic Products, Nutrition and Allergies on a request from the Commission relating to the evaluation of allergic foods for labeling purposes. (Request N° EFSA-Q-2003-016). 2004. *The EFSA Journal* 32: 1–197.

Quirce, S., Cuevas, M., DiezGomez, M., FernandezRivas, M., Hinojosa, M., Gonzalez, R., and Losada, E. 1992. Respiratory allergy to *Aspergillus*-derived enzymes in bakers' asthma. *J Allergy Clin Immunol* 90: 970–978.

Quirce, S. and Sastre, J. 1998.Occupational asthma. *Allergy* 53: 633–641.

Rietschel, R.L. and Flower, J.F. 1995. *Fisher's Contact Dermatitis*. Williams and Wilkins, Baltimore, MD.

Sainte-Laudy, J. 2001. Acetylsalicylic acid: Hypersensitivity, intolerance, or allergy? *Allergy Immunol (Paris)* 33(3): 120–126.

Scholl, I. and Jensen-Jarolim, E. 2004. Allergenic potency of spices: Hot, medium hot, or very hot. *Int Arch Allergy Immunol* 135(3): 247–261.

Sikora, M., Cartier, A., Aresery, M. et al. 2008. Occupational reactions to food allergens. In: *Food Allergy. Adverse Reactions to Foods and Food Additives*, 4th ed., D.D. Metcalfe, H.A. Sampson, R.A. Simon, Eds., pp. 223–250. Blackwell Publishing, New York.

Spergel, J.M. and Fiedler, J. 2005. Food allergy and additives: Triggers in asthma. *Immunol Allergy Clin North Am* 25(1): 49–67.

Stevenson, D.D. 2008. Tartrazine, azo, and non-azo dyes. In: *Food Allergy. Adverse Reactions to Foods and Food Additives*, 4th ed., D.D. Metcalfe, H.A. Sampson, and R.A. Simon, Eds., pp. 377–385. Blackwell Publishing, New York.

Taylor, S.L., Bush, R.K., and Nordlee, J.A. 2008. Sulfites. In: *Food Allergy. Adverse Reactions to Foods and Food Additives*, 4th ed., D.D. Metcalfe, H.A. Sampson, and R.A. Simon, Eds., pp. 353–368. Blackwell Publishing, New York.

Tuormaa, T.E.T. 1994. The adverse effects of food additives on health: A review of the literature with special emphasis on childhood hyperactivity. (Booklet). *J Orthomolec Med* 9(4): 225–243.

Uragoda, C.G. 1984. Asthma and other symptoms in cinnamon workers. *Br J Ind Med* 41: 224–227.

van Bever, H.P., Docx, M., and Stevens, W.J. 1989. Food and food additives in severe atopic dermatitis. *Allergy* 44(8): 588–594.

Vanhanen, M., Tuomi, T., Hokkanen, H., Tupasela, O., Tuomainen, A., Holmberg, P.C., Leisola, M., and Nordman, H. 1996. Enzyme exposure and enzyme sensitisation in the baking industry. *Occup Environ Med* 53(10): 670–676.

Vanhanen, M., Tuomi, T., Tiikkainen, U., Tupasela, O., Tuomainen, A., Luukkonen, R., and Nordman, H. 2001. Sensitisation to enzymes in the animal feed industry. *Occup Environ Med* 58(2): 119–123.

van Hengel, A.J. 2007. Declaration of allergens on the label of food products purchased on the European market. *Trends Food Sci Technol* 18(2): 96–100.

van Toorenbergen, A.W. and Dieges, P.H. 1985. Immunoglobulin E antibodies against coriander and other spices. *J Allergy Clin Immunol* 76: 477–481.

Weber, R.W. 2008a. Adverse reactions to the antioxidants butylated hydroxyanisole (BHA) and butylated hydroxytoluene (BHT). In: *Food Allergy. Adverse Reactions to Foods and Food Additives*, 4th ed., D.D. Metcalfe, H.A. Sampson, and R.A. Simon, Eds., pp. 386–393. Blackwell Publishing, Malden, MA/Oxford, U.K.

Weber, R.W. 2008b. Neurological reactions to foods and foods additives. In: *Food Allergy. Adverse Reactions to Foods and Food Additives*, 4th ed., D.D. Metcalfe, H.A. Sampson, and R.A. Simon, Eds., pp. 531–542. Blackwell Publishing, Malden, MA/Oxford, U.K.

White, I.R., Catchpole, H.E., and Rycroft, R.J. 1982. Rashes amongst persulphate workers. *Contact Dermatitis* 8: 168–172.

Woessner, K.M. 2008. Monosodium glutamate. In: *Food Allergy. Adverse Reactions to Foods and Food Additives*, 4th ed., D.D. Metcalfe, H.A. Sampson, and R.A. Simon, Eds., pp. 369–376. Blackwell Publishing, New York.

Worm, M., Ehlers, I., Sterry, W. et al. 2000. Clinical relevance of food additives in adult patients with atopic dermatitis. *Clin Exp Allergy* 30: 407–414.

Worm, M., Vieth, W., Ehlers, I. et al. 2001. Increased leukotriene production by food additives in patients with atopic dermatitis and proven food intolerance. *Clin Exp Allergy* 31: 265–273.

Wüthrich, B. 1993. Adverse reactions to food additives. *Ann Allergy* 71(4): 379–384.

# 15 Risk Analysis of Food Allergens

*Marielle Spanjersberg, Niels Lucas Luijckx,*
*and Geert Houben*

## CONTENTS

## 15.1  INTRODUCTION

Risk analysis is the process of identifying hazards, assessing the risk of these hazards, identifying management options to reduce risks, weighing these, choosing and implementing risk reduction measures, and communication of existing or potential risks. This process has been developed for chemical, physical, or biological hazards in or of food in general. For allergens, this process seemed less suitable until recently, because there was no sound risk assessment method. In this chapter, new developments are described allowing a clear risk analysis strategy for allergens in food (Figure 15.1). The structure of this chapter is based on the successive steps given in Figure 15.1.

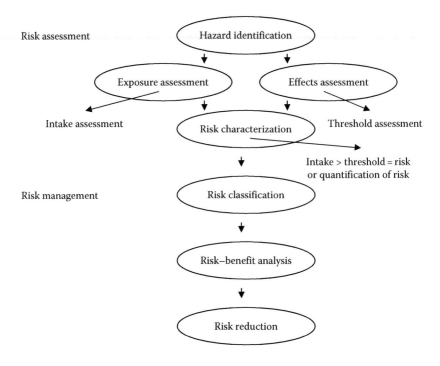

Risk assessment

Hazard identification

Exposure assessment

Effects assessment

Intake assessment

Risk characterization

Threshold assessment

Intake > threshold = risk
or quantification of risk

Risk management

Risk classification

Risk–benefit analysis

Risk reduction

Risk communication

**FIGURE 15.1**  Steps in the risk analysis process of food allergens.

## 15.2  RISK ASSESSMENT

Risk assessment is an empirically based process that estimates the risk of adverse health effects from exposure of an individual or population to a chemical, physical, or biological agent or property. The health risk assessment process involves the following steps: hazard identification, effects assessment (dose–response assessment), exposure assessment, and risk characterization (Van Leeuwen and Vermeire 2007).

### 15.2.1  Hazard Identification

A hazard is the inherent capacity of a substance to cause adverse effects in man or the environment under the conditions of exposure. In the area of food allergy, the hazard is a protein able to cause sensitization and, upon new exposure, an allergic reaction in subjects susceptible to that specific allergen. Food allergy often occurs due to food products that constitute important nutritional sources to man. Besides, we do not have much information on risk factors for the development of sensitization. Intervention strategies to prevent sensitization (the development of food allergy) thus are not feasible and practical yet. Management strategies for food allergy, therefore, mainly focus on the prevention and control of allergic reactions in sensitized subjects. In this chapter, risk analysis for the sensitization phase is therefore not further addressed and the chapter is restricted to considerations on risk assessment and risk management in the effect elicitation phase of food allergy.

Hazard is distinguished from risk: a substance that is toxic to humans is indeed a hazard but is not a risk as long as no human exposure occurs. If a hazard has been identified, the next steps of risk assessment become important.

## 15.2.2 Effects Assessment (Dose–Response Assessment)

In the effects assessment step the relationship between the level of exposure and the incidence, nature, and severity of an (adverse) effect following the exposure is determined. For most types of effects, it is assumed that there is a minimum dose or concentration below which adverse effects will not occur: the no effect level or threshold. To determine the threshold, different doses are tested, for most chemical hazards usually in laboratory animals. In toxicology, the highest tested dose without adverse effects is called the no observed adverse effect level (NOAEL). Based on the NOAEL established in an experimental study, a human limit value can be calculated, taking into account uncertainties and differences in experimental design and circumstances. Uncertainties and differences are accounted for by uncertainty factors (e.g., for interspecies differences, intraspecies variability, and exposure duration). For some types of substances, it is assumed that every level of exposure can result in adverse effects, in which case no threshold would exist. This, for instance, is assumed to apply for genotoxic carcinogens.

For food allergens, validated animal models for dose–response assessment are not available and human studies (double-blind placebo-controlled food challenges [DBPCFCs]) are the standard way to establish thresholds. It is practically impossible to establish the real population thresholds this way. Such population threshold can be estimated, but this is associated with major statistical and other uncertainties of low dose-extrapolation and patient recruitment and selection. As a matter of fact, uncertainties are of such order of magnitude that a reliable estimate of population thresholds is currently not possible. The result of the dose–response assessment can also be described as a threshold distribution rather than a single population threshold. Such distribution can effectively be used in probabilistic modeling as a tool in quantitative risk assessment (see Section 15.2.5)

## 15.2.3 Exposure Assessment

Exposure assessment determines the nature and extent of the exposure to a substance under varying conditions. In food allergy, this step requires information of the allergen concentration in the food and the rate of consumption of this type of food product. Uncertainty with respect to the exposure due to limited information and restrictions in the applied models and methods should be taken into consideration.

## 15.2.4 Risk Characterization

Risk characterization integrates the information derived from the effects assessment and the exposure assessment. If the exposure level is higher than the NOAEL (or LOED or the threshold), the conclusion is that there might be a health risk.

Traditionally, risk characterization is based on a deterministic approach, meaning that the risk is based on a point estimate, usually the worst case value for each input variable (worst-case NOAELs, assessment factors, and exposure levels). This worst-case approach is intended to ensure that even the most sensitive part of the population is protected under all conditions, and therefore generally overestimates the health risk. In the case of food allergens, the maximum consumption of a food may be multiplied by the maximum concentration of the allergen in this food. This results in the maximum estimate of the intake of the allergen. If this intake is higher than the lowest threshold observed, a possible reaction to the allergen cannot be ruled out.

For food allergens, a deterministic risk assessment will in many cases result in a conclusion that an allergic reaction in the most sensitive subjects cannot be excluded. However, there is no indication of the proportion of the population that might be at risk. Risk management interventions to reduce the risk will often require a major effort without reducing the risk completely down to zero. Without tools for quantifying the risks, a cost–benefit assessment for such risk management interventions can be made neither. The result of a deterministic risk assessment therefore often leads to inconclusive information. Therefore, there is a great need for quantitative information on the risks of allergens in food.

## 15.2.5  QUANTITATIVE RISK ASSESSMENT

In order to quantify the risk of food allergens, a method based on probabilistic techniques has been developed by TNO (Spanjersberg et al. 2007, Kruizinga et al. 2008).

In a probabilistic risk assessment, both variability and uncertainty in input variables can be taken into consideration. Variability represents the true heterogeneity in time, space, and of different members of a population. Examples of variability are interindividual variability in consumption and in sensitivity to, for instance, an allergen. Uncertainty is a lack of knowledge about the true value of the quantity. An example of uncertainty is associated with the limit of detection of an analytical method and the exploration of the threshold value outside the range of measurements. In contrast to the variability, uncertainty can be decreased, for example, by increasing the number of data points or using a more accurate method of analysis.

Both variability and uncertainty in threshold and exposure data can be taken into account by using probability distributions to represent the input variables instead of point estimates. The data are plotted in a cumulative distribution curve. For example, threshold data and intake data can be plotted as probability distributions. By combining the threshold distribution and the intake distribution, the output distribution will describe the probability that a part of the population will be exposed at such levels and under such circumstances that adverse effects may occur. Consequently, an approximation of the percentage of the population likely to experience adverse effects at various exposure levels can be made.

The schematic presentation (Figure 15.2) clearly shows the key characteristic of the probabilistic risk assessment approach: wherein worst-case modeling a point estimate (either a maximum or a mean) is chosen as the value for the input variable, in probabilistic modeling a data distribution is used.

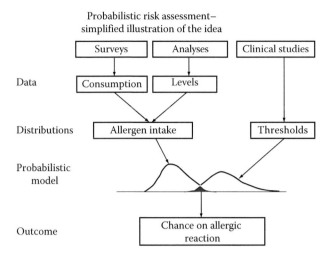

FIGURE 15.2   Schematic presentation of the probabilistic approach in food allergen risk assessment. (From Spanjersberg, M.Q.I. et al., *Food Chem. Toxicol.*, 45(1), 49, 2007. With permission.)

### 15.2.5.1   Probabilistic Modeling: How Does It Work?

The required data distributions (allergen concentration distribution in the product, product consumption distribution in the population, and allergen threshold distribution of a corresponding allergic population) are entered as specific statistical data distributions in a particular computer program that draws nonselected samples from these distributions. It thus repeatedly selects combinations of allergen intakes and thresholds: if the allergen intake exceeds the threshold, the result is recorded as an "allergic response" whereas an allergen intake lower than the threshold drawn leads to "no allergic response." This process is repeated numerous times (iterations). The percentage of expected allergic responses is determined. The above procedure is repeated for several times (runs) and the statistical characteristics of the distribution of the 25 percentages of allergic responses are calculated.

### 15.2.5.2   Prediction per Type of Allergic Response

In well-performed food challenge studies, the individual allergic reactions per dose are documented. Grouping the type of reaction, for instance distinction between subjective and objective allergic reactions, results in different threshold distributions, in this case a distribution for subjective and objective reactions, respectively (Figure 15.3).

Subjective symptoms (for instance, itch, nausea, abdominal pain, and dizziness) can only be reported by the subject being challenged and often occur at lower doses in comparison to objective reactions (e.g., urticaria, vomiting, diarrhea, and skin effects) that may occur with increasing doses and which can be verified independently by an outside observer. Other distinctions can be made as well, for instance oral effects, skin effects, gastrointestinal effects, etc.

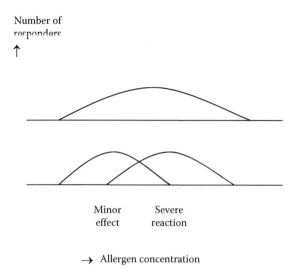

FIGURE 15.3    Distinction of the threshold distribution into type and/or severity.

Using these itemized distributions in the probabilistic model makes prediction of the type and/or severity of the expected allergic response in the population possible.

### 15.2.5.3    An Example of Quantitative Allergen Risk Assessment

A cow's milk protein allergic patient experienced an unexpected allergic reaction to dark chocolate sprinkles that contained no milk protein according to the packaging. Analysis of the concerning sample revealed the presence of milk protein, which explained the reaction of the patient. Since dark chocolate is known to be regularly cross-contaminated with cow's milk protein, due to the production of milk chocolate products in the same production line as the dark counterparts, the following question is raised: is the milk protein contamination level of unlabeled dark chocolate sprinkles to be considered a problem to the milk allergic population and if so, to which extent?

In order to investigate the potential problem, the concentrations of milk protein of the suspected sample, other batches of the same brand, and several other brands were determined. Together with appropriate milk protein threshold data (from a DBPCFC performed with cow's milk protein in adult milk allergic patients [Lam et al. submitted]) and consumption data of chocolate sprinkles (from a large-scale food consumption survey [Hulshof et al. 2004]), the risk of allergic reactions within the milk allergic population has been determined by using quantitative probabilistic risk assessment. The individual concentrations of the analyzed samples and the corresponding risks are shown in Figure 15.4. Obviously, with higher contamination level, the more persons are expected to respond.

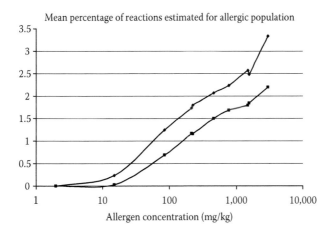

**FIGURE 15.4** Percentages of the milk protein allergic population expected to experience an allergic reaction after consuming unlabeled dark chocolate sprinkles (based on the calculated risks belonging to the individual samples analyzed). Upper curve: males, lower curve: females. Based on the milk protein concentrations of 10 samples from packagings not labeled as "may contain milk protein." Calculated using probabilistic modeling, 25 runs of 10,000 iterations for each simulation, process computerized in SAS.

## 15.3 RISK MANAGEMENT

Risk management is the part of the process where characterized risks are evaluated against options to reduce or avoid them. In general, aspects other than science (for instance cost, social responsibility, and (consumer) risk perception) are taken into account here.

The risk management process may involve the following steps: risk classification, risk-benefit analysis of risk reduction options, implementation of risk reduction measures, and monitoring these measures (Van Leeuwen and Vermeire 2007).

For allergen cross-contamination, no official regulation or guidance exists so industry depends on its own risk analysis or consultancy to set risk management options.

### 15.3.1 RISK CLASSIFICATION

In order to make justified risk management decisions, the first step is to classify the risks. This is often not an easy task. There is a balance between acceptability of a risk (both socially and regulatory based) and the chance that it occurs. In the case of allergen cross-contamination, this latter aspect is a crucial factor as risk management often focuses on reduction of the chance rather than avoidance.

If regulatory-based risk acceptability exists, the risk management process becomes easier and the focus is then on regulatory compliance. However, for allergen cross-contamination, no regulatory or policy guidelines exist (see Section 15.4).

Therefore, risk management decisions are currently based on common sense, a thorough analysis of the food production process, and the risk of the allergen as perceived by the company. Driven by fear for (legal) claims there may be a tendency to use a disclaimer (for instance "may contain") on the label when the chance of cross-contamination is realistic (Hefle et al. 2007). These disclaimers are not always based on sound risk analysis.

Based on knowledge of chance and effect (risk characterization), a first risk classification can be made. This will offer some insight into the priorities on risk avoidance or reduction, but it might leave a number of risks open for further risk analysis. Risk communication through the label or by other means then might become necessary.

### 15.3.2 RISK-BENEFIT ANALYSIS OF RISK REDUCTION OPTIONS

In the end, a food producing company will weigh all possible measures and consequences in a rough or more advanced costs–benefits assessment. Costs include the risk of liability claims. The benefit of reducing a risk is very difficult to quantify. Besides, constant monitoring is often required, so some extra cost will always remain. Without regulatory criteria, risk reduction is left to the companies' responsibility and standards. It is impossible within the scope of this chapter to address all aspects and factors to assess in a risk–benefit analysis of risk reduction options. However, since monitoring is a constant cost factor after implementation, we will illustrate how the probabilistic risk assessment described previously may also help in deciding about analytical techniques.

In Figure 15.5, an illustrative example is given. Further development of more sensitive analytical methods in the lower part of the concentration range does not

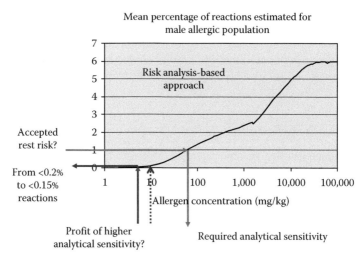

**FIGURE 15.5** Illustration of the use of probabilistic risk assessment data to decide on analytical performance.

automatically result in a relevant improvement in monitoring health risks (in red). The required analytical sensitivity can be estimated on the basis of an acceptable risk level (in green).

### 15.3.3  RISK REDUCTION

Risk reduction is often not a choice but simply required. Basically there are three risk management options: carry/accept the risk, transfer the risk (for instance insurance, but also labeling a disclaimer can be considered as a transfer of risk), or avoid or reduce the risk.

Avoidance is more or less the ultimate risk reduction strategy, but in practice this is most often impossible or unfeasible. Avoidance in the case of cross-contamination with food allergens means either dedicated location for production or stopping the use of the allergen in all products. However, this implies thorough chain control of cross-contamination in incoming goods and ingredients.

Good risk management requires good information management and implies thorough knowledge of products, processes, specifications of ingredients, and the (supply) chain, but most of all training and maintaining people in their work, awareness, and behavior.

For food allergen cross-contamination, several important risk reduction strategies are not difficult to list, and include

- Choosing ingredients and suppliers carefully
- Physical/building measures, including process design and production line design
- Storage management
- Careful planning of production
- Specified cleaning procedures

Other possible risk management measures range from control of recipes and specifications, awareness of the reuse of intermediate products in production (rework), and, in the case of carry over through the production line, discarding the first amount of product.

## 15.4  RISK COMMUNICATION (ALLERGEN DECLARATION AND PRECAUTIONARY LABELING)

The prevention of allergic reactions due to (hidden) allergens in food products is a matter of collective responsibility between authorities, food producers, and allergic consumers. There should be a balance between realistic and clear labeling of cross-contamination, patients' awareness of the risk for themselves, and possible other ways of communication by food producers directly to target groups.

As only strict avoidance of food allergens can prevent an allergic reaction, the allergic consumer relies on the allergy information on the packaging. Declaration of certain allergenic ingredients and products thereof used as ingredients, independent of the amounts used, is obligatory and clearly defined in EU legislation (directives 2003/89/EC and 2005/26/EC).

But an allergen can also be present due to cross-contamination, for instance if a production line cannot be cleaned completely after producing an allergen-containing product. In such cases, precautionary "may contain" labeling alerts to the possible presence of allergens. However, a directive or guidance for "may contain" labeling does not exist. Food industry therefore cannot rely on legal concentration levels that indicate when a product should be labeled in a precautionary way.

At present, many producers choose to label products in order to prevent insurance claims even if the chance of contamination and/or the potential health impact are negligible. In most EU countries, liability legislation and practice in court would probably require that a company demonstrates it has shown due diligence in reducing the risk before the disclaimer is accepted in court as such. Besides, precautionary labeling also leads to unnecessary limitation of consumer choice and devaluation of the allergen labeling information (Health Council of the Netherlands (GR) 2007). On the other hand, many products without precautionary labeling fill the shelves that indeed contain allergens as a cross-contamination, as shown by a recent survey of the Dutch Food and Consumer Product Safety Authority (VWA 2007).

Only in situations where cross-contamination is likely and/or when serious health risks are expected, "may contain" labeling should be adopted (Hefle et al. 2007). It is obvious that there is a need for more guidance on threshold levels and acceptability of risks.

In order to achieve uniform, transparent, and reliable allergy information on the label, quantitative risk assessment can be applied to set concentration levels for each major allergen and for different product categories that determine whether a product should be labeled precautionary or not.

## ACKNOWLEDGEMENTS

The authors would like to acknowledge Astrid Kruizinga and Monique Rennen for their contribution and editorial support.

## REFERENCES

Dutch Food and Consumer Product Safety Authority (Voedsel en Waren Autoriteit, VWA). Onderzoek naar de declaratie van allergenen op levensmiddelen. July 2007 [Report in Dutch].

Health Council of the Netherlands (Gezondheidsraad, GR). Voedselallergie. Report No. 2007/07 March 2007 [Report in Dutch].

Hefle, S.L., Furlong, T.J., Niemann, L., Lemon-Mule, H., Sicherer, S., and Taylor, S.L. 2007. Consumer attitudes and risks associated with packaged foods having advisory labeling regarding the presence of peanuts. *Journal of Allergy and Clinical Immunology* 120(1): 171–176.

Hulshof, K.F.A.M., Ocké, M.C., Van Rossum, C.T.M., Buurma-Rethans, E.J.M., Brants, H.A.M., Drijvers, J.J.M.M., and Ter Doest, D. 2004. Results of the Food Consumption Survey 2003. RIVM report 35003000/2004, TNO report V6000, [Report in Dutch].

Kruizinga, A.G., Briggs, D., Crevel, A., Knulst, A., Van den Bosch, L., and Houben, G.F. 2008. Probabilistic risk assessment model for allergens in food: Sensitivity analysis of the minimum eliciting dose and food consumption. *Food and Chemical Toxicology* 46(5): 1437–1443; doi: 10.1016/j.fct.09.109.

Lam, H.Y. et al. Cow's milk allergy in adults is rare but severe: Both casein and whey proteins are involved. *Submitted for publication*

Spanjersberg, M.Q.I., Kruizinga, A.G., Rennen, M.A.J., and Houben, G.F. 2007. Risk assessment and food allergy: The probabilistic model applied to allergens. *Food and Chemical Toxicology* 45(1): 49–54.

Van Leeuwen, C.J. and Vermeire, T. 2007. *Risk Assessment of Chemicals: An Introduction.* Springer, Dordrecht, the Netherlands. ISBN 9781402061011.

# Glossary

*Lucjan Jędrychowski*

The glossary has been limited to the basic terms occurring in this book and is prepared to help the reader understand the issues the book refers to. When the term is not included in the glossary, the readers are requested to refer to the specialist Web sites specified in the "glossary" group (the subchapter on the Web sites discusses this problem in greater detail).

**Allergy**, synonym of hypersensitivity—the term was first introduced by Pirquet in 1906. Allergies are inappropriate, pathologic, or exaggerated reactions of the immune system to substances (allergens) that in majority of people cause no symptoms. The symptoms of allergic diseases may be caused by exposure of the skin (SALT), the mucosa (MALT), the respiratory system (NALT and BALT), or the stomach and intestines (GALT) to allergens (particular food, food ingredients, particles of dust or pollen, or other substances). Qualitatively altered tissue reactivity caused by a specific allergen is based on immunological reaction triggered by forming specific antibodies or sensitive lymphocytes.

**Allergen**—a foreign substance which causes the immune system to produce specific antibodies—immunoglobulin E (IgE), immunoglobulin G (IgG), or sensitive lymphocytes against the substance and which induces an (pathological) allergic or hypersensitivity response. The IgE binds to receptors of the mast cells and basophiles. Upon re-exposure, the same foreign substance binds to IgE, causing chemical mediators to be released from the mast cells and basophiles, resulting in vasodilatation, itching, sneezing, wheezing, and other allergic symptoms.

**Anaphylaxis**, or anaphylactic shock, or anaphylactic reaction—a severe, frightening and life-threatening allergic reaction of the immune system occurring in response to an allergen. The symptoms may include heart rhythm and respiration disorders, lowered blood pressure, swelling, hives, and asthma like symptoms.

**Anergy**—a state of immune unresponsiveness to an allergen or antigen (e.g., of food origin). The mechanism is induced when the T cell's (T lymphocytes) antigen receptor is stimulated, effectively freezing T cell responses pending a "second signal" from the antigen-presenting cell. The delivery of the second signal by the antigen-presenting cell rescues the activated T cell from anergy, allowing it to produce the lymphokines necessary for the growth of additional T cells. Anergy is one of food-tolerance mechanisms.

**Angioedema**—an allergic symptom of skin swelling that results from a similar process causing urticaria (hives), but the swelling occurs beneath the skin instead of on the surface. Angioedema is characterized by the presence of fluid in subcutaneous tissues or submucosa, particularly of the face, eyes, lips, and sometimes tongue and throat, occurring in an anaphylactic reaction.

**Antibody**—a type of specific protein, also called an immunoglobulin, produced by lymphocytes to neutralize an antigen or foreign antigens (mainly proteins, micro-organisms—moulds, bacteria, viruses, pollens, dust mites, foods). Although many types of antibodies are protective, inappropriate or excessive formation of antibodies may lead to illness. When the organism forms immunoglobulin E (IgE) in the amount that exceeds normal level, allergic rhinitis, asthma, or eczema may result when the patient is again exposed to the substance which caused IgE antibody formation (allergen).

**Antigen**—a substance (chemical, toxin, protein, part of bacteria, virus, or pollen) which can trigger an immune response resulting in the production of antibodies against it as part of the body's defense against infection and/or disease. Many antigens are foreign proteins (those not naturally found in the body). An allergen is a special type of antigen which causes, among others, an IgE antibody response.

**Antihistamines**—a group of drugs which block the effects of histamine, a chemical released in body fluids during an allergic reaction. In rhinitis, antihistamines reduce itching, sneezing, and runny nose (allergy symptoms).

**Anti-inflammatory drugs**—drugs reducing the symptoms and signs of inflammation. In spite of not being a drug, immunotherapy ("allergy shots") reduces inflammation in both allergic rhinitis and allergic asthma.

**Asthma**—a chronic, inflammatory lung disease characterized by recurrent breathing problems. Patients with asthma have acute episodes when the air passages in their lungs get narrower and breathing becomes more difficult. Asthma episodes may be induced by allergens, although infections, exercise, cold air, and other factors are also important triggers.

**Bronchitis**—inflammation of the bronchi (lung airways) resulting in persistent cough that produces considerable quantities of sputum (phlegm). Bronchitis is more common in smokers and in the areas with high atmospheric pollution.

**Bronchodilators**—a group of drugs that widen the airways in the lungs.

**Bronchus**—a larger air passage that connects the trachea (windpipe) to the lungs. The plural form of "bronchus" is "bronchi."

**Cd**—parameter introduced by the authors expressing the product of temperature and time.

**Construct**—the DNA fragment used for transfer into a cell or tissue. It may consist of the gene or genes of interest, a marker gene, and appropriate control sequences as a single package. See also Transgene, Heritable construct, and Non-heritable construct.

**Contact dermatitis**—inflammation of the skin or rash caused by contact with various substances of a chemical, animal, or vegetable nature. The reaction may be an immunologic response or a direct toxic effect of the substance. Among the more common causes of a contact dermatitis reaction are detergents left on washed clothes, nickel (watch straps, bracelets and necklaces, and the fastenings on underclothes), chemicals in rubber gloves and condoms, certain cosmetics, plants such as poison ivy, and topical medications.

**Corticosteroids**—a group of anti-inflammatory drugs similar to the natural corticosteroid hormones produced by the cortex of the adrenal glands. The disorders that often improve upon corticosteroid treatment include asthma, allergic rhinitis, eczema, and rheumatoid arthritis.

**Digestive system**—the group of organs which breaks down food into chemical components that the body can absorb and use for energy and for building and repairing mechanisms in cells and tissues.

**Eczema**—inflammation of the skin, usually causing itching and sometimes accompanied by crusting, scaling, or blisters. A type of eczema often made worse by allergen exposure is termed "atopic dermatitis."

**EMBL**—the European Molecular Biology Laboratory (Heidelberg) Nucleotide Sequence Database (also known as EMBL-Bank). The database is produced in an international collaboration with GenBank (USA) and the DNA Database of Japan (DDBJ). The EMBL nucleotide sequence database is part of the Protein and Nucleotide Database Group (PANDA).

**Epinephrine**—a naturally occurring hormone, also called adrenaline, which increases the speed and force of heartbeats and thereby the work that can be done by the heart. It remains the drug of choice for anaphylaxis treatment.

**Expression product**—a product encoded by a specific RNA molecule. An RNA fragment may encode a protein, its sequence, and may have a regulatory or biological function.

**GM organism/genetically modified organism**—the term used interchangeably to recombinant-DNA organism; see Recombinant-DNA organism.

**Heritable construct**—a construct that is stably integrated into the genome and transmitted from generation to generation.

**Histamine**—a chemical mediator present in cells throughout the body that is released during an allergic reaction. Histamine is one of the substances responsible for the symptoms of inflammation and is the major reason for running nose, sneezing, and itching in allergic rhinitis.

**Hives**—see Urticaria.

**Immune system**—a collection of specific proteins, cells, and tissues that work to protect the body from foreign potentially harmful substances and microorganisms. The immune system plays a role in the control of lot of diseases, but also is the culprit behind the phenomena of allergies, hypersensitivity. There are some specific immune systems (see MALT, GALT, NALT, SALT).

**Immunoglobulins, or antibodies**—specific proteins produced by B-lymphocytes (the immune system cells). Immunoglobulins are present in blood and tissue fluids. Their function is to bind to substances in the body that are recognized as foreign antigens (often proteins on the surface of bacteria and viruses). This binding is a crucial event in the destruction of the microorganisms that bear antigens. Immunoglobulins also play a central role in allergies when they bind on one side to adipose cells and on the other to antigens, which are not necessarily a threat to health and provoke inflammatory reactions.

**Immunomodulators**—substances (nutrients, allergens, some food components, herbs, and drugs) that can affect the immune system function. There are two types of such substances depending on their effects: immunosuppressants and immunostimulators.

**Immunostimulators**—substances (nutrients, allergens, some food components, herbs, and drugs) which stimulate the immune system by inducing activation or increasing activity of any of its components. Immunostimulators, regarding their interacting specificity, can be divided into two groups: specific (antigens and vaccines which provide antigenic specificity in immune response) and nonspecific (such as adjuvants which act irrespective of antigenic specificity to augment the immune response of other antigen or stimulate the components of the immune system without antigenic specificity).

**Immunosuppressants**—substances (nutrients, allergens, some food components, herbs, and drugs) which are held responsible for immunosuppression of the immune system and which reduce the body's natural defenses against foreign invaders or antigens. An immunosuppressant may either be exogenous (e.g., immunosuppressive drugs), or endogenous (some hormones, e.g., testosterone).

**Immunotherapy**—a method of preventive and anti-inflammatory treatment of allergy to allergenic substances. Immunotherapy is highly effective in IgE-mediated diseases. It involves administering gradually increasing doses of the allergen which causes the immune system to become less sensitive by stimulating the production of a particular "blocking" antibody. Immunotherapy is accompanied by increases in IL-10 production and allergen-specific IgG, particularly the IgG4 isotype that blocks not only IgE-dependent histamine release from basophils but also IgE-mediated antigen presentation to T cells.

**Inflammation**—a state of tissue resulting from a protective tissue response to a chemical (but also mediators produced by sensitized adipose cells in response to allergen), physical injury, infection, or destruction of tissues, which serves to destroy, dilute, or wall off both the injurious agent and the injured tissues. The classical inflammation is manifested by pain, redness, swelling, heat, and functional disorders.

**Limit of detection (LOD)**—defined as the analyte concentration interpolated from a standard curve at a response level equivalent to zero concentration plus three standard deviations.

**Limit of quantitation (LOQ)**—the lowest and highest standard used in the analysis. (Expressed as the equivalent level [PPM] of the allergenic food present in the original sample, assuming that it has been extracted/diluted as in the kit instructions).

**Lymphocytes (T cells)**—a group of white blood cells of crucial importance to the adaptive part of the organism's immune system. There are many kinds of lymphocytes (Th 0, Th c, Th 1, Th 2, Th 17). Cytokines produced by T cells probably play a major role in orchestrating allergic inflammation. TH 1 cells produce IFN-γ and IL-2 but not IL-4 or IL-5 after activation. TH2 cells produce mainly IL-4, IL-13, and IL-5 but not IL-2 or IFN-γ. TH2 cells characterize human allergic responses and are present at mucosal surfaces during the late but not immediate response to an allergen exposure.

**Mast cells (B cells)**—cells play an important role in the body's allergic response when an allergen stimulates the release of antibodies which attach themselves to mast cells. Following subsequent allergen exposure, the mast cells release a lot of mediators including histamine (a chemical responsible for allergic symptoms) into the tissue.

**Marker genes**—used to determine when a piece of DNA has been successfully introduced into the organism cell. Marker genes are used either for selecting or for screening transformed cells.

**Non-heritable construct**—a construct which may be integrated into the genome of somatic cells but is not expected to be vertically transmitted, i.e., inherited across generations.

**RAST (RadioAllergoSorbent Test)**—a radiometry laboratory test used to detect IgE antibodies to specific allergens in blood.

**Recombinant-DNA organism**—an organism in which the genetic material has been changed through *in vitro* nucleic acid techniques, including recombinant deoxyribonucleic acid (DNA) and recombinant ribonucleic acid (RNA) and direct injection of nucleic acid into cells and organelles.

**Rhinitis**—inflammation of the mucous membrane that lines the nose (NALT). It is a frequent allergy symptom due to inhalant allergens (pollen, dust, or other airborne substances).

**Suppression**—the mechanisms of specific immunologic unresponsiveness or tolerance to foreign antigens (e.g., food antigens). The mechanism in the case of low doses of food antigens and occuring with mediation of regulatory cells (effector T-cells and CD4+ and CD25+, Tr1 and Th3 cells) and their soluble or cell surface-associated downregulatory cytokines (TGF-beta, IL-4 and IL-10). Their regulation by the major histocompatibility complex remains one of the central issues in immunology.

**Transgene**—a heritable genetic construct that has been integrated into the germline of an organism.

**Transgenic organism**—an organism containing a construct.

**Transfection**—the introduction of a nucleic acid construct into a cell(s) so that it remains intact and maintains its function.

**Threshold dose**—the lowest dose capable of eliciting an allergic reaction of organism—the synonym of the lowest observed adverse effect level (LOAEL) and minimal eliciting dose (MED).

**Urticaria, or hives**—a skin condition characterized by the development of itchy, raised white lumps surrounded by an area of red inflammation. See also Angioedema.

**Vectors**—vehicles for introducing recombinant-DNA constructs into recipient organisms or cells, such as plasmids, viruses, or a bacteria.

**wwPDB**, The Worldwide Protein Data Bank—a group which joined the wwPDB in 2006 and consists of organizations that act as deposition, data processing, and distribution centers for PDB data. The founding members are RCSB PDB (USA), PDBe (Europe), PDBj (Japan), and BMRB (USA). The mission of the wwPDB is to maintain a single Protein Data Bank Archive of macromolecular structural data freely and publicly available to the global community.

# Appendix: Information on Some Interesting Web Addresses on Allergy and Food Allergies

*Lucjan Jędrychowski*

Rapid IT development has enabled us to gain quick access to broad information in many fields of knowledge, for example, via the Internet. The dynamic growth of allergology sciences has generated a wealth of new information on this subject. Furthermore, improved diagnostics has contributed to better recognition of allergy-related intolerance cases. All the above developments have created a need for quick access to broad and varied information (Soeria-Atmadja et al. 2006).

Such information can be obtained on specialist Web pages (www), which have simplified access to a great wealth of information on allergy and intolerance for health professionals and consumers (Gendel 2002, Hileman et al. 2002, Zorzet et al. 2002, Nakamura et al. 2005). In compliance with the rules of "good practice" for Web page service (including technical and logical layout of a site, graphic presentation, visibility, and clarity of graphic and textual components), such Web sites gather useful information, often including explanation of basic terms used in a given field of science, in the form of a glossary (described below in greater detail). Some Web pages do not fulfill the requirements of "good practice" and are difficult to access or navigate, in which case it seems necessary to have some pre-orientation information.

The actual usefulness of Internet pages to a user can vary. Some Web pages are strictly scientific, mainly medical. Others provide more common knowledge and can be even commercial.

One undeniable advantage of specialist Web pages, these also contain glossaries, is the fact that the users can surf them, i.e., can use links to access other terms or can move back to any part of a given site. This means that it is possible to gain deep knowledge of a question one studies, which is often made easier owing to attached graphic presentations, photographs, or videos. The need expressed by Internet users to receive varied information has resulted in the creation of many specialist Internet pages, including specialist online allergen databases.

Among many Web pages on allergies, we can mention

- Educational and informational (with an aim of disseminating knowledge on allergy-related hypersensitivity—from sites directed to common consumers to pages addressed to medical scientists, and to users from any age group, from schoolchildren to adults), including a specifically distinguished sub-group of Web pages containing glossaries, whose aim is to explain the meaning of particular terms.

- Commercial (the aim is to promote health centers, treatments, tests, medications, and prophylactics methods among potential patients).
- Scientific (whose objective is to improve the knowledge in a specific area, i.e., terms related to allergens, recognition of mechanisms responsible for allergenic responses, medicine, biochemistry, genetics, spatial structure, or molecular biology).

The above division of Web pages and databases is not strict and unambiguous as they are cross-referenced by links.

Among specialist Web pages, allergen databases are an important item.

There are several Web sites that offer allergenicity testing of query amino acid sequences according to the FAO/WHO *in silico* protocol alone or as part of several interrogation formats:

AllerPredict—http://research.i2r.a-star.edu.sg/Templar/DB/Allergen/Predict/Predict.html, Structural Database of Allergenic Proteins (SDAP) (Ivanciuc et al. 2003)—http://fermi.utmb.edu/SDAP/sdap_who.html; AllerMatch (Fiers et al. 2004)—http://www.allermatch.org/; and Allergen Database for Food Safety (ADFS) (Nakamura et al. 2005)—http://allergen.nihs.go.jp/ADFS/.

All activities undertaken to organize and manage specialist databases, owing to their importance, are supported by various societies, scientific organizations or programs. Thus, such organizations often own their Web sites, which they consider a means for disseminating information about their actions.

As the existing databases are highly varied, it is almost impossible to give their exhaustive presentation (Gendel 2002, Hileman et al. 2002, Brusic et al. 2003, Gendel and Jenkins 2006, Radauer et al. 2008). Two Web pages, www.foodallergens.info and www.foodallergens.ifr.ac.uk, contain very good and broad general information about available databases on allergens. These databases are described in more detail by Gendel and Jenkins (2006).

Most of the databases, apart from the basic information on allergens, also offer graphic information, e.g., concerning a source of an allergen (plant, seed), information on botanic names, biochemical and physiological functions, etc. They also direct the user, via links, to other databases and Web pages holding similar information, or to relevant written references (e.g., databases Allergome, Informall, AllFam).

Although it is difficult to state firmly what character each database has, one can name some of the most popular ones and group them as

- General Information on allergy and allergens
  - AllAllergy—http://allallergy.net/
  - Allergome—http://www.allergome.org
  - allFam—http://www.meduniwien.ac.at/allergens/allfam/
  - www.foodallergens.info—informing about current scientific programs

- INFORMALL database (comprising information about Food Allergies for Consumers, Regulators, and Industry)—http://foodallergens.ifr. ac.uk/informall.html
- http://www.hon.ch/Library/Theme/Allergy/Glossary/allergy.html
- Allergen Nomenclature–List of allergens
  - IUIS Allergen Nomenclature Sub-Committee list (contains information on protein allergen nomenclature along with a list of allergens; it also gives a list of food allergens, new allergen forms, allergen nomenclature publications)—http://www.allergen.org
- Allergen sequences
  - AllergenOnline (FARRP) (intended for use as a tool for evaluating the safety of proteins included in foods through processing or genetic modification by classifying sequences into groups (allergen, putative allergen, insufficient evidence)—at present (2008) contains 1313 Peer Reviewed Sequences—http://allergenonline.com
  - AllerPredict—http://sdmc.i2r.a-star.edu.sg/Templar/DB/Allergen/
  - AllerMatch—http://www.allermatch.org/
  - Bioinformatics for Food Safety—http://www.iit.edu/~sgendel/fa.htm
  - Central Science Laboratory—http://www.csl.gov.uk/allergen/
  - International Immunogenetics Information System (integrated information system specializing in immunoglobulins (IG), T cell receptors (TR), and major histocompatibility complex (MHC) molecules of all vertebrate species)—http://imgt.cines.fr/
  - Structural database of allergen proteins—http://fermi.utmb.edu/SDAP/sdap_ver.html
  - Allergen sequence database at BISF—http://www.iit.edu/sgendel/fa.htm
- Allergen glossary—Among some major Web sites containing dictionaries and explanations of terms connected with allergies worth mentioning are
  - Health on the Net Foundation presents a detailed glossary of medical and scientific terms associated with allergies on the Web site http://healthonnet.org/Library/Theme/Allergy/Glossary/allergy.html
  - WebMD Medical Reference provided in collaboration with the Cleveland Clinic accessible at http://www.webmd.com/allergies/allergies glossary terms
  - American College of Allergy, Asthma and Immunology—ACAAI online—http://www.acaai.org/public/glossary/ and based on the latter dictionary:
  - http://www.healthatoz.com/healthatoz/Atoz/common/standard/transform.jsp?requestURI=/healthatoz/Atoz/dc/caz/resp/allr/allglossary.jsp
  - http://www.healthinforum.org/Allergy-Glossary-info-7493.html as well as others
  - http://www.ats-group.net/medical/dictionary-glossary-allergy.html
  - http://www.health24.com/medical/Condition_centres/777-792-797-1544,14124.asp
  - http://www.drgreene.com/21_1267.html

- http://www.allergytherapeutics.com/glossary.aspx
- http://www.webmd.com/allergies/living-with-0/chronic-allergies glossary
- http://findarticles.com/p/articles/mi_m1511/is_n3_v19/ai_20324752? tag=artBody;col1—created by National Institute of Allergy and Infectious Diseases (NIAID) A dictionary of allergology, translated into 75 languages
- http://www.projectallergy.com/allergy_glossary.cfm
- http://www.allergiesjr.com/glossary/3—for children
- http://www.hon.ch/Library/Theme/Allergy/Glossary/a.html

A richly illustrated dictionary of allergology edited by the University of Maryland Medical Centre seems to be an interesting source of information—http://www.umm.edu/careguides/000022.htm

Another Web site which can be of help to understand terms related to health and medical definitions of terms that appear in the Skin Test for Allergy article ishttp://www.medicinenet.com/skin_test_for_allergy/glossary.htm

Other very useful databases (mainly in terms of amino acid sequences in allergens) are the ones which characterize proteins (e.g., The UniProt Knowledgebase—http://expasy.org/sprot/. This database consists of

- UniProtKB/Swiss-Prot; a curated protein sequence database which strives to provide a high level of annotation (such as the description of the function of a protein, its domains structure, posttranslational modifications, variants, etc.)
- UniProtKB/TrEMBL; a computer-annotated supplement of Swiss-Prot that contains all the translations of EMBL nucleotide sequence entries not yet integrated in Swiss-Prot.

Other useful addresses, especially in the context of research on allergens in the fields of proteomics and genomics, are the databases on sequences of nucleotides corresponding to particular proteins or epitopes, e.g., The EMBL Nucleotide Sequence Database—http://www.ebi.ac.uk/embl/Access/, or the Protein and Nucleotide Database Group (PANDA)—http://www.ebi.ac.uk/panda/ or the database Ensembl—http://www.ensembl.org/index.html, http://www.ebi.ac.uk/ensembl/.

The above specification proves that databases differ in their aims and character. Some intend to collect general information on individual allergens, others focus on information regarding amino acid sequences, spatial structure of amino acids, similarities between epitopes, and biochemical functions (Gendel 2002, Soeria-Atmadja et al. 2006). There are also databases which—due to a large number of certain allergens—attempt at providing systematic groups (families) of allergens, using various criteria for this purpose, e.g., classical division of allergens into inhalatory, food, contact, plant and animal allergens, or biochemical functions, physiological functions (LTP, PR), phylogenetic origin, etc.

The fact that knowledge of allergen is developing very rapidly is confirmed by an equally dynamic growth of databases, with the database AllFam serving as an example. In just half a year (2008) AllFam increased its contents by 707 allergens, which were classified by sequence into 134 AllFam families to 954 allergens grouped in 140 families (Radauer et al. 2008). Another meaningful example of progressing development and improvement of the databases on allergens consists of the recent (The Allergome e-Newsletter-August 2008—allergome@allergome.org) modifications to the database ALLERGOME, which have equipped it with very helpful tools:

- The Allergenicity Scoring tool, which visualizes the overall current characterization status of the molecule, has been implemented for allergenic molecules.
- Connected with the Allergenicity Scoring tool is a new advanced search for molecule.
- The "AllergomeBlaster" which helps to
  - Compare allergenic sequences within the Allergome database and outside in Uniprot
  - Produce a report on sequence comparison
  - Obtain a Taxonomy tree using the out-linked NCBI Taxonomy Browser

Web server, "WebAllergen" has the similar function of comparing allergenic sequences and predicting the potential of allergenicity of proteins—http://weballergen.bii.a-star.edu.sg/

Other databases develop just as quickly. Apart from the dynamic development of the available databases, another fact worth noticing is that they become more and more accessible owing to the cross-referencing with links, e.g., the database ALLERTGENONLINE can direct you to

- International Union of Immunological Societies Allergen Nomenclature Sub-Committee—http://www.allergen.org
- Allergome, A database of allergenic molecules—http://www.allergome.org/
- The International ImMunoGeneTics database—http://imgt.cines.fr
- The biotechnology information for food safety database—http://www.iit.edu/~sgendel/fa.htm
- Swiss-prot protein knowledge database—http://www.expasy.ch/cgi-bin/lists?allergen.txt
- Gateway to all asthma, allergy, and intolerance information on the Web—http://allallergy.net/index.html
- Latex allergens—http://dmd.nihs.go.jp/latex/allergen-e.html
- The CSL allergen database compiled by the Molecular and Cellular Sciences Team—http://www.csl.gov.uk/allergen
- Protall—http://www.ifr.bbsrc.ac.uk/protall
- European allergy information resource center. European Bioinformatics Institute—http://www.ebi.ac.uk/

Another example of how a Web page can be expanded using thematic paths—links is an international Web site called Global Food Allergy Associations and Organizations—http://www.allergyfreepassport.com/refcenter/links/allergies.html (Table A.1). In many countries there are local (linguistically restricted) specialist

---

**TABLE A.1**

**Specification of Most Important National, International, and Topic Links from Global Food Allergy Associations and Organizations (http://www. allergyfreepassport.com/refcenter/links/allergies.html)**

| Country/Continent | Organization Name | Web Address |
|---|---|---|
| Australia | Allergy Unit: Royal Prince Alfred Hospital | http://www.cs.nsw.gov.au/rpa/allergy |
| | Anaphylaxis Australia Inc. | http://www.allergyfacts.org.au |
| | Australian Society of Clinical Immunology | http://www.allergy.org.au |
| Belgium | Allergie Preventie | http://www.astma-en-allergiekoepel.be |
| | Fondation pour la Prevention des Allergies | http://www.oasis-allergies.org/ |
| Canada | Allergy/Asthma Information Association | http://www.aaia.ca |
| | Allergy Directory | http://www.allergy-network.com/allergyuk |
| | Anaphylaxis Canada | http://www.anaphylaxis.ca |
| | Association Quebecoise des Allergies Alimentaires Canada | http://www.aqaa.qc.ca |
| | Canadian Society of Allergy and Clinical Immunology (CSACI) | http://www.csaci.medical.org |
| | Peanut Aware | http://www.peanutaware.com |
| Denmark | Astma-Allergi Forbundet | http://www.astma-allergi.dk |
| Europe | European Federation of Allergy and Airways Diseases Patients' Association (EFA) | http://www.efanet.org |
| Finland | Allergia-ja Astmaliitto | http://www.allergia.com |
| France | Association Francaise pour la Prevention des Allergies (AFPRAL) | http://www.prevention-allergies.asso.fr |
| Germany | Deutscher Allergie-und Asthmabund e.V. DAAB | http://www.daab.de |
| Greece | ANIKSI | http://www.allergyped.gr |
| Hungary | MAKIT Hungarian Society Of Allergology and Clinical Immunology | http://www.makit.hu |
| Italy | Federasma | http://www. federasma.org |
| The Netherlands | Nederlands Anafylaxis Netwerk | http://www.anafylaxis.net |
| | Stichting Voedsel Allergie | http://www.stichtingvoedselallergie.nl |
| New Zealand | Allergy New Zealand | http://www.allergy.org.nz |
| | Auckland Allergy Clinic Site | http://www.allergyclinic.co.nz |

## TABLE A.1 (continued)
## Specification of Most Important National, International, and Topic Links from Global Food Allergy Associations and Organizations (http://www. allergyfreepassport.com/refcenter/links/allergies.html)

| Country/Continent | Organization Name | Web Address |
|---|---|---|
| Norway | Norges Astma—og Allergiforbund (NAAF) | http://www.naaf.no |
| Singapore | Food Allergy—Singapore | http://www.foodallergysingapore.org/ |
| South Africa | Allallergy.net | http://www.allallergy.net |
| | Allergy Society of South Africa | http://www.allergysa.org |
| Spain | Asociacion Gallega de Asmaticos y Alergicos | http://www.accesible.org/asga |
| Sweden | Astma och Allergi Forbundet | http://www.astmaoallergiforbundet.se |
| Switzerland | aha! Schweizerisches Zentrum ftir Allergie, Haut und Asthma | http://www.ahaswiss.ch |
| The United Kingdom | Action Against Allergy | http://www.actionagainstallergy.co.uk |
| | Allergy Action | http://www.allergyaction.org |
| | Allergy Induced Autism | http://www.autismmedical.com |
| | The Allergy Site | http://www.theallergysite.co.uk |
| | British Allergy Foundation (BAF) Allergy UK | http://www.allergyuk.org |
| | Dairy Free | www.dairyfreeuk.com |
| | Food Allergy/ Intolerance Site | http://www.foodcanmakeyouill.co.uk |
| | Milk Free Kids | http://www.milkfree.org.uk |
| | No Cow's for Me Thanks | http://www.lactoseintolerance.co.uk |
| | Talk Allergy | www.talkallergy.com |
| The United States | Allergic Child | http://www.allergicchild.com |
| | Allergy and Asthma Network-Mothers of Asthmatics, Inc. | http://www.aanma.org |
| | Allergy Haven | http://www.allergyhaven.com/ |
| | Allergy Moms | http://allergymoms.com/index.php |
| | American Academy of Allergy, Asthma and Immunology | http://www.aaaai.org |
| | American Board of Allergy and Immunology | http://www.abai.org |
| | Asthma and Allergy Foundation of America (AAFA) | http://www.aafa.org |
| | Food Allergy and Anaphylaxis Alliance | http://www.foodallergyalliance.org |
| | Food Allergy and Intolerance Center | http://www.allergyhealthonline.com |
| | Food Allergy Anaphylaxis Network (FAAN) | http://www.foodallergy.org |
| | Food Allergy Connection | http://www.foodallergyconnection.org/ |
| | Food Allergy Info.com | http://foodallergyinfo.com/ |

(continued)

**TABLE A.1 (continued)**
**Specification of Most Important National, International, and Topic Links from Global Food Allergy Associations and Organizations (http://www.allergyfreepassport.com/refcenter/links/allergies.html)**

| Country/Continent | Organization Name | Web Address |
|---|---|---|
| | Food Allergy Initiative | http://www.foodallergyinitiative.org/ |
| | Food Allergy News for Kids | http://www.fankids.org |
| | Food Allergy News for Teens | http://www.fankids.org/FANTeen |
| | The Food Allergy Project | http://www.foodallergyproject.org/ |
| | Food Allergy Support Team | http://www. fastconnection.org |
| | Food Allergy Survivors Together | http://www.angelfire.com/mi/FAST |
| | Go Dairy Free | http://www.godairyfree.org/ |
| | Mothers of Children Having Allergies | http://www.mochallergies.org/ |
| | National Center for Complementary and Alternative Medicine | http://www.nccam.nih.gov |
| | National Institutes of Health | http://www.nih.gov |
| | Parents of Food Allergic Kids (POFAK) | http://www.kidswiuhfoodallergies.org/eve |
| | Peanut Allergy.com | http://www.peanutallergy.com/ |
| | Revolution Health Food Allergy Center | http://www.revolutionhealth.com/condi-tions/allergies/child-food-allergies/ |
| | Smart Foods Healthy Kids | http://www.smartfoodshealthykids.com/ |
| | World Allergy Organization (WAO-IAACI) | http://www.worldallergy.org |

databases. Some examples of such Web pages are given below. They are commercial and information Web sites which provide information about allergies in Poland (in Polish):

- http://www.alergia.org.pl—(information on journals covering the allergy problem)
- http://www.alergie.pl—(information on diagnosing and treatment of allergy, a list of clinical specialist practices)
- http://www.astma.edu.pl—a Web for patients with asthma (the pollen information), a discussion forum with clinical specialists
- http://www.alergen.info.pl—an allergological Web with information on pollen phase
- http://www.apsik.pl—a Web for parents of infants and children
- http://www.pik-net.pl/ikowal/azs/—a web for parents of infants and children with atopic skin inflammation

# REFERENCES

Brusic, V., Millot, M., Petrovsky, N., Gendel, S.M., Gigonzac, O., and Stelman, S.J. 2003 Allergen databases. *Allergy* 58(11): 1093–1100.

Fiers, M.W., Kleter, G.A., Nijland, H., Peijnenburg, A.A., Nap, J.P., and van Ham, R.C. 2004. Allermatch, a webtool for the prediction of potential allergenicity according to current FAO/WHO Codex alimentarius guidelines. *BMC Bioinform* 5: 133.

Gendel, S.M. 2002. Sequence analysis for assessing potential allergenicity. *Ann NY Acad Sci* 964: 87–98.

Gendel, S.M. and Jenkins, J.A. 2006. Allergen sequence databases. *Mol Nutr Food Res* 50(7): 633–637.

Hileman, R.E., Silvanovich, A., Goodman, R.E., Rice, E.A., Holleschak, G., Astwood, J.D., and Hefle, S.L. 2002. Bioinformatic methods for allergenicity assessment using a comprehensive allergen database. *Int Arch Allergy Immunol* 128: 280–291.

Ivanciuc, O., Schein, C.H., and Braun, W. 2003. SDAP: Database and computational tools for allergenic proteins. *Nucleic Acids Res* 31: 359–362.

Nakamura, R., Teshima, R., Takagi, K., and Sawada, J. 2005. Development of Allergen Database for Food Safety (ADFS): An integrated database to search allergens and predict allergenicity. *Kokuritsu Iyakuhin Shokuhin Eisei Kenkyusho Hokoku* 123: 32–36.

Radauer, C., Bublin, M., Wagner, S., Mari, A., and Breiteneder, H. 2008. Allergens are distributed into few protein families and possess a restricted number of biochemical functions. *J Allergy Clin Immunol* 121(4): 847–852.

Soeria-Atmadja, D., Lundell, T., Gustafsson M. G., and Hammerling U. 2006. Computational detection of allergenic proteins attains a new level of accuracy with in silico variable-length peptide extraction and machine learning. *Nucleic Acids Res* 34(13): 3779–3793.

Zorzet, A., Gustafsson, M., and Hammerling, U. 2002. Prediction of food protein allergenicity: A bioinformatic learning systems approach. *In Silico Biol* 2: 525–534.

# Index

## A

Abalone *(Haliotis midae),* 242
ABC, *see* Avidin–biotin complex
Acceptable Daily Intake, 368
Activating protein-1, 10, 56
ADCC, *see* Antibody-dependent cytotoxicity
ADFS, *see* Allergen Database for Food Safety
ADI, *see* Acceptable Daily Intake
AEDS, *see* Atopic eczema/dermatitis syndrome
*Aegilops tauschii,* 293
*Aeromonas hydrophila,* 330
AFM, *see* Atomic force microscopy
*A. fumigatus,* 327
AGA, *see* Antigliadin antibodies
AIF, *see* Apoptosis-inducing factor
AllFam database and bacterial
        allergens, 322
Allergen-containing food products
    European law, 85–86
    physicochemical and biochemical methods
        aptamers and aptazymes, 106
        atomic force microscopy, 106–107
        biosensors in protein and allergen
            analysis, 102–103
        immunometric methods, 94–101
        microarray-based proteomics, 104–105
        preliminary separation and purification,
            88–93
        protein arrays miniaturization, 105–106
    physicochemical and biochemical methods
        for, 87–88
Allergen Cor a 1.04 protein, role, 260; *see also*
        Hazelnut allergens
Allergen Database for Food Safety, 406
Allergenic hypersensitivity, 85
Allergens; *see also* Food allergens analysis;
        Microbiological allergens
    animal food allergens
        allergic reaction, 356
        animal tissue, 361
        insects, 359–361
        marine organisms, 356–359
    cereal allergens, biochemical properties,
        306–307
    crustacean allergens, 246–250
    definition, 4
    detection, 86
    egg allergens
        characteristics, 213, 215–218
        clinical cross-reactivity, 219

immunoreactivity and allergenicity
        changes, 218–219
fish allergens
    cross-reactivity, 227
    genetically modified, 227–229
    immunoreactivity and allergenicity
        changes, 226
    seafood allergens, features, 223–226
food allergens, 327–328, 387–388
    features, 185–190
    risk assessment, 388–393
    risk communication, 395–396
    risk management, 394–395
hazelnut allergens, 259–261
hidden allergens, 368, 371
lupine allergens, cross-reactivity, 274
microbiological allergens, characteristics,
        321–322
    allergens sources, 327–328
    bacteria, allergenic properties, 322–326
    food products, health benefits, 330–331
    microorganisms, application, 328–330
    mold allergens, 326–327
milk allergens
    characterization, 193–198
    immunoreactivity and allergenicity
        changes, 206–211
mold allergens, characteristics, 326–327
nut allergens
    background, 259
    biological and immunological properties,
        259–262
    cross-reactivity, 262–263
peanut allergens
    background, 267–268
    characteristic, 268–272
    cross reactivity, 273–274
    technological treatment and, 272–273
plant food allergens, 334–339
    α–amylase, 342–343
    BBE and chlorophyll binding proteins,
        350
    *Bet v* 1, 345–346
    cereal prolamins, cupin superfamily and
        germins, 343
    class I chitinases and hevein-like domain,
        346
    cystatins, 348
    expansins and glycoside hydrolases, 349
    IFR, 349
    kunitz-type protease inhibitors, 347–348

T - #0206 - 191219 - C2 - 234/156/20 - PB - 9780367385132